Manual
OF
Critical Care
Nursing

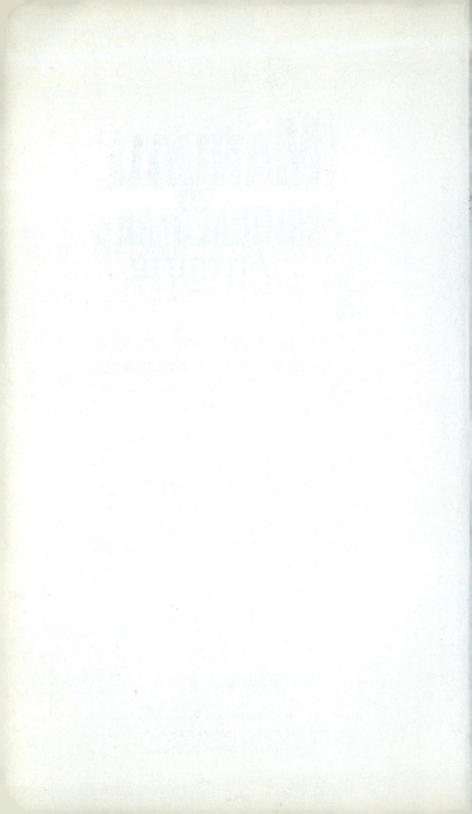

MANUAL

OF

CRITICAL CARE

Nursing

Nursing Interventions and Collaborative Management

THIRD EDITION

Edited by

Pamela L. Swearingen, RN
Special Project Editor

Janet Hicks Keen, RN, MS(N), CCRN, CEN
Consultant in Emergency, Trauma, and Critical Care Nursing
Staff Nurse, Level II
St. Joseph's Hospital of Atlanta
Atlanta, Georgia

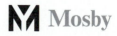 Mosby

St. Louis   Baltimore   Boston   Carlsbad   Chicago   Naples   New York
Philadelphia   Portland   London   Madrid   Mexico City   Singapore
Sydney   Tokyo   Toronto   Wiesbaden

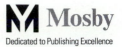
Mosby
Dedicated to Publishing Excellence

A Times Mirror
Company

Editor: Robin Carter
Developmental Editor: Jeanne Allison
Project Manager: Mark Spann
Production Editor: Melissa Martin
Designer: Kay Kramer
Manufacturing Supervisor: Karen Lewis
Cover art: AKA Design, Inc.

THIRD EDITION
Copyright © 1995 by Mosby–Year Book, Inc.

Printed in the United States of America
Composition by The Clarinda Company
Printing/binding by R.R. Donnelley & Sons Company

Mosby–Year Book, Inc.
11830 Westline Industrial Drive
St. Louis, Missouri 63146

ISBN 0-8151-7500-0

95 96 97 / 9 8 7 6 5 4 3 2 1

CONTRIBUTORS

Robert Aucker, PharmD, BCPS

Clinical Pharmacist
St. Joseph's Hospital of Atlanta
Atlanta, Georgia

Linda S. Baas, RN, PhD

Assistant Professor, College of Nursing and Health
Staff Nurse, CCU
University of Cincinnati Medical Center
Cincinnati, Ohio

Marianne S. Baird, RN, MN, CCRN

Clinical Nurse Specialist
St. Joseph's Hospital of Atlanta
Clinical Associate, Faculty at Emory University
  and Georgia State University
Atlanta, Georgia

Carol Barch, RN, MN, CCRN, CNRN, CFNP

Clinical Nurse Specialist
Department of Neurology
Emory University School of Medicine
Atlanta, Georgia

Mimi Callanan, RN, MSN

Epilepsy Clinical Nurse Specialist
Stanford Comprehensive Epilepsy Center
Stanford University Medical Center
Stanford, California

Alice Davis, RN, PhD, CNRN, CCRN

Assistant Professor
Nell Hodgson Woodruff School of Nursing
Emory University
Atlanta, Georgia

Patricia Hall, RN, PhD, CCRN
Clinical Nurse Specialist, Cardiac Services
Kennestone Hospital
Marietta, Georgia

Ursula Easterday Heitz, RN, MSN
Nursing Consultant
Nashville, Tennessee

Mima M. Horne, RN, MS, CDE
Diabetes Clinical Nurse Specialist
New Hanover Regional Medical Center
Adjunct Lecturer, School of Nursing
University of North Carolina–Wilmington
Wilmington, North Carolina

Cheri A. Howard, RN, MSN
Unit Director
Indiana University Medical Center
Indianapolis, Indiana

Marguerite M. Jackson, RN, MS, CIC, FAAN
Administrative Director
Medical Center Epidemiology Unit
Assistant Clinical Professor
Family and Preventive Medicine
University of California–San Diego
San Diego, California

Joyce Johnson, RN, PhD, CCRN
Assistant Professor
School of Nursing, College of Health Sciences
Georgia State University
Intensive Care Resource Nurse
Crawford Long Hospital
Atlanta, Georgia

Janet Hicks Keen, RN, MS(N), CCRN, CEN
Consultant in Emergency, Trauma, and Critical Care Nursing
Staff Nurse, Level II
St. Joseph's Hospital of Atlanta
Atlanta, Georgia
Clinical Faculty
Gordon College
Barnsville, Georgia

Dennis G. Ross, RN, MAE, PhD
Professor of Nursing
Castleton State College
Castleton, Vermont

Marilyn Sawyer Sommers, RN, PhD, CCRN

Associate Professor, College of Nursing and Health
Staff Nurse, Surgical ICU/Trauma
University of Cincinnati Medical Center
Cincinnati, Ohio

Johanna K. Stiesmeyer, RN, MS, CCRN

Cardiovascular Education Specialist
El Camino Hospital
Consultant, J.K. Stiesmeyer Nursing Educational Services
Mountain View, California

Nancy Stotts, RN, MN, EdD

Associate Professor
Department of Physiological Nursing
University of California–San Francisco
San Francisco, California

Ann Coghlan Stowe, RN, MSN

Chairperson, Department of Nursing
West Chester University
West Chester, Pennsylvania

Barbara Tueller Steuble, RN, MS

Education and Infection Control Coordinator
Amador Hospital
Jackson, California

Karen S. Webber, RN, MN

Assistant Professor, School of Nursing
Memorial University of Newfoundland
St. John's, Newfoundland, Canada

Patricia D. Weiskittel, RN, MSN

Renal Clinical Nurse Specialist
University of Cincinnati Medical Center
Cincinnati, Ohio

CONSULTANTS

Ellen Barker, RN, MSN, CNRN
Neuroscience Nursing Consultants
Newark, Delaware

Jacqueline J. Barrows, RN, HP (ASCP)
Haemonetics Corporation
Braintree, Massachusetts

Tally Bell, RN, MN, CCRN
HCA Wesley Medical Center
 and Wichita State University
Wichita, Kansas

Jean K. Berry, RN, PhD
University of Illinois
Chicago, Illinois

Carroll Conner Bouman, RN, MS, PhD(c)
University of Rochester
Rochester, New York

Patti Eisenberg, RN, MSN, CS
Jewish Hospital of St. Louis
 at Washington University Medical Center
St. Louis, Missouri

Peggy S. Gerard, RN, DNSc
Purdue University Calumet
Hammond, Indiana

Lisa Hopp, RN, PhD
Purdue University Calumet
Hammond, Indiana

PREFACE

Manual of Critical Care Nursing: Nursing Interventions and Collaborative Management was developed to provide nurses with a portable compendium of more than 75 clinical phenomena seen in critical care. The third edition features the addition of a chapter that discusses general concepts in caring for the critically ill and a chapter that focuses on multisystem trauma, to which major trauma and pelvic fractures have been added. This edition also has new sections on sedating and paralytic agents, alterations in consciousness, wound and skin care, pain, stroke, and heparin-induced thrombocytopenia. To the book's appendices, tables on major deep tendon reflexes and major superficial reflexes and a section on current infection prevention and control standards have been added.

Focusing on nursing diagnoses and interventions that are specific to each critical disorder, the book also provides a brief review of pathophysiology and discusses assessment data, diagnostic testing, and collaborative management. The order of presentation provides a hierarchy of information that enables the nurse to make nursing diagnoses and determine interventions specific to the individual patient. While patient teaching in critical care may, by necessity, be concentrated on immediate learning needs (for example, coughing, deep breathing, leg exercises), ideally the information provided in this text should be incorporated before discharge from the intensive care or step-down unit, verbally or *via* written instructions.

This edition has been thoroughly revised and updated. The outcome criteria are specific, positive statements that facilitate evaluation of care. New to this edition are timeframes for the outcome criteria, which have been reviewed for accuracy by an expert in quality improvement. Timeframes are provided as guidelines, since patients have their own unique response times, and to serve as reminders that Medicare and other third-party payors monitor the fine line between quality, cost-effective care and premature discharge, enabling nurses to set more realistic goals for nursing outcomes. In addition, the outcome timeframes may be different for CCU than for a step-down unit, and nurses should determine their applicability accordingly.

For clarity and consistency throughout the book, normal values are given for hemodynamic monitoring and other measurements. However, all values should be individualized to correspond to the patient's normal range of measurements. Although the book offers a host of interventions for each critical disorder, not all interventions are appropriate for every patient. It is the authors' intent that interventions that do apply to the individual patient be used in the development of a personalized care plan. In addition, nursing diagnoses and management techniques commonly used with critically ill patients are found in Chapter 1: "Nutritional Support," "Mechanical Ventilation," "Hemodynamic Monitoring," "Sedating and Paralytic Agents," "Alterations in Consciousness," "Wound and Skin Care," "Pain," "Prolonged Immobility," "Psychosocial Support," and "Psychosocial Support for the Patient's Family and Significant Others."

Only NANDA-approved nursing diagnoses are used in this manual. To promote consistency in the wording of nursing diagnoses among all nurses, we have followed closely the wording used by NANDA for its related factors. Readers who desire more information on disorders traditionally seen in the medical-surgical setting (for example, chronic obstructive pulmonary disease, renal calculi, diverticulosis, cancer) are encouraged to read *Manual of Medical-Surgical Nursing Care: Nursing Interventions and Collaborative Management,* third edition, edited by Pamela L. Swearingen (Mosby).

Manual of Critical Care Nursing was written to supplement critical care textbooks and assumes that the reader has a background in critical care pathophysiology and assessment parameters. The book can serve as a resource not only for clinicians but for academicians and students as well. The textual information and numerous tables will stimulate the clinician's recall of previously learned concepts. Academicians can use the book in teaching students how to apply theoretical concepts to clinical practice. Students will find the book an excellent tool in helping them assess the patient systematically, as well as prioritize nursing interventions. Our primary goal is to provide staff and students in critical care with a wealth of clinical information in a quick and easy-to-use format to help them apply nursing diagnoses in the critical care environment. Our reviewers believe that we have achieved this objective. We welcome comments from nurses who consult the book on a daily basis so that we can enhance its usefulness in future editions.

Pamela L. Swearingen

Janet Hicks Keen

Acknowledgements

We and the contributors would like to thank the many individuals whose input was valuable in the development of this manuscript. In particular, we wish to thank the following second edition contributors: Eva Kresge, RN, BSN; Ruth Kunkle, RN, MSN, CCRN; Patricia M. Roberts, RN, MSc, PhD; Judith K. Sands, RN, MS, EdD; and Andrea Walsh, RN, BSN, CD, CAC.

We are also grateful to Carol Monlux Swift, RN, BSN, for contributing the material on impaired verbal communication (originally published in *Manual of Medical-Surgical Nusing Care*, third edition), which has been added to the stroke section of this manual.

P. L. S.
J.H.K.

CONTENTS

1 GENERAL CONCEPTS IN CARING FOR THE CRITICALLY ILL

Nutritional support

The body adapts to starvation through a series of hormonal changes that compensate for the decreased intake of nutrients. If starvation is prolonged, the body uses its own substrate to optimize survival, with a resulting loss of skeletal muscle and adipose tissue. This state of protein-calorie malnutrition, marasmus, when complicated with severe stress, such as burns, serious injury, or sepsis, generates a neuroendocrine response—hypermetabolism, hypercatabolism, insulin resistance with hyperglycemia, and depletion of lean body mass. Studies indicate that patient outcomes for those with protein-calorie malnutrition are associated with an increased mortality and morbidity, including weakness, compromised immunity, decreased wound healing, infection, and organ failure. Consequently, the goal of therapy is to identify the pre-existing malnutrition, prevent further protein-calorie deficiencies, optimize the patient's current state, and reduce further morbidity.

NUTRITIONAL ASSESSMENT

Multiple sources of information are used, including any and all of the following: historical data, nutritional history, anthropometric data, bio-

1

chemical analysis of blood and urine, and duration of the disease process. With a critically ill individual, the nutritional history may be obtained from significant others.

NUTRITIONAL HISTORY A nutritional history identifies individuals who are or may be at risk for malnutrition during hospitalization. Investigate the adequacy of usual and recent food intake and, in particular, anything that has impaired adequate selection, preparation, ingestion, digestion, absorption, and excretion of nutrients before admission. Include the following in your history:

- Comprehensive review of usual dietary intake, including food allergies, food aversions, and use of nutritional supplements
- Recent unplanned weight loss or gain
- Chewing or swallowing difficulties
- Nausea, vomiting, or pain with eating
- Altered pattern of elimination (e.g., constipation or diarrhea)
- Chronic disease affecting utilization of nutrients (e.g., malabsorption, pancreatitis, diabetes mellitus)
- Recent trauma, surgery, or period of sepsis
- Use of medications (e.g., laxatives, antacids, antibiotics, antineoplastic drugs) and alcohol

Note excesses or deficiencies of nutrients and any special eating patterns (e.g., various vegetarian or prescribed diets), use of fad diets, or excessive supplementation.

PHYSICAL ASSESSMENT Most physical findings are not conclusive for particular nutritional deficiencies. Compare current assessment findings to past assessments, especially related to the following:

- Loss of muscle and adipose tissue
- Work and muscle endurance
- Changes in hair, skin, or neuromuscular function

ANTHROPOMETRIC DATA Anthropometrics is the measurement of the body or its parts. It is helpful to remember that 1 L of fluid equals approximately 2 lbs. Pounds and inches are converted to metric measurements using the following formulas:

Divide pounds by 2.2 to convert to kilograms (kg).
Divide inches by 39.37 to convert to meters (m).

- *Height:* Used to determine ideal weight and body mass index; if unavailable, obtain estimate from family or significant others, or compare patient's recumbent length with known mattress length.
- *Weight:* A readily available and practical indicator of nutritional status that can be compared to previous weight and ideal weight or used to calculate body mass index. Changes may reflect fluid retention (edema, third spacing), diuresis, dehydration, surgical resections, traumatic amputations, or weight of dressings or equipment. Use actual body weight to avoid overfeeding in starved patients and ideal body weight in patients who weigh >120% of ideal body weight. See Table 1-1.
- *Body mass index (BMI):* Used to evaluate adult weight. One calculation and one set of standards are applicable for both men and women:

$$\text{BMI (kg/m}^2) = \frac{\text{Weight (kg)}}{\text{Height (m)} \times \text{Height (m)}}$$

T A B L E 1 - 1   Height and weight guidelines for men and women

Height	Men (weight in lbs)			Women (weight in lbs)		
	Small frame	Medium frame	Large frame	Small frame	Medium frame	Large frame
4 ft 10 in	—	—	—	102-111	109-121	118-131
4 ft 11 in	—	—	—	103-113	111-123	120-134
5 ft	—	—	—	104-115	113-126	122-137
5 ft 1 in	—	—	—	106-118	115-129	125-140
5 ft 2 in	128-134	131-141	138-150	108-121	118-132	128-143
5 ft 3 in	130-136	133-143	140-153	111-124	121-135	131-147
5 ft 4 in	132-138	135-145	142-156	114-127	124-138	134-151
5 ft 5 in	134-140	137-148	144-160	117-130	127-141	137-155
5 ft 6 in	136-142	139-151	146-164	120-133	130-144	140-159
5 ft 7 in	138-146	142-154	148-168	123-136	133-147	143-163
5 ft 8 in	140-148	145-157	152-172	126-139	136-150	146-167
5 ft 9 in	142-151	148-160	156-176	129-142	139-153	149-170
5 ft 10 in	144-154	151-163	158-180	132-145	142-156	152-173
5 ft 11 in	146-157	154-166	161-184	135-148	145-159	155-176
6 ft	149-160	157-170	164-188	138-151	148-162	158-179
6 ft 1 in	152-164	160-174	168-192	—	—	—
6 ft 2 in	155-168	164-178	172-197	—	—	—
6 ft 3 in	158-172	167-182	176-202	—	—	—
6 ft 4 in	162-176	171-187	181-207	—	—	—

Data courtesy Metropolitan Life Insurance Company, 1983. For ages 25 through 59, with 5 lbs of indoor clothing for men and 3 lbs of indoor clothing for women and 1-in heels for both.

BMI values of 20-25 are optimum; values >25 indicate obesity; and values <20 indicate underweight status.

- *Triceps skinfold thickness (TSF):* Measured at the midpoint of the upper arm, which is located by taking half the distance between the olecranon and acromion process and grasping the skin and subcutaneous tissue at the back of the arm approximately 1 cm from the midpoint. Surgical calipers are used to measure the skinfold. Because of the variation among clinicians, the site of measurement, and the patient's position, age, and fluid status, it is difficult to use these measurements as a basis for evaluating patient status. Specially trained clinicians and dietitians should perform this assessment for more accurate results. A TSF measurement of <3 mm signals severely depleted fat stores.

DIAGNOSTIC TESTS

No laboratory test specifically measures nutritional status. Status can be estimated, however, using the following:

Protein status: Evaluated in the following tests, with normal values in parentheses: serum albumin (3.5-5.5 g/dl), transferrin (180-260 mg/dl), thyroxine-binding prealbumin (20-30 mg/dl), and retinol-binding protein (4-5 mg/dl). Normal values vary somewhat with different laboratory procedures and standards. Albumin and transferrin have relatively long half-lives of 19 and 9 days, respectively, whereas thyroxine-binding prealbumin and retinol-binding protein have very short half-lives of 24-48 h and 10 h, respectively. If hydration status is normal and anemia is absent, albumin and transferrin levels can be used as baseline indicators of adequacy of protein intake and synthesis. During protein-calorie malnutrition, however, the plasma albumin level, an indicator of visceral protein, is unchanged. For evidence of response to nutritional therapy, values for the short turnover proteins (i.e., thyroxine-binding prealbumin [although very expensive] and retinol-binding protein) are the most useful.

Nitrogen balance: If more nitrogen is taken in than excreted, nitrogen is said to be positive, and an anabolic state exists. If more nitrogen is excreted than taken in, nitrogen balance is said to be negative, and a catabolic state exists. Most nitrogen loss occurs through the urine, with a small, constant amount lost *via* skin and feces.

Nitrogen balance studies should be performed by specialists, because accurate measurement of 24-h food intake and urine output is required.

Creatinine-height index: Comparison of a patient's 24-h urinary creatinine excretion with a predicted urinary creatinine for individuals with the same height. This test evaluates body muscle mass. The quantity of creatinine produced is directly related to skeletal muscle wasting. The validity of results is affected by inaccuracies in the urine collection procedure and a lack of age-referenced norms.

ESTIMATING NUTRITIONAL REQUIREMENTS

The primary goal of nutritional support is to meet the needs for body temperature, metabolic processes, and tissue repair. Energy needs can be estimated using the following options:

Indirect calorimetry: Performed using a bedside metabolic cart. Specialized personnel are required to provide accurate results. Carts are an expense most units cannot justify.

Harris and Benedict equations: Determine basal energy expenditure (BEE). BEE can be calculated using the following equations developed by Harris and Benedict:

$$BEE \text{ (male)} = 66.5 + (13.8 \times W) + (5 \times H) - (6.8 \times A)$$

$$BEE \text{ (female)} = 655.1 + (9.6 \times W) + (1.9 \times H) - (4.7 \times A)$$

$$W = \text{weight (kg); } H = \text{height (cm); } A = \text{age (yr)}$$

Then multiply the BEE by a stress factor that is estimated from the degree of stress and the need for weight maintenance or repletion. Multiplying the BEE by 1.2-1.5 provides a range appropriate for most patients. The lower factor is appropriate for patients without significant stress, whereas the higher factor is appropriate for patients with higher levels of stress, such as major trauma or sepsis. Individuals with burns may require an even higher stress factor (e.g., 2-3 times the caloric requirements of the BEE).

Distribution of calories: A relatively normal distribution of calories usually is adequate. Percentages of total calories from carbohydrates, protein, and fat should equal approximately 50%, 15%, and 35%, respectively. To avoid overfeeding, 30-35 kcal/kg is appropriate for most critically ill patients.

- *Protein requirements:* Usually 1.5-2 g/kg/day.
- *Carbohydrate requirements:* Glucose administration of 5 mg/kg/min is a suitable amount. Carbohydrates provided in excess of this amount are not well utilized and may lead to hyperglycemia, excessive CO_2 production, hypophosphatemia, and fluid overload.
- *Fat requirements:* If protein and glucose are supplied as outlined, the remainder of needed calories can be supplied as fat. Fat can be administered in minimal quantities to satisfy needs for essential fatty acids, or it can be provided in larger quantities, as tolerated, to meet energy needs.

    Abnormal elevations in liver enzymes often occur in patients maintained on total parenteral nutrition (TPN) longer than 3 weeks. Usually the enzymes return to normal upon cessation of TPN. Giving cyclic TPN, in which the patient receives TPN for 12-16 h out of 24 h, may prevent enzyme elevation.

Vitamin and essential trace mineral requirements: In general, follow the Recommended Dietary Allowances (RDA) to provide minimum quantities of vitamins, minerals, and essential fatty acids. For specific patients, supplement specific vitamins or minerals needed in increased amounts for existing disease states (e.g., zinc and vitamins A and C for burns; thiamine, folate, and B_{12} for history of chronic alcohol ingestion).

Fluid requirements: Many factors affect fluid balance. All sources of intake (oral, enteral, intravenous, and medications), as well as output (urine, stool, drainage, emesis, fluid shifts, and respiratory and evaporative losses), must be considered.

Special diets for organ-specific pathology: Costly, and the metabolic advantages of some products remain unproven.

- *Hepatic failure:* Branched-chain amino acids in combination with reduced aromatic amino acid concentrations are used to alleviate encephalopathy secondary to hepatic failure. General use for the critically ill has not been shown to affect outcome.
- *Renal disease:* High percentages of essential amino acids are used to improve nitrogen use and decrease urea formation.
- *Respiratory disease:* A low-protein and low-carbohydrate diet decreases CO_2 production and, consequently, the work of breathing.

NUTRITIONAL SUPPORT MODALITIES

Cost, safety, and convenience have been the rationale for enteral over parenteral nutritional support, but the potential physiologic benefits are a more compelling argument. The gastrointestinal (GI) system, believed by many to be dormant during stressful events, is metabolically, immunologically, and bacteriologically active. Studies indicate that enteral feedings prevent passage of bacteria from the GI tract into the lymphatic system and other organs, reducing a major source of sepsis and possible organ failure while fostering wound healing and immunocompetence.

Enteral formulas: Composed of a wide variety of standard and modular formulas. Also see Table 1-2.

- **Standard:** Include blended whole food diets, which are less costly but have problems that include possible bacterial growth, solids that settle out, variation in nutrient composition, and the necessity of a large-bore tube for the viscous solution; and commercial formulas, which are sterile, homogenous, and suitable for small-bore feeding tubes, and have a fixed nutrient composition.
- **Modular:** Consist of a single nutrient that may be combined with other modules (nutrients) to form a package tailor-made for an individual's specific deficits (e.g., carbohydrate, fat, protein, and vitamin modules).

Nutritional composition

- **Carbohydrates:** The most easily digested and absorbed component in enteral formulas; 80% of all carbohydrates are broken down and absorbed as simple glucose in the normal intestine.

    Lactase: An enzyme that aids in the digestion of lactose and is most commonly deficient in African Americans, Asians, Native Americans, and Jews. A secondary form also may be found in individuals for whom large amounts of lactose are given in a milk-based diet. Symptoms include watery diarrhea, abdominal cramps, flatulence, fullness, nausea, stool with a pH of <6, and stool that tests positive for glucose.

    Fiber: Now included in many commercial preparations because it is claimed to be helpful in controlling blood glucose, reducing hyperlipidemia, and controlling bowel disorders, such as diverticula. These preparations are highly viscous and require a large-bore feeding tube, such as a 10 French (10 Fr) or an infusion pump. Begin the infusion slowly to reduce transient symptoms of gas and abdominal distention.

T A B L E 1 - 2   **Types of enteral formulations**

Enteral formula	Description
Blended diets	
Compleat, Compleat Modified, Vitaneed	Nutritionally complete, requiring complete digestive capabilities; composed of natural food groups including meat, vegetables, milk, and fruit
Milk-based formulas	
Meritene, Sustagen, Carnation Instant (if mixed with milk)	Nutritionally adequate diet for general nutritional support
Lactose-free formulas	
Ensure, Entrition 1, Isocal, Osmolite	Nutritionally adequate, liquid preparation; used for general nutritional support; isoosmolar or hypoosmolar; all except Osmolite low in residue
Elemental or chemically defined formulas	
Criticare	Nutrients tailored for specific needs (e.g., low-sodium, lactose-free, high-nitrogen diet); 40% protein supplied as small peptides; nutritionally adequate; used for general nutritional support
Travasorb HN	Nutritionally adequate; used for general nutritional support; contains additional hydrolyzed protein that is readily digested and absorbed
Specialty formulas	
Hepatic failure	
Hepatic Travasorb	Nutritionally complete; contains a greater ratio of branched-chain to aromatic amino acids while restricting total amino acid concentrations and adding nonprotein calories
Hepatic-Aid II	Nutritionally incomplete powder formula with essential nutrients in easily digestible form; high in branched-chain amino acids; low in aromatic amino acids and methionine
Renal failure	
Renal Travasorb	Contains no electrolytes, lactose, or fat-soluble vitamins; high in calories; contains mostly essential amino acids; restricted total protein content may reduce or postpone the need for dialysis
Amin-Aid	Nutritionally incomplete powder supplement with essential nutrients and minimal electrolytes in readily digestible form
Respiratory insufficiency	
Pulmature	Nutritionally complete; contains a higher proportion of fat to carbohydrates; reduces CO_2 production
Modular formulas	Offers highly flexible tailoring of nutrients (e.g., fat [Lipomul], protein [Pro Mod], and carbohydrates [Moducal]) for specific needs

Modified from Webber KS: Providing nutritional support. In Swearingen PL, editor: *Manual of medical-surgical nursing care,* ed 3, St Louis, 1994, Mosby.

- **Protein:** Three forms commonly are used:

  Polymeric: Protein found in complete and original form (e.g., commercial and blenderized whole food diets that require normal levels of pancreatic enzyme).

  Hydrolyzed: Protein that has broken down into smaller forms to assist absorption. It is helpful in short bowel syndrome or pancreatic insufficiency.

  Elemental: Protein that requires no further digestion and is ready for absorption. It is most useful in hepatic and renal disorders.

- **Fat:** Two forms are the primary sources:

  Long-chain triglycerides (LCT): A major source of essential fatty acids, fat-soluble vitamins, and calories.

  Medium-chain triglycerides (MCT): Foster the absorption of fat but have fewer side effects of nausea and vomiting, abdominal distention, and diarrhea.

Types of feeding tubes and sites

- **Stomach:** Easiest for tube placement, simulates normal GI function, and may be used for intermittent or continuous feedings. The stomach is the site best reserved for patients who are alert, with intact gag and cough reflexes. Entry site is nasal, oral, or stomach.

  Small bore: Soft polyurethane or silicone with or without tungsten tip; designed for long-term use; size 6-12 Fr; length 36-45 in. Trade names include Keofeed, Dobhoff. Some nasoenteric feeding tubes have a Y port added, allowing irrigation and medication administration without disconnecting the administration set. Examples include Flexiflow, Ross.

  Large bore: Stiff, polyvinyl chloride; size 10-18 Fr; used for short-term feeding of highly viscous fluids. One trade name is Levine.

  Combination: A soft silicone tube may be contained within a stiff outer tube that is removed, leaving the inner soft tube in place, or the tube may have a rigid guidewire that is removed after insertion. This tube is easier to place.

  Gastrostomy: A soft tube inserted directly into the stomach either temporarily or permanently. Problems include site difficulties, leakage, mobility, and catheter occlusion and expulsion.

  Percutaneous endoscopic gastrostomy (PEG) tube: Soft tube inserted into the stomach *via* the esophagus and then drawn through the abdominal skin using a stab incision.

- **Small bowel:** Used for patients with diminished protective pharyngeal reflexes; the small bowel is less affected than the stomach and colon by postoperative ileus. Tube placement is more difficult. Elemental formulas often are required for easier absorption. Continuous feedings are tolerated better inasmuch as the continuous drip approximates normal function. Entry sites are nasal, oral, duodenum, and jejunum.

  Small bore: See "Stomach" above. Some tubes have one port for feeding into the jejunum and a second port that allows for aspiration and decompression of the stomach.

  Duodenum/jejunum: Minimizes risk of vomiting and aspiration compared with gastric feedings. A jejunostomy tube is soft, inserted into the jejunum, and not easily dislodged. Needle catheter (Witzel) jejunostomy is an alternative method of nutrient delivery and often is placed at the time of surgery.

Infusion rates: See Table 1-3.

Management of complications: See Table 1-4.

Parenteral nutrition (PN):   The postinjury metabolic stress response is said to peak at 3-4 days. Initiating nutritional support within 48 h, once the patient is stabilized, can decrease morbidity in a previously well-nourished person who is critically ill by supplying nutrients to prevent catabolism of skeletal and visceral protein stores.

Parenteral nutrition provides some or all nutrients by peripheral venous catheter (PVC) or central venous catheter (CVC) to meet total nutritional needs in patients who cannot be given enteral support or to supplement patients who cannot absorb enough calories using the GI tract. Parenteral nutrition is more expensive and has more complications than enteral nutrition.

- *Parenteral solutions:*   These solutions are derived from combinations of dextrose, amino acids, fat, electrolytes, vitamins, and trace elements. Total nutrient admixtures (TNA) are formulated by combining dextrose, fat, and amino acids in one container; or, alternately, dextrose and amino acids are combined and a separate delivery device is used for fat. An in-line filter cannot be used with TNA because it would trap lipid molecules.

  Carbohydrates: Dextrose solutions 5%-50% are used to meet part of the patient's energy needs. When hypertonic solutions are infused, insulin demand and CO_2 and O_2 consumption are increased, which may lead to respiratory distress and hypermetabolism.

T A B L E 1 - 3   **Methods and rates of administration for enteral products**

Type	Example	Comments
Bolus	250-400 ml 4-6×/day	May cause cramping, bloating, dumping; not recommended
Intermittent	120 ml isotonic formula with 30-50 ml H_2O flush over 30-60 min	Starting regimen
	Advancement: Increase formula q8-12h by 60 ml if residual <½ volume of previous feeding	Should not exceed 30 ml/min; may cause cramping, nausea, bloating, diarrhea, aspiration
Continuous	40-50 ml/h, full strength, isotonic formula	Starting regimen
	Advancement: Increase by 25 ml q8h; if serum albumin levels <2.5 g/dl or initial loose stools, dilute formula to 150 mOsm	

Modified from Webber KS: Providing nutritional support. In Swearingen PL, editor: *Manual of medical-surgical nursing care,* ed 3, St Louis, 1994, Mosby.

T A B L E 1 - 4   Management of complications in the tube-fed patient

Complication/ possible causes	Suggested management strategy
Nausea and vomiting	
Fast rate	Decrease rate
Fat intolerance	Fat should compose no more than 30%-40% of total intake
Lactose intolerance	As prescribed, change to lactose-free product
Hyperosmolality	Dilute feeding
Delayed gastric emptying	See **Risk for aspiration,** p. 16
Product odor	Mask with flavoring
Blocked tube	
Viscous formula/medications; inadequate flushing	Flush tube with 50-150 ml water after each feeding/medication administration. Flush q4h with 30 ml water. Do not instill crushed medications in small-bore tubes. Substitute liquid preparations after consulting a pharmacist and attending physician, or crush into a very fine powder and dissolve in 30 ml water. Incompatibilities between drugs and feeding formulas are possible. Blocked tubes may be cleared with proteolytic enzyme papain (Adolph's Meat Tenderizer) and pancreatic enzyme (Viokase). A device called Intro-Reducer has been designed to clear blocked soft feeding tubes, but its efficacy has not been documented.

Protein: Synthetic crystalline essential and nonessential amino acid formulations are available in concentrations of 3%-15%. Special amino acid formulations for specific disorders are available (see "Estimating Nutritional Requirements," p. 4).

Fat: Lipid 10%-20% is an isotonic solution providing essential fatty acids and a source of concentrated calories. For best use and tolerance, lipids should be infused with carbohydrates and protein over no less than 8 h. The most common symptoms of an adverse reaction include febrile response, chills and shivering, and pain in the chest and back. A second type of adverse reaction occurs with prolonged use of IV fat emulsions and may result in a transient increase in liver enzymes, kernicterus, eosinophilia, and thrombophlebitis. Keep the infusion rate 1 ml/min for the first 15-30 min and then increase it to 80-100 ml/h for the remainder of the first infusion.

Selection of feeding site

CVC: Used for infusion of large amounts of nutrients or electrolytes with smaller fluid volumes (hypertonic solutions) than with pe-

T A B L E 1 - 5   Catheters used in parenteral nutrition

Catheter	Description
Subclavian/jugular	
Single lumen	Soft, flexible, silicone catheter; considered less irritating and less thrombotic but kinks easily. Some catheters have a microbial cuff, providing a physical and chemical barrier to bacterial migration. Multiple uses for specimen retrieval, feeding, and medication administration increase the risk of infection, especially in compromised patients.
Multilumen	Dedication of one lumen in a multilumen catheter is common practice, enabling other lumen(s) to be used for medication administration and laboratory monitoring.
Right atrial (e.g., Hickman, Broviac)	Composed of silicone rubber with plastic external segment; usually implanted in OR. For long-term use.
Implantable (e.g., Infuse-a-Port, Port-a-Cath)	Usually implanted in OR. Designed for repeated access, making repeated venipuncture unnecessary.
Peripheral devices	
Dual lumen	Short-term use. Allows dedication of one lumen for nutritional support while reserving second lumen for incompatible medications.

Modified from Webber KS: Providing nutritional support. In Swearingen PL, editor: *Manual of medical-surgical nursing care,* ed 3, St Louis, 1994, Mosby.

ripheral parenteral nutrition. The solution usually is delivered through a large-diameter vein (e.g., superior vena cava *via* the subclavian or jugular vein). The volume of blood flow rapidly dilutes the hypertonic solutions and decreases the irritation of vein walls. However, there are more complications with CVC than with the peripheral route.

PVC: The need for low osmolality of solutions (<800 mOsm/L) can limit usefulness. However, combining solutions of dextrose, amino acids, and lipids lowers the osmolality, providing a concentrated energy source that can be delivered through a peripheral vein, usually of the hand or forearm. This method is usually reserved for individuals who need partial or total nutritional support for short periods and for whom CVC access is unavailable.

Types of catheters: See Table 1-5.

Monitoring infusion rates: Using an infusion pump, PN is given at a consistent rate, with gradual acceleration of the infusion rate on initiation or deceleration on cessation over a 3-day period to avoid wide fluctuations in blood glucose. A typical rate is 50-100 ml/h, which increases 25-50 ml/h/day, depending on the patient's status.

Managing complications: See Table 1-6.

T A B L E 1 - 6   Management of complications in patients receiving parenteral nutrition

Potential complications	Management strategy
Pneumothorax	Ensure that x-ray is done immediately after insertion. Determine placement of catheter before initiating feeding by monitoring for diminished or unequal breath sounds, tachypnea, dyspnea, and labored breathing.
Subclavian artery injury	If pulsatile, bright red blood returns into the syringe, assist physician with immediate removal of the needle, and apply pressure for 10 min anteriorly and posteriorly at the point of penetration.
Catheter occlusion	If solution is infusing sluggishly, flush line with heparinized saline. Check to see if line is kinked. If line is occluded, try to aspirate clot, and contact physician, who may prescribe a thrombolytic agent.

Electrolyte imbalances occurring in both enteral and parenteral nutrition: See Table 1-7.

TRANSITIONAL FEEDING

A period of adjustment is needed before discontinuing nutritional support. Taper nutritional supplements for patients receiving enteral and parenteral nutrition as oral intake increases. Patients receiving parenteral nutrition may have some mucosal atrophy of the bowel and need a period of adjustment before the bowel can fully resume its usual functions of digestion and absorption.

NURSING DIAGNOSES AND INTERVENTIONS (FOR PATIENTS RECEIVING ENTERAL AND PARENTERAL NUTRITION)

Altered nutrition: Less than body requirements related to inability to ingest, digest, or absorb nutrients

Desired outcome: Within 7 days of initiating parenteral/enteral nutrition, patient has adequate nutrition as evidenced by level or steady weight gain of ¼-½ lb/day; improved or normal measures of protein stores (serum albumin 3.5 g/dl, transferrin 180-260 mg/dl, thyroxine-binding prealbumin 20-30 mg/dl, and retinol-binding protein 4-5 mg/dl); state of nitrogen balance as measured by nitrogen balance studies; presence of wound granulation; and absence of infection (see **Risk for infection,** p. 17).

- Ensure nutritional screening and assessment of patient within 72 h of admission; document. See guidelines, p. 1. Reassess weekly.
- Monitor electrolytes, BUN, and blood sugar daily until stabilized. Ensure that serum albumin, transferrin, or prealbumin and trace elements are monitored weekly. Document.
- Weigh patient daily.
- Record I&O carefully, tracking fluid balance trends.

T A B L E 1 - 7 Electrolyte imbalances occurring in enteral and parenteral nutrition

Sodium: Daily requirement is 60-150 mEq. Sodium is the primary extracellular cation in maintaining concentration and volume of extracellular fluid.

Complication	Pathophysiology/strategy
Hypernatremia	In protein-calorie malnutrition, patients have increased sodium owing to extravascular volume expansion and intravascular volume depletion. Monitor sodium levels as depletion resolves, edema decreases, and diuresis occurs. Hypernatremia also occurs in patients receiving hypertonic tube feedings without adequate water supplements. **Sources:** Amino acid solutions contain varying amounts of sodium (up to 70 mEq/L); some antibiotics (e.g., sodium penicillin) also have a high sodium content (31-200 mEq/dl). Corticosteroids may cause sodium retention, and blood products can contain increased levels (130-160 mEq/L).
Hyponatremia	Can be a problem in patients with gastric suctioning and in those receiving diuretic agents or those with syndrome of inappropriate antidiuretic hormone. **Replacement:** TPN solutions can replace sodium by using acetate, phosphate, or chloride salt form, depending on underlying disease state. In patients with renal failure, the phosphate form should not be used. In acidemia, the acetate form is preferred to correct the imbalance.

Continued.

T A B L E 1 - 7   **Electrolyte imbalances occurring in enteral and parenteral nutrition—cont'd**

Potassium: Daily requirement is 50-100 mEq. Potassium is the major intracellular cation required for neurotransmission, protein synthesis, cardiac and renal function, and carbohydrate metabolism.

Complication	Pathophysiology/strategy
Hyperkalemia	May be caused by excessive parenteral or enteral potassium supplementation or increased tissue catabolism, especially in renal insufficiency. **Sources:** Amino acid solutions contain potassium. Elevated potassium levels occur in patients receiving angiotensin-converting enzyme inhibitors, heparin, cyclosporin, and potassium-sparing diuretics.
Hypokalemia	May occur during anabolism (tissue synthesis) in patients being refed. Potassium shifts into the intracellular space, and patients require supplementation. It also may occur in patients with high GI losses or increased loss from diuretics. Potassium levels in patients with acid-base disorders may be misleading: potassium decreases by 0.4-1.5 mEq/L for every increase in pH of 0.1. **Replacement:** In daily TPN solutions, 80-120 mEq may be given to patients without renal problems. Potassium can be replaced using acetate, phosphate, and chloride forms, depending on the underlying disease state, but it should be titrated separately to avoid potential waste of TPN solutions. Infusion rates >0.5 mEq/kg/h are associated with cardiac irregularities.

Phosphorus: Daily requirement is 2.5-4.5 mg/dl. Phosphorus is required for release of oxygen from hemoglobin in the form of 2,3-diphosphoglycerate and for bone deposition, calcium regulation, and synthesis of carbohydrates, fats, and protein.

Complication	Pathophysiology/strategy
Hyperphosphatemia	Occurs in catabolic stress, renal failure, and hypocalcemia. Treatment involves ingestion of aluminum antacids, which bind phosphate in the intestine. **Sources:** Phosphorus-rich solutions, antacids, diuretic agents, and steroids.

| Hypophosphatemia | A complication often found in malnourished patients on refeeding; it has a high mortality rate. As the patient receives fluids containing dextrose, phosphorus shifts rapidly into the intracellular space, causing hypophosphatemia. **Replacement:** Phosphate-rich TPN solutions. |

Magnesium: Daily requirement is 18-30 mEq. Magnesium is required for carbohydrate and protein metabolism and enzymatic reactions.

Complication	Pathophysiology/strategy
Hypermagnesemia	Transient elevations can occur with use of diuretics or extracellular volume depletion. **Source:** Magnesium-containing antacids.
Hypomagnesemia	Low levels commonly occur in patients with severe malnutrition or lower GI losses and in those given insulin for hyperglycemia. For anabolism to occur, 2 mEq of magnesium per gram of nitrogen is required. **Replacement:** Parenteral magnesium.

Calcium: Daily requirement is 1,000-1,500 mg. Calcium is a necessary ingredient of cells that play a major role in neurotransmission.

Complication	Pathophysiology/strategy
Hypercalcemia	Occurs in thiazide diuretic use, prolonged immobilization, and decreased excretion. **Source:** Side effect of diuretic use.
Hypocalcemia	May occur from reduced total body calcium or reduced ionized calcium. It also occurs in the presence of hyperphosphatemia. A deficit can be misleading, inasmuch as serum calcium is bound to protein and varies with changing albumin levels. Further, in acidosis, a lower pH results in release of more calcium from protein, which elevates serum calcium levels. The opposite is true as pH rises. **Replacement:** Calcium-rich parenteral solutions.

- Administer formula within 10% of prescribed rate. Check volume infused and rate hourly.
- Ensure that patient receives the prescribed amount of calories.

Risk for aspiration related to GI bleeding, delayed gastric emptying, and site of feeding tube

Desired outcome: Patient is free of aspiration problems as evidenced by auscultation of clear lung sounds, VS within patient's baseline, and absence of signs of respiratory distress.

- Check x-ray for position of feeding tube before each feeding. Insufflation with air and aspiration of stomach contents do not confirm placement of feeding tubes. Mark and secure tubing for future reference.
- Assess respiratory status q4h, observing respiratory rate and effort and presence of adventitious breath sounds.
- Monitor for fever of unexplained origin q4h.
- Auscultate bowel sounds, percuss abdomen, and assess abdominal contour and girth q8h. Consult physician if bowel sounds are absent, the abdomen becomes distended, or nausea and vomiting occur.
- Elevate HOB ≥30 degrees during and for 1 h after feeding. If this is not possible or comfortable for patient, turn patient into a slightly elevated right side-lying position to enhance gravity flow from the greater stomach curve to the pylorus.
- Consult physician if residual feeding is >50% of the hourly feed. Hold the feeding for 1 h and recheck residual.
- Stop tube feeding ½-1h before chest physical therapy, suctioning, or placing patient supine.
- Discuss with physician the possibility of placing feeding tube well beyond the pylorus.
- As prescribed, administer metoclopramide HCl or other agents that promote gastric motility.

Diarrhea (or risk for same) related to bolus feeding, lactose intolerance, bacterial contamination, osmolality intolerance, medications, and low fiber content

Desired outcome: Patient has formed stools within 24-48 h of intervention.

General

- Assess abdomen and GI status, including bowel sounds, distention, consistency and frequency of bowel movements, cramping, skin turgor, and other indicators of hydration.
- Monitor I&O status carefully.

Specific problems

- Bolus feeding: Switch to intermittent or continuous feeding method.
- Lactose intolerance: As prescribed, switch to lactose-free products.
- Bacterial contamination
  - Obtain stool sample for culture and sensitivity.
  - Use clean technique in handling feeding tube, enteral products, and feeding sets.
  - Change all equipment q24h.
  - Refrigerate all opened products but discard after 24 h.
  - Discard feedings hanging for >8 h.

- Osmolality intolerance
  - Determine osmolality of feeding formula. Most are isotonic (plasma osmolality 300 mOsm). If hypertonic, reduce rate. If problem continues, dilute to ½ formula and ½ water but maintain rate.
- Medications
  - Monitor use of antibiotics, antacids, antidysrhythmics, aminophylline, H_2-receptor blocker, potassium chloride, and use of sorbitol in liquid medications.
  - As prescribed, administer *Lactobacillus acidophilus* to restore GI flora or use tincture of opium to decrease GI motility.
- Low fiber content: Add bulk-forming agents (psyllium or fiber preparations).

Impaired tissue integrity (or risk for same) related to mechanical irritant (presence of enteral tube)
Desired outcome: At time of discharge from critical care, patient's tissue is intact with absence of erosion around orifices, excoriation, skin rash, or mucous membrane breakdown.
Gastric/enteral tube
- Assess skin for irritation or tenderness q8h.
- Use a small-bore tube if possible.
- If long-term support is needed, discuss potential for using gastrostomy or jejunostomy tube with physician.
- Give ice chips, chewing gun, or hard candies prn if permitted.
- Apply petrolatum ointment to lips q2h.
- Brush teeth and tongue q4h.
- Alter position of tube daily to avoid pressure on underlying tissue. Use hypoallergenic tape to anchor tube.
Gastrostomy tube
- Assess site for erythema, drainage, tenderness, and odor q4h.
- Monitor placement of tube q4h.
- Secure tube so there is no tension on patient's tissue and skin.
- Wash skin with soap and water daily; pat dry.
Jejunostomy tube
- Assess site for erythema, drainage, tenderness, and odor q4h.
- Secure tube so there is no tension. Coil tube on top of dressing if necessary.
- Cleanse skin with half-strength solution of hydrogen peroxide and water; rinse hydrogen peroxide from skin; dry. Apply povidone-iodine ointment around insertion site daily and prn.
- Dress site with split 4×4s and tape with paper or hypoallergenic tape.

Risk for infection related to invasive procedures or malnutrition
Desired outcome: Patient is free of infection as evidenced by temperature and VS within normal limits, total lymphocytes 25%-40% (1,500-4,500 μl), WBC count ≤11,000 μl, and absence of the clinical signs of sepsis, including erythema and swelling at insertion site, chills, fever, and glucose intolerance.
- Ensure adequate nutritional support, based on individual needs. For guidelines, see p. 1.
- Twice weekly and prn, monitor total lymphocyte count, WBC count, and differential for values outside normal range.

- Check blood glucose q6h for values outside normal range.
- Examine catheter insertion site(s) q8h for erythema, swelling, or purulent drainage.
- Use meticulous sterile technique when changing central line dressing, containers, or lines.
- Avoid using central line that is being used for nutritional support for blood drawing, pressure monitoring, or administration of medications or other fluids.
- Change all administration sets within the time frame established by agency.
- Culture specimens from the catheter tip and exit site prn.
- Take blood specimens for culture, if sepsis is suspected, and administer antibiotics as prescribed.
- Hang fat emulsion for the time frame established by agency.

Altered cardiopulmonary tissue perfusion (or risk for same) related to interruption of arterial flow (air embolus)
Desired outcome: Patient has adequate cardiopulmonary tissue perfusion as evidenced by VS, ABG values, and arterial oximetry within normal limits and absence of dyspnea, tachypnea, cyanosis, chest pain, tachycardia, and hypotension.

- Check chest x-ray to determine catheter position.
- Position patient in Trendelenburg position when changing tubing or when neck vein catheters are inserted or removed.
- Teach patient Valsalva maneuver (if possible) for implementation during tubing changes.
- Use Luer-Lok connectors on all connections.
- Tape all tubing connections longitudinally to prevent disconnection.
- Use occlusive dressing over insertion site for 24 h after catheter is removed to prevent air entry *via* catheter-sinus tract.
- Monitor patient for chest pain, tachycardia, tachypnea, cyanosis, and hypotension.
- If air embolus is suspected, clamp the catheter and turn patient to left side-lying Trendelenburg position to trap air in the right ventricle. Ensure adequate oxygenation. Consult physician immediately.

Risk for fluid volume deficit related to failure of regulatory mechanisms, hyperglycemia, and hyperglycemic hyperosmotic nonketotic syndrome (HHNK)
Desired outcome: Patient's hydration status is adequate as evidenced by baseline VS, glucose <300 mg/dl, balanced I&O, urine specific gravity 1.010-1.025, and electrolytes within normal limits.

- Weigh patient daily; monitor I&O hourly.
- Consult physician for urine output <1 ml/kg/h.
- Check urine specific gravity; consult physician for value >1.035.
- Monitor serum osmolality and electrolytes daily and prn; consult physician for abnormalities.
- Monitor for circulatory overload during fluid replacement.
- Monitor for indicators of hyperglycemia. Perform finger stick q6h prn until blood glucose is stable. Administer insulin (usually a sliding scale) as prescribed to keep blood glucose levels <200 mg/dl.
- Assess rate and volume of nutritional support hourly. Reset to prescribed rate as indicated.

- Provide 1 ml free water for each calorie of enteral formula provided (or 30-50 ml/kg body weight).

ADDITIONAL NURSING DIAGNOSES

For other nursing diagnoses and interventions, see "Fluid and Electrolyte Disturbances," Chapter 10, which includes discussion of the electrolyte abnormalities listed in Table 1-7.

Mechanical ventilation

To ensure optimal care of the patient who requires mechanical ventilation, the practitioner must have adequate knowledge of the equipment and processes involved in mechanical ventilation. An in-depth discussion of the entire process is beyond the scope of this book; therefore it is assumed that the reader has basic knowledge on which to build.

TYPES OF VENTILATORS

Three categories of ventilators are used to deliver oxygen and artificial respiration.

Volume cycled: Most widely used ventilator. It is designed to deliver a preset volume of gas (tidal volume). The machine continues to deliver the predetermined tidal volume independent of changes in airway resistance or lung compliance. The ventilator is equipped with safety valves that can be set to terminate inspiration when peak pressures are excessive. Generally these pressure limits are set at 10-20 cm H_2O pressure over the patient's normal delivery pressure. The sophisticated design permits variable modes of delivery (see below). Refer to agency policy regarding alarm limits.

Pressure cycled: Terminates inspiration once a preset pressure is reached, at which time the patient exhales passively. When airway resistance increases because of mucous secretions or bronchospasm, the inspiratory cycle may terminate before adequate tidal volume is delivered. This ventilator is used only for stable patients with normal lung compliance.

Negative pressure: Intrapleural pressure ranges from -2 to -10 cm H_2O. The positive pressure ventilators already discussed generate 5-10 cm H_2O pressure to deliver a breath. Negative pressure ventilators generate subatmospheric pressure to the thorax and trunk to initiate respiration and do not require intubation for use. The iron lung, chest cuirass shell, and poncho chest shell are examples. There has been a resurgence of interest in and use of these devices for long-term home therapy.

MODES OF MECHANICAL VENTILATION

Controlled mechanical ventilation (CMV):   Delivers a preset tidal volume at a preset rate, ignoring the patient's own ventilatory drive. Its use is restricted to patients with CNS dysfunction, drug-induced paralysis or sedation, or severe chest trauma for whom negative pressure–driven respiratory effort is contraindicated. This is the simplest but least frequently used mode.

Assist-control ventilation (ACV):   Delivers a preset tidal volume when the patient initiates a negative pressure respiratory effort (inspiration). With adequate tidal volume delivery, work of breathing is decreased and alveolar ventilation improves. Machine sensitivity can be adjusted to prevent hyperventilation in patients whose respiratory rate increases because of mild anxiety or neurologic factors. If hyperventilation cannot be controlled, the patient may need to be changed to the mode that follows.

Synchronized intermittent mandatory ventilation (SIMV):   Delivers a preset tidal volume at a preset rate. In addition, the patient can breathe spontaneously (at his or her own rate and tidal volume) between ventilator breaths from an oxygen reservoir that is attached to the machine. The ventilator is synchronized to deliver the mandatory breath when the patient initiates inspiratory effort. Optimally, this mode prevents breath stacking caused by exhaling against machine-delivered inspirations. This is considered the standard mode of ventilation.

Positive end-expiratory pressure (PEEP):   Frequently used in conjunction with mechanical ventilation to improve ventilatory function of the lungs, thereby increasing Pao_2. PEEP increases functional residual capacity (FRC) and compliance and decreases dead space ventilation and shunt fraction by applying a given pressure at the end of expiration. This pressure counteracts small airway collapse and keeps alveoli open so that gas exchange can occur across the alveolar-capillary membrane. Areas of the lungs that are poorly ventilated normally can participate in adequate gas exchange, thereby decreasing shunting. This mechanism is effective for atelectatic alveoli, as well as for alveoli that are filled with fluid, but it does not improve lung function if the problem is one of poor perfusion. Generally, PEEP pressures range from 2.5 to 10 cm H_2O. Higher pressures (>35 cm H_2O) may be used if the patient can tolerate the increase and if the condition warrants. Application of this pressure increases intrathoracic pressure and compromises the patient's hemodynamic status by decreasing venous return, right ventricular filling pressures, and cardiac output. These mechanisms may cause or potentiate hypotension and shock, particularly in patients with volume depletion. PEEP also can cause pneumothorax if used at levels >10 cm H_2O or if lung compliance is diminished. **Note:** Continuous positive airway pressure (CPAP) functions in the same manner as PEEP but is a mode used independently of mechanically delivered breaths and is continuous throughout the respiratory cycle.

High-frequency ventilation and oscillation: An alternative mode of ventilation in which small tidal volumes are delivered at high rates. The resulting lower airway and intrathoracic pressures may reduce the risk of complications secondary to barotrauma and circulatory depression, which are associated with the high peak airway pressures of conventional ventilatory modes. Tidal volume is low and minute ventilation is high, making this the ideal mode for ventilation of patients with major airway disruption. High-frequency ventilation requires the use of special ventilators and a specially designed ET tube. The three basic mechanisms that are used are discussed in Table 1-8.

T A B L E   1 - 8   High-frequency jet ventilation

Mode	Rate	Tidal volume	Mechanism
High-frequency positive pressure ventilation (HFPPV)	60-100 cpm	3-6 ml/kg	Pneumatically controlled valve connected to high-pressure gas source; pulses gas into airway, while additional gases are entrained into the airway *via* a humidification circuit
High-frequency jet ventilation (HFJV)	100-200 cpm	50-400 ml	Gas under pressure is propelled through a narrow cannula (inserted in ET tube) while additional gases are entrained through a humidifier
High-frequency oscillations (HFO)	>200 cpm (800-3,000 vibrations/min)	50-80 ml	Gas is oscillated through ET tube *via* a piston; gas flows over the connection, and PEEP is created *via* resistant tubing on the outflow port; gas exchange occurs primarily by diffusion

cpm, Cycles per minute.

Inverse ratio ventilation (IRV):   Technique in which the inspiratory phase is prolonged and the expiratory phase is shortened. Normal I/E ratio is 1:2-4. During IRV the I/E ratio is increased to >1:1 (e.g., 2:1), thereby promoting alveolar recruitment, which improves oxygenation at lower levels of PEEP. The patient may require administration of a paralyzing agent and sedation to minimize the discomfort associated with this unusual breathing pattern.

COMPLICATIONS RELATED TO MECHANICAL VENTILATION

Barotrauma: Can occur when ventilatory pressures increase intrathoracic pressure, causing damage to major vessels or organs in the thorax and referring damage to the abdomen.

Tension pneumothorax: Develops when pressurized air enters the thoracic cavity. The high pressure of positive pressure ventilation may blow a hole in diseased or fragile lung tissue, leading to this life-threatening complication. In addition to the usual indicators of pneumothorax, sudden and sustained increases in peak inspiratory pressure will develop in the patient during mechanical ventilation.

Caution: If it is suspected that a pneumothorax has developed, disconnect the ventilator and manually ventilate using 100% oxygen while an assistant notifies physician. Prepare for immediate emergency chest tube placement.

Gastrointestinal complications: Peptic ulcers with profound hemorrhage may develop as a result of physiologic pressures and stress. Antacids, histamine H_2-receptor antagonists (e.g., cimetidine), and sucralfate (Carafate) routinely are administered to prevent these ulcers from developing. In addition, gastric dilatation can occur as a result of the large amounts of air swallowed in the presence of an artificial airway. If it is left untreated, paralytic ileus, vomiting, and aspiration may develop. Extreme dilatation can compromise respiratory effort because of the restriction of diaphragmatic movement. Treatment includes insertion of a gastric tube and application of intermittent suction to the GI tract.

Hypotension with decreased cardiac output: Develops as a result of decreased venous return secondary to increased intrathoracic pressure. Generally, this phenomenon is transient and is seen immediately after the patient has been placed on mechanical ventilation. PEEP, especially at levels >20 cm H_2O, may increase the incidence and severity of this phenomenon because of the significant increase in intrathoracic pressure that occurs with its use. The goal for fluid therapy when PEEP is used is to maintain the least intravascular volume that allows for adequate cardiac output to perfuse vital organs. Monitor HR and BP hourly, or more frequently if the patient is unstable. Monitor cardiac output as prescribed *via* flow-directed pulmonary artery (Swan-Ganz) catheter. See "Hemodynamic Monitoring," p. 30, for details regarding cardiac output.

Increased intracranial pressure: Occurs as a result of decreased venous return, which causes pooling of blood in the head. See "Craniocerebral Trauma," p. 123, for additional information.

Fluid imbalance: Increased production of antidiuretic hormone (ADH) occurs as a result of increased pressure on baroreceptors in the thoracic aorta, which causes the system to react as if the body were volume depleted. ADH stimulates the renal system to retain water. Patients may need diuretics if signs of hypervolemia are present. Be alert to new symptoms of dependent edema or adventitious breath sounds.

Anxiety: Many individuals experience anxiety related to discomfort associated with loss of control over their ventilatory process and the perception that their health status is threatened. Hypoxemia and air hunger, if present, contribute to anxiety and prompt rapid, shallow, and often irregular respiratory efforts. Coordinated and effective ventilation may not be possible with severe anxiety and agitation. For these patients, aggressive sedation with potent pharmacologic agents may be necessary to reduce the work of breathing and facilitate effective mechanical ventilation. See "Sedating and Paralytic Agents," p. 40.

WEANING THE PATIENT FROM MECHANICAL VENTILATION

The weaning process can involve any of the following: oxygen, PEEP, mechanical ventilation, and the artificial airway. Successful weaning depends more on the patient's overall condition than on the technique

T A B L E 1 - 9 Pulmonary function parameters for the patient being weaned from mechanical ventilation

Pulmonary function	Optimal parameters	Definition
Minute ventilation	$\leq$10 L/min	Tidal volume $\times$ respiratory rate; if adequate, means patient is breathing at a stable rate with adequate tidal volume
Negative inspiratory force	≥ -20 cm H_2O	Measures respiratory muscle strength. Maximum negative pressure that patient is able to generate to initiate spontaneous respirations; indicative of patient's ability to initiate inspiration independently
Maximum voluntary ventilation	$\geq 2 \times$ resting minute ventilation	Measures respiratory muscle endurance. Indicates patient's ability to sustain maximal respiratory effort
Tidal volume	5-10 ml/kg	Indicates patient's ability to ventilate lungs adequately
Arterial blood gases	$Pao_2 \geq$60 mm Hg $Paco_2 \leq$45 mm Hg pH 7.35-7.45 **or** patient's baseline	
Fractional concentration of inspired oxygen (Fio_2)	$\leq$0.40	

used. Physiologic factors (cardiovascular status, levels of fluids and electrolytes, and acid-base and nutritional status, as well as comfort and sleep pattern) and emotional factors (fear, anxiety, coping skills, general emotional state, and ability to cooperate) are important and must be evaluated both before and during the weaning process. In addition, pulmonary function parameters must be met before the weaning process is begun (Table 1-9). Goals for the weaning process are listed in Table 1-10. Traditionally three methods are employed for weaning the patient from mechanical ventilation.

T-piece adapter: Patient is taken off the ventilator and initiates spontaneous respiratory effort for increasingly longer periods of time. In this manner the patient builds strength and endurance for independent respiratory effort. Continuous positive airway pressure (CPAP) may be added to prevent alveolar collapse, thus allowing for more efficient gas exchange.

T A B L E 1 - 1 0   Goals for weaning

RR	<25 breaths/min
Tidal volume (V_T)	At least 3-5 ml/kg
HR/BP	Within 15% of baseline
Arterial pH	≥7.35
Pao_2	≥60 mm Hg and stable
$Paco_2$	≤45 mm Hg and stable
O_2 saturation	≥90%
Cardiac dysrhythmias	None
Use of accessory muscles of respiration	None

Intermittent mandatory ventilation: Ventilator-generated breaths are decreased gradually while patient builds strength and endurance. This is the most widely accepted method for patients receiving long-term ventilatory support. If multiple failures at weaning occur, the T-piece method may be used, starting with 1-2 min off the ventilator, followed by 58-59 min on, with a gradual reversal of this ratio until the patient breathes independently.

Pressure support ventilation (PSV): Assists the patient's normal breathing pattern with positive airway pressure applied during inspiration; 3-5 cm H_2O pressure support is added to SIMV (see p. 20), which significantly decreases the work of breathing through the demand flow system. Patients control their rate, inspiratory time, tidal volume, and inspiratory flow rate. When the patient stops inspiring, the positive pressure stops. The amount of pressure support is gradually decreased as the patient is weaned from the ventilator.

TROUBLESHOOTING MECHANICAL VENTILATOR PROBLEMS

The most important assessment factor in troubleshooting a mechanical ventilator is the effect on the patient. Regardless of which alarm sounds, always assess the patient first to evaluate his or her physiologic response to the problem. (See Tables 1-11 and 1-12 for processes that contribute to high-pressure and low-pressure alarm situations.)

NURSING DIAGNOSES AND INTERVENTIONS

Impaired gas exchange (or risk for same) related to altered oxygen supply secondary to nonphysiologic tidal volume distribution associated with mechanical ventilation

Desired outcome: Patient has adequate gas exchange as evidenced by Pao_2 >60 mm Hg, $Paco_2$ 35-45 mm Hg, Spo_2 ≥92%, Svo_2 ≥60%, and RR 12-20 breaths/min.

• Observe for, document, and report any changes in patient's condition consistent with increasing respiratory distress. (See "Clinical Presentation," p. 264, in "Acute Respiratory Failure.")
• Position patient to allow for maximal alveolar ventilation and comfort. Remember that in normal situations, the dependent lung receives more ventilation and more blood flow than the nondependent lung; however, during mechanical ventilation the dependent portion

T A B L E   1 - 1 1   Processes contributing to high-pressure alarm situations

Increased airway resistance	Decreased lung compliance
Patient requires suctioning	Pneumothorax, pulmonary edema, atelectasis, worsening of underlying disease process
Kinks in ventilator circuitry	
Water or expectorated secretions in circuitry	
Patient coughs or exhales against ventilator breaths	
Patient biting ET tube	
Bronchospasm	
Herniation of airway cuff over end of artificial airway	
Change in patient position that restricts chest wall movement	
Breath stacking	

T A B L E   1 - 1 2   Processes contributing to low-pressure alarm situations

Patient disconnected from machine
Leak in airway cuff
    Insufficient air in cuff
    Hole or tear in cuff
    Leak in one-way valve of inflation port
Leak in circuitry
    Poor fittings on water reservoirs
    Dislodged temperature-sensing device
    Hole or tear in tubing
    Poor seal in circuitry connections
Displacement of airway above vocal cords
Loss of compressed air source

of the lung receives less distribution of tidal volume than do the non-dependent areas. Follow body positioning protocol:

- □ Analyze Spo_2, Svo_2, and ABG results with patient in different positions to determine adequacy of ventilation.
- □ Use postural drainage principles where appropriate.
- □ In unilateral lung disease, position patient with healthy lung down.
- □ In bilateral lung disease, position patient in right lateral decubitus position, inasmuch as the right lung has more surface area. If ABG results show that the patient tolerates left lateral decubitus position, alternate between the two positions.
- Turn patient q2h or more frequently if signs of deteriorating pulmonary status occur.

- Auscultate over artificial airway to assess for leaks.
- Assess ventilator for proper functioning and parameter settings, including Fio_2, tidal volume, rate, mode, peak inspiratory pressure, sigh volume and rate, and temperature of inspired gases. In addition, ensure that circuits are tight and alarms are set.
- Keep ventilator circuitry free of condensed water and expectorated secretions, because these fluids may obstruct the flow of gases to and from the patient.
- Monitor serial ABG results. Be alert for decreases in Pao_2 or increases in $Paco_2$ with concomitant decrease in pH (<7.35), which can signal inadequate gas exchange. Also observe for decreased $Paco_2$ (<35 mm Hg) with increased pH (>7.45), which may signal mechanical hyperventilation. Notify physician of dysrhythmias, which can occur even with modest alkalosis if the patient has heart disease or is receiving inotropic medications (see Appendix 7). Arrange for ABG analysis when change in patient's condition warrants.
- Keep manual resuscitator at bedside for ventilation in case of malfunctioning equipment.

Ineffective airway clearance (or risk for same) related to altered anatomic structure secondary to presence of ET or tracheostomy tube
Desired outcome: Patient maintains a patent airway as evidenced by absence of adventitious breath sounds or signs of respiratory distress such as restlessness and anxiety.

- Assess and document breath sounds in all lung fields at least q2h. Note quality and presence or absence of adventitious sounds.
- Monitor patient for restlessness and anxiety, which can signal early airway obstruction.
- Using sterile technique, suction patient's secretions, based on assessment findings, to maintain patency of airway. Document amount, color, and consistency of tracheobronchial secretions. Report significant changes (e.g., increase in production of secretions, tenacious secretions, bloody sputum) to physician. In addition, document patient's tolerance to suctioning procedure.
- Maintain artificial airway in a secure and proper alignment.
- Maintain correct temperature (32°-36° C [89.6°-96.8° F]) of inspired gas. Cold air irritates airways, and hot air may burn fragile lung tissue.
- Maintain humidification of inspired gas to prevent drying of tracheal mucosa. In addition, without humidification, tracheobronchial secretions may become thick and tenacious, creating mucous plugs that place patient at risk for development of atelectasis and infection.

Ineffective breathing pattern (or risk for same) related to anxiety secondary to use of mechanical ventilation
Desired outcome: Patient exhibits stable RR of 12-20 breaths/min (synchronized with ventilator) and absence of restlessness, anxiety, lethargy, and/or sounding of high-pressure alarm.

- Monitor for evidence that patient is fighting ventilator: frequent sounding of high-pressure alarm when patient breathes against mechanical inspiration or mismatch of patient's respiratory rate and ventilator cycle.

- Monitor respiratory rate and quality, and monitor for signs of respiratory distress (e.g., tachypnea, hyperventilation, anxiety, restlessness, lethargy, and cyanosis, which is a late sign).
- Teach patient technique for progressive muscle relaxation (see **Health-seeking behavior,** p. 323). Stay with patient until the respirations are under control. Reassure patient that he or she will be able to synchronize respirations with the ventilator once he or she relaxes.
- Administer prescribed pain medication or sedation when prescribed for restlessness, which increases O_2 demand and consumption, thus interfering with adequate ventilation.

Risk for infection related to increased environmental exposure (contaminated respiratory equipment), tissue destruction (during intubation or suctioning), and invasive procedures (intubation, suctioning, presence of ET tube)

Desired outcome: Patient is free of infection as evidenced by normothermia, WBC count $\leq$11,000 μl, clear sputum, and negative sputum culture results.

- Assess patient for signs and symptoms of infection, including temperature $>38°$ C (100.4° F), tachycardia (HR >100 bpm), erythema of tracheostomy, and foul-smelling sputum. Document all significant findings.
- To minimize the risk of cross-contamination, wash hands before and after contact with the respiratory secretions of any patient (even though gloves were worn) and before and after contact with patient who is undergoing intubation.
- Recognize that bacteria and spores can be introduced easily during suctioning. Follow standard techniques:
  - Use aseptic technique during suctioning process, including use of sterile catheter, gloves, and suctioning or lavage solutions.
  - Suction tracheobronchial tree before the oropharynx to avoid introducing oral pathogens into tracheobronchial tree.
  - Never store or reuse a single-use suction catheter. Consider use of closed system for suctioning.
  - Change suction cannisters and tubing within the time frame established by agency. Change cannisters and tubing between patients.
  - Tightly recap saline bottle used for suctioning. Be sure bottle is marked with date and time; dispose of unused portion within the time frame established by agency.

Note: Wear gloves on both hands when handling secretions to protect yourself from transmission of herpesvirus, which can cause herpetic whitlow (infection of the fingertip with herpesvirus).

- To reduce the risk of infection caused by trauma or cross-contamination, perform suctioning on an "as needed" basis rather than routinely.
- Use sterile gloves when performing tracheostomy care to prevent colonization of stoma with bacteria from practitioner's hands.
- Provide oral hygiene at least q4-8h to prevent overgrowth of normal flora and aerobic gram-negative bacilli.

- Recognize ways that water reservoirs and ventilator equipment can be potential sources of contamination by following these precautions:
  - Use sterile fluids in all humidifiers and nebulizers.
  - Change all ventilatory circuitry within the time frame established by agency or sooner if soiled with secretions.
  - Empty condensed water or expectorated secretions in tubes into attached traps—not back into patient.
  - Empty water traps on tubing during each ventilator check.
  - When disconnecting patient from ventilatory circuits, keep end of connectors sterile by placing them on opened sterile gauze pads.
  - Keep connectors on manual resuscitator bags clean and free of secretions between use. Although there are no data suggesting that bags be changed with any frequency when used for only one patient, they should not be used between patients without sterilization.
- Maintain appropriate seal on artificial airway cuff to prevent aspiration of oral secretions.
- Keep cuff sealed and HOB elevated 30-45 degrees for patients receiving continuous gastric feedings. Monitor patient for reflux of feedings, as well as for signs of intolerance to feedings (absence of bowel sounds, abdominal distention, residual feedings >100 ml), which can precipitate vomiting and result in pulmonary aspiration of gastric contents.
- Be aware of special risk factors for patients with tracheostomy tubes and intervene accordingly:
  - Maintain tracheostomy tube in a secure and proper alignment to avoid irritation of stoma from too much movement.
  - Change tracheostomy ties q24h or more frequently if heavily soiled with secretions or wound exudate.
  - Perform stoma care at least q8h, using aseptic technique until stoma is completely healed. Keep area around stoma dry at all times to prevent maceration and infection. Change stoma dressing as needed to keep it dry.
  - Avoid use of cotton-filled gauze or other material that may shed small fibers. Patient may aspirate fibers, which in turn can lead to infection.
  - Use aseptic technique (including use of sterile gloves and drapes) when changing tracheostomy tube.
- Culture secretions or wound drainage; administer antibiotics as prescribed.

Anxiety related to actual or perceived threat to health status as a result of need for or presence of mechanical ventilation

Desired outcome: Within 12 h of initiation of mechanical ventilation, patient relates the presence of emotional comfort and exhibits a decrease in irritability, with an HR within patient's normal range.

- Because the general public equates ventilator placement with a hopelessly chronic, vegetative state, reassure patient and significant others that ventilatory support may be a temporary measure until the underlying pathophysiologic process has resolved. At that time the patient may be weaned from the ventilator.
- Reassure patient that he or she will not be left alone.

- Explain all procedures to patient and significant others before they are initiated. Inform patient of his or her progress.
- Describe and point out the alarm system, explaining that it will alert staff in the event of an accidental disconnection.
- Provide patient with mechanism for communication (e.g., picture board, erasable marker board, pen and paper). See **Impaired verbal communication,** p. 89, in "Psychosocial Support."

Impaired gas exchange (or risk for same) related to altered oxygen supply secondary to weaning from mechanical ventilation

Desired outcomes: Patient has adequate gas exchange as evidenced by Pao_2 >60 mm Hg, $Paco_2$ <45 mm Hg, Spo_2 ≥92%, Svo_2 ≥60%, and pH 7.35-7.45 (or values within 10% of patient's baseline).

- Maintain patient in a comfortable position to enhance ventilation. Many patients find that semi-Fowler's position promotes effective respirations.
- Observe for indicators of hypoxia, including tachycardia, tachypnea, cardiac dysrhythmias, anxiety, and restlessness.
- Assess and record VS q15min for the first hour of weaning, then hourly if patient is stable. Report significant findings to physician, such as increased respiratory effort, hyperventilation, anxiety, lethargy, cyanosis.
- Check patient's tidal volume after the first 15 min of weaning and as needed. Optimally, it will be within 5-10 ml/kg.
- Obtain specimen for ABG analysis 20 min after weaning has been initiated or as prescribed. As available, monitor Spo_2 and Svo_2 for values outside normal range.

Anxiety related to perceived threat to health status secondary to weaning process

Desired outcome: Within 4 h of initiation of weaning process, patient expresses the attainment of emotional comfort and is free of the signs of harmful anxiety as evidenced by HR ≤100 bpm, RR ≤20 breaths/min, and BP within patient's normal range.

- Before weaning process is initiated, discuss plans for weaning with patient and significant others. Explain that patient's condition will be assessed at frequent intervals during the weaning procedure. Provide time for questions and answers about the procedure.
- Stay with patient during the initial phase of weaning, keeping patient informed of progress being made. Provide positive feedback for positive efforts.
- Teach patient progressive muscle relaxation technique, which may reduce anxiety and fear and thus relax chest muscles. (See **Health-seeking behavior,** p. 323.)
- Instruct patient to take deep breaths if he or she is capable of doing so. This may provide the confidence of knowing that he or she can initiate and sustain respirations independently.
- Leave call light within patient's reach before leaving bedside. Reassure patient that help is nearby.

ADDITIONAL NURSING DIAGNOSES

Also see nursing diagnoses and interventions under "Prolonged Immobility," p. 78; "Psychosocial Support," p. 88; and "Psychosocial Support for the Patient's Family and Significant Others," p. 100.

Hemodynamic monitoring

Many critically ill adults have a history of cardiovascular disease or are at risk for cardiovascular complications; therefore it is important to be able to assess cardiac function and related factors influencing cardiovascular functioning. There are four major cardiac mechanisms that determine cardiac output (CO), which is the amount of blood ejected from the heart over 1 min. These mechanisms are preload, afterload, contractility, and heart rate.

Preload: Can be defined as the degree of myocardial fiber stretch at the end of diastole just before contraction. Starling's law of the heart describes the concept of preload: the greater the stretch of the myocardial muscle, the greater the force of contraction. However, if the stretch is excessive, contractility will diminish. This mechanism enables the heart to pump varying volumes of blood and to keep the output of the two ventricles matched. Preload is a function of the volume of blood delivered to the ventricle and the compliance (ability to stretch) of the ventricle at end diastole. Factors that affect ventricular volume include venous return, circulating blood volume, and atrial contractility. Factors that affect ventricular compliance include the stiffness and thickness of the cardiac muscle. Any problem that influences one of these factors will result in a change in preload, with a concomitant change in CO. Clinically, preload is described as ventricular end-diastolic pressure (VEDP), because pressure in the ventricle correlates closely with volume. Right ventricular diastolic (filling) pressure is reflected by the right atrial pressure (RAP) or the central venous pressure (CVP). Left ventricular diastolic (filling) pressure is reflected by the left atrial (LA), pulmonary artery diastolic (PAD), or pulmonary artery wedge (PAW) pressure measurements.

Afterload: Refers to the tension that develops within the ventricular myocardium during systole. In order for the heart to eject its contents, it must overcome any resistant forces. The pulmonary, aortic, and arterial pressures are the main impediments to flow for the right and left ventricles. Other resistant forces include blood viscosity, vascular resistance, distensibility of the vascular system, and the valves themselves. Because vascular resistance plays a major role in determining pressure, afterload is evaluated by calculating the pulmonary vascular resistance (PVR) for right ventricular afterload and systemic vascular resistance (SVR) for left ventricular afterload. The significance of these measures is that the higher the afterload, the greater the myocardial wall tension and the greater the work of the heart to overcome resistance to flow. This work is achieved at the expense of oxygen utilization. In the abnormal heart in which there is diminished coronary blood flow, an increased afterload may result in ischemic myocardial injury and possible infarction.

Contractility: Refers to the inherent capacity of the myocardium to contract. This mechanism functions independently of variations in preload and afterload. Although contractility cannot be measured directly, a change can be inferred when there is a decreased CO, and other variables that affect CO (i.e., preload, afterload, heart rate) remain the same. Several factors positively influence contractility: sympathetic stimulation, calcium, positive inotropic agents such as digitalis and amrinone, and beta-adrenergic drugs. Factors such as acidemia, hypoxia, beta-blocker drugs, and antidysrhythmic drugs decrease it.

Heart rate (HR): Alterations in HR affect myocardial functioning profoundly. Slight increases in HR with a constant stroke volume (SV) result in increased CO. Very rapid rates are associated with a reduction in CO as diastolic time is shortened, resulting in decreased coronary perfusion and reduced ventricular filling time. Bradycardia usually results in decreased CO unless there are increases in SV because of longer ventricular filling times.

Hemodynamic monitoring refers to the specialized methods of evaluating cardiovascular performance. It provides information about cardiac performance, tissue perfusion, blood volume, tissue oxygenation, and vascular tone. Indirect methods of hemodynamic monitoring include measurement of arterial pressure *via* manual or automated BP cuff or Doppler test and measurement of CO with an echo Doppler device. Direct methods of measuring hemodynamic values include those obtained by arterial, central venous, and pulmonary artery catheters. This section focuses on direct methods of hemodynamic monitoring. Normal hemodynamic values with derived parameters are found in Table 1-13.

DIRECT HEMODYNAMIC MEASUREMENT

Arterial catheters: Generally inserted *via* the radial artery, because this artery is readily accessible and collateral blood flow is usually adequate. The arterial pressure waveform is displayed on a bedside monitor for continuous observation of systolic, diastolic, and mean arterial pressures. The appearance of the arterial waveform is influenced by clinical conditions and mechanical factors. In hypertensive and hyperdynamic states, there is a steep rate of rise in the pressure waveform, as well as a high peak systolic pressure. In shock states or severe heart failure, the waveform is damped with a slow rate of rise. Dysrhythmias, such as PVCs, usually result in small, irregular waveforms associated with each abnormal contraction. Mechanical factors that influence the waveform include overdamping, catheter whip, and inaccurate calibration/zeroing (Table 1-14). Complications of arterial catheters include arterial thrombosis with ischemia, infection, exsanguination, and infiltration. Continuous observation of the arterial line insertion site for infection and leakage is an important nursing responsibility.

Systolic blood pressure: Determined by (1) the amount of blood ejected by the ventricle per beat (stroke volume), (2) wall compliance of the arterial system, and (3) peripheral resistance. Elevations in systolic pressure often reflect changes in vascular compliance, such as the hypertension seen in individuals with vascular atherosclerosis. A decrease in systolic pressure will be seen with heart disorders that result in decreased stroke volume or with the use of arterial vasodilators such as nitroprusside, nitroglycerine, and nifedipine.

Diastolic blood pressure: Determined by (1) volume of blood within the arterial system, (2) compliance of the arterial wall, and (3) peripheral resistance. Because coronary artery blood flow occurs during diastole and a drop in diastolic pressure may result in ischemia of the

TABLE 1-13   Hemodynamic formulas

Parameter	Formula	Normal values
Cardiac output (CO)	$\dfrac{O_2 \text{ consumption}}{\text{A-V}O_2 \text{ difference}}$	4-7 L/min
Cardiac index (CI)	$\dfrac{CO}{\text{Body surface area (BSA)}}$	2.5-4 L/min/m^2
Coronary perfusion pressure (CPP)	Diastolic BP $-$ PAWP	50-70 mm Hg
Stroke volume (SV)	$\dfrac{CO}{HR} \times 1{,}000$	55-100 ml/beat
Stroke volume index (SVI)	$\dfrac{SV}{BSA}$	30-60 ml/beat/m^2
Arterial oxygen content (CaO_2)	(Hgb $\times$ 1.34) $\times$ SaO_2	18-20 ml/vol%
Venous oxygen content (CvO_2)	(Hgb $\times$ 1.34) $\times$ SvO_2	15.5 ml/vol%
Oxygen delivery (DO_2)	CaO_2 $\times$ CO $\times$ 10	800-1,000 ml/min
Oxygen delivery index (DO_2I)	CaO_2 $\times$ CI $\times$ 10	500-600 ml/min/m^2
Arteriovenous oxygen content difference (C[a-v]O_2)	CaO_2 $-$ CvO_2	4-6 ml/vol%
Oxygen consumption ($\dot{V}O_2$)	CO $\times$ 10 $\times$ C(a-v)O_2	200-250 ml/min
Oxygen consumption index ($\dot{V}O_2$I)	CI $\times$ 10 $\times$ C(a-v)O_2	115-165 ml/min/m^2
Systemic vascular resistance (SVR)	$\dfrac{\text{MAP} - \text{RAP}}{CO} \times 80$	900-1,200 dynes/sec/cm^{-5}
Pulmonary vascular resistance (PVR)	$\dfrac{\text{PAM} - \text{PAWP}}{CO} \times 80$	60-100 dynes/sec/cm^{-5}

subendocardium, diastolic BP is an important measure, particularly when vasodilating drugs are administered.

Mean arterial pressure (MAP): The average pressure within the arterial tree throughout the cardiac cycle. It can be calculated by the following formula:

$$\text{MAP} = \frac{\text{Systolic BP} + 2 \text{ (Diastolic BP)}}{3}$$

Normal value is 70-105 mm Hg. MAP reflects the average force that pushes blood through the systemic circulation throughout the cardiac cycle; therefore it is an important indicator of tissue blood flow. Because MAP is the product of CO $\times$ SVR, an increase in CO or SVR

T A B L E 1 - 1 3   Hemodynamic formulas—cont'd

Parameter	Formula	Normal values
Left ventricular stroke work index (LVSWI)	SVI × (MAP − PAWP) × 0.136	40-75 g/m^2/beat
Right ventricular stroke work index (RVSWI)	SVI × (MPAP − RAP) × 0.136	4-8 g/m^2/beat
Mean arterial pressure (MAP)	$\dfrac{\text{Systolic BP} + 2(\text{Diastolic BP})}{3}$	70-105 mm Hg
Mean pulmonary artery pressure (MPAP, PAM)	$\dfrac{\text{PAS} + 2(\text{PAD})}{3}$	10-15 mm Hg
Mixed venous oxygen saturation (Svo$_2$)	$(CO × Cao_2 × 10) − \dot{V}o_2$	60%-80%
Central venous pressure (CVP)		2-6 mm Hg
Right atrial pressure (RAP)		4-6 mm Hg
Left atrial pressure (LAP)		8-12 mm Hg
Right ventricular pressure (RVP)		25/0-5 mm Hg
Pulmonary artery systolic pressure (PAS)		20-30 mm Hg
Pulmonary artery diastolic pressure (PAD)		8-15 mm Hg
Pulmonary artery wedge pressure (PAWP)		6-12 mm Hg

will increase MAP, and a decrease in either value will decrease MAP.
Central venous catheters: CVP is the measurement of systemic venous pressure at the level of the right atrium (RA). CVP can be measured by a catheter that is threaded into the jugular, subclavian, or other large vein or by a separate port of a PA catheter. Normal value is 2-6 mm Hg. Because 60% of the blood volume is contained in the venous bed, the CVP is valuable in assessing fluid volume excess or deficit. In addition, it provides information regarding right ventricular (RV) function and venous tone. Disease processes that may increase CVP include right ventricular failure, cardiac tamponade, fluid volume overload, pulmonary hypertension, tricuspid valve disease, and chronic left ventricular failure. Usually, decreased CVP is caused by hypovolemia; however, venodilatation due to sepsis, drugs, or neurogenic causes also may decrease CVP.

T A B L E   1 - 1 4   **Mechanical problems affecting hemodynamic measurements**

Problem	Waveform appearance	Cause
Overdamping*	Smaller than usual with a slow rise; diminished or absent dicrotic notch (arterial and pulmonary artery catheters)	Air bubbles in system Thrombus formation Lodging of catheter against vessel wall Kinking or knotting of catheter or tubing Loose connection in tubing or transducer Incorrect calibration Spontaneous catheter migration into a near-wedged position (PA catheter only)
Catheter whip	Erratic, "noisy" waveform with highly variable and inaccurate pressures	Spurious movement of the catheter tip within the vessel lumen (may require repositioning) Catheter too long for vessel (arterial)
No waveform	Complete absence of waveform	Large leak in the system, usually with blood backing up into the tubing Loose or cracked transducer or air in transducer Stopcock turned to wrong position Catheter tip or lumen totally occluded by clot Inadequate pressure (<300 mm Hg) on pressure bag Defective transducer or amplifier
Inability to obtain a wedged reading (PA catheter only)	Absence of wedge waveform after balloon inflation	Balloon rupture Retrograde catheter slippage

*Whenever the amplitude of an arterial or PA waveform decreases, the patient first should be assessed for hypovolemia or shock.

Pulmonary artery catheters: Inserted *via* the jugular, subclavian, or femoral vein and passed through the right side of the heart into the pulmonary artery, where the tip of the catheter is positioned in the pulmonary capillary bed. This catheter provides valuable information that can be used in the assessment or treatment of life-threatening illness or injury during which assessment of blood volume, heart function, and tissue oxygenation is essential. Assessment data that may be de-

TABLE 1-15 Abnormal pulmonary artery pressures

Hemodynamic pressure	Normal range	Clinical conditions
PAS	20-30 mm Hg	*Increased:* right ventricular failure, constrictive pericarditis, cardiac tamponade, CHF, pulmonary hypertension (primary or related to lung disease) *Decreased:* hypovolemia, preload reduction
PAD*	8-15 mm Hg	*Increased:* left ventricular failure, mitral stenosis, left-to-right shunts, pulmonary hypertension (primary or related to lung disease) *Decreased:* hypovolemia, preload reduction
PAWP†	6-12 mm Hg	*Increased:* left ventricular failure, cardiac tamponade, mitral valve regurgitation, acute ventricular septal defect, fluid volume overload *Decreased:* hypovolemia, afterload reduction

*PAD may exceed PAWP by ≥5 mm Hg in patients with pulmonary hypertension, hypoxemia, acidosis, pulmonary emboli, and other lung disease.

†PAWP >PAD signals a mechanical problem (i.e., overwedging or improper identification of PAD).

rived from this catheter include RAP; right ventricular pressure (RVP); PAP, including systolic, diastolic, and mean pressures; PAWP; CO; core body temperature; and Svo_2. Other calculated hemodynamic and oxygen transport variables may be derived using PA catheter measurements (see Table 1-13). Abnormal pulmonary artery pressures are discussed in Table 1-15. Although the risk of major complications with this catheter is low (3%), it is important for the nurse to be familiar with the possibilities: ventricular or atrial dysrhythmias, pulmonary ischemia or infarction, pulmonic valve injury, endocarditis, tricuspid valve damage, pulmonary artery rupture, infection, and emboli (thrombotic, air, balloon).

Right atrial pressure: This is essentially the same as CVP. With the PA catheter, RAP can be monitored continuously and displayed on a bedside screen. In addition, the catheter lumen can be used for fluid or drug administration. Normal mean RAP is 4-6 mm Hg.

Right ventricular pressure: Measured during catheter insertion only and can provide information about the function of the right ventricle and the tricuspid and pulmonic valves. Normal RVP is 25/0-5 mm Hg. Elevation of right ventricular systolic pressure may be seen in pulmonic stenosis, pulmonary hypertension, or ventricular septal defect (VSD) with left-to-right shunt. Elevation of right ventricular diastolic pressure may occur with right ventricular failure, cardiac tamponade, or constrictive pericarditis. It is important for the nurse to identify the normal right ventricular waveform because a complication of the PA catheter is redirection of the catheter tip into the right ventricle, causing ventricular ectopy.

Pulmonary artery pressure: Used to evaluate left-sided heart function and pulmonary vascular disease. Normal PAP is 20-30/8-15 mm Hg. In patients with healthy pulmonary vasculature, the PAD pressure corresponds closely to the PAWP and reflects the left ventricular end-diastolic pressure (LVEDP). A significant difference (i.e., >5 mm Hg) between the PAD and PAWP is seen with pulmonary disease or a pulmonary embolus. When this occurs, PA systolic and diastolic pressures are elevated, whereas the PAWP remains normal. Specific disease states that elevate PAP include pulmonary hypertension, pulmonary embolism, hypoxia, left ventricular failure because of valve disease, MI, cardiomyopathy, and left-to-right intracardiac shunt. A decreased PAP is seen with hypovolemia and pharmacologic preload reduction.

Pulmonary artery wedge pressure: Reflects the LVEDP and is used to evaluate cardiac performance. Normal mean PAWP is 6-12 mm Hg. An elevated PAWP may be seen with left ventricular failure, acute mitral regurgitation, acute VSD, and acute cardiac tamponade. A decreased PAWP is seen with hypovolemia and afterload reduction. PEEP/CPAP >10 cm H_2O may result in falsely elevated PAP and PAWP. However, patients should not be disconnected from the ventilator to measure PAP and PAWP, because significant hypoxemia and inaccurate measurements can result. Correlation of measured pressures with the respiratory cycle may improve the accuracy of these measurements.

Cardiac output: The volume of blood in liters ejected by the heart each minute and the product of the stroke volume (SV) and heart rate (HR). Normal value is 4-7 L/min. SV is the volume of blood ejected by the heart per beat. Normal SV is 55-100 ml/beat. To compare individual differences in CO in relation to body size, the CO is divided by the body surface area (BSA) to obtain the value known as the *cardiac index (CI)*. Normal CI is 2.5-4 L/min/m^2.

Systemic vascular resistance: The major factor that determines left ventricular afterload and therefore is the clinical measurement used to evaluate it. The formula for SVR is the following:

$$SVR = \frac{(MAP - RAP)}{CO} \times 80$$

Normal value for SVR is 900-1,200 dynes/sec/cm^{-5}. Any factor that increases SVR will increase the workload of the heart; therefore measures are taken (e.g., vasodilator therapy) to keep SVR within normal limits.

Pulmonary vascular resistance: The clinical measure of right ventricular afterload. The formula for PVR is the following:

$$PVR = \frac{PAM - PAWP}{CO} \times 80$$

The normal value is 60-100 dynes/sec/cm^{-5}. PVR may be elevated as a result of mitral or aortic valve disease, congenital heart disease, long-standing left ventricular heart failure, hypoxia, COPD, or pulmonary embolus. Drugs also may affect the PVR (e.g., norepinephrine and the prostaglandins increase it, whereas isoproterenol, nifedipine, sodium nitroprusside, and acetylcholine decrease it).

Mixed venous oxygen saturation: Can be measured with the use of mixed venous blood samples from the distal port of the PA catheter or by continuous monitoring *via* a fiberoptic PA catheter. Svo_2 is the average percentage of Hgb bound with oxygen in the venous blood and is reflective of the patient's ability to balance oxygen supply and demand at tissue level. Normal range for Svo_2 is 60%-80%. Very low levels (<30%) usually are associated with lactic acidosis and a poor prognosis. Measurement of Svo_2 is valuable in the critical care setting because it can aid in the diagnosis and treatment of many life-threatening conditions. With continuous monitoring it can be used to evaluate the effects of medical and nursing interventions on tissue oxygen use. Four factors affect the oxygen supply-demand relationship and Svo_2 values: arterial oxygen saturation (Sao_2), CO, Hgb, and oxygen consumption (Vo_2). If the Svo_2 value changes by more than 10% and the change is sustained for more than 10 min, the nurse should evaluate each of the aforementioned factors and determine which are affecting Svo_2 (see Table 1-16).

Left atrial catheters: Inserted into the left atrium during cardiac surgery and brought through the chest wall or epigastric area. Left atrial pressure (LAP) is the most direct measure of LVEDP and may be indicated for the cardiac surgery patient with significant pulmonary hypertension. During connection to a transducer, a continuous display of left atrial pressure is possible. The normal value for LAP is 8-12 mm Hg. Because the catheter enters directly into the left atrium, the patient is at great risk for air or tissue emboli. An in-line air filter should be added to the flush system to reduce the risk of air emboli. If the waveform pattern dampens, aspirate until blood is seen. If there is no blood return, consult physician but do not flush.

NURSING DIAGNOSES AND INTERVENTIONS

Knowledge deficit: Rationale for hemodynamic monitoring and procedure for catheter insertion

Desired outcome: Within 24 h of catheter placement, patient verbalizes knowledge of the rationale for hemodynamic monitoring, procedure for insertion of lines, and sensations that are experienced during and after the procedure.

- Assess patient's knowledge about hemodynamic monitoring. As indicated, explain to patient that hemodynamic monitoring is useful in guiding therapy and that the PA catheter can measure pressures in and near the heart.
- Teach patient about the insertion procedure, emphasizing that a local anesthetic agent will be used, he or she will not be able to move during the procedure, frequent x-rays will be taken, and a dressing will be applied to the insertion site.
- Explain the sensations that may be felt during the procedure: a stick from the local anesthetic, pressure as the catheter advances, coldness from the cleansing solution, burning from the injection of lidocaine, claustrophobia from drapes over the face, dull pushing and pulling sensations in the neck, and coldness from the injection of cardiac output iced solution (if used).

T A B L E   1 - 1 6   Factors affecting mixed venous oxygen saturation

Factor	Effect on Svo_2	Clinical examples
Arterial oxygen saturation		
↑ Sao_2	↑ Svo_2	Supplemental oxygen
↓ Sao_2	↓ Svo_2	Reduced oxygen supply (i.e., ARDS, ET suctioning, removal of supplemental oxygen)
Cardiac output		
↑ CO	↑ Svo_2	Administration of inotropes to increase contractility
↓ CO	↓ Svo_2	Dysrhythmias, increased SVR, MI
Hemoglobin		
↓ Hgb	↓ Svo_2	Hemorrhage, hemolysis, severe anemia in patients with cardiovascular disease
Oxygen consumption		
↑ $\dot{V}o_2$	↓ Svo_2	States in which metabolic demand exceeds oxygen supply (e.g., shivering, seizures, hyperthermia, hyperdynamic states)
↓ $\dot{V}o_2$	↑ Svo_2	States in which there is failure of peripheral tissue to extract or use oxygen: · Significant peripheral arteriovenous shunting: cirrhosis, renal failure · Redistribution of blood away from beds where oxygen extraction occurs: sepsis, acute pancreatitis, major burns · Blockage of oxygen uptake or utilization: cyanide poisoning (including nitroprusside toxicity), carbon monoxide poisoning
Mechanical problems	Artifactitious ↑ Svo_2	Wedged PA catheter

- Instruct patient to report any anxiety or discomfort that occurs during the procedure, because medications can be given as necessary.

Risk for infection related to presence of invasive hemodynamic catheters

Desired outcome: Patient is free of infection as evidenced by normothermia, WBC count ≤11,000 μl, negative culture results, and absence of erythema, heat, swelling, or purulent drainage at the insertion site.

- On a daily basis, monitor temperature for elevations >37° C (99° F); WBC count for elevation; and catheter insertion site for erythema, tenderness to the touch, local warmth, and purulent drainage.
- As prescribed, obtain culture of any suspicious drainage and report positive findings.
- Use normal saline rather than D_5W for hemodynamic flush solution.

- Change hemodynamic tubing, transducer, and flush solution according to hospital protocol.
- Maintain closed system to transducer and for flush solution. Keep all external openings and stopcocks securely capped at all times.
- Use closed system for cardiac output injectate.
- Maintain occlusive, dry sterile dressing over insertion site.
- Change dressing per agency protocol, using aseptic technique.
- Record date of catheter insertion and ensure that catheter is changed per agency protocol.
- If infection occurs, send catheter tip for culture and sensitivity test.

Altered cardiopulmonary tissue perfusion (or risk for same) related to interrupted blood flow secondary to migration of PA catheter into a wedged position, overwedging of balloon, continuous wedge position, or local vascular thrombosis

Desired outcomes: Within 2 h of this diagnosis, patient has adequate pulmonary perfusion as evidenced by normal PA waveform and RR 12-20 breaths/min with normal depth and pattern (eupnea).

- Monitor PA waveform continuously. Report any change in configuration, particularly if the waveform becomes decreased in amplitude and flattened in appearance (see Table 1-14).
- Assess patient for interrupted pulmonary arterial blood flow as evidenced by acute onset of pleuritic chest pain, SOB, tachypnea, and hemoptysis.
- On a daily basis, evaluate position of catheter *via* chest x-ray. Look for wedge-shaped infiltrate, which could signal impaired pulmonary tissue perfusion.
- Exercise care in taking PAWP measurements. Prolonged and repeated readings can cause trauma to the vessel wall. Another common problem is overwedging the catheter. Monitor PA waveform when wedging balloon. Inject enough air to obtain a wedge configuration but no more than the amount recommended by catheter manufacturer. Never pull back on syringe to remove air; disconnect syringe and allow passive deflation of balloon.
- Consider following trends of PAD pressures rather than those of PAWP. Verify correlation of PAD to PAWP q4-8h. Be aware that PAD may exceed PAWP by ≥ 5 mm Hg in patients with acidosis, hypoxemia, pulmonary emboli, lung disease, and associated pulmonary hypertension.
- Consult physician if PA waveform remains in wedged position after balloon deflation.
- Pay special attention to PA waveform when patient moves about (e.g., when being taken to x-ray department or getting up and into a chair).

Altered peripheral tissue perfusion (involved extremity) related to interrupted blood flow secondary to presence of arterial catheter or thrombosis caused by catheter

Desired outcome: Within 2 h of this diagnosis, patient has adequate perfusion to affected extremity as evidenced by brisk capillary refill (<2 sec), natural color, warm skin, normal sensation, and the ability to move the fingers.

- On a continuous basis, monitor capillary refill, color, temperature, sensation, and movement. Be alert to indicators of ischemia and teach them to the patient, stressing the importance of notifying staff members promptly should they occur.

- Maintain arterial line on continuous flush at 3 ml/h with heparinized normal saline (1 U heparin/ml saline or flush solution recommended by agency); ensure that pressure bag remains inflated at 300 mm Hg.
- Ensure tight connections of tubing throughout the system.
- Support patient's wrist or appropriate extremity with arm board or other supportive device to prevent flexion and movement of the catheter.

Risk for injury related to potential for insertion complications secondary to ventricular irritability, patient movement during insertion procedure, or difficult anatomy

---

Note: With PA or CVP catheter insertion, the following complications may occur: carotid artery puncture, air embolism, right ventricular perforation, hemorrhage, thoracic duct injury, pneumothorax, and cardiac tamponade. With PA catheter insertion, ventricular dysrhythmias may occur.

Desired outcome: Patient has no complications from PA or CVP catheter insertion as evidenced by normal sinus rhythm on ECG, BP within patient's normal range, HR ≤ 100 bpm, RR ≤ 20 breaths/min with normal pattern and depth (eupnea), normal breath sounds, and absence of adventitious breath sounds or muffled heart sounds.

- During preprocedure teaching, caution patient about the importance of remaining still during insertion of catheter. Provide sedation as prescribed.
- Perform a baseline assessment, monitoring BP, HR, RR, breath sounds, heart sounds, and ECG. Perform a postprocedure assessment, comparing it with baseline findings. Be alert to decreased BP, pulsus paradoxus (see Table 2-7, p. 155), increased HR or RR, diminished or absent breath sounds, and muffled heart sounds, as well as dysrhythmias on ECG. Report significant findings.
- After the procedure, obtain a chest x-ray as prescribed.
- Keep lidocaine at bedside for immediate IV injection if patient has sustained ventricular dysrhythmias.
- Administer prophylactic lidocaine to patients at high risk (those with electrolyte disorders, acidosis, or myocardial ischemia) as prescribed.

Sedating and paralytic agents

Most, if not all, critically ill patients experience some degree of anxiety. Patients requiring critical care are severely ill or injured, and this realization alone promotes symptoms of anxiety in all but those who are deeply obtunded. Extreme anxiety, when outwardly expressed as agitation, restlessness, and increased random motor movement, may be termed "agitation syndrome."

Anxiety and agitation in critically ill patients are prompted by emotional factors, including fear, loss of physical control, life-threatening

T A B L E 1 - 1 7　Pathologic conditions contributing to agitation

Addison's crisis	Intracranial bleeding
Anxiety disorder	Cerebral vasospasm
Delirium tremens	Cerebral edema
Developmental disability	Infection
Drug intoxication	Meningitis
Fear	Encephalitis
Encephalopathy	Brain abscess
Hepatic	Sepsis syndrome
Metabolic	Opiate withdrawal
Uremic	Organic brain syndrome
Hypercarbia	Pain, inadequately controlled
Hypoglycemia	Partial drug-induced paralysis
Hyponatremia	Antibiotic (e.g., aminoglycosides)
Hypoxemia	Electrolyte disorders (e.g., hypophosphatemia)
ICU crisis	Sedative withdrawal
Impaired cerebral perfusion	Sleep deprivation
Cerebral thrombosis	Steroid psychosis
Subarachnoid hemorrhage	

illness, inability to communicate (e.g., mechanical ventilation), and feelings of helplessness. Common pathophysiologic factors contributing to agitation syndrome include hypoxemia, impaired cerebral perfusion, infection, alcohol withdrawal, and encephalopathy (see Table 1-17). Environmental factors such as noise, temperature extremes, and sleep interruption add to anxiety and agitation. Unrelieved stress, manifested in the form of anxiety or agitation, retards healing and can increase mortality.

Optimally, potential causes of agitation syndrome will be identified and alleviated or appropriately managed using nonpharmacologic methods. However, administration of potent drugs sometimes is necessary to relieve anxiety or agitation that is refractory to nonpharmacologic measures. The section "Psychosocial Support" suggests nonpharmacologic nursing interventions that should be used along with pharmacotherapy. The remainder of this section discusses use of sedatives in situations in which nonpharmacologic interventions are not entirely effective.

If pharmacologic sedation is necessary, the ultimate goal should be to reduce anxiety and produce a calm but communicative state. Generally this is best accomplished by administering frequent, incremental doses of sedatives just until the desired effects are achieved. Close monitoring, individualized dosing, and titration to desired effect are essential in avoiding oversedation and toxicity in critically ill patients. Major organ dysfunction, use of multiple medications, tissue catabolism, and other factors render critically ill patients particularly vulnerable to the toxic effects of many sedatives. Excessive sedation has been

T A B L E 1 - 1 8   Nerve stimulation in relationship to percent blockage

Number of twitches	Percent blockage
4	0-50%
3	60%-70%
2	70%-80%
1	80%-90%
None	>90%

associated with delayed diagnosis of neurologic events, muscle wasting, and nosocomial complications, such as deep vein thrombosis, compression injury, and pneumonia. Since clinical conditions frequently change and drug requirements vary, sedatives should be withdrawn periodically (usually daily) to enable evaluation of the patient's underlying mental status.

ASSESSMENT

Anxiety: Subjective characteristics include increased tension, apprehension, fear, shakiness, uncertainty, distress, and feelings of helplessness. Objective findings include cardiovascular excitation, superficial vasoconstriction, pupil dilatation, increased perspiration, restlessness, poor eye contact, tremors, extraneous motor movement, and facial tension.

Pain: Subjective description of pain by the patient. Use visual analog scale, numerical scale, and "happy faces" or other coded method to establish baseline and evaluate pain control. Objective findings include autonomic responses such as changes in BP and HR, increased or decreased RR, pupil dilatation, increased perspiration, guarding, moaning, crying, restlessness, facial grimace, and rigid muscle tone.

Neuromuscular blockade: The level or depth of paralysis may be quantified using a device called a peripheral nerve stimulator. Typically a technique called the "train-of-four" (TOF) is chosen because it imposes the least discomfort. The TOF setting on the peripheral nerve stimulator will deliver four signals along the nerve path. The muscle response is then measured to evaluate how many signals are blocked compared with the number actually delivered. In the absence of neuromuscular blockade, the muscle should move four times equally in response to four signals. As receptors are loaded with neuromuscular blocking agents (NMBAs), fewer muscle contractions are seen. See Table 1-18.

COLLABORATIVE MANAGEMENT

A variety of therapeutic options are available to produce sedation in critically ill patients (Table 1-19). Alleviation of pain as a stimulus for anxiety/agitation is essential. Appropriate analgesics must be used for patients in whom pain is a component of agitation.

Opiate analgesics: Reliably relieve pain, are readily titrated, and

T A B L E 1 - 1 9   Classes of drugs used for sedation

Drug class	Specific agent
anesthetics	propofol
antihistamines	diphenhydramine
	hydroxyzine
antipsychotics	haloperidol
	chlorpromazine
	thorazine
barbiturates	phenobarbital
	pentobarbital
benzodiazepines	midazolam
	diazepam
	lorazepam
	clonazepam
miscellaneous	paraldehyde
	scopolamine

have significant sedative effects. Morphine is widely used in intermittent bolus dosing and as a continuous infusion. Other opiates commonly used include meperidine (Demerol) and fentanyl citrate (Sublimaze). When used in combination with sedatives, less of both medications is required.

Benzodiazepines: Relieve anxiety, promote sleep, and produce sedation by specific depressant effect on gamma-aminobutyric acid (GABA) and other nonspecific CNS depressant effects. Benzodiazepines produce muscle relaxation, which has the beneficial effect of reducing dosage requirements when NMBAs are used to induce paralysis. Dose-related effects on mental status range from relief of anxiety to sedation and coma. All benzodiazepines promote amnesia by preventing memory consolidation. This effect is particularly useful in patients undergoing unpleasant procedures. Midazolam (Versed) is reported to be superior to other benzodiazepines in preventing recall. Safety, ease of use, lack of paradoxic agitation, lack of recall, and reversibility with flumazenil make benzodiazepines attractive choices for sedation in many critical care situations. Table 1-20 describes specific characteristics of the widely used benzodiazepines.

- *Lorazepam (Ativan):*   Most commonly given as an intermittent bolus, but sometimes used as a continuous infusion. Lorazepam has no active metabolites; therefore in patients with advanced age or hepatic failure, drug effects do not seem to accumulate.
- *Diazepam (Valium):*   First drug of this class to be used, is inexpensive but has a long half-life, which causes prolonged sedation and may increase length of stay in ICU. An active metabolite may result in prolonged sedative effects (up to 200 h after a given dose). Diazepam should be avoided in patients with liver dysfunction or severe heart failure because of reduced hepatic clearance. Limited solubility in water restricts use to intermittent bolus injections. A

T A B L E   1 - 2 0   Benzodiazepine characteristics

Benzodiazepines		Lorazepam (Ativan)	Diazepam (Valium)	Midazolam (Versed)
Dosage	**Intermittent**	0.5-1 mg, q1-2h	2.5-5 mg, q3-4h	0.15-0.35 mg/kg, q1-2h
	Continuous	0.25-2 mg/h 4-35 μg/min	N/A	0.03-0.22 mg/kg/h 0.5-4 μg/kg/min
Pharma-cokinetics	**Metabolism**	Hepatic	Hepatic	Hepatic
	Active metabolites	None	Yes	Yes
	Excretion	Renal	Renal	Renal
	Half-life (in hours)	10-20	20-200	2-5*

*Several studies have shown midazolam's half-life to approach that of lorazepam in critically ill patients.

lipid suspension form of diazepam is now available. This formulation is less irritating to veins and may be used as a continuous IV infusion.
- *Midazolam (Versed):*   Short acting and rapidly metabolized, which makes this drug particularly useful for short procedures, such as bronchoscopies and endoscopies. Because of its short half-life, continuous infusions are required to maintain sedation for longer periods. With prolonged metabolization in critically ill patients, this drug may lead to extended sedation and difficulty with extubation, particularly in patients with sepsis or hepatic impairment.
- *Chlordiazepoxide (Librium):*   Sometimes used to manage agitation associated with alcohol withdrawal, a common inducer of agitation in the critically ill. When physiologically unstable patients are admitted to critical care, it is not always possible to obtain a clear history of alcohol use. The first clue may come 24-48 h later, when the patient becomes agitated and restless. However, because of chlordiazepoxide's relatively long half-life and several long-lived active metabolites, it is a poor choice for sedation and delirium tremens prophylaxis when compared to newer benzodiazepines that are safer and easier to titrate. Lorazepam (Ativan) generally is preferred because of its relatively short duration and simple metabolism.

Anesthetic agents: Although there is no absolute definition of anesthesia, there are four general components: analgesia, amnesia, absence of pathologic reflexes (e.g., vagal response to pain), and lack of purposeful movement. Once restricted to surgical settings, forms of anesthesia increasingly are employed in critical care areas. Anesthesia can be accomplished *via* use of a single agent or by several combinations of drugs. Many anesthetics are restricted to use by or with the direct supervision of an anesthesiologist; however, one anesthetic, propofol (Diprivan), recently has been approved by the FDA for use in critical care settings.
- *Propofol:*   A lipid suspension that is administered as a titratable, continuous infusion to provide a desired level of sedation to intu-

T A B L E   1 - 2 1   **Propofol (Diprivan) characteristics**

*Dosage**		1-3 mg/kg/h 5-50 µg/kg/min
Pharmacokinetics	**Metabolism**	Hepatic
	Metabolites	None
	Excretion	Renal
	Half-life	1.5-2 h
Cardiovascular effects		Minimal: 15% ↓ BP and MAP (short lived ≈ 15 min) (cause: ↓ SVR and [-] inotrope)

*Propofol is a sedative-hypnotic at the above recommended dosages but is classified chemically as an anesthetic.

bated, mechanically ventilated patients (Table 1-21). Patients awaken promptly and with remarkably clear mental function after sedation with propofol. Extubation time is more predictable because recovery time generally is <10 min. Recovery time after prolonged infusion is not increased, in contrast to some benzodiazepines. Hemodynamic changes (e.g., vasodilatation, decreased MAP) can be minimized by adequate hydration and slow increases in the infusion rate. As with other potent sedatives, the patient should be allowed to awaken daily to evaluate the underlying mental status.

Antipsychotics: Have been used to reduce agitation in disoriented and agitated patients. Patients should be well hydrated to avoid hypotension associated with parenteral use of these drugs.

- *Haloperidol lactate (Haldol):*   A butyrophenone antipsychotic that is especially helpful in managing ICU psychosis and during withdrawal of sedatives. Incremental bolus doses or continuous infusions are used. IV route is considered investigational but has been widely used in critically ill patients because onset of action is rapid and extrapyramidal side effects occur less frequently than with the IM route.
- *Chlorpromazine (Thorazine):*   A phenothiazine sometimes used as a sedative, particularly if the patient also displays evidence of psychosis. Chlorpromazine produces alpha-receptor blockade, and hypotension is likely. For this reason, and because it generally is less potent than haloperidol, chlorpromazine is not used frequently in critically ill patients.

Neuromuscular blocking agents: Used when longer periods of complete paralysis are necessary in intubated, mechanically ventilated patients. All possible causes of agitation (e.g., pain, fear, suctioning, hypoxemia) must be investigated thoroughly before neuromuscular blockade is initiated. NMBAs generally are used in the following situations: (1) to decrease oxygen consumption in patients who otherwise are unable to obtain satisfactory oxygen saturation; (2) to alleviate specific medical conditions (e.g., status asthmaticus, tetanus, malignant hyperthermia, status epilepticus, ARDS); (3) to immobilize patients for surgical and invasive procedures; and (4) to manage increased intra-

cranial pressure. There are, however, alternative means for managing many of the above situations.
- *Depolarizing NMBAs:* Succinylcholine (Anectine) is the only depolarizing NMBA with widespread clinical use. It is used to produce rapid, brief paralysis, most often during emergent intubation. Long-term blockade is not practical because of rapid tachyphylaxis and desensitization of receptors to blocking effects.
- *Nondepolarizing NMBAs:* The class of NMBAs most commonly used in the critically ill patient. The most common agents used are pancuronium (Pavulon), vecuronium (Norcuron), and atracurium (Tracrium). See Table 1-22. There are many drugs and certain physiologic states that can augment or antagonize neuromuscular blockage in the critically ill patient (Table 1-23). These should be assessed continuously throughout the course of therapy.

Clinicians should determine a therapeutic endpoint or goal for paralysis and titrate neuromuscular blockade to achieve that goal. Examples of such therapeutic endpoints are decreases in peak inspiratory pressure, decreases in oxygen consumption, and inability to move. Monitoring the degree of neuromuscular blockade is essential. This can be done by using a peripheral nerve stimulator (see "Assessment"). Another commonly used method is providing a "drug holiday," to enable return of neuromuscular function in order to assess muscle strength. NMBAs provide no analgesia or anxiolysis. The need for adequate analgesia and anxiolysis cannot be overemphasized.

NURSING DIAGNOSES AND INTERVENTIONS

Anxiety related to actual or perceived threat of death, change in health status, threat to self-concept or role, unfamiliar people or environment, or the unknown

Desired outcome: Within 4-6 h of initiating therapy, patient's anxiety is diminished as evidenced by verbalization of same, HR ≤100 bpm, RR ≤20 breaths/min, and decrease in restlessness and extraneous motor movement.
- Carefully assess for and correct factors contributing to anxiety (Table 1-17).
- Evaluate adequacy of pain control. Administer opiate or other analgesics in small doses at frequent intervals.
- Initiate nonpharmacologic measures to reduce anxiety (see Table 1-36, p. 73).
- Administer short-acting benzodiazepine in small doses at frequent intervals. Monitor carefully for excessive sedation and respiratory depression. Have flumazenil (Romazicon) immediately available for reversal of drug effects.
- If anxiety is profound and associated with sensory/perceptual alterations (e.g., hallucinations), consider use of antipsychotic agent. Ensure adequate hydration before use, and monitor closely for hypotension.

Impaired gas exchange (or risk for same) related to decreased oxygen supply secondary to decreased ventilatory drive occurring with sedative use and CNS depression or secondary to decreased chest wall movement occurring with residual neuromuscular blockade

Desired outcome: Within 1 h of intervention, patient has adequate

T A B L E 1 - 2 2 Neuromuscular blocking agent characteristics

Neuromuscular blocking agents		Pancuronium (Pavulon)	Vecuronium (Norcuron)	Atracurium (Tracrium)
Dosage	Intermittent	0.04-0.1 mg/kg q1h prn	0.01-0.015 mg/kg q15min	0.1 mg/kg q15min
	Continuous	1-1.6 µg/kg/min	0.8-1.2 µg/kg/min	5-15 µg/kg/min
Pharmacokinetics	Metabolism	Renal > Hepatic	Hepatic > Renal	Plasma
	Excretion	Renal	Renal (15%)	Plasma
			Biliary (30%-50%)	Renal
				Biliary
	Metabolites (active or toxic)	Yes	Yes	No
	Half-life (elimination)	132-257 min (2-4 h)	80-97 min	20-30 min
Cardiovascular effects		Moderate ↑ HR ↓ BP ↑ CO	Minimal <1% ↑ HR ↓ BP	Minimal ↑ HR ↓ BP

Important comments:
1. Pancuronium is by far the most cost-effective paralytic agent, followed by vecuronium.
2. Atracurium offers an advantage in that it does not rely on the kidneys or the liver for metabolism or excretion from the body and therefore will not accumulate in those patients with renal or hepatic insufficiency.

T A B L E   1 - 2 3   Drugs and physiologic conditions that affect NMBAs

Drugs that augment neuromuscular blockade

aminoglycoside antibiotics	lidocaine
bretylium	procainamide
calcium channel blockers	propranolol
clindamycin	quinidine
cyclosporin	vancomycin

Drugs that antagonize neuromuscular blockade

anticholinesterase agents	phenytoin
azathioprine	ranitidine
carbamazepine	theophylline
corticosteroids	

Physiologic conditions that increase neuromuscular blockade

acidosis	hypokalemia
dehydration	hyponatremia
hypercalcemia	hypothermia
hypermagnesemia	myasthenia gravis
hypocalcemia	

Physiologic conditions that decrease neuromuscular blockade

alkalosis	hypernatremia
hyperkalemia	decreased peripheral perfusion

gas exchange as evidenced by orientation to time, place, and person; Pao_2 $\geq$80 mm Hg; $Paco_2$ 24-30 mm Hg; Spo_2 $\geq$90; and RR 12-20 breaths/min with normal depth and pattern (eupnea).

- Assess patient's respiratory rate, depth, and rhythm at least qh when heavily sedated. Fully sedated patients require continuous direct monitoring until VS are stable and protective reflexes (e.g., gag reflexes) are present.
- If NMBAs are used, assess depth of paralysis using peripheral nerve stimulator. Titrate dose to maintain desired level of paralysis (Table 1-18).
- Continuously monitor Spo_2 *via* pulse oximetry. Alternatively, monitor chest wall movement *via* apnea monitor. Have appropriate antidote (e.g., naloxone for opiates, flumazenil for benzodiazepines, and pyridostigmine and atropine for NMBAs) and airway management equipment immediately available.
- Position patient to promote full lung expansion. Encourage deep breathing at frequent intervals.

Knowledge deficit: Lack of recall related to interrupted memory consolidation secondary to benzodiazepine use

Desired outcome: Within 12 h of cessation of benzodiazepine therapy, patient recalls information essential to self-protection and self-care.

- Remind patient that recall of unpleasant procedures (e.g., cardioversion, endoscopy) will be diminished and that this is a desired effect of the medication.

- Reinforce necessary information (e.g., NPO instructions, need to call for assistance when changing positions, and need for deep breathing) at frequent intervals until comprehension is demonstrated.
- Review outcome or findings of procedure with patient as necessary until patient expresses satisfactory understanding.

Alterations in consciousness

Consciousness is a state of awareness of self and the environment that consists of two components: content (cognition and affect) and arousal (appearance of wakefulness). Changes in content and arousal due to physiologic, psychologic, or environmental factors alter the state of consciousness, resulting in a broad spectrum of behavioral manifestations such as coma, confusion, and agitation. Factors precipitating various alterations in consciousness are listed in Table 1-24. Because of the many complications and safety issues surrounding it, impaired consciousness in the hospitalized patient is associated with longer hospital stays and higher morbidity and mortality rates.

ASSESSMENT

HISTORY AND RISK FACTORS

- *Age:* Elders more prone to alterations in consciousness.
- *Cardiovascular status:* Disorders that lower cardiac output and procedures that cause postcardiotomy delirium, intraaortic balloon pump sequelae, states of lowered perfusion (lowered MAP), and dysrhythmias.
- *Pulmonary disorders:* Those causing hypoxia and hypoxemia.
- *Drug therapy:* Sedation, analgesia, drug toxicity, drug interactions.
- *Cerebral disorders:* Deteriorating brain condition, such as an expanding lesion; degree of brain injury sustained (mild-severe).
- *Surgical factors:* Nature and extent of surgery and anesthesia time.
- *Perceptual/sensory factors:* Sleep deprivation, sensory overload, sensory deprivation, impaired sensation (hypesthesia, decreased hearing or vision), and impaired perception (inability to interpret environmental stimuli).
- *Metabolic factors:* Changes in glucose level, hypermetabolism, hypometabolism.
- *Fluid and electrolyte disturbances:* Sodium and potassium imbalances, hypovolemia.

CLINICAL PRESENTATION

- *Confusion:* A state of reduced wakefulness or awareness manifested by alternating periods of hyperirritability and drowsiness. Daytime drowsiness is contrasted with nighttime agitation. Confusion often begins as a clouding of consciousness, characterized by attention deficit. In confusion, there is disorientation to time and place, but disorientation to self is rare. Patients have difficulty following commands, misjudge or misinterpret sensory stimuli (pull at tubes and dressings), appear distracted, have memory impairment, and communicate inappropriately (yelling, swearing, and using nonsensical speech).
- *Delirium:* A transient alteration in mental state that develops along

---

T A B L E   1 - 2 4   Factors precipitating alterations in consciousness

---

Confusion
    Age
    Aggressive and dominant personality
    Anesthesia time
    Cardiac dysrhythmia
    Body temperature
    Cerebral disorders
    Fluid and electrolyte disorders
    Drugs
    Metabolic disturbances
    Pulmonary disorders
    Number of intensive care days
    Sleep deprivation

Delirium
    Cerebral disorders
    Metabolic disorders
    Toxins
    Electrolyte imbalances
    End-stage disease (renal, liver)
    Pulmonary disorders
    Impaired communication
    Withdrawal syndromes
    Drugs
    Neuropsychiatric disorders

Stupor
    Diffuse organic cerebral dysfunction
    Confused with the catatonic behavior of schizophrenia or severe depres-
        sive reaction

Coma
    Central nervous system dysfunction
        Cerebral structural changes (brain injury)
        Cerebrovascular impairment (hemorrhage, ischemia, or edema)
    Metabolic conditions

Vegetative state (coma vigil)
    Coma related to cerebral or metabolic disorders

Locked-in syndrome
    Supranuclear motor deefferentation related to brainstem injury

---

the continuum of clouding of consciousness, confusion, global cognitive impairment, and psychosis. Delirium is characterized by disorientation to time, place, and person; disorganized thinking; fear; irritability; misinterpretation of sensory stimuli; altered psychomotor activity; altered sleep-wake cycles; memory impairment; hallucinations; and dreamlike delusions. Lucid intervals alternate with episodes of delirium. Clinical variants of delirium include the hyperactive-hyperalert form, hypoactive-hypoalert form, and a combination form that includes lethargy and agitation.

- *Stupor:* Characterized by deep sleep with responsiveness only to vigorous and repeated stimuli with return to unresponsiveness when the stimulus is removed. Stupor usually is related to diffuse organic cerebral dysfunction but may be confused with the catatonic behavior of schizophrenia or the behavior associated with a severe depressive reaction.
- *Coma:* Manifestation of an alteration in arousal and diminished awareness of self and environment to such an extent that no understandable response to external stimuli or inner need is elicited. There is no language spoken, no covert or overt attempt to communicate, and no eye opening, and motor responses to noxious stimuli do not result in recognizable defensive movements. The extent of coma, however, is difficult to quantify because limits of consciousness are difficult to define and self-awareness can only be inferred from appearance and actions. Coma occurs when normal central nervous system (CNS) function is disrupted by cerebral structural changes (brain injury), cerebrovascular impairment (hemorrhage, ischemia, or edema), or metabolic conditions (hepatic encephalopathy).
- *Vegetative state:* Also called coma vigil, this state is a subacute or chronic condition that follows brain injury and is characterized by a return of wakefulness (eyes are open and sleep patterns may be observed) but without observable signs of cognitive function (unable to follow commands, offers no comprehensible sounds, displays no localization to stimuli). The vegetative state follows a coma, usually is permanent, and can persist for many years because the autonomic and vegetative functions necessary for life have been preserved.
- *Locked-in syndrome:* Characterized by paralysis of all four extremities and the lower cranial nerves but with preservation of consciousness. Associated with supranuclear motor deefferentation (disruption of the pathways of the brainstem motor neurons), this condition prevents the patient from communicating by word or body movement. This condition can be distinguished from a vegetative state or akinetic mutism because patients are left with the capacity to communicate through lateral eye movement and eye blinking. Patients give appropriate signs of being aware of themselves and their environment but often demonstrate disrupted sleep patterns.

PHYSICAL ASSESSMENT Requires a thorough evaluation of mental/emotional status, cranial nerve function, motor function, sensory function, and reflex activity. Baseline neurologic findings elicited from each component of the examination must be documented. When alterations in consciousness are manifested, the mental/emotional component of the examination is of particular importance. Minimally, the purpose of the assessment is to determine the extent of wakefulness and cognition through observed responses, such as eye opening, movement of the head and body, verbalization, and ability to follow commands. However, these observations alone will not fully discriminate the subtle differences in altered states of arousal and should be accompanied by in-depth assessment of the mental status and incorporate cognitive testing, as well. A variety of testing techniques and tools are available for use.

- *Mental status testing:* A subjective assessment requiring patient cooperation for maximal results. See Table 1-25.

T A B L E 1 - 2 5 Mental status component of the neurologic examination

1. General appearance
2. Behavior (with and without stimulation)
3. Language and speech characteristics (organization, coherence, and relevance)
4. Mood and affect
5. Judgment
6. Abstract thinking
7. Orientation (time, place, person)
8. Attention and concentration
9. Memory (recent and remote)
10. Cognition (following commands, fund of knowledge, interpretation of information, and problem solving)

T A B L E 1 - 2 6 Mini mental status examination

1. What is the year, season, date, day, month (5 points)
2. Where are we: state, county, town, hospital, room (5 points)
3. Name three objects (3)
4. Count backward by sevens (e.g., 100, 93, 86, 79, 72) (5 points)
5. Repeat same three objects from number 3 above (3 points)
6. Name a pencil and watch (2 points)
7. Follow a three-step command (3 points)
8. Write a sentence (1 point)
9. Follow the command "close your eyes" (1 point)
10. Copy a design (e.g., two hexagons) (1 point)

- *Mini mental status examination:* Objective neuropsychologic tool that measures orientation, recall, attention, calculation, and language. Scores less than 23 (total 25) indicate cognitive dysfunction. Patient participation is necessary to complete this examination. See Table 1-26.
- *Glasgow coma scale:* Quantitative, three-part scale that assesses the best eye opening, motor, and verbal responses. Scores range from 3-15, with 3 being unresponsive and 15 being awake, alert, and oriented. Patients who are unable to cooperate can be evaluated using this scale. See Appendix 3.
- *Rancho Los Amigos cognitive functioning scale (RLA):* An eight-level scale that describes levels of cognitive functioning from unresponsive to sensory stimuli to purposeful/appropriate actions. Patients who are unable to cooperate can be evaluated using this scale. See Table 1-27.

DIAGNOSTIC TESTS

Neurodiagnostic testing: See "Craniocerebral Trauma," p. 130.
Neuropsychologic testing: Although not a routine part of critical

T A B L E 1 - 2 7 Cognitive rehabilitation goals*

Level	Response	Goal/intervention
I	None	*Goal:* Provide sensory input to elicit responses of increased quality, frequency, duration, and variety.
II	Generalized	
III	Localized	
		Intervention: Give brief but frequent stimulation sessions, and present stimuli in an organized manner, focusing on one sensory channel at a time; for example:
		Visual: Intermittent television, family pictures, bright objects.
		Auditory: Tape recordings of family or favorite song, talking to patient, intermittent TV or radio.
		Olfactory: Favorite perfume, shaving lotion, coffee, lemon, orange.
		Cutaneous: Touch or rub skin with different textures such as velvet, ice bag, warm cloth.
		Movement: Turn, ROM exercises, up in chair.
		Oral: Oral care, lemon swabs, ice, sugar on tongue, peppermint, chocolate.
IV	Confused, agitated	*Goal:* Decrease agitation and increase awareness of environment. This stage usually lasts 2-4 wk.
		Interventions: Remove offending devices (e.g., nasogastric [NG] tube, restraints), if possible.
		Do not demand patient follow-through with task.
		Provide human contact unless this increases agitation.
		Provide a quiet, controlled environment.
		Use a calm, soft voice and manner around patient.

Continued.

care, it should be anticipated and planned for during the recovery phase for patients with brain injury or alterations in consciousness. This testing serves as a comprehensive baseline for rehabilitation by evaluating higher cortical function, such as memory and language.

COLLABORATIVE MANAGEMENT

For confusion: Underlying physiologic imbalances or drug interactions are determined and corrected. Once these are eliminated, care

T A B L E 1 - 2 7   Cognitive rehabilitation goals—cont'd

Level	Response	Goal/intervention
V VI	Confused, inappropriate Confused, appropriate	*Goal:* Decrease confusion and incorporate improved cognitive abilities into functional activity. *Interventions:* Begin each interaction with introduction, orientation, and interaction purpose. List and number daily activity in the sequence in which it will be done throughout the day. Maintain a consistent environment. Provide memory aids (e.g., calendar, clock). Use gentle repetition, which aids learning. Provide supervision and structure. Reorient as needed.
VII VIII	Automatic, appropriate Purposeful	*Goal:* Integrate increased cognitive function into functional community activities with minimal structuring. *Interventions:* Enable practicing of activities. Reduce supervision and environmental structure. Help patient plan adaptation of ADL and home living skills to home environment.

*Adapted from Rancho Los Amigos Hospital, Inc, Levels of Cognitive Functioning (scale based on behavioral descriptions or responses to stimuli). From Swift CM: Neurologic disorders. In Swearingen PL, editor: *Manual of medical-surgical nursing care, ed 3,* St Louis, 1994, Mosby.

should focus on eliminating sensory/perceptual deficits (use of hearing aid and eye glasses) and reorientation techniques that include orientation to self and environment.

For delirium: Underlying physiologic imbalances, drug interactions, and sensory/perceptual impairment are determined and corrected. Reorientation techniques to self and environment also are instituted. Neuropsychologic evaluation should be performed and appropriate drug therapy initiated (see "Sedating and Paralytic Agents," p. 40).

For coma: Determination of cognitive function based on the RLA score should guide interventions. Low-level cognitive function (RLA I, II, and III) requires initiation of a sensory stimulation program, while RLA IV (confused/agitated) requires a structured program that minimizes stimulation. A rehabilitation consultation that includes physical, occupational, and speech therapy evaluations enables a plan of care that prevents or minimizes problems related to the injury, such as spasticity or swallowing disorders, or complications of immobility, such as disuse syndrome, contractures, and pressure ulcers.

For locked-in syndrome: Establishment of a communication pattern is a critical element. A mental health consultation should be obtained to assist in intervening with the psychologic sequelae that could accompany this syndrome. A rehabilitation consultation (see "Coma," above) also is indicated. Sleep-wake cycle disturbances should be minimized by providing a normal day/night routine to the greatest extent possible.

For vegetative state: Neurodiagnostic and neuropsychologic testing should confirm this diagnosis. Although the long-term prognosis is not optimistic for the majority of these patients, supportive care, which minimizes such complications as pressure ulcers and aspiration, is essential. A stimulation program for low-level cognitive function, including visual, auditory, tactile, gustatory, and vestibular stimuli, may be initiated.

NURSING DIAGNOSES AND INTERVENTIONS

Sensory/perceptual alterations related to physiologic changes, psychologic changes, environmental changes, sensory deprivation, sensory overload, and drug interactions

Desired outcome: Within 48 h of this diagnosis, patient's level of arousal and cognition improves and patient responds consistently and appropriately to stimuli.

- Eliminate environmental causes of sensory/perceptual deficit.
  - □ Assess patient for potential causes of sensory/perceptual deficits. For the hearing- or vision-impaired patient, wearing eye glasses or hearing aids will decrease misinterpretation of visual and auditory stimuli.
  - □ Assess environment for potential causes of disorientation and confusion. Maintain day/night environment as much as possible. Keep clocks and calendars within patient's field of vision.
- Develop a plan of care consistent with sensory/perceptual deficit.
  - □ Assess patient for sensory deprivation and sensory overload. Decrease or increase stimulation based on RLA assessment (see Table 1-27) and patient's needs. For example, agitated and confused individuals require structure and reorientation interventions, while those who are comatose or stuporous require stimulation techniques.
  - □ Orient patient to time, place, and person during all interactions. Explain procedures in terms patient can understand.
  - □ Teach significant others reorientation and sensory stimulation strategies and provide liberal visitation to facilitate their assistance.
  - □ Assess underlying cause of confusion or delirium before using sedation, antianxiolytic, analgesic, or antipsychotic drug therapy (see "Sedating and Paralytic Agents," p. 40). Also see "Psychosocial Support," p. 90, for this nursing diagnosis.

Impaired verbal communication related to neurologic deficits

Desired outcome: Within 24 h of this diagnosis, patient communicates needs and feelings and exhibits decreased frustration and fear related to communication barriers.

- Determine underlying cause of impaired communication, including physiologic (cortical, brainstem, or cranial nerve injury) or psychologic (depression, fear, or anger).

- When communicating with these patients, use their name, face them, use eye contact if they are awake, speak clearly, and use a normal tone of voice.
- Be alert to nonverbal messages, especially eye movement, blinking, facial expressions, and head and hand movements. Attempt to validate these signals with the patient.
- Assure patient that you are attempting to find methods that promote communication if patient's needs cannot always be understood.
- For the patient who does not respond to or acknowledge verbal stimulation, continue communication attempts anyway.
- Teach significant others methods of communication and encourage them to continue attempts at communication.
- Brainstem-evoked potentials and immittance audiometry (hearing test) can provide useful information related to a patient's ability to receive and process auditory stimuli. Detection and treatment of otitis media in patients who have ET tubes will increase hearing.
- Obtain a speech therapy consultation to assess nature and severity of communication impairment and assist in developing a communication plan. Special attention is required for individuals with locked-in syndrome.
- Obtain a mental health consultation to assist with patient who is angry, frustrated, and fearful owing to the communication impairment.

Impaired physical mobility related to perceptual or cognitive impairment or imposed restrictions of movement

Desired outcome: By the time of discharge from the critical care unit, patient demonstrates ROM and muscle strength within 10% of baseline parameters.

- Assess muscle strength and tone to determine type of interventions required. Consult physical therapy and occupational therapy for evaluation and treatment plan.
- Manage decreased muscle tone (flaccidity):
  - Maintain body alignment and positioning.
  - Perform passive ROM and stretching exercises.
  - Avoid prolonged periods of limb flexion.
  - Apply splints and other adaptive devices to maintain functional position of the extremities.
  - Turn patient q2h.
  - Consider chair sitting as the patient stabilizes.
- Manage increased muscle tone (spasticity):
  - Avoid supine position; use side-lying, semiprone, prone, and high Fowler's positions.
  - Position limbs opposite flexion posture.
  - Use skeletal muscle relaxant, such as baclofen (Lioresal), as prescribed for decreasing tone.
- Monitor calcium and alkaline phosphatase levels. Increased levels can lead to the development of heterogenous ossification, which often is seen with states of impaired mobility, such as spinal cord injury. See "Fluid and Electrolyte Disturbances," p. 667.
- Maintain patient's skin integrity. See "Wound and Skin Care," p. 57.
- Prevent pulmonary complications in the following ways:
  - Encourage coughing and deep breathing if patient is able, or suction as needed.

- Assess swallowing ability before initiating oral feedings. Obtain dysphagia consultation (usually from a speech therapist) if swallowing reflexes are impaired.
- Initiate enteral feeding protocol for patients with feeding tubes to prevent aspiration. See "Nutritional Support," p. 1.

ADDITIONAL NURSING DIAGNOSES

Also see the following: "Nutritional Support," p. 12; "Sedating and Paralytic Agents," p. 46; "Prolonged Immobility," p. 17; and **Risk for disuse syndrome,** p. 138, in "Craniocerebral Trauma."

Wound and skin care

A wound is a disruption of tissue integrity caused by trauma, surgery, or an underlying medical disorder. Wound management is directed at preventing infection and/or deterioration in wound status and promoting healing.

Wounds closed by primary intention

Clean surgical or traumatic wounds whose edges are closed with sutures, clips, or sterile tape strips are referred to as wounds closed by primary intention. Impairment of healing most frequently manifests as dehiscence, evisceration, infection, or delayed healing. Individuals at high risk for disruption of wound healing include those who are obese, diabetic, elderly, malnourished, receiving steroids, immunosuppressed, or undergoing chemotherapy or radiation therapy.

ASSESSMENT

Optimal healing: Immediately after injury, the incision line is warm, reddened, indurated, and tender. After 1 or 2 days, wound fluid on the incision line dries, forming a scab that subsequently falls off and leaves a pink scar. After 7-9 days a healing ridge, a palpable accumulation of scar tissue, forms. In patients who undergo cosmetic surgery, scab formation and a healing ridge are purposely avoided to minimize scar formation. See Table 1-28.

Impaired healing: Lack of an adequate inflammatory response manifested by absence of initial redness, warmth, and induration or inflammation that persists or occurs after the fifth postinjury day; continued drainage from the incision line 2 days after injury (when no drain is present); absence of a healing ridge by the ninth day after injury; presence of purulent exudate. See Table 1-28.

DIAGNOSTIC TESTS

WBC with differential: To assess for infection.

Gram's stain of drainage: If infection is suspected, to identify the offending organism and aid in the selection of preliminary antibiotics.

Culture and sensitivity of tissue by biopsy or swab: To determine optimal antibiotic. Infection is said to be present when there are 10^5 organisms per gram of tissue or presence of fever and drainage.

T A B L E 1 - 2 8   Assessment of healing by primary intention

Expected findings	Abnormal findings
Edges well approximated	Edges not well approximated
Good inflammatory response (redness, warmth, induration, pain) initially postinjury	Decreased or absent inflammatory response, or inflammatory response that persists or occurs after the fifth day
No drainage (without drain present) 48 h after closure	Drainage continues >48 h after closure
Healing ridge present by postoperative day 7-9	No healing ridge present by postoperative day 9; hypertrophic scar or keloid

From Stotts NA: Managing wound care. In Swearingen PL, editor: *Manual of medical-surgical nursing care,* ed 3, St Louis, 1994, Mosby.

COLLABORATIVE MANAGEMENT

Application of a sterile dressing in surgery: To protect wound from external contamination or trauma, or to provide pressure. Usually, surgeon changes the initial dressing.

Regular (house) diet: To promote positive nitrogen state for optimal wound healing.

Multivitamins, especially C: To promote tissue healing.

Minerals, especially zinc and iron: May be prescribed, depending on patient's serum levels.

Supplemental oxygen: Empirically, 2-4 L/min in high-risk patients. After injury, wound Po_2 is low and administration of oxygen may promote healing.

Insulin: As needed to control glucose levels in individuals with diabetes mellitus (DM).

Local or systemic antibiotics: Given when infection is present and sometimes used prophylactically.

Incision and drainage: To drain pus when infection is present and localized. This allows healing by secondary intention. Often, the wound is irrigated with antiinfective agents such as dilute Dakin's solution.

NURSING DIAGNOSES AND INTERVENTIONS

Impaired tissue integrity: Wound, related to altered circulation, metabolic disorders (e.g., DM), alterations in fluid volume and nutrition, and medical therapy (chemotherapy, radiation therapy, and steroid administration)

Desired outcome: Patient exhibits the following signs of wound healing: well-approximated wound edges; good initial postinjury inflammatory response (erythema, warmth, induration, pain); no inflammatory response after the fifth day postinjury; no drainage (without drain present) 48 h after closure; healing ridge present by postoperative day 7-9.

- Assess wound for indications of impaired healing, including absence of a healing ridge, presence of drainage or purulent exudate, and delayed or prolonged inflammatory response. Monitor VS for signs of infection, including elevated temperature and HR. Document findings.
- Follow proper infection-control techniques when changing dressings. If a drain is present, keep it sterile, maintain patency, and handle it gently to prevent it from becoming dislodged. If wound care will be necessary after hospital discharge, teach the dressing change procedure to patient and significant others.
- For persons with DM, perform serial monitoring of blood glucose and administer insulin to keep glucose level <200 mg/dl.
- Explain to patient that deep breathing promotes oxygenation, which enhances wound healing. If indicated, provide incentive spirometry at least 4 times a day. Stress the importance of position changes and activity as tolerated to promote ventilation. Splint incision as needed.
- Monitor perfusion status by checking BP, HR, capillary refill time in the tissue adjacent to incision, moisture of mucous membranes, skin turgor, volume and specific gravity of urine, and I&O.
- For nonrestricted patients, ensure a fluid intake of at least 2-3 L/day.
- Encourage ambulation or ROM exercises as allowed to enhance circulation to the wound.
- To promote positive nitrogen state, which enhances wound healing, provide a diet with adequate protein, vitamin C, and calories. Encourage between-meal supplements. If patient complains of feeling full with 3 meals a day, give more frequent small feedings.

Surgical or traumatic wounds healing by secondary intention

Wounds healing by secondary intention are those with tissue loss or heavy contamination that form granulation tissue and contract in order to heal. Most often, impairment of healing is caused by increased contamination and impairment of perfusion, oxygenation, and nutrition, which results in a delay in the healing process. Individuals at risk for impaired healing include those who are obese, diabetic, malnourished, elderly, taking steroids, immunosuppressed, or undergoing radiation or chemotherapy.

ASSESSMENT

Optimal healing: Initially, the wound edges are inflamed, indurated, and tender. At first, granulation tissue on the floor and walls is pink, progressing to a deeper pink and then to a beefy red; it should be moist. Epithelial cells from the tissue surrounding the wound gradually migrate across the granulation tissue. As healing occurs, the wound edges become pink, the angle between surrounding tissue and the wound becomes less acute, and wound contraction occurs. Occasionally a wound has a tract or sinus that gradually decreases in size as healing occurs. The time frame for healing depends on the size and location of the wound, as well as on the patient's physical and psychologic status. See Table 1-29.

T A B L E   1 - 2 9   **Assessment of healing by secondary intention**

Expected findings	Abnormal findings
Initially postinjury, wound edges inflamed, indurated, and tender; with epithelialization, edges become pink	Initially postinjury, decreased inflammatory response or inflammation around the wound continues after the fifth postinjury day; epithelialization slowed or mechanically disrupted so not continuous around wound
Granulation tissue initially avascular and moist and then turns pink; becomes beefy red over time	Granulation tissue remains pale or is excessively dry or moist
No odor present	Odor present
No exudate or necrotic tissue present	Exudate or necrotic tissue present

From Stotts NA: Managing wound care. In Swearingen PL, editor: *Manual of medical-surgical nursing care,* ed 3, St Louis, 1994, Mosby.

Impaired healing: Exudate appears on the floor and walls of the wound and does not abate as healing progresses. It is important to note the distribution, color, odor, volume, and adherence of the exudate. The skin surrounding the wound should be assessed for signs of tissue damage, including disruption, discoloration, and increasing pain. When a drain is in place, the volume, color, and odor of the drainage should be evaluated. See Table 1-29.

DIAGNOSTIC TESTS

CBC with WBC differential: To assess hematocrit (Hct) level and for presence of infection. Increased WBC count signals infection, while a decrease occurs with immunosuppression. Watch the differential for a shift to the left, which indicates infection. Monitor the lymphocyte count; $\leq$1,800 μl is a sign of malnutrition. For optimal healing, the Hct should be >20%.

Gram's stain of drainage: To determine the offending organism, if present, and aid in the selection of the preliminary antibiotic.

Tissue biopsy or culture and sensitivity of drainage: To determine presence of infection and the optimal antibiotic, if appropriate.

Ultrasound, sonogram, or sinogram: To determine wound size, especially when abscesses or tracts are suspected.

COLLABORATIVE MANAGEMENT

Débriding enzymes: To soften and remove necrotic tissue; for example, fibrinolysin plus desoxyribonuclease (Elase).

Dressings: To provide débridement, keep healthy wound tissue moist, or provide antiseptic agent to decrease wound surface bacterial counts. See Table 1-30.

Hydrophilic agents: To remove contaminants and excess exudate; for example, dextran beads or paste (Envisan) or polymer flakes (Bard Absorption Dressing).

T A B L E 1 - 3 0 Dressings used for wound care

Dressing	Advantages	Limitations
Dry to dry* (insert dry and remove dry)	Highly absorbent; débridement	Excessively drying to tissue; disruption of new tissues; painful removal
Wet to dry* (insert wet and remove dry)	Good absorption but not as absorptive as dry to dry; good débridement	Drying of tissues but not as much as dry to dry; disruption of new tissue; painful removal
Moist to moist* (insert and remove moist)	Provides topical antiinfective agent; no wound desiccation; good débridement; not painful; inexpensive	Less effective removal of exudate; if excessively wet, can cause tissue maceration; if it dries out, dressing must be moistened before removal
Xeroform gauze	Provides topical antiseptic; keeps tissue hydrated; minimal pain with removal	Can cause tissue maceration if excessively moist
Porcine skin dressing	Can provide topical antibiotic; keeps tissue hydrated; not painful when removed; often used before closure of wound with tissue grafts	Expensive; usually stored in refrigerator until use

Continued.

Hydrotherapy: To soften and remove debris mechanically.

Wound irrigation with or without antiinfective agents: To dislodge and remove bacteria and loosen necrotic tissue, foreign bodies, and exudate. Antiinfective agents work locally to kill organisms.

IV fluids: To ensure adequate perfusion for patients unable to take adequate oral fluids.

Topical or systemic vitamin A: As needed to reverse adverse effects of steroids on healing. Use is limited to 7-10 days.

Drain(s): To remove excess tissue fluid or purulent drainage.

Surgical débridement: To remove dead tissue and reduce debris and fibrotic tissue.

Skin graft: To provide coverage of wound if necessary.

Tissue flap: To fill tissue defect and provide wound closure with its own blood supply.

Regular diet, supplemental oxygen, multivitamins and minerals, insulin, and incision and drainage: See discussion, "Wounds Closed by Primary Intention," p. 58.

T A B L E   1 - 3 0   Dressings used for wound care—cont'd

Dressing	Advantages	Limitations
Transparent dressing (e.g., Op-Site, Tegaderm, Bioocclusive)	Prevents loss of wound fluid; protects wound from external contamination; minimal pain with removal; protects from friction and fluid loss	Must withdraw excessive drainage and reseal dressing; appearance of drainage erroneously suggests infection
Hydrocolloid dressing (e.g., Duoderm, Restore, Intact)	Maintains moist wound surface while minimizing pooling; easy to apply; minimal pain with removal	Cannot directly assess wound without removing dressing; "melts" when used under radiant heat; limited absorption
Hydrophilic gel (e.g., Vigilon, Intrasite Gel)	Maintains moist wound surface; nonadherent; absorbs some exudate; compatible with topical medications; easy to apply; minimal pain with removal	Causes maceration when in direct contact with normal tissue; expensive; may require frequent changing; provides minimal absorption of exudate
Alginates (e.g., Sorbsan)	Physiologic; maintains moisture; painless	Not good for dry wounds
Foams (e.g., Lyofoam, Allevin)	Maintains moist wound surface; insulates wound; nonadherent	Poor barrier; opaque; not good for wounds with copious viscous drainage

*All dressings are sterile, coarse mesh gauze without cotton fiberfill and are covered with a dry sterile outer layer to prevent ingress of organisms. When moisture is prescribed, it is provided with an antiinfective agent or physiologic solution.

From Stotts NA: Managing wound care. In Swearingen PL, editor: *Manual of medical-surgical nursing care,* ed 3, St Louis, 1994, Mosby.

NURSING DIAGNOSES AND INTERVENTIONS

Impaired tissue integrity: Wound, related to presence of contaminants, metabolic disorders (e.g., DM), medical therapy (e.g., chemotherapy or radiation therapy), altered perfusion, immunosuppression, or malnutrition

Desired outcomes: Patient's wound exhibits the following signs of healing: initially postinjury wound edges are inflamed, indurated, and tender; with epithelialization edges become pink within 1 wk of injury; granulation tissue develops (identified by pink tissue that becomes beefy red) within 1 wk of injury; and there is absence of odor, exudate, or necrotic tissue. Patient or significant other successfully demonstrates wound care procedure before hospital discharge, if appropriate.

• Monitor for the following signs of impaired healing: initially postinjury decreased inflammatory response or inflammatory response that lasts >5 days; epithelialization slowed or mechanically disrupted and noncontinuous around the wound; granulation tissue remaining pale or excessively dry or moist; presence of odor, exudate, and/or necrotic tissue.

- Apply prescribed dressings (see Table 1-30). Insert dressing into all tracts to promote gradual closure of those areas. Ensure good hand-washing before and after dressing changes, and dispose of contaminated dressings appropriately.
- When a drain is used, maintain its patency, prevent kinking of the tubing, and secure the tubing to prevent the drain from becoming dislodged. Use aseptic technique when caring for drains.
- To help prevent contamination, cleanse the skin surrounding the wound with a mild disinfectant (e.g., soap and water). Do not use friction with cleansing if tissue is friable.
- If irrigation is prescribed for reducing contaminants, use high-pressure irrigation with a 35 ml syringe with an 18-gauge needle. If the tissue is friable or the wound is over a major organ or blood vessel, use extreme caution with the irrigation pressure. To remove contaminants effectively, use a large volume of irrigant (e.g., 100-150 ml).
- Topically applied antiinfective agents, such as neomycin and iodophors, are absorbed by the wound and can produce systemic side effects. When these agents are used, be alert to side effects such as toxicity to cells in the wound, nephrotoxicity, and acidosis.
- When a hydrophilic agent such as Debrisan or Bard Absorption Dressing is prescribed, remove it with high-pressure irrigation. If the agent were to be removed with a 4×4 or surgical sponge, the friction would disrupt capillary budding and delay healing.
- When topical enzymes are prescribed, use them on necrotic tissue only and follow package directions carefully. Be aware that some agents, such as povidone-iodine, deactivate the enzymes. Protect surrounding undamaged skin with zinc oxide or aluminum hydroxide paste.
- Teach patient or significant other the prescribed wound care procedure, if indicated.

Pressure ulcers

Pressure ulcers result from a disruption in tissue integrity and are most often caused by excessive tissue pressure or shearing of blood vessels. High-risk patients include the elderly and those who have decreased mobility, decreased LOC, impaired sensation, debilitation, incontinence, sepsis/elevated temperature, or malnutrition.

ASSESSMENT

High-risk individuals should be identified upon admission assessment, with daily assessments during hospitalization, using a standard assessment schema. When pressure ulcers are present, their severity can be graded on a scale of I to IV:

Grade I: Nonblanchable erythema of intact skin. In dark-skinned individuals, heat may be the only indication of a grade I pressure ulcer.

Grade II: Partial-thickness skin loss that involves epidermis and/or dermis; seen as an abrasion, blister, or shallow crater.
Grade III: Full-thickness skin loss that involves subcutaneous tissue but does not extend through fascia.
Grade IV: Full-thickness injury that involves muscle, bone, or supporting structures.
See "Surgical or Traumatic Wounds Healing by Secondary Intention," p. 59, for other assessment data.

DIAGNOSTIC TESTS

See "Diagnostic Tests," p. 60, in "Surgical or Traumatic Wounds Healing by Secondary Intention."

COLLABORATIVE MANAGEMENT

Debriding enzymes: To soften and remove necrotic tissue.
Dressings: To provide débridement, keep healthy tissue moist, or apply an antiinfective agent. See Table 1-30.
Hydrophilic agents: To remove contaminants and excess moisture.
Wound irrigation with antiinfective agents: To reduce contamination.
Hydrotherapy: To soften and remove debris mechanically.
Diet: Adequate protein and calories to promote positive nitrogen state for rapid wound healing.
Supplemental vitamins and minerals: As needed.
Supplemental oxygen: Usually 2-4 L/min to promote wound healing for high-risk patients or those with delayed wound healing.
Surgical débridement: Removal of devitalized tissue with a scalpel to reduce the amount of debris and fibrotic tissue.
Tissue flap: Provides closure of wound as well as its own blood supply.
Cultured keratinocytes: Provide cover for the wound in the form of a sheet of skin cells grown from a biopsy of the patient's own skin.
Growth factors: Naturally occurring proteins that stimulate new cell formation (e.g., platelet-derived growth factor, insulin).
Hyperbaric oxygen: Used with difficult wounds to support oxidative processes in healing.

NURSING DIAGNOSES AND INTERVENTIONS

Impaired tissue integrity (or risk for same) related to excessive tissue pressure, shearing forces, or altered circulation
Desired outcomes: Patient's tissue remains intact. Following interventions/instructions, patient participates in preventive measures and verbalizes understanding of the rationale for these interventions.
• Identify individuals at risk and systematically assess skin over bony prominences daily; document.
• Establish and post a position-changing schedule.
• Assist patient with position changes. There is an inverse relationship between pressure and time in ulcer formation; therefore, heavier patients need to change position more frequently. Position changes include turning the bed-bound patient q1-2h, as well as having the wheelchair-bound patient (who is able) perform pushups in the chair

q15min to ensure periodic relief from pressure on the buttocks. Use pillows or foam wedges to keep bony prominences from direct pressure. In addition, patients with a history of previous tissue injury will require pressure relief measures more frequently. Because high Fowler's position results in increased shearing, use low Fowler's position and alternate supine position with prone and 30-degree elevated side-lying positions.

- For immobile patients, totally relieve pressure on heels by raising them off the bed surface *via* pillows that are inserted under the length of the lower leg.
- Minimize friction on tissue during activity. Friction causes shearing of vessels, which leads to tissue disruption. Lift rather than drag patient during position changes and transferring; use a draw sheet to facilitate patient movement. Do not massage over bony prominences, inasmuch as this can result in tissue damage.
- Minimize skin exposure to moisture. Cleanse at the time of soiling and at routine intervals. Use moisture barriers and disposable briefs as needed.
- Use a mattress that reduces pressure, such as foam, alternating air, gel, or water.
- To enhance circulation, encourage patient to maintain current level of activity.

Impaired tissue integrity: Presence of pressure ulcer, with increased risk for further breakdown related to altered circulation and presence of contaminants or irritants (chemical, thermal, or mechanical)

Desired outcomes: Stages I and II are healed within 7-10 days; stages III and IV may require months to heal. Following intervention/instructions, patient verbalizes causes and preventive measures for pressure ulcers and successfully participates in the plan of care to promote healing and prevent further breakdown.

- Evaluate grade of pressure ulcer (see "Assessment," p. 63).
- Maintain a moist physiologic environment to promote tissue repair and minimize contaminants. Change dressings as prescribed.
- Be sure patient's skin is kept clean with regular bathing, and be especially conscientious about washing urine and feces from the skin. Soap should be used and then thoroughly rinsed from the skin.
- If the patient has excessive perspiration, ensure frequent bathing and change bedding as needed.
- To absorb moisture and prevent shearing when the patient is moved, apply heel and elbow covers as needed.
- Use lamb's wool to keep the areas between the toes dry. Change wool periodically, depending on the amount of moisture present.
- Do not use a heat lamp because it increases the metabolic rate of the tissues, resulting in increased demand for blood flow in an area with impaired perfusion. As a result, ulcer diameter and depth can be increased.
- Teach patient and significant others the importance of and measures for preventing excess pressure as a means of preventing pressure ulcers.
- Provide wound care as needed (described under "Surgical or Traumatic Wounds Healing by Secondary Intention," p. 59).

ADDITIONAL NURSING DIAGNOSES

See "Surgical or Traumatic Wounds Healing by Secondary Intention" for **Impaired tissue integrity,** p. 62.

Pain

PATHOPHYSIOLOGY

Critically ill patients endure substantial pain from pathologic conditions, injury, and such therapeutic interventions as surgery and multiple invasive diagnostic procedures. Even seemingly unconscious patients experience pain. The pain experience is compounded by fear, anxiety, and barriers to communication. In addition, pain control assumes a low priority when juxtaposed against respiratory or hemodynamic instability, either of which is common in critical care areas. The presence of pain is a significant stressor for critically ill patients and contributes to other problems such as confusion, inadequate ventilation, immobility, sleep deprivation, depression, and immunosuppression.

Pain is a subjective experience based in part on anatomic and physiologic functioning and modulated by psychologic factors. Because of the subjective nature of the pain experience, it is the patient, not the nurse, who must describe the intensity of pain. In order to alleviate discomfort, the nurse must believe the patient's pain description. When selecting the most appropriate interventions for patients experiencing pain, the nurse must evaluate anticipated and actual psychophysiologic effects of the intervention and consider other accompanying conditions, as well as the setting in which the treatment occurs. Despite the availability of effective analgesics and many new pain control technologies, many critically ill patients continue to be treated inadequately for pain.

Characteristic pain patterns develop according to the area affected and the underlying pathophysiologic process. Superficial structures, such as subcutaneous tissue, ligaments, tendons, and parietal pleura, contain numerous small pain fibers. Pain resulting from stimulation of these areas usually is well localized and often described as pricking and burning. Pain associated with deeper visceral structures is often poorly localized and usually described as aching, although it may be sharp or burning. Pain associated with muscle injury is similar to visceral pain and is mediated through the same deep sensory systems. Acute ischemia causes burning or aching pain distal to the area of vascular occlusion. This characteristic pain is believed to be caused by the release of metabolic byproducts associated with tissue hypoxia.

Patients expect that pain will be controlled. Failure to control pain interferes with therapeutic goals, such as mobility and ventilation, and erodes trust in health care providers. Factors contributing to inadequate pain control include failure to accurately assess pain intensity, attitudes toward the behaviors and personality traits of individuals experiencing pain, belief that the administration of opioid analgesics could lead to iatrogenic addiction, and concern for respiratory depression. Nurses have an ethical obligation to relieve pain and suffering and thus reduce the associated physiologic and psychologic risks of untreated pain.

ASSESSMENT

A thorough baseline assessment, whenever possible, is important in accurately evaluating and managing pain. Frequent, brief assessments are necessary postoperatively and during acute episodes of pain until the pain is well controlled.

HISTORY AND RISK FACTORS Question patient regarding previous or current pain; usual ways in which pain is described and expressed; previously used pharmacologic and nonpharmacologic methods of pain control; previous history of chemical dependence, including alcohol use; attitudes and beliefs toward pain and use of opioid, anxiolytic, or other medications; typical coping responses for pain or stress; and expectations regarding pain management.

SUBJECTIVE PRESENTATION Because pain is subjective, only the patient can evaluate pain intensity accurately. One or more of several pain assessment tools should be used to assist the patient in rating pain. Comparisons of the patient's ratings before and after a given intervention are used to guide therapy. In addition to the self-report measurement tools that follow, the patient should be asked to describe the nature of the pain (e.g., dull, sharp, pressure, cramping), location, and aggravating and relieving factors.

Numerical rating scale (NRS): Patient ranks pain numerically, usually from 1-5 or 1-10.

Visual analog scale (VAS): Patient marks a 10 cm line to indicate pain intensity.

Adjective rating scale (ARS): Patient selects an adjective that best describes the pain intensity.

OBJECTIVE PRESENTATION Used to supplement self-reports or used exclusively if the patient is unconscious or has other profound communication barriers.

Physiologic: Increases in HR, BP, and RR all associated with untreated pain. Other physiologic responses associated with autonomic stimulation are listed in Table 1-31.

Behavioral: Social, cultural, and environmental factors affect reactions to pain. A number of nonverbal indicators are listed in Table 1-32.

VITAL SIGNS AND HEMODYNAMICS With untreated pain, usually reflect autonomic stimulation (e.g., elevated HR and RR and increased SVR

T A B L E   1 - 3 1   Autonomic indicators of pain

Diaphoresis, pallor

Vasoconstriction

Increased systolic and diastolic BP

Increased pulse rate ($>$100 bpm)

Pupillary dilatation

Change in respiratory rate (usually increased to $>$20 breaths/min)

Muscle tension or spasm

Decreased intestinal motility, evidenced by nausea, vomiting, abdominal distention, and possibly ileus

Endocrine imbalance, evidenced by sodium and water retention and mild hyperglycemia

T A B L E   1 - 3 2 **Nonverbal indicators of pain**

Skeletal muscle tension	Psychic reactions
Facial grimace, tension	Short attention span
Guarding or splinting of the affected part	Irritability
Restlessness	Anxiety
Increase in motor activity	Sleep disturbances
Decrease in motor activity	Anger
	Crying
	Fearfulness
	Withdrawal

and BP). IV opiate analgesics promptly reduce SVR directly as a result of vasodilatation and indirectly as a result of pain relief.

COLLABORATIVE MANAGEMENT

Opioid agonists: Centrally acting analgesics that bind with receptors in the CNS and other tissues, thus blocking pain sensation and causing various other effects, including feelings of well-being, vasodilatation, and respiratory depression. They are used to manage moderate to severe acute pain. For the most effective therapy, titrate in small increments to produce the desired analgesia with minimal side effects. Patient-controlled analgesia (PCA) pumps, continuous peripheral or epidural infusions, and small frequent IV bolus dosing are effective methods used for patients in critical care areas. Opioid tolerance, physiologic or psychologic dependence, and addiction are unusual when opioids are used to manage acute pain in patients without a history of chemical dependency. Parenteral opioids may cause hypotension in patients with hypovolemia. Restore fluid volume before or concurrent with administration. Dose-related respiratory depression is a significant disadvantage, particularly in patients with chronic hypoxia, debilitation, or advanced age. Naloxone (Narcan) should be immediately available to reverse respiratory depression. See Table 1-33 for equianalgesic doses of narcotic analgesics and Table 1-34 for uses of opioid and opioid agonist-antagonist analgesia.

- *Morphine:*   Most frequently used opioid; considered "first-line" therapy for moderate to severe acute pain. Vasodilatory effects are beneficial for patients with left ventricular failure, pulmonary hypertension, or pulmonary edema. Rapid IV injection may trigger histamine release with related increases in SVR and decreases in CO/CI and MAP. Histamine-related bronchospasm may occur in patients with asthma. Ventilatory depression is possible, and IV bolus injection may result in an episode of sudden apnea. Epidural administration results in reduced responsiveness of the respiratory center in the brainstem to carbon dioxide. This results in a gradual increase in $Paco_2$, respiratory pauses, delayed expiration, and possible respiratory acidosis.
- *Hydromorphone (Dilaudid):*   Highly effective opioid; substitute analgesic for patient with morphine allergy or intolerance.

T A B L E   1 - 3 3   Equianalgesic doses of narcotic analgesics

Class/name	Route	Equianalgesic dose (mg)*	Average duration (h)
Morphine-like agonists			
codeine	IM, SC	130†	3
	PO	180†	3
hydromorphone (Dilaudid)	IM, SC	1.5-2	4
	PO	6-7.5	4
levorphanol (Levo-Dromoran)	IM, SC	2	6
	PO	4	6
morphine	IM, SC	10	4
oxycodone (Percodan)	PO	30†	4
oxymorphone (Numorphan)	IM, SC	1-1.5	4
	Rectal	10	4
Meperidine-like agonists			
fentanyl (Sublimaze)	IV, IM, SC	0.1-0.2	1‡
meperidine (Demerol)	IM, SC	100	3
Methadone-like agonists			
methadone (Dolophine)	IM, SC	10	6
	PO	10-20	6
propoxyphene (Darvon)	PO	130-250†	4
Mixed agonist-antagonist§			
buprenorphine (Buprenex)	IM	0.3-0.6	4
butorphanol (Stadol)	IM, SC	2-3	3
nalbuphine (Nubain)	IM, SC	10-20	4
pentazocine (Talwin)	IM	30-60	3
	PO	10-200†	3

Modified from Baumann T, Lehman M: Pain management. In DiPiro J et al, editors: *Pharmacotherapy: a pathophysiologic approach,* New York, 1988, Elsevier Science Publishing; and Young L, Koda-Kimble M, editors: *Applied therapeutics: the clinical use of drugs,* ed 5, Vancouver, Wash, 1992, Applied Therapeutics.
*Recommended starting dose; actual dose must be titrated to patient response.
†Starting doses lower (codeine 30 mg, oxycodone 5 mg, meperidine 50 mg, propoxyphene 65-130 mg, pentazocine 50 mg).
‡Respiratory depressant effects persist longer than analgesic effects.
§Mixed agonist-antagonist analgesics may precipitate withdrawal in patients with opiate dependency.

- ***Meperidine (Demerol):***   Indicated for brief courses (i.e., <48 h) in patients with allergy or intolerance to morphine, hydromorphone, or other opiates. Its toxic metabolite, normeperidine, is a cerebral irritant and may cause seizures.
- ***Fentanyl:***   Potent synthetic opioid. IV preparation is especially use-

T A B L E 1 - 3 4 Use of opioid and opioid agonist-antagonist analgesia

Route	Commonly prescribed medications	Advantages	Disadvantages
Continuous IV infusion	morphine, fentanyl (Sublimaze), hydromorphone (Dilaudid)	· Useful for severe, predictable pain · Relieves pain with lower doses than IV bolus · Avoids peaks and valleys of pain present with IV bolus and IM injections	· Requires frequent observation to monitor flow rate · VS must be monitored often, especially respiratory status · Weaning necessary
IV bolus	morphine, fentanyl, hydromorphone, meperidine (Demerol)	· Useful for severe, intermittent pain (i.e., for procedures, treatments) · Rapid onset of action	· Relatively short duration of pain relief · Fluctuating levels · Possibility of excessive sedation as drug levels peak
Patient-controlled analgesia (PCA); may be delivered IV or SC	morphine, fentanyl, buprenorphine (Buprenex)	· Useful for moderate to severe pain · Enables titration by patient for effective analgesia without excessive sedation · Relief of pain with lower dosages of medication · Immediate delivery of medication	· Pumps necessary to deliver drug are expensive · Patient must have clear mental status · Health care provider resistance to self-administration by patient

		Advantages	Disadvantages
Epidural and intrathecal	morphine, fentanyl, local anesthetics (e.g., bupivacaine)	· Patient's sense of self-control lowers anxiety · Less nursing time spent preparing medications · Provides greater analgesia with less CNS depression than parenteral narcotics · Enables direct binding of narcotics to opioid receptor sites in the spinal cord, thereby minimizing CNS depression · Directly blocks pain impulse transmission to central cortex when anesthetics are used	· Difficult to assess patency and placement · Significant infection risk
IM/SC injection	meperidine, morphine, pentazocine (Talwin), nalbuphine (Nubain), butorphanol (Stadol), buprenorphine	· Useful for moderate to severe pain · Longer duration of action than with IV route · Faster pain relief than with oral medication · SC route useful for patients with poor IV access and little muscle mass	· Variable absorption and fluctuating levels, especially in hypotensive and edematous patients · Possibility of excessive sedation as drug levels peak · Potential delay in administration

ful in critical care because of minimal cardiovascular effects, short duration of action, and rapid onset of action. Duration of action increases with repeated doses.

Caution: A fentanyl patch may be used for continuous analgesia, usually with supplemental doses of morphine or other opiate titrated to produce analgesia, but only should be used for patients with opiate tolerance. Respiratory depression with hypoventilation occurs, as with morphine.

Opioid agonist-antagonists: Stimulate and antagonize opiate receptors to varying degrees, depending on agent and dose. They may precipitate withdrawal in patients receiving opiates on a regular basis. See Tables 1-33 and 1-34.
- *Pentazocine (Talwin):*   Predominately agonist effects but with weak antagonist activity. It may cause increased MAP, LVEDP, and mean PAP, thus increasing myocardial workload.
- *Butorphanol (Stadol):*   Adverse effects reported in patients with CHF or acute MI. It may be useful in decreasing side effects associated with epidural morphine.

Nonsteroidal antiinflammatory drugs (NSAIDs):   Diminish the effects of prostaglandins, rendering afferent receptors less sensitive to bradykinin, histamine, and serotonin, which in turn decreases pain receptor stimulation. Most NSAIDs are given orally (e.g., ibuprofen, aspirin), but injectable NSAIDs such as ketorolac are available. Prostaglandin inhibition decreases platelet adhesiveness and may result in bleeding complications. See Table 1-35.
- *Ketorolac (Toradol):*   Effective for short-term use in relieving mild to moderate pain. There is a minimal effect on ventilation, and the drug has been effective when given on an alternate schedule with morphine or other opiate analgesic during ventilator weaning of postoperative patients. There is a possibility of renal toxicity, which limits use to patients with normal renal function. Bleeding complications are more likely with high-dose therapy and in older adults.

Other pharmacologic interventions: Sedatives and anxiolytics (e.g., midazolam [Versed]) often used to reduce anxiety associated with pain and to promote amnesia when painful procedures are planned. Spinal analgesia with a local anesthetic agent may be used with epidural opiates. Intermittent or continuous local neural blockade, such as intercostal nerve block, is used for specific localized pain.

T A B L E   1 - 3 5   Common nonnarcotic and nonsteroidal antiinflammatory analgesics

acetaminophen (Tylenol, Tempra)
acetylsalicylic acid (aspirin)
ibuprofen (Motrin, Advil, Nuprin)
indomethacin (Indocin)
ketorolac (Toradol)
naproxen (Naprosyn, Anaprox, Aleve)

Nonpharmacologic interventions: Include sensory, emotional, and cognitive interventions, such as massage, relaxation, distraction, and guided imagery. These interventions are used for mild pain and anxiety and as adjuncts to pharmacologic management of moderate to severe pain. See Table 1-36.

T A B L E   1 - 3 6   Common nonpharmacologic methods of pain control

Physical therapies/modalities
- *Massage:* To relax muscular tension and increase local circulation. Back and foot massage are especially relaxing.
- *ROM exercises (passive, assisted, or active):* To relax muscles, improve circulation, and prevent pain related to stiffness and immobility.
- *Heat/cold applications:* To alter pain threshold, reduce muscle spasm, and decrease vascular congestion, particularly in the area of injury. Cold decreases initial tissue injury response. Heat facilitates clearance of tissue toxins and fluids.
- *Transcutaneous electrical nerve stimulation (TENS):* A battery-operated device used to send weak electric impulses *via* electrodes placed on the body. The sensation of pain is reduced during and sometimes after treatment.

Emotional interventions
- *Prevention and control of anxiety:* Limiting anxiety reduces muscle tension and increases the patient's pain tolerance. Anxiety and fear contribute to autonomic stimulation and pain responses. Progressive relaxation exercises and encouraging slow, controlled breathing may be helpful.
- *Promoting self-control:* Feelings of helplessness and lack of control contribute to anxiety and pain. Techniques such as PCA and promoting self-helping behaviors contribute to feelings of self-control.

Cognitive interventions
- *Preparatory information:* Preparing the patient by explaining what can be expected, thereby reducing stress and anxiety. Preoperative teaching is an example of this technique.
- *Patient education:* Teaching methods for preventing or reducing pain. Examples include suggesting comfortable postoperative positions, methods of ambulation, and splinting of incisions when coughing.
- *Distraction:* Encouraging patient to focus on something unrelated to the pain. Examples include conversing, reading, watching television or videos, listening to music, relaxation techniques (see **Health-seeking behavior,** p. 323.)
- *Humor:* Can be an excellent distraction and may help the patient cope with stress.
- *Guided imagery:* The patient employs a mental process that uses images to alter a physical or emotional state. This technique promotes relaxation and decreases pain sensations.
- *Biofeedback:* The patient learns conscious control of physiologic processes that normally are controlled unconsciously. Muscle tension and chronic or episodic pain may be reduced.

Many of these techniques may be taught to and implemented by the patient and significant others.

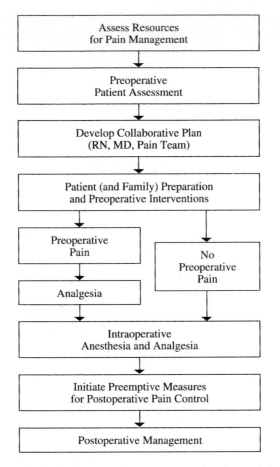

Figure 1-1: Pain treatment flow chart: preoperative and intraoperative phases. (From the Acute Pain Management Guideline Panel: *Acute pain management: operative or medical procedures and trauma, clinical practice guideline,* AHCPR Pub No 92-0032, Agency for Health Care Policy and Research, Public Health Service, Rockville, Md, 1992, US Department of Health and Human Services.)

NURSING DIAGNOSES AND INTERVENTIONS

Pain related to biophysical injury secondary to pathology; surgical, diagnostic, or treatment interventions; or trauma

Desired outcomes: Within 2 h of initiating therapy, patient's subjective evaluation of discomfort improves, as documented by a pain scale. Patient does not exhibit nonverbal indicators of pain (Table 1-32). Autonomic indicators (Table 1-31) are diminished or absent. Verbal responses, such as crying or moaning, are absent.

• Develop a systematic approach to pain management for each patient. The primary nurse should collaborate with the surgeon, anesthesi-

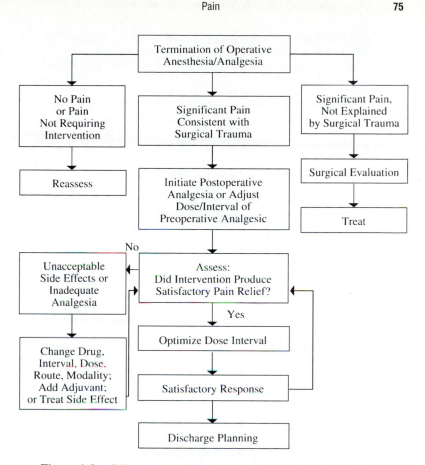

Figure 1-2: Pain treatment flow chart: postoperative phase. (From the Acute Pain Management Guideline Panel: *Acute pain management: operative or medical procedures and trauma, clinical practice guideline,* AHCPR Pub No 92-0032, Agency for Health Care Policy and Research, Public Health Service, Rockville, Md, 1992, US Department of Health and Human Services.)

ologist, and patient for optimal management of pain. See Figures 1-1 and 1-2[13] for pain treatment flow charts for preoperative and postoperative patients.

- Monitor patient at frequent intervals for the presence of discomfort. Use a formal method of assessing pain. One method is to have the patient rate discomfort on a scale of 0 (no discomfort) to 10 (worst pain). Other methods may be used, but the method selected should be used consistently.
- Evaluate patients with acute and chronic pain for nonverbal indicators of discomfort (see Table 1-32).
- Evaluate patients with acute pain for autonomic indicators of dis-

comfort (Table 1-31). Be aware that patients with chronic pain (>6 mo duration) will not exhibit an autonomic response.

- Evaluate health history for evidence of alcohol and drug (prescribed and nonprescribed) use. Individuals with a history of chemical dependence may require a higher dose for effective analgesia. Persons with evidence of chronic or acute hepatic insufficiency require a reduced dose and careful selection of appropriate analgesics. Consult pain control team if available. All care providers must be consistent in setting limits while providing effective pain control through pharmacologic and nonpharmacologic methods. Psychiatric or mental health consultation may be necessary.

    Be aware that some opioid agonist-antagonist analgesics (e.g., butorphanol, buprenorphine, pentazocine) have strong narcotic antagonist activity and may trigger withdrawal symptoms in individuals with opiate dependency.

- Administer opioid and related mixed agonist-antagonist analgesics as prescribed (Table 1-34). Monitor for side effects, such as respiratory depression, excessive sedation, nausea, vomiting, and constipation. Be aware that meperidine (Demerol) may produce excitation, muscle twitching, and seizures, especially in conjunction with phenothiazines. Do not administer mixed agonist-antagonist analgesics concurrently with morphine or other pure agonists, because reversal of analgesic effects may occur.

- Assess patients receiving opioid analgesics at frequent intervals for evidence of excessive sedation when awake or respiratory depression (i.e., RR <10 breaths/min or Sao_2 $<90\%$-92%). In the presence of respiratory depression, reduce the amount or frequency of the dose as prescribed. Have naloxone (Narcan) readily available to reverse severe respiratory depression. **Note:** Due to respiratory depression and excessive sedation, older adults and individuals with asthma, COPD, and other respiratory disorders should be monitored closely when receiving opiate analgesics.

- If the patient is receiving epidural or intrathecal narcotic, monitor closely for side effects and complications.

- Check patient's analgesia record for the last dose and amount of medication given during surgery and in the postanesthesia recovery room. Be careful to coordinate timing and dose of postoperative analgesics with previously administered medication.

- Administer nonnarcotic and nonsteroidal antiinflammatory agents (Table 1-35) as prescribed for relief of mild to moderate pain or on alternating schedule with opiate analgesics for moderate to severe pain. NSAIDs are especially effective when pain is associated with inflammation and soft-tissue injury. Ketorolac (Toradol) may be given IM or IV when oral agents are contraindicated. Monitor for excessive bleeding, gastric irritation, and renal compromise in patients receiving NSAIDs.

- Administer prn analgesics before pain becomes severe. Prolonged stimulation of pain receptors results in increased sensitivity to painful stimuli and will increase the amount of drug required to relieve pain.

- Administer intermittently scheduled or supplemental analgesics before painful procedures (suctioning, chest tube removal), ambulation, and at bedtime, scheduling them so that their peak effect is achieved at the inception of the activity or procedure.

- Augment analgesic therapy with sedatives and tranquilizers to prolong and enhance analgesia. Avoid substituting sedatives and tranquilizers for analgesics.
- Wean patient from opioid analgesics by decreasing dosage or frequency of the drug. When changing route of administration or medication, be certain to employ equianalgesic doses of the new drug (Table 1-33).
- Augment action of medication by employing nonpharmacologic methods of pain control (Table 1-36). Many of these techniques may be taught to and implemented by the patient and significant others.
- Maintain a quiet environment to promote rest. Plan nursing activities to enable long periods of uninterrupted rest at night.
- Evaluate for and correct nonoperative sources of discomfort (i.e., position, full bladder, infiltrated IV site).
- Position patient comfortably, and reposition at frequent intervals to relieve discomfort due to pressure and improve circulation.
- Sudden or unexpected changes in pain intensity can signal complications such as internal bleeding or leakage of visceral contents. Carefully evaluate the patient and consult the surgeon immediately.
- Document efficacy of analgesics and other pain control interventions, using the pain scale or other formalized method.

Ineffective breathing pattern related to neuromuscular impairment secondary to central respiratory depression

Desired outcome: Patient exhibits effective ventilation within 30 min of this diagnosis as evidenced by relaxed breathing, RR 12-20 breaths/min with normal depth and pattern (eupnea), clear breath sounds, normal color, Pao_2 ≥80 mm Hg, pH 7.35-7.45, $Paco_2$ 35-45 mm Hg, HCO_3^- 22-26 mEq/L, and Spo_2 ≥92%.

- Assess and document respiratory rate and depth qh. Note signs of respiratory compromise, including RR <10 or >26; shallow or grunting respirations; use of accessory muscles of respiration; prolonged inspiratory/expiratory ratio; pallor or cyanosis; decreased vital capacity; and increased residual volume. Consult physician for evidence of respiratory compromise.
- Monitor Spo_2 and ABG values. Consult physician for decreased Spo_2 (<90%-92%) or increased $Paco_2$ (>45 mm Hg).
- Assess and document LOC q1-2h.
- Use apnea monitor as indicated.
- Keep naloxone (Narcan) at patient's bedside during and for 24 h after epidural or intrathecal administration.
- Maintain IV access for immediate administration of naloxone to reverse respiratory depression.
- Respiratory depression may persist for as long as 24 h after the last dose of epidural morphine. Monitor for respiratory depression during and for 24 h after patient's receipt of epidural or intrathecal opioids.

Urinary retention related to inhibition of reflex arc secondary to opioid action

Desired outcomes: Within 4 h of this diagnosis, complete bladder emptying is achieved. Overflow incontinence is absent.

- Monitor for symptoms of urinary retention: bladder distention, frequent voiding of small amounts of urine, sensation of bladder fullness, residual urine, dysuria, and overflow incontinence.
- Monitor I&O precisely.
- Catheterize bladder intermittently or insert indwelling catheter as prescribed.
- Administer IV naloxone as prescribed.

Risk for impaired skin integrity related to itching secondary to alteration in sensory modulation from opioid effects

Desired outcome: Patient's skin remains intact.

- Administer diphenhydramine or hydroxyzine as prescribed.
- Maintain comfortably cool environment.
- Apply cool, moist compresses.
- If relief from the above measures is inadequate, administer small amounts of IV naloxone as prescribed.

Prolonged immobility

NURSING DIAGNOSES AND INTERVENTIONS

Activity intolerance related to prolonged bed rest, generalized weakness, and an imbalance between oxygen supply and demand

Desired outcome: Within 48 h of discontinuing bed rest, patient exhibits cardiac tolerance to low-intensity exercise as evidenced by HR $\leq$20 bpm over resting HR, systolic BP $\leq$20 mm Hg over or under resting systolic BP, Svo_2 $\geq$60%, RR $\leq$20 breaths/min, normal sinus rhythm, warm and dry skin, and absence of crackles, murmurs, and chest pain.

- Perform ROM exercises bid to qid on each extremity. Individualize the exercise plan on the basis of the following guidelines:
  - *Mode or type of exercise:* Begin with passive exercises, moving the joints through the motions of abduction, adduction, flexion, and extension. Progress to active assisted exercises in which you support the joints while the patient initiates muscle contraction. When the patient is able, supervise him or her in active isotonic exercises, during which the patient contracts a selected muscle group, moves the extremity at a slow pace, and then relaxes the muscle group. Have the patient repeat each exercise 3-10 times.

Caution: Avoid isometric exercises in cardiac patients. Stop any exercise that causes muscular or skeletal pain. Consult with a physical therapist for necessary modifications.

  - *Intensity:* Begin with 3-5 repetitions as tolerated by the patient. Assess exercise tolerance by measuring HR and BP at rest, peak exercise, and 5 min after exercise. If HR or systolic BP increases >20 bpm or >20 mm Hg over the resting level, decrease the number of repetitions. If HR or systolic BP decreases >10 bpm or >10 mm Hg at peak exercise, this could be a sign of left ventricular failure, denoting that the heart cannot meet this workload. For other adverse signs and symptoms, see "Assessment," which follows.

T A B L E 1 - 3 7   Physiologic effects of bed rest (deconditioning)

Increased HR and BP for submaximal workload
Decrease in functional capacity
Decrease in circulating volume
Orthostatic hypotension
Reflex tachycardia
Modest decrease in pulmonary function
Increase in thromboemboli
Loss of muscle mass
Loss of muscle contractile strength
Deficient protein state
Negative nitrogen state

- □ *Duration:* Begin with 5 min or less of exercise. Gradually increase the exercise to 15 min as tolerated.
- □ *Frequency:* Begin exercises bid-qid. As the duration increases, the frequency can be reduced.
- □ *Assessment of exercise tolerance:* Be alert to signs and symptoms that the cardiovascular and respiratory systems are unable to meet the demands of the low-level ROM exercises. Excessive SOB may occur if (1) transient pulmonary congestion occurs secondary to ischemia or left ventricular dysfunction; (2) lung volumes are decreased; (3) oxygen-carrying capacity of the blood is reduced; or (4) there is shunting of blood from the right to the left side of the heart without adequate oxygenation. If cardiac output does not increase to meet the body's needs during modest levels of exercise, systolic BP may fall; the skin may become cool, cyanotic, and diaphoretic; dysrhythmias may be noted; crackles may be auscultated; or a systolic murmur of mitral regurgitation may occur. If the patient tolerates the exercise, increase the intensity or number of repetitions each day. See Table 1-37 for physiologic effects of bed rest (deconditioning).
- Ask patient to rate perceived exertion (RPE) experienced during exercise, basing it on the following scale developed by Borg (1982):
  0 Nothing at all
  1 Very weak effort
  2 Weak (light) effort
  3 Moderate
  4 Somewhat stronger effort
  5 Strong effort
  7 Very strong effort
  9 Very, very strong effort
  10 Maximal effort
  The patient should not experience a RPE >3 while performing ROM exercises. Reduce the intensity of the exercise and increase the frequency until an RPE of ≤3 is attained.
- As the patient's condition improves, increase activity as soon as possible to include sitting in a chair. Assess for orthostatic hypotension, which can occur as a result of decreased plasma volume and diffi-

culty in adjusting immediately to postural change. Prepare the patient for this by increasing the amount of time spent in high Fowler's position and moving the patient slowly and in stages. (For additional information about activity progression, see Table 4-1, p. 274.)
- Increase activity level by having patient perform self-care activities such as eating, mouth care, and bathing as tolerated.
- Teach significant others the purpose and interventions for preventing deconditioning. Involve them in the patient's plan of care.
- To help allay fears of failure, pain, or medical setbacks, provide emotional support to patient and significant others as patient's activity level is increased.

Risk for disuse syndrome related to mechanical or prescribed immobilization, severe pain, or altered LOC
Desired outcome: Patient displays full ROM without verbal or nonverbal indicators of *pain.*

Note: ROM exercises should be performed every day for all immobilized patients with *normal* joints. Modification may be required for patients with flaccidity (i.e., immediately following CVA or spinal cord injury) to prevent subluxation; or for patients with spasticity (i.e., during the recovery period for patients with CVA or spinal cord injury) to prevent an increase in spasticity. Consult with physical therapist or occupational therapist for assistance with modifying the exercise plan for these patients. In addition, be aware that ROM exercises are contraindicated for patients with rheumatologic disease during the inflammatory phase and for joints that are dislocated or *fractured.*

- Be alert to the following areas that are especially prone to joint contracture: *shoulder,* which can become "frozen" to limit abduction and extension; *wrist,* which can "drop," prohibiting extension; *fingers,* which can develop flexion contractures that limit extension; *hips,* which can develop flexion contractures that affect the gait by shortening the limb or develop external rotation or adduction deformities that affect the gait; *knees,* in which flexion contractures can develop to limit extension and alter the gait; and *feet,* which can "drop" as a result of plantarflexion, which limits dorsiflexion and alters the gait.
- Ensure that patient changes position at least q2h. Post a turning schedule at patient's bedside. Position changes not only will maintain correct body alignment, thereby reducing strain on the joints, but also will prevent contractures, minimize pressure on bony prominences, and promote maximal chest expansion.
  □ Try to place patient in a position that achieves proper standing alignment: head neutral or slightly flexed on the neck, hips extended, knees extended or minimally flexed, and feet at right angles to the legs. Maintain this position with pillows, towels, or other positioning aids.
  □ To prevent hip flexion contractures, ensure that the patient is prone or side-lying, with the hips extended for the same amount of time patient spends in the supine position.
  □ When the HOB must be elevated 30 degrees, extend the patient's shoulders and arms, using pillows to support the position, and allow the fingertips to extend over the edge of the pillows to maintain normal arching of the hands.

Caution: Because elevating the HOB promotes hip flexion, ensure that patient spends equal time with the hips in extension (see intervention, "To prevent hip flexion . . .," above.

> □ When patient is in the side-lying position, extend the lower leg from the hip to help prevent hip flexion contracture.
> □ When able to place patient in the prone position, move patient to the end of the bed and allow the feet to rest between the mattress and footboard. This not only will prevent plantarflexion and hip rotation, but also will prevent injury to the heels and toes. Place thin pads under the angles of the axillae and lateral aspects of the clavicles to prevent internal rotation of the shoulders and maintain anatomic position of the shoulder girdle.

- To maintain the joints in neutral position, use the following as indicated: pillows, rolled towels, blankets, sandbags, antirotation boots, splints, and orthotics. When using adjunctive devices, monitor the involved skin at frequent intervals for alterations in integrity, and implement measures to prevent skin breakdown.
- Assess for footdrop by inspecting the feet for plantarflexion and evaluating patient's ability to pull the toes upward toward the nose. Although feet posture naturally in plantarflexion, be particularly alert to the patient's inability to pull the toes up. To prevent footdrop, foam boots or "high top" tennis shoes may be used to support the feet. Document this assessment daily.
- Teach patient the rationale and procedure for ROM exercises, and have patient return the demonstrations, if able. Review **Activity intolerance,** earlier, to ensure that patient does not exceed his or her tolerance. Provide passive exercises for patients unable to perform active or active-assistive exercises. In addition, incorporate movement patterns into care activities, such as position changes, bed baths, getting the patient on and off the bed pan, or changing the patient's gown. Ensure that joints especially prone to contracture are exercised more stringently.
- Perform and document limb girth measurements, dynamography (hand-grip device that measures muscle strength), ROM, and exercise baseline limits to assess patient's existing muscle mass and strength and joint motion.
- Explain to patient that muscle atrophy occurs because of disuse or failure to use the joint, often due to immediate or anticipated pain. Eventually, disuse may result in a decrease in muscle mass and blood supply and a loss of periarticular tissue elasticity, which in turn can lead to increased muscle fatigue and joint pain with use.
- Emphasize the importance of maintaining or increasing muscle strength and periarticular tissue elasticity through exercise. If unsure about patient's complicating pathology, consult with physician about the appropriate form of exercise for patient.
- Explain the need to participate maximally in self-care as tolerated to help maintain muscle strength and enhance a sense of participation and control.
- For *non*cardiac patients needing greater help with muscle strength, assist with resistive exercises (e.g., moderate weightlifting to in-

crease the size, endurance, and strength of the muscles). For patients in beds with Balkan frames, provide the means for resistive exercise by implementing a system of weights and pulleys. First, determine patient's baseline level of performance on a given set of exercises, and then set realistic goals with the patient for repetitions. For example, if the patient can do 5 repetitions of lifting a 5-lb weight with the biceps muscle, the goal may be to increase the repetitions to 10 within 1 wk, to an ultimate goal of 20 within 3 wk and then advance to 7½-lb weights.

- If the joints require rest, isometric exercises can be used. With these exercises, teach patient to contract a muscle group and hold the contraction for a count of 5 or 10. The sequence is repeated for increasing numbers or repetitions until an adequate level of endurance has been achieved. Thereafter, maintenance levels are performed.
- Provide a chart to show patient's progress, and combine this with large amounts of positive reinforcement. Post the exercise regimen at the bedside to ensure consistency by all health care personnel.
- Provide periods of uninterrupted rest between exercises/activities to enable patient to replenish energy stores.
- Seek a referral to a physical therapist (PT) or occupational therapist (OT) as appropriate.

Altered oral mucous membrane related to ineffective oral hygiene
Desired outcome: Patient's oral mucosa, lips, and tongue are intact within 24 h before discharge from intensive care unit.

- Assess patient's oral mucous membrane, lips, and tongue q2h, noting presence of dryness, exudate, swelling, blisters, and ulcers.
- If patient is alert and able to take oral fluids, offer frequent sips of water or ice chips to alleviate dryness.
- Perform mouth care q2-4h, using a soft-bristled toothbrush to cleanse the teeth and a moistened cloth or sponge-tipped applicator to moisten crusty areas or exudate on tongue and oral mucosa. For patient with intubation, suction mouth continuously during oral hygiene to remove fluid and debris.
- Apply lip balm q2h and prn to prevent cracking of lips.
- If indicated, use an artificial saliva preparation to assist in keeping mucous membrane moist.
- As appropriate, have patient wear dentures as soon as he or she is able, to improve communication and enhance comfort.

Note: If it is necessary to put fingers in patient's mouth, wear gloves on both hands. This practice will reduce the risk of acquiring herpetic whitlow (infection of fingertip).

Self-care deficit related to cognitive, neuromuscular, or musculoskeletal impairment; or related to activity intolerance secondary to prolonged bed rest
Desired outcome: Patient's physical needs are met by patient, nursing staff, or significant others.

- Assess patient's ability to perform self-care on the basis of functional status (e.g., comatose state, hemiplegia, sensory or motor deficit, alterations in vision).
- If patient is comatose, meet all patient's physical needs, including

bathing, oral hygiene, feeding, elimination. Involve significant others in the plan of care. Explain all procedures to patient and significant others before performing them.

- For patient who is not comatose, collaborate with him or her on a plan of care that promotes as much self-care as patient is capable of providing. Schedule care activities around the periods of time patient has the most energy to meet his or her needs. Use assessment criteria for activity tolerance, p. 78, to evaluate patient's tolerance of the activity.
- If patient is alert, keep toiletries and other necessary items within his or her reach.
- Do not rush patient; allow adequate time for performance of self-care activities.
- Encourage patient; reinforce the value of progress that is made.
- As appropriate, consult with occupational therapy department regarding use of assistive devices such as long-handled tools.
- If visual impairment exists, place all objects within patient's field of vision. If diplopia is present, apply an eye patch and alternate it between patient's eyes q2-3h.

Altered peripheral tissue perfusion related to interrupted arterial and venous flow secondary to prolonged immobility

Desired outcomes: By discharge from the ICU, patient has adequate peripheral circulation as evidenced by normal skin color and temperature and adequate distal pulses ($>2+$ on a 0-4+ scale) in peripheral extremities.

- Identify patients at high risk for tissue impairment: individuals with altered LOC, immobility, hypothermia, hyperthermia, cachexia, hypoalbuminemia, inability to perform ADL, or advanced age.
- Identify patients at risk for deep vein thrombosis (DVT), including those with chronic infection and a history of peripheral vascular disease and smoking, as well as the aged, obese, and anemic.
- Teach patient that pain, redness, swelling, and warmth in the involved area and coolness, unnatural color or pallor, and superficial venous dilatation distal to the involved area are all indicators of DVT and should be reported to a staff member promptly if they occur.
- Monitor for the same indicators listed earlier, along with routine VS checks. If patient is asymptomatic for DVT, assess for a positive Homans' sign: Flex the knee 30 degrees and dorsiflex the foot. Pain elicited with the dorsiflexion may be a sign of DVT, and patient should be referred to physician for further evaluation. Additional signs of DVT may include fever, tachycardia, and elevated ESR. Normal ESR (Westergren method) in males under 50 years is 0-15 mm/h, over 50 years 0-20 mm/h; in females under 50 years it is 0-20 mm/h, over 50 years 0-30 mm/h.
- Teach patient calf-pumping (ankle dorsiflexion-plantarflexion) and ankle-circling exercises. Instruct patient to repeat each movement 10 times, performing each exercise hourly during extended periods of immobility, provided that patient is free of symptoms of DVT. Help promote circulation by performing passive ROM or encouraging active ROM exercises.
- Encourage deep breathing, which increases negative pressure in the lungs and thorax to promote emptying of large veins.

- When not contraindicated by peripheral vascular disease, ensure that patient wears antiembolic hose or pneumatic sequential compression stockings. Remove them for 10-20 min q8h and inspect underlying skin for evidence of irritation or breakdown. Reapply hose after elevating patient's legs at least 10 degrees for 10 min.
- Instruct patient not to cross the feet at the ankles or knees while in bed because doing so may cause venous stasis. If patient is at risk for DVT, elevate the foot of the bed 10 degrees to increase venous return.
- Patients at risk for DVT may require pharmacologic interventions such as aspirin, sodium warfarin, or heparin. Administer medication as prescribed, and monitor appropriate laboratory values (e.g., PT, PTT). Educate patient to self-monitor for and report bleeding (epistaxis, bleeding gums, hematemesis, hemoptysis, melena, hematuria, and ecchymoses).
- In patients prone to DVT, acquire bilateral baseline measurements of the midcalf, knee, and midthigh and record them on patient's Kardex. Monitor these measurements daily and compare them to the baseline measurements to rule out extremity enlargement caused by DVT.

Altered cerebral tissue perfusion (orthostatic hypotension) related to interrupted arterial flow to the brain secondary to prolonged bed rest
Desired outcome: When getting out of bed, patient has adequate cerebral perfusion as evidenced by HR <120 bpm and BP ≥90/60 mm Hg immediately after position change (or within 20 mm Hg of patient's normal range), dry skin, normal skin color, and denial of vertigo and syncope, with return of HR and BP to resting levels within 3 min of position change.

- Assess patient for factors that increase the risk of orthostatic hypotension because of fluid volume changes (recent diuresis, diaphoresis, or change in vasodilator therapy), altered autonomic control (diabetic cardiac neuropathy, denervation post heart transplant, or advanced age), or severe left ventricular dysfunction.
- Explain the cause of orthostatic hypotension and measures for preventing it.
- Application of antiembolic hose, which are used to prevent DVT, may be useful in preventing orthostatic hypotension once the patient is mobilized. For patients who continue to have difficulty with orthostatic hypotension, it may be necessary to supplement the hose with elastic wraps to the groin when the patient is out of bed. Ensure that these wraps encompass the entire surface of the legs.
- When patient is in bed, provide instructions for leg exercises as described under **Activity intolerance,** p. 78.
- Prepare patient for getting out of bed by encouraging position changes within necessary confines. It is sometimes possible and advisable to use a tilt table to reacclimate patient to upright positions.
- Follow these guidelines for mobilization:
  - Check the BP in any high-risk patient for whom this will be the first time out of bed.
  - Have the patient dangle legs at the bedside. Be alert to indicators of orthostatic hypotension, including diaphoresis, pallor, tachycardia, hypotension, and syncope. Question patient about the presence of lightheadedness or dizziness.

□ If indicators of orthostatic hypotension occur, check the VS. A drop in systolic BP of 20 mm Hg and an increased pulse rate, combined with symptoms of vertigo and impending syncope, signal the need for return to a supine position.

□ If leg dangling is tolerated, have patient stand at the bedside with two staff members in attendance. If no adverse signs or symptoms occur, have patient progress to ambulation as tolerated.

Constipation related to less than adequate fluid or dietary intake and bulk, immobility, lack of privacy, positional restrictions, and use of narcotic analgesics

Desired outcomes: Within 24 h of this diagnosis, patient verbalizes knowledge of measures that promote bowel elimination. Patient relates the return of his or her normal pattern and character of bowel elimination within 3-5 days of this diagnosis.

• Assess patient's bowel history to determine normal bowel habits and interventions that are used successfully at home.

• Monitor and document patient's bowel movements, diet, and I&O. Be alert to the following indications of constipation: fewer than patient's usual number of bowel movements, abdominal discomfort or distention, straining at stool, and patient complaints of rectal pressure or fullness. Fecal impaction may be manifested by oozing of liquid stool and confirmed *via* digital examination.

• Auscultate each abdominal quadrant for at least 1 min to determine the presence of bowel sounds. Normal sounds are clicks or gurgles occurring at a rate of 5-34/min. **Note:** Bowel sounds are decreased or absent with paralytic ileus. High-pitched rushing sounds may be heard during abdominal cramping, indicating an intestinal obstruction.

• If a rectal impaction is suspected, use a gloved, lubricated finger to remove stool from the rectum. This stimulation may be adequate to stimulate bowel movement. Oil-retention enemas may soften impacted stool.

• Unless contraindicated, encourage a high-roughage diet and a fluid intake of at least 2-3 L/day. Individualize fluid intake according to physiologic state for patients with renal, hepatic, or cardiac disorders.

• Maintain patient's normal bowel habits whenever possible by offering the bed pan; ensuring privacy; and timing medications, enemas, or suppositories so that they take effect at the time of day the patient normally has a bowel movement. Provide warm fluids before breakfast and encourage toileting to gain advantage of gastrocolic or duodenocolic reflexes.

• To promote peristalsis, maximize patient's activity level within the limitations of endurance, therapy, and pain.

• Consult physician for pharmacologic interventions as necessary. To help prevent rebound constipation, make a priority list of interventions to ensure minimal disruption of patient's normal bowel habits. The following is a suggested hierarchy of interventions:

□ Bulk-building additives (psyllium)
□ Mild laxatives (apple or prune juice, milk of magnesia)
□ Stool softeners (docusate sodium or docusate calcium)
□ Potent laxatives and cathartics (bisacodyl, cascara sagrada)
□ Medicated suppositories
□ Enemas

- Discuss the role narcotic agents and other medications have in constipation. Teach alternative methods of pain control (see p. 73).

Diversional activity deficit related to prolonged illness and hospitalization

Desired outcome: Within 24 h of intervention, patient engages in diversional activities and relates the absence of boredom.

- Be alert to patient indicators of boredom, including wishing for something to read or do, daytime napping, and expressed inability to perform usual hobbies because of hospitalization.
- Assess patient's activity tolerance as described on p. 78.
- Collect a database by assessing patient's normal support systems and relationship patterns with significant others. Question patient about his or her interests, and explore diversional activities that may be suitable for the hospital setting and patient's level of activity tolerance.
- Personalize the patient's environment with favorite objects and photographs of significant others.
- Provide low-level activities commensurate with patient's tolerance. Examples include books or magazines pertaining to patient's recreational or other interests, television, or writing for short intervals.
- Initiate activities that require little concentration and proceed to more complicated tasks as patient's condition allows. For example, if reading requires more energy or concentration than patient is capable of, suggest that significant others read to patient or bring in audiotapes of books, such as those marketed for the visually impaired.
- Encourage discussion of past activities or reminiscence as a substitute for performing favorite activities during convalescence.
- As patient's endurance improves, obtain appropriate diversional activities, such as puzzles, model kits, handicrafts, and computerized games and activities; encourage patient to use them.
- Encourage significant others to visit within limits of patient's endurance and to involve patient in activities that are of interest to him or her, such as playing cards or backgammon. Encourage significant others to stagger their visits throughout the day.
- Spend extra time with patient.
- Suggest that significant others bring in a radio, or, if appropriate, a TV, if not part of the standard room.
- If appropriate for patient, arrange for hospital volunteers to visit, play cards, read books, or play board games.
- As appropriate for patient who desires social interaction, consider relocation to a room in an area of high traffic.
- As patient's condition improves, assist him or her with sitting in a chair near a window so that outside activities can be viewed. When patients are able, provide opportunities to sit in a solarium so that they can visit with other patients. If the physical condition and weather permit, take patient outside for brief periods of time.
- Request consultation from social services, OT, pastoral services, and psychiatric nurse for interventions as appropriate.
- Increase patient's involvement in self-care to provide a sense of purpose, accomplishment, and control. Performing in-bed exercises (e.g., deep breathing, ankle circling, calf pumping), keeping track of

I&O, and similar activities can and should be accomplished routinely by these patients.

Altered sexuality pattern related to actual or perceived physiologic limitations on sexual performance secondary to disease, therapy, or prolonged hospitalization

Desired outcome: Within 72 h of this diagnosis, patient relates satisfaction with sexuality and/or understanding of the ability to resume sexual activity.

- Assess patient's normal sexual function, including the importance placed on sex in the relationship, frequency of interaction, normal positions used, and the couple's ability to adapt or change to meet requirements of patient's limitations.
- Identify patient's problem diplomatically and clarify it with patient. Indicators of sexual dysfunction can include regression, acting-out with inappropriate behavior such as grabbing or pinching, sexual overtures toward the hospital staff, self-enforced isolation, and other similar behaviors.
- Encourage patient and significant other to verbalize feelings and anxieties about sexual abstinence or hurting the patient. Develop strategies collaboratively among the patient, significant other, and yourself.
- Encourage acceptable expressions of sexuality by the patient. For example, in a woman this can involve wearing makeup, jewelry, and her own clothing.
- Inform patient and significant other that it is possible to have time alone together for intimacy. Provide that time accordingly by putting a "Do Not Disturb" sign on the door, enforcing privacy by restricting staff and visitors from the room. Encourage caressing, touching, and kissing.

Altered role performance: Dependence versus independence

Desired outcome: Within 48 h of this diagnosis, patient collaborates with care givers in planning realistic goals for independence, participates in own care, and takes responsibility for self-care.

- Encourage patient to be as independent as possible within limitations of the endurance, therapy, and pain. Be aware, however, that temporary periods of dependence are appropriate, inasmuch as they enable the person to restore energy reserves needed for recovery.
- Ensure that all health care providers are consistent in conveying their expectations of eventual independence.
- Alert patient to areas of overdependence, and involve him or her in collaborative goal setting to achieve independence.
- Do not minimize patient's expressions of feelings of depression. Allow patient to express emotions, while providing support, understanding, and realistic hope for a positive role change.
- If indicated, provide self-help devices to increase patient's independence with self-care.
- Provide positive reinforcement when patient meets or advances toward goals.

Psychosocial support

Psychosocial support of patients and their families/significant others is an integral component of any care plan or care map. Founded on principles of holistic care, in which body, mind, and spirit operate in tandem, this section addresses psychosocial care within the context of the individual's primary social structure. Considerable overlap will be noted between nursing diagnoses for the patient and those for the family. Nursing interventions should occur simultaneously for both the patient and the family/significant others.

NURSING DIAGNOSES AND INTERVENTIONS

Knowledge deficit: Current health status and therapies
Desired outcome: Before any medical or nursing intervention and within the 24-h period before discharge from the critical care unit, patient verbalizes understanding of current health status and interventions.
- Assess current level of knowledge about health status.
- Assess cognitive and emotional readiness to learn.
- Recognize barriers to learning, such as ineffective communication, neurologic deficit, sensory alterations, fear, anxiety, or lack of motivation.
- Assess learning needs and establish short- and long-term goals.
- Use individualized verbal or written information to promote learning and enhance understanding. Give simple, direct instructions. If indicated, use audiovisual tools to supplement information.
- Encourage significant others to reinforce correct information about diagnosis and therapies.
- As appropriate, facilitate referral of neurologically impaired patient to neurologic clinical nurse specialist or other specialist as appropriate.
- Encourage interest about health care information by involving patient in planning care. Explain rationale for care.
- Interact frequently with patient to evaluate comprehension of information given. Ask patient to repeat what has been explained. Individuals in crisis often need repeated explanations before information can be understood. Also be aware that many individuals may not understand seemingly simple medical terms (e.g., "terminal," "malignant," "constipation").
- As appropriate, assess understanding of informed consent. Assist patient to use information received to make informed health care decisions (e.g., about invasive procedures, surgery, resuscitation).
- Assess understanding of right to self-determination; provide information as indicated. If requested, assist patient with executing an advance directive for health care.

Anxiety related to actual or perceived threat of death, change in health status, threat to self-concept or role, unfamiliar people and environment, or the unknown
Desired outcomes: Within 1-2 h of intervention, anxiety is absent or reduced as evidenced by patient's verbalization of same, HR ≤ 100 bpm, RR ≤ 20 breaths/min, and an absence of or decrease in irritability and restlessness.

- Engage in honest communication; provide empathetic understanding. Actively listen and establish an atmosphere that enables free expression.
- Assess level of anxiety. Be alert to verbal and nonverbal cues:
  - *Mild:* Restlessness, irritability, increase in questions, focusing on the environment.
  - *Moderate:* Inattentiveness, expressions of concern, narrowed perceptions, insomnia, increased HR.
  - *Severe:* Expressions of feelings of doom; rapid speech; tremors; poor eye contact; preoccupation with the past; inability to understand the present; possible presence of tachycardia, palpitations, nausea, and hyperventilation.
  - *Panic:* Inability to concentrate or communicate, distortion of reality, increased motor activity, vomiting, tachypnea.
- For severe anxiety or panic state, refer to psychiatric clinical nurse specialist, case manager, or other health-team members as appropriate.
- If hyperventilation occurs, encourage slow, deep breaths by having patient mimic your own breathing pattern.
- Validate the nursing assessment of anxiety with the patient. ("You seem distressed; are you feeling uncomfortable now?")
- After an episode of anxiety, review and discuss the thoughts and feelings that led to the episode.
- Identify coping behaviors currently being used (e.g., denial, anger, repression, withdrawal, daydreaming, or drug or alcohol dependence). Review coping behaviors used in the past. Assist in using adaptive coping to manage anxiety.
- Encourage expression of fears, concerns, and questions. ("I know this room looks like a maze of wires and tubes; please let me know when you have any questions.")
- Reduce sensory overload by providing an organized, quiet environment (see **Sensory/perceptual alterations,** p. 90).
- Introduce self and other health care team members; explain each individual's role as it relates to the plan of care or care map.
- Teach relaxation and imagery techniques. See **Health-seeking behavior,** p. 323.
- Enable support persons to be in attendance whenever possible.
- Engage in and promote awareness of touch to significant others when appropriate. Kinds of touch are described in Table 1-38.

Impaired verbal communication related to neurologic or anatomic deficit, psychologic or physical barriers (e.g., tracheostomy, intubation), or cultural or developmental differences

Desired outcome: At the time of intervention, patient communicates needs and feelings and relates decrease in or absence of frustration over communication barriers.

- Assess etiology of impaired communication (e.g., tracheostomy, cerebrovascular accident, cerebral tumor, Guillain-Barré syndrome).
- Along with patient and significant others, assess patient's ability to read, write, and comprehend English. If patient speaks a language other than English, collaborate with English-speaking family member or interpreter to establish effective communication.

T A B L E   1 - 3 8   Kinds of touch

Instrumental touch
  · Task or procedure related
  · May be negatively perceived but accepted as impersonal
Affective touch
  · Expressive, personal
  · Caring
  · Comforting
  · May be positively or negatively perceived
  · Influenced by cultural patterns
Therapeutic touch
  · A deliberate intervention to accomplish a purpose
  · Massage
  · Acupressure
  · Use of space around the individual to mobilize energy fields

---

- When communicating, use eye contact; speak in a clear, normal tone of voice; and face the patient.
- If patient is unable to speak because of a physical barrier (e.g., tracheostomy, wired mandibles), provide reassurance and acknowledge frustration. ("I know this is frustrating for you, but please do not give up. I want to understand you.")
- Provide slate, word cards, pencil and paper, alphabet board, pictures, or other device to assist patient with communication. Adapt the call system to meet the patient's needs. Document the meaning of the patient's signals in response to questions.
- Explain the source of the communication impairment to significant others; teach them effective communication alternatives (see preceding intervention).
- Be alert to nonverbal messages, such as facial expressions, hand movements, and nodding of the head. Validate meanings with the patient.
- Recognize that the inability to speak may foster maladaptive behaviors. Encourage patient to communicate needs; reinforce independent behaviors.
- Be honest; do not relate understanding if you are unable to interpret patient's communication.

Sensory/perceptual alterations related to therapeutically or socially restricted environment; psychologic stress; altered sensory reception, transmission, or integration; or chemical alteration

Desired outcomes: At the time of intervention, patient verbalizes orientation to time, place, and person; relates the ability to concentrate; and expresses satisfaction with the degree and type of sensory stimulation being received.

- Assess factors contributing to the sensory/perceptual alteration.
  - *Environmental:* Excessive noise in the environment; constant, monotonous noise; restricted environment (immobility, traction, isolation); social isolation (restricted visitors, impaired communication); therapies.

□ *Physiologic:* Altered organ function, sleep or rest pattern disturbance, medication, previous history of altered sensory perception.
- Determine the appropriate sensory stimulation needed; plan care accordingly.
- Control factors that contribute to environmental overload. For example, avoid constant lighting (maintain day/night patterns); reduce noise whenever possible (e.g., decrease alarm volumes, avoid loud talking, keep room door closed, provide ear plugs).
- Provide meaningful sensory stimulation:
  □ Display clocks, large calendars, and meaningful photographs and objects from home.
  □ Depending on patient's preferences, provide a radio, music, reading materials, and tape recordings of family and significant others. Earphones help block out external stimuli.
  □ Position patient toward window when possible.
  □ Discuss current events, time of day, holidays, and topics of interest during patient care activities.
  □ As needed, orient patient to surroundings. Direct patient to reality as necessary.
  □ Establish personal contact by touch to help promote and maintain contact with the real environment.
  □ Encourage significant others to communicate with patient frequently, using a normal tone of voice.
  □ Convey concern and respect. Introduce yourself and call patient by name.
  □ Stimulate vision with mirrors, colored decorations, and pictures.
  □ Stimulate sense of taste with sweet, salty, and sour substances if appropriate.
  □ Encourage use of eye glasses and hearing aids.
- Inform patient before initiating interventions and using equipment.
- Encourage participation in health care planning and decision making whenever possible. Allow for choice when possible.
- Assess sleep-rest pattern to evaluate its contribution to the sensory/perceptual disorder. Ensure that patient attains at least 90 min of uninterrupted sleep as frequently as possible. For more information, see next nursing diagnosis.

Sleep pattern disturbance related to environmental changes, illness, therapeutic regimen, pain, immobility, or psychologic stress

Desired outcomes: After discussion, patient identifies factors that promote sleep. Within 8 h of intervention, patient attains 90 min periods of uninterrupted sleep and verbalizes satisfaction with ability to rest.
- Assess usual sleeping patterns (e.g., bedtime routine, hours of sleep per night, sleeping position, use of pillows and blankets, napping during the day, nocturia).
- Explore relaxation techniques that promote rest/sleep (e.g., imagining relaxing scenes, listening to soothing music or taped stories, using muscle relaxation exercises).
- Identify causative factors and activities that contribute to insomnia, adversely affect sleep patterns, or awaken patient. Examples include pain, anxiety, depression, hallucinations, medications, underlying illness, sleep apnea, respiratory disorder, caffeine, fear, or medical or nursing interventions.

TABLE 1-39 Nonpharmacologic measures to promote sleep

Activity	Example(s)
Mask or eliminate environmental stimuli	Use eyeshields, ear plugs
	Play soothing music
	Dim lights at bedtime
	Mask odors from dressings/drainage; change dressing or drainage container as indicated
Promote muscle relaxation	Encourage ambulation as tolerated throughout the day
	Teach and encourage in-bed exercises and position changes
	Perform back massage at bedtime
	If not contraindicated, use a heating pad
Reduce anxiety	Ensure adequate pain control
	Keep patient informed of his or her progress and treatment measures
	Avoid overstimulation by visitors or other activities immediately before bedtime
	Avoid stimulant drugs (e.g., caffeine)
Promote comfort	Encourage patient to use own pillows, bedclothes if not contraindicated
	Adjust bed; rearrange linens
	Regulate room temperature
Promote usual presleep routine	Offer oral hygiene at bedtime
	Provide warm beverage at bedtime
	Encourage reading or other quiet activity
Minimize sleep disruption	Maintain quiet environment throughout the night
	Plan nursing activities to allow long periods (at least 90 min) of undisturbed sleep
	Use dim lights when checking on patient during the night

- Organize procedures and activities to allow for 90 min periods of uninterrupted rest/sleep. Limit visiting during these periods.
- Whenever possible, maintain a quiet environment by providing ear plugs or decreasing alarm levels. The use of "white noise" (e.g., low-pitched, monotonous sounds; electric fan; soft music) may facilitate sleep. Dim the lights for a period of time q24h by drawing the drapes or providing blindfolds.
- If appropriate, limit daytime sleeping. Attempt to establish regularly scheduled daytime activity (e.g., ambulation, sitting in chair, active ROM), which may promote nighttime sleep.
- Investigate and provide nonpharmacologic comfort measures that are known to promote sleep (Table 1-39).

Fear related to separation from support systems, unfamiliarity with environment or therapeutic regimen, or loss of sense of control
Desired outcomes: Following intervention, patient communicates

fears and concerns and relates the attainment of increased psychologic and physical comfort.

- Assess perceptions of the environment and health status and determine contributing factors to feelings of fear. Evaluate verbal and nonverbal responses.
- Acknowledge fears. ("I understand that this equipment frightens you, but it is necessary to help you breathe.")
- Provide opportunities for expression of fears and concerns. ("You seem very concerned about receiving more blood today.") Listen actively. Recognize that anger, denial, occasional withdrawal, and demanding behaviors may be coping responses.
- Encourage asking of questions and gathering of information about the unknown. Provide ongoing information about equipment, therapies, and routines according to patient's ability to understand.
- To promote an increased sense of control, encourage participation in the plan of care whenever possible. Provide continuity of care by establishing a routine and arranging for consistent care givers whenever possible. Appoint a primary nurse or care manager as appropriate.
- Discuss with health care team members the appropriateness of medication therapy for fear or anxiety that is disabling.
- Explore patient's desire for spiritual or psychologic counseling. Make referrals as appropriate.
- Collaborate with physician about a visit by another individual with the same disorder.

Ineffective individual coping related to health crisis, sense of vulnerability, or inadequate support systems

Desired outcomes: Within 24 h of this diagnosis, patient verbalizes feelings, identifies strengths, and begins using positive coping behaviors.

- Assess patient's perceptions and ability to understand current health status.
- Establish honest communication. ("Please tell me what I can do to help you.") Assist with identifying strengths, stressors, inappropriate behaviors, and personal needs.
- Support positive coping behaviors. ("I see that reading that book seems to help you relax.")
- Provide opportunities for expression of concerns; gather information from nurses and other support systems. Provide explanations about prescribed routine, therapies, and equipment. Acknowledge feelings and assessment of current health status and environment.
- Identify factors that inhibit ability to cope (e.g., unsatisfactory support system, knowledge deficit, grief, fear).
- Recognize maladaptive coping behaviors (e.g., severe depression, drug or alcohol dependence, hostility, violence, suicidal ideations). Confront these behaviors. ("You seem to be requiring more pain medication. Are you experiencing more physical pain, or does it help you to remove yourself from reality?") Refer patient to case manager, psychiatric liaison, clinical nurse specialist, or clergy, as appropriate.
- As patient's condition allows, assist with reducing anxiety. See **Anxiety,** p. 88.

T A B L E   1 - 4 0   Stages of grieving

Protest stage	Denial: "No, not me"
	Disbelief: "But I just saw her this morning"
	Anger
	Hostility
	Resentment
	Bargaining to postpone loss
	Appeal for help to recover loss
	Loud complaints
	Altered sleep and appetite
Disorganization	Depression
	Withdrawal
	Social isolation
	Psychomotor retardation
	Silence
Reorganization	Acceptance of loss
	Development of new interests and attachments
	Restructuring of life-style
	Return to preloss level of functioning

- Help reduce sensory overload by maintaining an organized, quiet environment. See **Sensory/perceptual alterations,** p. 90.
- Encourage regular visits by significant others. Encourage them to engage in conversation with patient to help minimize patient's emotional and social isolation.
- Assess significant others' interactions with patient. Attempt to mobilize support systems by involving them in patient care whenever possible.
- As appropriate, explain to significant others that increased dependency, anger, and denial may be adaptive coping behaviors used by patient in early stages of crisis until effective coping behaviors are learned.

Anticipatory grieving related to perceived potential loss of physiologic well-being (e.g., expected loss of body function or body part, changes in self-concept or body image, or terminal illness)

Desired outcomes: Following interventions, patient and significant others/family express grief, participate in decisions about the future, and communicate concerns to health care team members and to one another.

- Assess factors contributing to anticipated loss.
- Assess and accept patient's behavioral response. Expect reactions such as disbelief, denial, guilt, anger, and depression. Determine stage of grieving as described in Table 1-40.
- Assess spiritual, religious, and sociocultural expectations related to loss. ("Is religion an important part of your life? How do you and your family/significant other[s] deal with serious health problems?") Refer to the clergy or community support groups as appropriate.
- Encourage patient and family/significant other(s) to share their con-

cerns. ("Is there anything you'd like to talk about today?") Also, respect their desire not to speak.
- Demonstrate empathy. ("This must be a very difficult time for you and your family.") Touch when appropriate (see Table 1-38).
- In selected circumstances, provide an explanation of the grieving process. This approach may assist in better understanding and acknowledging feelings.
- Assess grief reactions of patient and family/significant other(s) and identify a potential for dysfunctional grieving reactions (e.g., absence of emotion, hostility, avoidance). If the potential for dysfunctional grieving is present, refer to case manager, psychiatric clinical nurse specialist, clergy, or other as appropriate.
- When appropriate, assess patient's wishes about tissue donation.

Dysfunctional grieving related to loss of physiologic well-being or fatal illness
Desired outcomes: Within 24 h of this diagnosis, patient expresses grief, explains the meaning of the loss, and communicates concerns with family/significant other(s). The patient completes necessary self-care activities.
- Assess grief stage (see Table 1-40) and previous coping abilities. Discuss patient's feelings, the meaning of loss, and goals. ("How do you feel about your condition/illness? What do you hope to accomplish in these next few days/weeks?")
- Acknowledge and permit anger; set limits on the expression of anger to discourage destructive behavior. ("I understand that you must feel very angry, but for the safety of others, you may not throw equipment.")
- Identify suicidal behavior (e.g., severe depression, statements of intent, suicide plan, previous history of suicide attempt). Ensure safety and refer to case manager, psychiatric clinical nurse specialist, psychiatrist, clergy, or other support system.
- Encourage patient and family/significant other(s) to participate in ADL and diversional activities. Identify physiologic problems related to loss (e.g., eating or sleeping disorders) and intervene accordingly.
- Collaborate with physician about a visit by another individual with the same disorder, if appropriate.

Powerlessness related to health care environment or illness-related regimen
Desired outcomes: Within 24 h of this diagnosis, patient makes decisions about self-care and therapies and relates an attitude of realistic hope and a sense of self-control.
- Assess personal preferences, needs, values, and attitudes.
- Before providing information, assess knowledge and understanding of the state of health and necessary interventions.
- Recognize expressions of fear, lack of response to events, and lack of interest in information, any of which may signal a sense of powerlessness.
- Evaluate medical and nursing interventions and adjust them, as appropriate, to support patient's sense of control. For example, if the patient always bathes in the evening to promote relaxation before bedtime, modify the care plan or map to include an evening bath rather than follow the hospital routine of giving a morning bath.

- Assist patient to identify and demonstrate activities that can be performed independently.
- Whenever possible, offer alternatives related to routine hygiene, diet, diversional activities, visiting hours, or treatment times.
- Ensure privacy and preserve territorial rights whenever possible. For example, when distant relatives and casual acquaintances request information about the patient's status, refer them to the patient or a family member who can provide acceptable amounts of information.
- Discourage patient's dependency on staff. Avoid overprotection and parenting behaviors.
- Assess support systems; enable significant others to be involved in care whenever possible.
- Offer realistic hope for the future. If appropriate, encourage direction of thoughts beyond the present.
- Provide referrals to clergy and other support systems as appropriate.

Spiritual distress related to separation from spiritual/religious/cultural supports or challenged belief and value system

Desired outcomes: Within 24 h of this diagnosis, patient verbalizes spiritual or religious beliefs and expresses hope for the future, the attainment of spiritual or religious support, and the availability of the requisites for resolving conflicts.

- Assess spiritual or religious beliefs, values, and practices. ("Do you have a religious preference? How important is it to you? Are there any religious or spiritual practices you wish to participate in while in the hospital?")
- Inform patient and family/significant other(s) of the availability of spiritual aids, such as a chapel or religious services.
- Present a nonjudgmental attitude toward patient's religious or spiritual beliefs and values. Attempt to create an environment that is conducive to free expression.
- Identify available support systems that may assist in meeting the patient's religious or spiritual needs (e.g., clergy, patient's fellow church members, support groups).
- Be alert to comments related to spiritual concerns or conflicts. ("I don't know why God is doing this to me." "I'm being punished for my sins.")
- Use active listening and open-ended questioning to assist in resolving conflicts related to spiritual issues. ("I understand that you want to be baptized. We can arrange to do that here.")
- Provide privacy and opportunities for religious practices, such as prayer and meditation.
- If spiritual beliefs and therapeutic regimens are in conflict, provide honest, concrete information to encourage informed decision making. ("I understand that your religion discourages receiving blood transfusions. Do you understand that by refusing blood your condition is more difficult to treat?")

Social isolation related to altered health status, inability to engage in satisfying personal relationships, altered mental status, or altered physical appearance

Desired outcome: Within 24 h of this diagnosis, patient demonstrates interaction and communication with others.

- Assess factors contributing to social isolation:

- ▫ Restricted visiting hours
- ▫ Absence of or inadequate support system
- ▫ Inability to communicate (e.g., presence of endotracheal tube/tracheostomy)
- ▫ Physical changes that affect self-concept
- ▫ Denial or withdrawal
- ▫ Critical care environment
- Recognize patients at higher risk for social isolation: the older adult, disabled, chronically ill, economically disadvantaged.
- Assist with identification of feelings associated with loneliness and isolation. ("You seem very sad when your family leaves the room. Can you tell me more about your feelings?")
- Determine need for socialization and identify available and potential support systems. Explore methods for increasing social contact (e.g., tapes of loved ones, more frequent visitations/hospital volunteers, scheduled interaction with nurse or support staff).
- Provide positive reinforcement for socialization that lessens feelings of isolation and loneliness. ("Please continue to call me when you need to talk to someone. Talking will help both of us to better understand your feelings.")
- Facilitate patient's ability to communicate with others (see **Impaired verbal communication,** p. 89).

Body image disturbance related to loss or change in body parts or function or physical trauma

Desired outcomes: Before hospital discharge, patient acknowledges body changes and demonstrates movement toward incorporating changes into self-concept. Maladaptive responses, such as severe depression, are absent.

- Establish open, honest communication. Promote an environment that is conducive to free expression. ("Please feel free to talk to me whenever you have any questions.") Assess indicators suggesting body image disturbance as listed in Table 1-41.
- When planning care, be aware of interventions that may influence body image (e.g., medications, procedures, and monitoring).

T A B L E   1 - 4 1   **Indicators suggesting body image disturbance**

Nonverbal indicators

   Missing body part—internal or external (e.g., splenectomy or amputated extremity)

   Change in structure (e.g., open, draining wound)

   Change in function (e.g., colostomy)

   Avoidance of looking at or touching body part

   Hiding or exposing body part

Verbal indicators

   Expression of negative feelings about body

   Expression of feelings of helplessness, hopelessness, or powerlessness

   Personalization or depersonalization of missing or mutilated part

   Refusal to acknowledge change in structure or function of body part

- Assess knowledge of patient's pathophysiologic process and current health status. Clarify any misconceptions.
- Discuss the loss or change with the patient. Recognize that what may seem to be a small change may be of great significance to the patient (e.g., arm immobilizer, catheter, hair loss, ecchymoses, facial abrasions).
- Explore expressions of concern, fear, and guilt. ("I understand that you are frightened. Your face looks very different now, but you will see changes and it will improve. Gradually you will begin to look more like yourself.")
- Encourage patient and family/significant other(s) to interact with one another. Help family/significant other(s) to support the patient's feelings related to the changed body part or function. ("I know your son looks very different to you now, but it would help if you speak to him and touch him as you would normally.")
- Encourage gradual participation in self-care activities as the patient becomes physically and emotionally able. Allow for some initial withdrawal and denial behaviors. For example, when changing dressings over traumatized part, explain what you are doing but do not expect the patient to watch or participate initially.
- Discuss the potential for reconstruction of the loss or change (i.e., surgery, prosthesis, grafting, physical therapy, cosmetic therapies, organ transplant).
- Recognize manifestations of severe depression (i.e., sleep disturbances, change in affect, change in communication pattern). As appropriate, refer to case manager, psychiatric clinical nurse specialist, clergy, or support group.
- Help patient attain a sense of autonomy and control by offering choices and alternatives whenever possible. Emphasize strengths and encourage activities that interest patient.
- Offer realistic hope for the future.

Risk for violence related to sensory overload, suicidal behavior, rage reactions, neurologic disease, perceived threats, toxic reaction to medications, or substance withdrawal
Desired outcome: Patient does not harm self or others.

- Assess factors that may contribute to or precipitate violent behavior (e.g., medication reactions, inability to cope, suicidal behavior, confusion, hypoxia, substance withdrawal, and preictal and postictal states).
- Attempt to eliminate or treat causative factors. For example, provide patient teaching, reorient patient, ensure delivery of prescribed oxygen therapy, and reduce or prevent sensory overload (see **Sensory/perceptual alterations,** p. 90).
- Assess for history of physical aggression, family violence, and substance abuse as maladaptive coping behaviors.
- Monitor for early signs of increasing anxiety and agitation (i.e., restlessness, verbal aggressiveness, inability to concentrate). Assess for body language that is indicative of violent behavior: clenched fists, rigid posture, increased motor activity.
- Approach patient in a positive manner and encourage verbalization of feelings and concerns. ("I understand that you are frightened. I will be here from 3 PM to 11 PM to care for you.")

- Offer as much personal and environmental control as the situation allows. ("Let's discuss the care you will need today. What fluids would you like to drink? Would you prefer a bath in the morning or evening?")
- Help patient distinguish reality from altered perceptions. Orient to time, place, and person. Alter the environment to promote reality-based thought processes (e.g., provide clocks, calendars, pictures of loved ones, familiar objects).
- For acute confusion that becomes aggressive, do not attempt to re-orient patient, and avoid arguing. Instead, avoid supporting illusions by stating "I believe that you (see, hear) that; however, I do not (see, hear) that." Use nonthreatening mannerisms, facial expressions, and tone of voice.
- Initiate measures that prevent or reduce excessive agitation:
  □ Reduce environmental stimuli (e.g., alarms, loud or unnecessary talking).
  □ Before touching patient, explain interventions, using short, con-cise statements.
  □ Speak quietly (but firmly, as necessary) and project a caring at-titude. ("We are very concerned for your comfort and safety. Can we do anything to help you feel more relaxed?")
  □ Avoid crowding (i.e., of equipment, visitors, health care person-nel) in patient's personal environment.
  □ Avoid direct confrontation.
- Explain and discuss patient's behavior with family/significant oth-er(s). Acknowledge frustration, concerns, fears, and questions. Re-view safety precautions with family/significant others (Table 1-42).

T A B L E 1 - 4 2   Safety precautions in the event of violent behavior

Patient safety
- Remove harmful objects from the environment, such as heavy objects, scissors, tubing.
- Apply padding to side rails according to agency protocol.
- If available, use bed alarms.
- Use restraints as necessary and prescribed. Monitor patient's neurovas-cular status at frequent intervals.
- Set limits on patient's behavior, using clear and simple commands.
- As prescribed, consider chemical sedation when unable to control pa-tient's behavior with other means.
- Explain safety precautions to patient and family/significant others.

Care giver safety
- Place patient in bed closest to nursing station. Maintain visibility at all times by keeping door open.
- Alert hospital security department when risk of violence is present.
- Do not approach a violent patient without adequate assistance from others.
- Never turn your back on a violent patient.
- Maintain a calm, matter-of-fact tone of voice.
- Monitor security measures at frequent intervals.
- Remain alert.

Hopelessness related to prolonged isolation or activity restriction, failing or deteriorating physiologic condition, long-term stress, or loss of faith in God or belief system
Desired outcomes: Before hospital discharge, patient verbalizes hopeful aspects of health status and relates that feelings of despair are absent or lessened.
- Develop open, honest communication with the patient. Actively listen, provide empathetic understanding of fears and doubts, and promote an environment that is conducive to free expression.
- Assess patient's and family's/significant others' understanding of health status and prognosis; clarify any misperceptions.
- Assess for indicators of hopelessness: unwillingness to accept help, pessimism, withdrawal, lack of interest, silence, loss of gratification in roles, previous history of hopeless behavior, hypoactivity, inability to accomplish tasks, expressions of incompetence, closing eyes and turning away.
- Provide opportunities for the patient to feel cared for, needed, and valued by others. For example, emphasize importance of relationships. ("Tell me about your grandchildren." "It seems that your family loves you very much.")
- Support significant others who seem to spark or maintain patient's feelings of hope. ("Your husband's mood seemed to improve after your visit.")
- Recognize factors that promote sense of hope (i.e., discussions about family members, reminiscing about better times).
- Explore patient's coping mechanisms; assist with expanding positive coping behavior (see **Ineffective individual coping,** p. 93).
- Assess spiritual foundation and needs (see **Spiritual distress,** p. 96).
- Promote anticipation of positive events (i.e., mealtime, grandchildren's visits, bath time, extubation, discontinuation of traction).
- Help patient recognize that although there may be no hope for returning to original life-style, there *is* hope for a new, but different life.
- Avoid insisting that the patient assume a positive attitude. Encourage hope for the future, even if it is the hope for a peaceful death.
- Set realistic, attainable goals and reward achievement.

Psychosocial support for the patient's family and significant others

NURSING DIAGNOSES AND INTERVENTIONS

Altered family processes related to situational crisis (patient's illness)
Desired outcome: Following intervention, family/significant others demonstrate effective adaptation to change/traumatic situation as evidenced by seeking external support when necessary and sharing concerns.
- Assess character of family/significant others: social, environmental, ethnic, and cultural factors; relationships; and role patterns. Identify developmental stage. Be aware that other situational or maturational

crises may be ongoing, such as an elderly parent or teenager with a learning disability.

- Assess previous adaptive behaviors. ("How do you react in stressful situations?") Discuss observed conflicts and communication breakdown. ("I noticed that your brother would not visit your mother today. Has there been a problem we should be aware of? Knowing about it may help us better care for your mother.")
- Acknowledge the family's/significant others' involvement in patient care and promote strengths. ("You were able to encourage your wife to turn and cough. That is very important to her recovery.") Encourage participation in patient care conferences. Promote frequent, regular patient visits.
- Provide information and guidance related to the patient. Discuss the stresses of hospitalization and encourage discussions of feelings, such as anger, guilt, hostility, depression, fear, or sorrow. ("You seem to be upset since having been told that your husband is not leaving the hospital today.") Refer to clergy, case manager, clinical nurse specialist, or social services as appropriate.
- Evaluate interactions among patient and family/significant others. Encourage reorganization of roles and priority setting as appropriate. ("I know your husband is concerned about his insurance policy and seems to expect you to investigate it. I'll ask the financial counselor to talk with you.")
- Encourage family/significant others to schedule periods of rest and activity outside the critical care unit and to seek support when necessary. ("Your neighbor volunteered to stay in the waiting room this afternoon. Would you like to rest at home? I'll call you if *anything* changes.")

Family coping: Potential for growth, related to use of support systems and referrals and choosing experiences that optimize wellness

Desired outcomes: At the time of the patient's diagnosis, family/significant others express their intent to use support systems and resources and identify alternative behaviors that promote communication and strengths. Family/significant others express realistic expectations and do not demonstrate ineffective coping behaviors.

- Assess relationships, interactions, support systems, and individual coping behaviors. Permit movement through stages of adaptation. Encourage further positive coping.
- Acknowledge expressions of hope, future plans, and growth among family members/significant others.
- Encourage development of open, honest communication. Provide opportunities in a private setting for interactions, discussions, and questions. ("I know the waiting room is very crowded. Would you like some private time together?")
- Refer the family/significant others to community or support groups (e.g., ostomy support group, head injury rehabilitation group).
- Encourage exploration of outlets that foster positive feelings, for example, periods of time outside the hospital area, meaningful communication with the patient or support individuals, and relaxing activities (e.g., showering, eating, exercising).

Ineffective family coping: Compromised, related to inadequate or incorrect information or misunderstanding, temporary family disorgani-

zation and role change, exhausted support systems, unrealistic expectations, fear, or anxiety

Desired outcomes: Following intervention, family/significant others
verbalize feelings, identify ineffective coping patterns, identify
strengths and positive coping behaviors, and seek information and support from the nurse or other support systems.

- Establish open, honest communication. Assist in identifying
  strengths, stressors, inappropriate behaviors, and personal needs. ("I
  understand your mother was very ill last year. How did you manage
  the situation?" "I know your loved one is very ill. How can I help
  you?")
- Assess for ineffective coping (e.g., depression, substance abuse, violence, withdrawal) and identify factors that inhibit effective coping
  (e.g., inadequate support system, grief, fear of disapproval by others,
  knowledge deficit). ("You seem to be unable to talk about your husband's illness. Is there anyone with whom you can talk about it?")
- Assess knowledge regarding patient's current health status and therapies. Provide information frequently and allow sufficient time for
  questions. Reassess understanding at frequent intervals.
- Provide opportunities in a private setting to talk and share concerns
  with nurses or other health care providers. If appropriate, refer to
  psychiatric clinical nurse specialist for therapy.
- Offer realistic hope. Help family/significant others to develop realistic expectations for the future and to identify support systems that
  will assist them with planning for the future.
- Reduce anxiety by encouraging diversional activities (e.g., period of
  time outside of hospital) and interaction with outside support systems. ("I know you want to be near your son, but if you would like
  to go home to rest, I will call you if *any* changes occur.")

Ineffective family coping: Disabling, related to unexpressed feelings,
ambivalent family relationships, or disharmonious coping styles among
family members/significant others

Desired outcomes: Before hospital discharge, family/significant others verbalize feelings, identify sources of support as well as ineffective coping behaviors that create ambivalence and disharmony, and do
not demonstrate destructive behaviors.

- Establish open, honest communication and rapport. ("I am here to
  care for your mother and to help you, as well.")
- Identify ineffective coping behaviors (e.g., violence, depression, substance abuse, withdrawal). ("You seem to be angry. Would you like
  to talk to me about your feelings?") Refer to psychiatric clinical
  nurse specialist, clergy, or support group as appropriate.
- Identify perceived or actual conflicts. ("Are you able to talk freely
  among yourselves?" "Are your brothers and sisters able to help and
  support you during this time?")
- Encourage healthy functioning. For example, facilitate open communication and encourage behaviors that support cohesiveness. ("Your
  mother enjoyed your last visit. Would you like to see her now?")
- Assess knowledge about patient's current health status. Provide opportunities for questions; reassess understanding at frequent intervals.
- Assist with developing realistic goals, plans, and actions. Refer to

clergy, case manager, psychiatric nurse, social services, financial counseling, and family therapy as appropriate.

- Encourage family/significant others to spend time outside of the hospital and to interact with support individuals. Respect the need for occasional withdrawal.
- Include the family/significant others in the patient's plan of care. Offer them opportunities to become involved in patient care, for example, ROM exercises, patient hygiene, and comfort measures (e.g., back rub).

Fear related to patient's life-threatening condition and/or knowledge deficit

Desired outcome: Following intervention, family/significant others relate that fear has been lessened.

- Assess fears and understanding related to the patient's clinical situation. Evaluate verbal and nonverbal responses.
- Acknowledge the fears. ("I understand these tubes must frighten you, but they are necessary to help nourish your son.")
- Assess history of coping behavior. ("How do you react to difficult situations?") Determine resources and significant others available for support. ("Who/what usually helps during stressful times?")
- Provide opportunities for expression of fears and concerns. Recognize that anger, denial, withdrawal, and demanding behavior may be adaptive coping responses during initial period of crisis.
- Provide information at frequent intervals about patient's status and the therapies and equipment used. Demonstrate a caring attitude.
- Encourage use of positive coping behaviors by identifying the fear(s), developing goals, identifying supportive resources, facilitating realistic perceptions, and promoting problem solving.
- Recognize anxiety and encourage family/significant others to describe their feelings. ("You seem very uncomfortable tonight. Can you describe your feelings?")
- Be alert to maladaptive responses to fear: potential for violence, withdrawal, severe depression, hostility, and unrealistic expectations of staff or of patient's recovery. Provide referrals to psychiatric clinical nurse specialist or other as appropriate.
- Offer *realistic* hope, even if it is the hope for the patient's peaceful death.
- Explore desires for spiritual, religious, or psychologic counseling.
- Assess your own feelings about the patient's life-threatening illness. Acknowledge that your attitude and fear may be reflected to the family/significant others.
- For other interventions, see previous nursing diagnoses: **Altered family processes; Ineffective family coping:** Compromised; and **Ineffective family coping:** Disabling.

Knowledge deficit: Patient's current health status or therapies

Desired outcome: Following intervention, family/significant others verbalize knowledge and understanding about the patient's current health status or therapies.

- At frequent intervals, inform the family/significant others about the patient's current health status, therapies, and prognosis. Use individualized verbal, written, and audiovisual strategies to promote understanding.

- Evaluate family/significant others at frequent intervals for understanding of information that has been provided. Adjust teaching as appropriate. Some individuals in crisis need repeated explanations before comprehension can be assured. ("I have explained many things to you today. Would you mind summarizing what I've told you so that I can be sure you understand your husband's status and what we are doing to care for him?")
- Encourage family/significant others to relay correct information to the patient. This also reinforces comprehension for family/significant others and patient.
- Ask if needs for information are being met. ("Do you have any questions about the care your mother is receiving or about her condition?")
- Help family/significant others use the information they receive to guide health care decisions (e.g., regarding patient's surgery, resuscitation, organ donation).
- Promote active participation in patient care when appropriate. Encourage family/significant others to seek information and express feelings, concerns, and questions.

Selected Bibliography

Acute Pain Management Guideline Panel: *Acute pain management: operative and medical procedures and trauma, clinical practice guideline,* AHCPR Pub No 92-0032, Agency for Health Care Policy and Research, Public Health Service, Rockville, Md, 1992, US Department of Health and Human Services.

American Association of Cardiovascular and Pulmonary Rehabilitation: *Guidelines for cardiac rehabilitation programs,* Champaign, Ill, 1991, Human Kinetic Books.

American Psychiatric Association: *Diagnostic and statistical manual of mental disorders,* ed 3, Washington, DC, 1987, The Association.

Arbour R: Weaning a patient from a ventilator, *Nursing* 23(2):52-56, 1993.

Armstrong D, Crisp C: Pharmacoeconomic issues of sedation, analgesia, and neuromuscular blockade in critical care, *New Horizons* 2(1):85-93, 1994.

A.S.P.E.N. Board of Directors: Guidelines for use of parenteral and enteral nutrition in adult and pediatric patients, *J Parenter Enter Nutr* 17(4):1SA-25SA, 1993.

Baas L, editor: *Essentials of cardiac nursing,* Rockville, Md, 1991, Aspen.

Bird R, Makela E: Alcohol withdrawal: what is the benzodiazepine of choice? *Ann Pharmacotherapy* 28:67-71, 1994.

Borg GV: Psychophysical basis of perceived exertion, *Med Sci Sports Exerc* 14:377-381, 1982.

Bouley G: The experience of dyspnea during weaning, *Heart Lung* 21(5):471-476, 1992.

Bragg CL: Practical aspects of epidural and intrathecal narcotic analgesia in the intensive care unit, *Heart Lung* 18(6):599-608, 1989.

Bridges E: Transition from ventilatory support: knowing when the patient is ready to wean, *Crit Care Nurs Quart* 15(1):14-20, 1992.

Briones T: Pressure support ventilation: new ventilatory technique, *Crit Care Nurse* 12(4):51-60, 1992.

Chernow B: *The pharmacologic approach to the critically ill patient,* ed 3, Baltimore, 1994, Williams & Wilkins.

Cuzzell JZ: Choosing a wound dressing: a systematic approach, *AACN Clin Issues Crit Care Nurs* 3(1):566-577, 1990.

Davidson J: Neuromuscular blockade: indications, peripheral nerve stimulation, and other concurrent interventions, *New Horizons* 2(1):75-84, 1994.

Durbin CG: Sedation in the critically ill patient, *New Horizons* 2(1):64-74, 1994.

Edes TE, Walk BE, Austin JL: Diarrhea in tube-fed patients: feeding formula not necessarily the cause, *Am J Med* 88(2):91-93, 1990.

Ellender P: The use of neuromuscular blocking agents in ICU patients, *Hospital Pharmacy* 29(1):36-44, 1994.

Folstein M, Folstein S, McHugh P: Mini-mental state, a practical method for grading the cognitive state of patients for clinicians, *J Psychiatr Res* 12(5):189-198, 1975.

Gianino S, St John RE: Nutritional assessment of the patient in the intensive care unit, *Crit Care Nurs Clin North Am* 5(1):1-16, 1993.

Gillman PH: Continuous measurement of cardiac output: a milestone in hemodynamic monitoring, *Focus Crit Care* 19(2):155-158, 1992.

Gujol M: A survey of pain assessment and management practices among critical care nurses, *Am J Crit Care Nurs* 3(2):123-127, 1994.

Hall P: Critical care nursing: psychosocial aspects of care. In Burrell L, editor: *Adult nursing in hospital and community settings,* Norwalk, Conn, 1992, Appleton & Lange.

Halm M: The effectiveness of support groups in reducing anxiety for family members of critically ill patients. In *Proceedings of the Sixteenth Annual National Teaching Institute,* Newport Beach, Calif, 1989, AACN.

Hansen-Flaschen J et al: Use of sedating drugs and neuromuscular blocking agents in patients requiring mechanical ventilation for respiratory failure—a national survey, *JAMA* 266(20):2870-2875, 1991.

Hayden R: Trend-spotting with an Svo_2 monitor, *Am J Nurs* 93(1):26-33, 1993.

Hayter J: The rhythm of sleep, *Am J Nurs* 80(4):457, 1980.

Hofgren K et al: Initial pain course and delay to hospital admission in relation to myocardial infarct size, *Heart Lung* 18(3):274-280, 1989.

Inaba-Roland K, Maricle R: Assessing delirium in the acute care setting, *Heart Lung* 21(2):48-55, 1992.

Interqual: The ISD-A review system with adult ISD criteria, August 1992, North Hampton, NH, and Marlboro, MA, Interqual, Inc.

Jeejeebhoy KN, Detsky AS, Baker JP: Assessment of nutritional status, *J Parenter Enter Nutr* 14(5):193S-196S, 1990.

Kim MJ, McFarland GK, McLane AM: *Pocket guide to nursing diagnosis,* ed 6, St Louis, 1995, Mosby.

Knebel A: Weaning from mechanical ventilation: current controversies, *Heart Lung* 20(4):321-331, 1991.

Konstantinides NN, Lehmann S: The impact of nutrition on wound healing, *Crit Care Nurse* 13(5):25-44, 1993.

Krasner D: *Chronic wound care,* King of Prussia, Pa, 1990, Health Management Publications.

La Van FB, Hunt TK: Oxygen and wound healing, *Clin Plast Surg* 17(3):463-472, 1990.

Lipowski Z: Transient cognitive disorders (delirium and acute confusional states) in the elderly, *Am J Psychiatry* 140(11):1426-1436, 1983.

Maklebust J, Sieggreen M: *Pressure ulcers: guidelines for prevention and nursing management,* West Dundee, Ill, 1991, S-N Publications.

Malacrida R et al: Pharmacokinetics of midazolam administered by continuous intravenous infusion to intensive care patients, *Crit Care Med* 20(8):1123-1126, 1991.

Malkmus D, Booth B, Kodimer C: *Rehabilitation of the head-injured adult, comprehensive cognitive management,* Downey, Calif, 1980, Professional Staff Association of the Ranchos Los Amigos Hospital.

Marcuard SP, Stegall KS: Unclogging feeding tubes with pancreatic enzyme, *J Parenter Enter Nutr* 14(2):198-200, 1990.

Mason H: Morphine sulfate, transdermal fentanyl citrate, and ketorolac tromethamine: effects on postoperative pulmonary function, *Am J Crit Care Nurs* 2(1):61-64, 1993.

Max M: Improving outcomes of analgesic treatment: is education enough? *Ann Intern Med* 113(11):885-889, 1990.

Maxam-Moore V: Analgesics for cardiac surgery patients in critical care: describing current practice, *Am J Crit Care Nurs* 3(1):31-39, 1994.

McMahon MM, Farnell MB, Murray MJ: Nutritional support of critically ill patients, *Mayo Clin Proc* 68:911-920, 1993.

Metheny J: Minimizing respiratory complications of nasoenteric tube feedings: state of the science, *Heart Lung* 22(3):213-223, 1993.

Mlynczak B: Assessment and management of the trauma patient in pain, *Crit Care Nurs Clin North Am* 1(1):55-65, 1989.

Moore EE, Moore FA: Immediate enteral nutrition following multisystem trauma: a decade perspective, *J Am Coll Nutr* 10(6):633-648, 1991.

Murray M, Plevak D: Analgesia in the critically ill patient, *New Horizons* 2(1):56-63, 1994.

Norris SO, Provo B, Stotts NA: Physiology of wound healing and risk factors that impeded the healing process, *AACN Clin Issues Crit Care Nurs* 3(1):542-552, 1990.

Olsson GL et al: Nursing management of patients receiving epidural narcotics, *Heart Lung* 18(2):130-137, 1989.

Owen A: *Pocket guide to critical care monitoring,* St Louis, 1992, Mosby.

Ozuna J, Brennan D: Impaired physical mobility. In Cammermyer M, Appledorn C, editors: *Core curriculum for neuroscience nursing,* Chicago, 1993, American Association of Neuroscience Nurses.

Pasero C, McCaffery M: Unconventional PCA: making it work for your patient, *Am J Nurs* 93(9):38-41, 1993.

Pesola GR: Room-temperature thermodilution cardiac output: proximal injectate lumen vs proximal infusion lumen, *Am J Crit Care* 2(2):132-133, 1993.

Plum F, Posner J: *The diagnosis of stupor and coma,* ed 3, Philadelphia, 1980, FA Davis.

Pressure ulcers in adults: prediction and prevention, Washington, DC, 1992, US Department of Health and Human Services, Agency for Health Care Policy Research.

Puntillo K: Dimensions of procedural pain and its analgesic management in critically ill surgical patients, *Am J Crit Care Nurs* 3(2):116-122, 1994.

Renner L, Meyer L: Injectate port selection affects accuracy and reproducibility of cardiac output measurements with multiport thermodilution pulmonary artery catheters, *Am J Crit Care* 3(1):55-61, 1994.

Rodneaver G et al: Wound healing and wound management: focus on débridement, *Adv in Wound Care* 7(1):22-39, 1994.

Sanders KM et al: Low incidence of extrapyramidal symptoms in treatment of delirium with intravenous haloperidol and lorazepam in the intensive care unit, *J Intensive Care Medicine* 4(3):201-204, 1989.

Sanders KM, Stern TA: Management of delirium associated with use of the intra-aortic balloon pump, *Am J Crit Care* 2(5):371-377, 1993.

Seshadri V, Meyer-Tettambel OM: Electrolyte and drug management in nutritional support, *Crit Care Nurs Clin North Am* 5(1):31-36, 1993.

Shinners PA, Pease MO: A stabilization period of 5 minutes is adequate when measuring pulmonary artery pressures after turning, *Am J Crit Care* 2(6):474-477, 1993.

Shoemaker W: Monitoring and management of acute circulatory problems: the expanded role of the physiologically oriented critical care nurse, *Am J Crit Care* 1(1):38-53, 1992.

Snider BS: Use of muscle relaxants in the ICU: nursing implications, *Crit Care Nurse* 13(6):55-60, 1993.

Stotts NA: Impaired wound healing. In Carrieri VK et al, editors: *Pathophysiologic phenomena in nursing,* ed 2, Philadelphia, 1993, Saunders.

Stotts NA: Managing wound care. In Swearingen PL, editor: *Manual of medical-surgical nursing care,* ed 3, St Louis, 1994, Mosby.

Stillwell S: *Mosby's critical care nursing reference,* St Louis, 1992, Mosby.

Talbot JM: Guidelines for the scientific review of enteral food products for special medical purposes, *J Parenter Enter Nutr* 15(3):99S-174S, 1991.

Teasdale G, Jennett B: Assessment of coma and impaired consciousness: a practical scale, *Lancet* 2:81, July 6, 1974.

Tess M: Acute confusional states in critically ill patients: a review, *J Neurosci Nurs* 23(6):398-402, 1991.

Tittle M, McMillan S: Pain and pain-related side effects in an ICU and on a surgical unit: nurses' management, *Am J Crit Care Nurs* 3(1):25-30, 1994.

Vender J: Sedation, analgesia, and neuromuscular blockade in critical care: an overview, *New Horizons* 2(1):2-7, 1994.

Webber KS: Providing nutritional support. In Horne MM, Swearingen PL, editors: *Pocket guide to fluid, electrolyte, and acid-base balance,* ed 2, St Louis, 1993, Mosby.

Webber KS: Providing nutritional support. In Swearingen PL, editor: *Manual of medical-surgical nursing care,* ed 3, St Louis, 1994, Mosby.

Wenger N, Hellerstein HK: *Rehabilitation of the cardiac patient,* ed 3, New York, 1992, Wiley & Sons.

Winslow EH: Cardiovascular consequences of bed rest, *Heart Lung* 14(3):236-246, 1985.

Young L, Koda-Kimble M, editors: *Applied therapeutics: the clinical use of drugs,* ed 5, Vancouver, Wash, 1992, Applied Therapeutics.

2 MULTISYSTEM TRAUMA

Major trauma

PATHOPHYSIOLOGY

Each year in the United States injuries result in over 150,000 deaths due to intentional or unintentional causes. Injuries are the leading cause of death in the United States for all persons < age 44 and result in more lost years of potential life than any other cause. Aggressive public education and other prevention measures are necessary to reduce the staggering burden posed by trauma: lost lives, lifetime disability, enormous health care costs, and lost wages. Rapid transport to a trauma center and immediate resuscitation must occur within 1 h of the initial injury to maximize the chance of survival and limit the disabling consequences of major trauma.

Mechanisms of injury: Certain injuries can be predicted based on a knowledge of the object producing the injury (e.g., motor vehicle, handgun); type of energy released (e.g., kinetic, thermal, chemical); force of energy (e.g., velocity of vehicle or missile); and use of protective devices (e.g., seatbelts, air bags, helmets).

Types of injury: *Blunt injuries* occur without interruption of skin integrity. The degree of injury is related to the transfer of energy causing tissue deformation and the responsiveness of the anatomic structure involved. For example, hollow organs (e.g., stomach, bladder), which tend to be compressible when force is applied, are less likely to rupture than solid organs (e.g., liver, spleen), which are less compressible. Common causes of blunt injury are vehicular collisions and falls.

Penetrating injuries are produced from the motion of foreign objects that penetrate tissue, causing direct damage. Indirect damage may occur because of tissue deformation associated with energy transference from the penetrating object into the surrounding tissues. As a missile penetrates tissue, the surrounding tissue is briefly displaced, creating a temporary cavity. This process is called cavitation and is responsible for the massive tissue damage caused by high-velocity missiles. Usually injury inflicted by stab wounds follows a more predictable pattern and involves less tissue destruction than does injury from gunshot wounds.

Oxygen delivery and consumption: Massive fluid shifts related to tissue damage and blood loss create a severe fluid volume deficit. Profound hypovolemic shock ensues unless replacement of estimated blood and fluid loss is initiated rapidly and maintained until the bleeding is controlled. An oxygen debt is created by a profound imbalance between oxygen supply and demand that develops as a consequence of the hypovolemia and inadequate cellular tissue perfusion.

After initial restoration of circulating fluid volume, the body develops a hyperdynamic circulatory state, which is associated with improved survival and fewer complications. The hyperdynamic circulatory state compensates for the oxygen debt incurred during the initial traumatic injury. This phase generally peaks at 48-72 h and diminishes within 7-10 days. An inability to achieve and maintain a hyperdynamic state as measured by a higher than normal cardiac index (CI), oxygen delivery (Do_2), and oxygen consumption (Vo_2) is associated with higher mortality and shock-related organ failure (Bishop, 1993).

Neuroendocrine stress response: To sustain functioning, the brain, blood, and bone marrow require glucose as an energy source. Immediately after major trauma, the central nervous system (CNS) triggers a series of reactions that promote compensation. Catecholamines such as epinephrine and norepinephrine are released. These hormones mobilize glycogen stores, increase available glucose, suppress pancreatic insulin secretion, and enhance peripheral use of glucose, resulting in a net increase in blood glucose. Glycogen stores are rapidly depleted (in <24 h), and energy is then generated from the breakdown of fat and protein. Breakdown of muscle tissue and viscera creates a negative nitrogen balance. Occasionally, subclinical adrenal insufficiency becomes clinically apparent following severe injury; exogenous steroids are administered if standard resuscitative measures fail to correct shock.

The centrally mediated release of antidiuretic hormone (ADH) promotes water absorption in the distal tubules, which increases intravascular volume and diminishes urinary output. The renin-angiotensin complex is stimulated, and aldosterone is released. The aldosterone promotes sodium and water reabsorption and contributes to intravascular volume.

Systemic inflammatory response syndrome: In patients who sustain major trauma, the inflammatory response is triggered by direct trauma as well as by the presence of foreign bodies such as road dirt, missiles, and catheters. In addition, an increase in circulating levels of catecholamines triggers the release and production of white blood cells. When widespread inflammation is present, the term systemic inflammatory response syndrome (SIRS) is used. Although the hemodynamic response and clinical findings associated with SIRS are similar to those with sepsis, the term sepsis should be used only when an infection is documented.

Multiple organ dysfunction syndrome: The overwhelming inflammation associated with SIRS ultimately can lead to multiple organ dysfunction syndrome (MODS). MODS is a major cause of late mortality in polytrauma patients and accounts for up to 10% of all trauma deaths. Sepsis or direct organ injury, if present, adds to the likelihood of MODS. In addition, inadequate initial resuscitation or inability to achieve and maintain a compensatory hyperdynamic state contributes to the development of organ failure in trauma patients. The presence of endotoxin, tumor necrosis factor, interleukin-1, and other mediators of sepsis is associated with hypotension, acidosis, circulatory collapse, and resulting MODS. New therapies are directed against these mediators. Major organs affected by MODS include the lungs, kidneys, liver, and the CNS.

Coagulopathy: Massive blood transfusion is associated with abnormal hemostasis due to fluid resuscitation with stored blood, which is deficient in some coagulation factors and platelets. Replacement of clotting components with fresh-frozen plasma and platelet transfusions, as appropriate, helps prevent transfusion-related coagulopathies. Disseminated intravascular coagulopathy (DIC) is a severe acquired bleeding disorder that may be triggered by massive trauma and SIRS. Factors contributing to the development of DIC in the polytrauma patient include impaired tissue perfusion, capillary stasis, hypotension, hypoxemia, and acidemia. The presence of DIC in patients with major trauma is a grave complication because of the surgical nature of most major injuries.

Hypothermia: Multiple factors increase the likelihood of hypothermia in major trauma. Exposed body surface area or viscera may occur at the scene of injury or during the initial resuscitation. Cold blood and room-temperature resuscitation fluids lower the core body temperature. Prolonged exposure to cool temperatures in resuscitation or operative areas is an additional factor. When present, central thermoregulatory failure due to CNS injury, intoxication, or hypoperfusion contributes to hypothermia. Mild hypothermia may help preserve the function and viability of major organs, particularly when tissue perfusion is diminished due to injury, shock, or surgical clamping of arteries. However, severe hypothermia creates significant physiologic alterations, including CNS depression, dysrhythmias, acidosis, and electrolyte imbalances.

Psychologic response: Victims of major trauma sustain life-threatening injuries. The patient often is aware of the situation and fears death. Even after the physical condition stabilizes, the patient may have a prolonged or severe reaction triggered by the trauma.

ASSESSMENT

Preservation of the patient's survival and optimization of the chance for life without disability depend on fast and accurate determination of the extent of all major injuries. It is essential to perform a complete and rapid assessment with the patient's clothing removed.

HISTORY AND RISK FACTORS

Mechanism of injury: A knowledge of the events leading to the injury can predict certain patterns of injury. For example, an unrestrained driver in an automobile collision typically sustains injuries to the cranium, face, cervical vertebrae, torso, and lower extremities. High-velocity gunshot wounds typically result in large, ragged exit wounds with massive internal injury along the missile path due to cavitation.

Intoxicants: Acute alcohol intoxication is a common finding with blunt and penetrating trauma. Other intoxicants may be involved as well. The presence of intoxicants produces neurologic and pupillary changes that may be incorrectly attributed to CNS injury. In addition, acute alcohol or drug intoxication causes cardiovascular, hematologic, and ventilatory changes that compound injury-related alterations. Finally, intoxicants dull the pain response and may obscure important signs that are useful for accurate diagnosis of intraabdominal and other injuries.

Preexisting medical conditions: Chronic health conditions such as hypertension, diabetes, COPD, cerebrovascular disorders, renal failure, and immune disorders produce physiologic alterations that increase the susceptibility for injury and impair physiologic responses to injury. Use of prescribed and illicit drugs should be determined. For example, beta-blocking medications inhibit sympathetic stimulation and limit the patient's ability to compensate for hypovolemia by increasing the HR. Individuals with insulin-dependent diabetes may require additional insulin to respond to transient hyperglycemia. Chronic opiate use increases tolerance to opiates, and greater than usual amounts may be necessary for analgesia. An accurate history is necessary in order to plan interventions that prevent acute withdrawal from opiates, alcohol, or other substances.

Last meal: Information regarding time, quantity, and type of food or beverage ingested is necessary for planning care to prevent vomiting and reduce the risk of aspiration.

Tetanus immunization: Tetanus immunization history is important to determine the need for tetanus vaccine or immunoglobin (Table 2-1).

INITIAL SUBJECTIVE PRESENTATION Mild tenderness to severe pain may be present, with the pain either localized to the site of injury or diffuse. Pain may be referred, particularly if abdominal structures are involved. Dyspnea, SOB, agitation, restlessness, and anxiety are associated with impaired tissue perfusion and oxygenation. Nausea and vomiting may occur, and the conscious patient who has sustained blood loss often complains of thirst, an early sign of hemorrhagic shock. Slurred speech and poor coordination are present with intoxication.

INITIAL OBJECTIVE PRESENTATION Varies according to site of injury, blood loss, and involved structures. For posterior examination, ensure that spinal alignment is maintained while turning patient. General findings are listed below.

Inspection: Abrasions and ecchymoses suggest mechanism of injury and involvement of underlying structures. Ecchymoses may take hours to days to develop, depending on rate of blood loss. Absence of external evidence of injury does not exclude the possibility of serious in-

TABLE 2-1 Tetanus prophylaxis in routine wound management—United States, 1985

History of adsorbed tetanus toxoid (doses)	Clean, minor wounds		All other wounds*	
	Td†	TIG	Td†	TIG
Unknown or <3	Yes	No	Yes	Yes
≥3‡	No§	No	No‖	No

Modified from Centers for Disease Control: *MMWR* 34(27):422, 1985.

Td, Tetanus and diphtheria (toxoid); *TIG,* tetanus immunoglobulin.

*Such as, but not limited to, wounds resulting from missiles, crushing, burns, and frostbite.

†For children <7 yr: DPT (DT, if pertussis vaccine is contraindicated) is preferred to tetanus toxoid alone. For persons ≥7 yr, Td is preferred to tetanus toxoid alone.

‡If only three doses of *fluid* toxoid have been received, a fourth dose of toxoid, preferably an adsorbed toxoid, should be given.

§Yes, if >10 yr since last dose.

‖Yes, if >5 yr since last dose. (More frequent boosters are not needed and can accentuate side effects.)

ternal injury. Protrusion of bone fragments and viscera may be present. Entrance and exit wounds (if present) should be determined with penetrating injuries. Protruding instruments should not be removed because additional harm and renewed bleeding may occur.

Auscultation: Diminished or absent breath sounds, distant heart sounds, diminished or absent bowel sounds.

Palpation: Weak and irregular pulse, cool and clammy skin, subcutaneous emphysema over area of injury, swelling and point tenderness over injured area.

Percussion: Dullness over blood-filled areas or internal hematomas.

MODS: Findings vary according to specific organs involved. Initially fever, flushing, tachypnea, warm skin, bounding pulses, S_4 gallop, and diuresis may be found and are consistent with a hypermetabolic state. Later findings are consistent with impaired tissue perfusion. CNS findings include lethargy, confusion, hyporeflexia, and coma. Pulmonary manifestations include tachypnea, hypoxemia, and diminished breath sounds. Cardiovascular findings include diminished peripheral pulses, pallor, and cool, moist skin. Gastrointestinal and genitourinary systems may demonstrate diminished or absent bowel sounds and diminished urinary output. Jaundice may be present. Hematologic alterations result in excessive bleeding from venipunctures, superficial injuries, abnormal bruising, and possible hematomas.

VITAL SIGNS AND HEMODYNAMICS

Initial: Widely variable, according to catecholamine response, volume status, and drugs administered. Increased RR and compensatory tachycardia are typical. The absence of tachypnea suggests CNS injury or severe intoxication. Patients taking beta-blocking medications may not experience tachycardia, and HR may remain within normal limits despite serious blood loss. BP may be normal, slightly elevated, or diminished, depending on blood loss. In young adults, compensatory responses maintain a normal BP until major blood loss occurs. If left untreated, hypotension with MAP <70 mm Hg occurs, sometimes very rapidly, depending on volume of blood lost. Diminished CVP, PAP, and CO/CI reflect hypovolemia and should be corrected immediately. SVR is elevated due to hypovolemia and catecholamine release.

Hyperdynamic phase: After fluid volume resuscitation, a hyperdynamic circulatory state compensates for the oxygen debt incurred during the initial traumatic injury. Increases in CO/CI are present. Do_2 is greatly increased because of hypermetabolism and other factors such as pain, agitation, infection, and tachycardia. Vo_2 may be double the normal of 250-300 ml/min. Svo_2 usually is >80%. SVR is <900 dynes/sec/cm^{-5} during this phase. If hyperdynamic metabolic needs are not supported by oxygen administration, aggressive fluid resuscitation, and other measures as necessary, MODS may ensue.

MODS: Failure of compensatory mechanisms results in decreasing CO/CI and increasing PAWP as heart failure ensues. Svo_2 may be low (<60%), reflecting abnormally high oxygen extraction, or somewhat higher (60%-80%), reflecting precapillary shunting. An Svo_2 value of <50% is considered critical and requires immediate intervention. SVR is often >1,200 dynes/sec/cm^{-5}. The patient may require pressor support to maintain MAP >70 mm Hg.

DIAGNOSTIC TESTS

CBC: Serial determination of Hct/Hgb reflects the amount of blood lost. If drawn immediately after the injury, Hct/Hgb levels may be normal, but serial levels will reveal dramatic decreases during resuscitation and as extravascular fluid mobilizes during the recovery phase. Leukocytosis is expected with a moderate to high total WBC count. Later, an increase in WBCs or a shift to the left reflects the anticipated inflammatory response and may signal infection.

Blood chemistries: Glucose is elevated initially due to catecholamine release and insulin resistance. Ionized calcium levels decline due to metabolic alterations associated with impaired tissue perfusion and binding with citrate from stored blood. Baseline levels of electrolytes, enzymes, and other chemistries are drawn for later comparison and to guide therapy.

MODS: Venous lactate levels may be elevated if tissue perfusion is inadequate and anaerobic metabolism is present. If precapillary shunting is present or cardiac output is diminished, arterial lactate levels may be normal; however, venous samples will reflect the acidosis by elevation >5-15 mg/dl, the normal level.

ABG analysis: May show pH <7.35 and HCO_3^- <22 mEq/L due to metabolic acidosis, which is present if inadequate tissue oxygen delivery leads to anaerobic metabolism and excess lactate production. Decreased Pao_2 is present if ventilation is compromised by pulmonary injury or altered LOC.

Oximetry: Continuous pulse oximetry is used to assess oxygen saturation. Oxygen therapy should be titrated to maintain Spo_2 of ≥92%-94%, according to individual injuries and preexisting medical conditions.

Type and cross-match: To determine presence of antigens so that recipient and donor blood are compatible. If blood loss is very rapid, requiring immediate transfusion, O-negative (without major antigens) blood or type-specific blood is used until a full cross-match can be performed.

Blood alcohol, toxicology screen: To check for the presence of alcohol or other intoxicant, if suspected. Positive results are used to guide therapy and prevent acute withdrawal symptoms.

Urinalysis: To check for the presence of blood or bacteria due to upper or lower urinary tract injury.

X-rays: Performed to check for the presence of fractures, abnormal air or fluids, and foreign objects and to determine location of large organs. With polytrauma patients, cervical spine, chest, abdomen, pelvic, and extremity x-rays usually are necessary.

CT scan: To detect presence of soft tissue injury, hematomas, and subtle fractures.

Caution: Because of the risk of rapid deterioration, the patient should be accompanied by an experienced nurse during the time it takes to perform the scan. Appropriate monitoring and resuscitation equipment must be readily available.

COLLABORATIVE MANAGEMENT

Airway management: A patent airway must be secured, by intubation or cricothyroidotomy, if necessary. If cervical spine injury is suspected, the cervical spine is stabilized during the procedure by maintaining constant in-line positioning with gentle traction. Nasal intubation is preferred to the oral route because there is less manipulation of the cervical spine. However, the success of a particular method depends on the individual patient and the experience of the clinician. Cricothyroidotomy is indicated when other means of intubation are not possible or are contraindicated.

Oxygen: All trauma patients require supplemental oxygen due to the initial blood loss and reduced oxygen carrying capacity of the blood and because of greatly increased tissue demand for oxygen during the hypermetabolic phase. High-flow oxygen by mask is indicated initially. Subsequent oxygen therapy should be titrated according to ABG values and continuous pulse oximetry. Mechanical ventilation is often required because of direct injury or ventilatory impairment associated with MODS.

Fluid management: Underresuscitation of trauma patients during the initial 48-72 h may lead to shock, MODS, and death. Two or more large-bore ($\geq$16 gauge) short catheters must be placed to maximize rapid delivery of fluids and blood. Use of IV tubing with an exceptionally large internal diameter (trauma tubing), absence of stopcocks, use of external pressure, and dilution of packed RBCs to decrease viscosity are techniques used to promote rapid fluid volume therapy. When rapid infusion of large amounts of fluid is required, all fluid should be warmed to body temperature to prevent hypothermia. Crystalloids can be stored in a blanket warmer. Rapid warmer/infusor devices are available for administration of blood products. A combination of crystalloids, colloids, and blood products is necessary for most major trauma patients. As soon as available, fluid requirements should be estimated according to hemodynamic parameters derived from PA measurements. A hyperdynamic state is supported during the initial 72 h and until stable. Fluid requirements for patients with significant craniocerebral trauma are very precise (see p. 131).

Crystalloids: Balanced salt solutions such as 0.9% NaCl (normal saline) or lactated Ringer's (LR) are commonly used. These solutions are inexpensive and convenient to store, but intravascular retention is poor. Sustained use of normal saline can lead to hyperchloremic metabolic acidosis; therefore LR is generally preferred except when administered simultaneously through the same IV line as blood products. Normal saline is used with blood products, instead, because the ionized calcium in LR can interact with the citrate anticoagulant in banked blood and cause clot formation.

Colloids: These do not readily cross capillary walls and therefore do not pass between the tissue compartments as easily as crystalloids. The osmotic force generated by the large molecular weight (colloid) substances results in increased plasma osmotic pressure and promotes intravascular fluid retention. Albumin, dextran, and hetastarch are colloid substances in current use. Colloids are generally used as a supplement to crystalloid therapy.

Packed red blood cells (PRBCs):   Some degree of blood loss is associated with most injuries, and massive transfusion is sometimes necessary. Massive transfusion is defined as replacement of one half of the patient's blood volume at one time or complete replacement of the patient's blood volume over 24 h. If blood loss is very rapid during the initial resuscitation, immediate transfusion with O-negative (without major antigens) blood may be required. When bleeding continues, type-specific blood is used until a full cross-match can be performed. The patient must be properly and permanently identified with trauma alias or name, if known, to prevent transfusion errors. Complications of massive transfusion are numerous. Hypocalcemia caused by calcium binding with citrate in stored PRBCs results in depressed myocardial contractility, particularly in hypothermic patients or in those with impaired liver function. One ampule of 10% calcium chloride should be administered after every 4 U of PRBCs. Abnormal hemostasis may occur, since stored PRBCs are deficient in some coagulation factors and platelets. Replacement of clotting components with fresh-frozen plasma and platelet transfusions, as appropriate, will help prevent transfusion-related coagulopathies.

Autotransfusion: Shed blood is filtered and reinfused into the patient. Shed blood is captured from chest tube drainage or the operative field and reinfused immediately. Various techniques are used to capture and reinfuse the blood. Advantages of autotransfusion include reduced risk of disease transmission, absence of incompatibility problems, and ready availability of blood. Disadvantages include risk of blood contamination and presence of naturally occurring factors that promote anticoagulation.

Pneumatic antishock garment (PASG, military antishock trousers [MAST]):   Traditionally used to stabilize patients with hypovolemic shock. The inflatable trousers and optional inflatable abdominal compartment increase external pressure, resulting in an increase in MAP and splinting of fractures. Their use is controversial because an increase in BP, which formerly was believed to be caused by an auto-transfusion effect, is now deemed to be caused by an increase in SVR. Pulmonary compromise and increased intracranial pressure (IICP) may result from use of PASGs, particularly when the abdominal compartment is inflated. Uncontrolled thoracic bleeding is a clear contraindication. Other reported contraindications include severe head injury and possible diaphragmatic rupture. Once in place, the garment should be deflated slowly and systematically, with frequent assessments of VS and concurrent fluid resuscitation.

Gastric intubation: Permits gastric decompression, aids in removal of gastric contents, and is necessary to prevent vomiting and possible aspiration.

Urinary drainage: An indwelling catheter is inserted to obtain a specimen for urinalysis and to monitor hourly urine output. See "Renal and Lower Urinary Tract Trauma," p. 161, for precautions.

Pharmacotherapy

Antibiotics: Broad-spectrum antibiotics are used initially to prevent infections. More specific antimicrobial agents are used when results from culture and sensitivity tests are available.

Opiate analgesia: Because opiates alter the sensorium, making evaluation of the patient's condition difficult, they are seldom used in the early stages of injury. Short-acting sedatives such as midazolam (Versed) may be used during procedures. Opiates are used after the patient has had a full surgical evaluation and during the immediate postoperative period. The IV route is preferred because of its reliable effects and ease of control. Opiate tolerance is increased in chronic users, and larger than usual amounts of analgesics may be required. Use of mixed agonist/antagonists (e.g., butorphanol [Stadol], nalbuphine [Nubain], pentazocine [Talwin]) may trigger acute withdrawal in chronic opiate users. Such agents should be avoided in these individuals.

Tetanus prophylaxis: Tetanus immunoglobin and tetanus toxoid are considered on the basis of CDC recommendations (see Table 2-1).

Nutrition therapy: Complex nutritional needs must be met because of the hypermetabolic state associated with major trauma. Parenteral nutrition usually is necessary because of one or more of the following factors: postoperative status, ileus, and injury to the GI tract. When present, infection and sepsis contribute to the negative nitrogen state and increased metabolic needs. Prompt initiation of nutrition therapy is essential for rapid healing and prevention of complications. For more information, see "Nutritional Support," p. 1.

Surgery: Need for surgery depends on the type and extent of injuries. The surgical team is coordinated by the trauma surgeon. When several specialty surgeons are required because of injuries to various systems, the order of surgeries is coordinated carefully to preserve life and limit the potential for disability. Areas of rapid blood loss are addressed first.

NURSING DIAGNOSES AND INTERVENTIONS

Fluid volume deficit related to active loss secondary to physical injury

Desired outcomes: Within 12 h of this diagnosis, patient becomes normovolemic as evidenced by MAP ≥70 mm Hg, HR 60-100 bpm, normal sinus rhythm on ECG, CVP 2-6 mm Hg, PAWP 6-12 mm Hg, CI ≥2.5 L/min/m², SVR 900-1,200 dynes/sec/cm⁻⁵, urinary output ≥0.5 ml/kg/h, warm extremities, brisk capillary refill (<2 sec), and distal pulses >2+ on a 0-4+ scale.

- Monitor BP q15min, or more frequently in the presence of obvious bleeding or unstable VS. Be alert to changes in the MAP of >10 mm Hg. Even a small but sudden decrease in BP signals the need to consult the physician, especially with the trauma patient in whom the extent of injury is unknown.
- Monitor HR, ECG, and cardiovascular status q15min until volume is restored and VS are stable. Check ECG to note HR elevations and myocardial ischemic changes (i.e., ventricular dysrhythmias and ST-segment changes), which can occur because of dilutional anemia in susceptible individuals.
- In the patient with evidence of volume depletion or active blood loss, administer pressurized fluids rapidly through several large-caliber (≥16 gauge) catheters. Use short, large-bore IV tubing (trauma tubing) to maximize flow rate. Avoid use of stopcocks, because they slow the infusion rate. Fluids should be warmed to prevent hypothermia.

Caution: Evaluate patency of IV catheters continuously during rapid-volume resuscitation.

- Measure PA pressures q1-2h or more frequently if there is ongoing blood loss. Measure CO/CI and calculate SVR and PVR q4-8h, or more often in unstable patients. Be alert to low or decreasing CVP and PAWP. An elevated HR, along with decreased PAWP, decreased CO/CI, and increased SVR suggests inadequate fluid resuscitation. During the hyperdynamic phase, calculate Do_2 and $\dot{V}o_2$ and support higher than normal values by oxygen and fluid administration, conservation of energy, and other measures according to individual patient. Anticipate higher than normal CO/CI and lower than normal SVR. Mild to moderate pulmonary hypertension may occur in patients with thoracic injury, smoke inhalation, or adult respiratory distress syndrome (ARDS). Patients at high risk for developing ARDS include those with direct injury to the chest, sepsis, or massive blood transfusion.
- Measure urinary output q1-2h. Be alert to output <0.5 ml/kg/h for 2 consecutive hours. Low urine output usually reflects inadequate intravascular volume in the patient with abdominal trauma.
- Monitor for physical indicators of hypovolemia, including cool extremities, capillary refill >2 sec, and absent or decreased amplitude of distal pulses.
- Estimate ongoing blood loss. Measure all bloody drainage from tubes or catheters, noting drainage color (e.g., coffee-ground, burgundy, bright red [Table 2-13]). Note the frequency of dressing changes due to saturation with blood to estimate amount of blood loss *via* wound site.
- Administer oxygen to maximize tissue delivery of oxygen. Use continuous pulse oximetry to assess for adequate oxygenation. Evaluate ABG results as available.

Pain related to physical injury secondary to external trauma or surgery

Desired outcomes: Within 2 h of this diagnosis, patient's subjective evaluation of discomfort improves, as documented by a pain scale. Nonverbal indicators of discomfort, such as grimacing, are absent.

- Evaluate patient for presence of preoperative and postoperative pain. Preoperative pain is anticipated and is a vital diagnostic aid. Use a pain scale with the patient to rate discomfort and effectiveness of strategies to relieve pain. Devise alternative methods to communicate with patients with endotracheal tubes or other barriers to communication.
- Administer narcotics and other analgesics as prescribed. Avoid preoperative administration of opiate analgesics until the patient has been evaluated thoroughly by a trauma surgeon. Once prescribed, inform patient of the availability of analgesics. Postoperatively, administer prescribed analgesics promptly before the pain becomes severe. Analgesics are helpful in relieving pain, as well as in aiding in the recovery process by promoting greater ventilatory excursion. Be aware that substance abuse often is involved in traumatic events; victims therefore may be drug or alcohol users, with a higher than average tolerance to narcotics. These same persons may suffer symptoms of alcohol or narcotics withdrawal that need recognition and treatment. In addition, recognize that narcotic analgesics can decrease GI motility and may delay return to normal bowel functioning. Document the degree of pain relief obtained, using the pain scale.
- Supplement analgesics with nonpharmacologic maneuvers (e.g., positioning, back rubs, distraction) to aid in pain reduction.
- See Chapter 1, p. 74, for additional pain intervention.

Altered protection related to clotting factor alterations or decreased hemoglobin level

Desired outcomes: Patient is free of symptoms of bleeding as evidenced by absence of bleeding at venipuncture sites, mucous membranes, catheter insertion sites, incisions, and GI tract. Coagulation profiles return to normal by the time of transfer from ICU.

- Obtain blood for coagulation and related studies: PT, PTT, Hct, Hgb, fibrinogen levels, and FDPs.
- Observe for bleeding at venipuncture sites, mucous membranes, catheter insertion sites, incisions, and GI tract. Test gastric drainage, emesis, and stool for the presence of occult blood.
- Administer H_2-receptor antagonists and/or sucralfate (Carafate) as prescribed to reduce gastric acid and prevent erosion of gastric mucosa.
- Avoid IM injections and multiple venipunctures. Use IV route for medication administration.
- If DIC is present, see "Disseminated Intravascular Coagulation," p. 608, for treatment.

Risk for infection related to inadequate primary defenses secondary to physical trauma or surgery; related to inadequate secondary defenses due to decreased hemoglobin or inadequate immune response; related to tissue destruction and environmental exposure; and related to multiple invasive procedures

Desired outcome: Patient is free of infection as evidenced by core or rectal temperature $<37.8°$ C ($100°$ F); HR #100 bpm; orientation to time, place, and person; and absence of unusual redness, warmth, or drainage at surgical incisions and drain sites.

- Monitor VS for evidence of infection, noting temperature increases and associated increases in heart and respiratory rates. An elevated CO and a decreased SVR suggest sepsis. Consult surgeon if these are new findings. See Tables 10-1 and 10-2, pp. 625 and 626, for hemodynamic profiles of early and late septic shock. Also refer to "Shock," p. 623.
- Evaluate orientation and LOC q2-4h.
- Ensure patency of all surgically placed tubes or drains. Irrigate or attach to low-pressure suction as prescribed. Promptly report unrelieved loss of tube patency.
- Evaluate incisions and wound sites for evidence of infection: unusual redness, warmth, delayed healing, and purulent or unusual drainage.
- Note color, character, and odor of all drainage. Consult physician and culture drainage if it is foul smelling or abnormal.
- Administer parenteral antibiotics in a timely fashion. Reschedule antibiotics if a dosage is delayed for more than 1 h. Recognize that failure to administer antibiotics on schedule may result in inadequate blood levels and treatment failure.
- Administer tetanus immunoglobulin and tetanus toxoid as prescribed (see Table 2-1). Ensure that patient receives a wallet card to document tetanus immunization, if given.
- Change dressings as prescribed, using aseptic technique. Prevent cross-contamination from various wounds by changing one dressing at a time.

Impaired tissue integrity related to mechanical factors (including physical injury); altered circulation secondary to hemorrhage or direct vascular injury; nutritional deficit secondary to hypermetabolic state; and impaired physical mobility

Desired outcome: Patient has adequate tissue integrity as evidenced by wound healing within an acceptable time frame according to extent of injury.

- On admission, clean and irrigate all cutaneous injuries with 0.9% NaCl, or use some other procedure according to individual prescription or hospital protocol.
- Assess all wounds, fistulas, and drain sites q4-8h for signs of irritation, infection, and ischemia. Inspect for healing and presence of granulation tissue q8h.
- Identify infected and devitalized tissue. Aid in the removal of eschar by irrigation or wound packing, or prepare patient for surgical débridement.
- Turn patient q1-2h. Identify need for specialty bed in patients with multiple risk factors for impaired tissue integrity.
- Promptly change all dressings that become soiled with drainage or blood.
- Protect the skin surrounding tubes, drains, or fistulas, keeping the areas clean and free from drainage. If necessary, apply ointments, skin barriers, or drainage pouches to protect the surrounding skin. Consult wound specialist as necessary.

- Ensure adequate protein and calorie intake for tissue healing (see **Altered nutrition,** below).
- See "Wound and Skin Care," p. 57, for more information.

Hypothermia related to exposure at the scene of injury, temporary loss of temperature regulatory mechanisms due to shock or CNS ischemia, surgical exposure of abdominal viscera, and administration of large volumes of unwarmed fluid or blood

Desired outcomes: Patient's temperature remains or returns to normal within 24 h of this diagnosis. Complications of hypothermia are avoided as evidenced by normal sinus rhythm on ECG; patient oriented to time, place, and person; Pao_2 $\geq$80 mm Hg; and absence of prolonged bleeding from wounds, incisions, and venipuncture sites.

- Warm all fluids administered during the initial resuscitation phase and until the patient postoperatively approaches normothermia. Prewarm crystalloids so that they are ready for immediate use. Because standard blood warmers are ineffective in rapid warming of large volumes of blood, avoid their use if blood loss is massive, inasmuch as serious hypotension may occur due to the delay caused by the slow passage of blood through the warmer. Rapid-volume infusers are invaluable for immediate warming of large volumes (i.e., 800-1,200 ml/min) of blood and fluids as they are infused.
- Keep ambient room temperature in trauma receiving, surgical, and critical care areas as warm as possible. Keep patient dry and cover head to reduce heat loss.
- Avoid unnecessary exposure of the patient. Keep patient covered with warmed blankets whenever possible.
- Monitor core temperature *via* rectal or esophageal probe, urinary catheter attachment, or PA catheter until normothermia is attained.
- Be aware that vasodilatation during rewarming can result in an intravascular fluid volume deficit (see **Fluid volume deficit,** p. 117).
- Be aware that vasodilatation during rewarming necessitates evaluation and frequent titration of vasoactive infusions.
- Monitor for and promptly report serious dysrhythmias (i.e., atrial fibrillation with rapid ventricular response, ventricular dysrhythmias, and AV conduction block), which are associated with severe or prolonged hypothermia.
- Be aware that hypothermia compromises cortical functioning, and the patient may be confused, disoriented, or somnolent, or may have other neurologic derangements. These symptoms may make it difficult to evaluate concurrent head injury.
- Monitor ABG values at frequent intervals for evidence of hypoxemia. Hypothermia causes a shift to the left in the oxyhemoglobin dissociation curve and may impair oxygen unloading to peripheral tissue.
- Because DIC may develop several days after a hypothermic episode, monitor for excessive bleeding from wounds, surgical incisions, and venipuncture sites and promptly report the presence of serious or progressive thrombocytopenia. (See "Disseminated Intravascular Coagulation," p. 608).

Altered nutrition: Less than body requirements related to increased need secondary to hypermetabolic posttrauma state and possible decreased intake secondary to direct injury or surgical disruption of GI tract or ileus

Desired outcome: Within 5 days of this diagnosis, patient has adequate nutrition as evidenced by maintenance of baseline body weight and state of nitrogen balance on nitrogen studies.

- Collaborate with physician, dietitian, and pharmacist to estimate patient's metabolic needs on the basis of type of injury, activity level, and nutritional status before injury.
- Consider patient's specific injuries and preexisting medical condition when planning nutrition.
- Monitor serum markers of nutritional status: prealbumin, transferrin, albumin.
- Do not start enteral feeding until bowel function returns (i.e., bowel sounds are present, and patient experiences hunger).
- Recognize that opiates decrease GI motility and may cause nausea and vomiting.
- Weigh patient daily to evaluate trend. Be alert to steady decreases in weight, and evaluate loss by assessing and comparing with volume status and fluid shifts.
- Collect 24 h urine for urea nitrogen value, as prescribed, to evaluate nitrogen balance.
- For additional information, see "Nutritional Support," p. 1.

Fear related to potentially threatening situation (serious injuries, hospitalization) and supported by presence of pain, unfamiliarity, and noxious environmental stimuli present in critical care area; communication barrier (e.g., intubation); and sensory impairment from direct injuries

Desired outcome: Within 24 h of this diagnosis, patient exhibits decreased symptoms of fear: apprehension, tension, nervousness, tachycardia, superficial vasoconstriction, aggressiveness, and withdrawal.

- Assess level of fear and understanding of present condition.
- Plan care to provide as restful an environment as possible.
- Provide information regarding nursing care, treatment plan, and progress. It is often necessary to repeat information because injury, stress, and fear can interfere with comprehension.
- Promote visits by family members and significant others.
- Offer to consult hospital chaplain or patient's clergy member as desired by patient.
- Assess and promote patient's usual coping strategies. It may be helpful to interview family members.
- Provide referral to support groups for trauma patients and family members.
- See this diagnosis in "Psychosocial Support," p. 92, for more information.

Risk for injury related to potential for use of alcohol or illicit drugs; or related to propensity for thrill-seeking behaviors

Desired outcomes: The potential for postdischarge use of alcohol or illicit drugs is identified by the time of hospital discharge. The potential for thrill-seeking behaviors is evaluated by the time of hospital discharge.

- Evaluate preinjury status regarding use of intoxicants.
- Assess for preinjury patterns of thrill-seeking behaviors.

- Initiate early referral to social services or discharge planner if need of rehabilitation is anticipated.
- Refer patients and family members to appropriate rehabilitation program or counseling as indicated. Immediately following serious injury, the patient and family members are very impressionable, making this period an ideal time to begin addressing behaviors that place that patient at risk for additional injury.
- Initiate injury prevention education. Provide instructions on proper seat belt application (across the pelvic girdle rather than across soft tissue of the lower abdomen), firearm safety, injury prevention for infants and children, and other factors suitable for the persons involved.

Posttrauma response related to unanticipated serious physical injury or event resulting in physical trauma

Desired outcome: By the time of hospital discharge, patient verbalizes that the psychosocial impact of the event has decreased; cooperates with treatment plan; and does not exhibit signs of severe stress reaction, such as display of inconsistent affect, suicidal or homicidal behavior, or extreme agitation or depression.

- Evaluate mental status at systematic intervals during the acute and recovery periods. Be alert to indicators of severe stress reaction such as display of affect inconsistent with statements or behavior, suicidal or homicidal statements or actions, extreme agitation or depression, and failure to cooperate with instructions related to care.
- Anticipate some reexperience of traumatic event. Reassure patient and significant others that this is common.
- Consult with specialist such as psychologist, psychiatric nurse clinician, or pastoral counselor if patient displays signs of severe stress reaction, as described in the first intervention.
- Consider organic causes that may contribute to posttraumatic stress response (e.g., severe pain, alcohol intoxication or withdrawal, electrolyte imbalance, metabolic encephalopathy, or impaired cerebral perfusion).
- For other psychosocial interventions, see "Psychosocial Support," p. 88.

ADDITIONAL NURSING DIAGNOSES

Also see the following as appropriate: "Nutritional Support," p. 12; "Hemodynamic Monitoring," p. 37; "Sedating and Paralytic Agents," p. 46; "Alterations in Consciousness," p. 55; "Wound and Skin Care," p. 58; "Pain," p. 74; "Prolonged Immobility," p. 78; "Psychosocial Support," p. 88; "Psychosocial Support for the Patient's Family and Significant Others," p. 100; other trauma discussions in this chapter; and "Shock," p. 623.

Craniocerebral trauma

PATHOPHYSIOLOGY

Trauma to the head from blunt and penetrating forces can result in injury to the brain, support structures, blood vessels, and cranium in any combination. Blunt injuries to the brain and cranium are caused by acceleration, deceleration, and rotational forces (e.g., vehicular collisions, falls, and high-impact sports). Penetrating injuries occur from piercing forces that traverse the cranium and, ultimately, damage underlying brain tissue and support structures.

Outcome following head trauma is variable but can be predicted to some extent based on the type of lesion, severity of injury, and length of coma. However, age, preinjury medical status, mechanism of injury, intracranial pressure, and brainstem integrity are important factors influencing outcome.

Injuries are classified as primary or secondary. Primary injuries involve direct injury to the cranium or brain structures, whereas changes in brain structure as a result of the direct injury are classified as secondary.

Primary injuries

Linear skull fractures: Nondisplaced, associated with low-velocity impact.

Basilar skull fractures: Linear, involving the base of the cranium's anterior, middle, and posterior fossae.

Depressed skull fractures: Characterized by depression of the skull over the point of impact; may be comminuted (usually closed without direct brain penetration), compressed, or compound (open).

Concussion: Diffuse, axonal brain injuries classified as mild (no loss of consciousness, possible brief episodes of confusion or disorientation); moderate (brief loss of consciousness, transient focal neurologic deficits); or severe (prolonged loss of consciousness with sustained neurologic deficits lasting <24 h).

Contusion: Bruising of the brain tissue often associated with lacerations and capillary hemorrhages. Contusions can be described as *coup* if the brain injury is directly beneath the site of impact or *contrecoup* if the brain injury is opposite the site of impact.

Diffuse axonal injuries (DAI):   Diffuse areas of white matter that have been torn or sheared; usually not detected by CT scan.

Secondary injuries

Epidural hematomas: Commonly occur following a temporal linear skull fracture that lacerates the middle meningeal artery below it or from fractures of the sagittal and transverse sinuses. The hematoma develops rapidly in the space between the skull and dura.

Subdural hematomas: Bleeding from the veins between the dura and the arachnoid spaces; classified as acute, subacute, and chronic.

Subarachnoid hemorrhage: Seen over the convexities of the brain and in the basal cisterns; indicative of bleeding into the ventricular system.

Intracranial hematomas: Generally result from injury to the small arteries and veins within the subcortical white matter of the temporal and frontal lobes; usually associated with petechiae, contusions, and edema.

Herniation syndromes: Processes whereby a portion of the brain is displaced through openings within the intracranial cavity. Herniation occurs when there is a pressure difference between the supratentorial and infratentorial compartments. When herniation occurs, the vascular system is compressed, destroyed, or lacerated, resulting in ischemia, necrosis, and ultimately death. Several herniation syndromes may occur, and each has specific characteristics.

- **Cingulate herniation:** Occurs because of a unilateral hemispheric increase in ICP. It is best described as a shift to the side opposite the increased hemispheric pressure, as noted on CT scan. Cingulate herniation compresses the anterior cerebral artery and internal cerebral vein, contributing further to the development of cerebral edema, ischemia, and IICP. Associated neurologic deficits may include decreased LOC and unilateral or bilateral lower extremity weakness or paralysis.
- **Uncal herniation:** Life-threatening emergent situation that occurs when an expanding lesion of the middle or temporal fossa forces the tip (uncus) of the temporal lobe toward the midline, causing it to protrude over the edge of the tentorium cerebelli and compress the oculomotor nerve (III) and the posterior cerebral artery. During this process the uncus may be lacerated, and the midbrain is compressed and pushed against the tentorial edge. In addition to the fixed and dilated pupil on the side of herniation, there is deterioration of LOC and further elevation in ICP.
- **Transtentorial (central) herniation:** Occurs with expanding lesions of the frontal, parietal, or occipital lobes or with severe, generalized cerebral edema. Subcortical structures, including the basal ganglia and diencephalon (thalamus and hypothalamus), herniate through the tentorium cerebelli causing compression of the midbrain and posterior cerebral arteries bilaterally. Often, cingulate and uncal herniation precede this life-threatening process.

Table 2-2 describes the clinical features of uncal and central herniation syndromes. It is important to note, however, that many of these manifestations may occur too rapidly to be observed, and changes in respiratory patterns will not be seen in critically ill patients who are mechanically ventilated.

- **Transcranial (extracranial) herniation:** Occurs when intracranial contents under pressure are forced through an open wound, surgical site, or cranial vault fracture. While the resultant loss of brain volume lowers ICP and may prevent intracranial herniation, this is an ominous sign and the patient is at risk for infection, further brain injury, and death.

Changes in intracranial pressure dynamics (IPD)

IPD is based on the volume-pressure relationship within the cranium (Munro-Kellie hypothesis). Three volumes exist within the fixed, rigid cranial vault: the brain, blood, and cerebrospinal fluid (CSF). Under normal conditions these volumes exert a pressure that is <15 mm Hg. When any of these volumes increases, pressure increases and compensatory mechanisms (shunting of CSF into the intrathecal space or vasoconstriction to reduce blood volume) are activated to reduce the volume. In addition, the brain requires a constant blood supply to maintain normal function. With brain injury, the intrinsic compensatory mechanisms are damaged or overwhelmed, and functions that serve to maintain cerebral perfusion are compromised. Extrinsic measures are

T A B L E   2 - 2   Assessment of central and uncal herniations

Criteria	Diencephalic		Midbrain/upper pons	Lower pons/upper medulla
	Early	Late		
Central herniation				
Respiratory pattern	Deep sighs, yawning	Cheyne-Stokes	Hyperventilation that is sustained and regular	Shallow, rapid, irregular
Pupils: size/reaction	Small; react to bright light; small range of contraction	Small; react to bright light; small range of contraction	Midpositioned; irregularly shaped; fixed reaction to light	Midpositioned; fixed
Oculocephalic/oculovestibular responses (doll's head maneuver/ice water caloric)	Full conjugate or slightly roving eye movements; full conjugate lateral; ipsilateral response to ice water ear irrigation	Same as early; nystagmus absent	Impaired; may be dysconjugate	No response
Motor responses				
At rest	Contralateral paresis, which may worsen	Motionlessness	Abnormal extension posturing	Flaccidity
To stimulus	Bilateral Babinski's	Abnormal flexion posturing	Rigidity	Bilateral Babinski's

Uncal herniation

	Early third nerve	Late third nerve
Respiratory pattern	Normal	Hyperventilation that is regular and sustained
Pupils: size/reaction	Moderate dilatation; ipsilateral to primary lesion; sluggish constriction; brisk contralateral pupillary reaction	Widely dilated and fixed ipsilateral pupil
Oculocephalic/oculovestibular responses (doll's head maneuver/ice water caloric)	Present or dysconjugate, full conjugate, slow ipsilateral eye movement or dysconjugate due to contralateral eye not moving medially	Impaired or absent; Full lateral movement with contralateral eye; absence of medial movement with ipsilateral eye
Motor response to stimulus	Contralateral extensor plantar reflex	Ipsilateral hemiplegia; abnormal posturing; absence of all responses

Modified from Plum F, Posner J: *Diagnosis of stupor and coma*, ed 3, Philadelphia, 1980, Davis.

necessary to maintain the normal pressure-volume relationship and preserve cerebral perfusion pressure (CPP). Table 6-3, p. 449, lists indicators of IICP. Treatment of derangements in IPD is based on the relationship between ICP and CPP and is stated simply:

$$CPP = MAP - ICP$$

MAP is calculated using the following equation:

$$MAP = \frac{Systolic\ BP + 2(Diastolic\ BP)}{3}$$

The goal of treatment is to maintain CPP >60 mm Hg and reduce ICP to <15 mm Hg.

ASSESSMENT

Baseline physical examination data should include assessment of mental status, cranial nerves, motor status, sensory status, and reflexes. Thereafter, continuous neurologic assessment should be based on the clinical status of the patient. Ideally, a complete neurologic assessment should be performed. However, many components of the examination require patients to follow commands. For patients unable to follow commands, the neurologic assessment should be tailored individually to the patient's abilities and redesigned as necessary. The Glasgow Coma Scale (Appendix 3) and Cognitive Rehabilitation Goals (Rancho Los Amigos Scale, Table 1-27, p. 53) should be part of the neurologic assessment. Record specific patient responses to stimuli and the type of stimuli required to produce the response. The following are assessment findings related to specific injuries.

Epidural hematoma/linear skull fracture: Scalp lacerations, swelling, tenderness, and ecchymosis. Classic epidural signs are loss of consciousness, followed by a lucid interval and then rapid deterioration. Ipsilateral pupil dilatation and contralateral weakness, followed by brainstem compression, occur if treatment is not initiated emergently.

Basilar skull fracture: Dural tears resulting in rhinorrhea and otorrhea are common. Anterior fossa injuries are associated with periorbital ecchymosis (raccoon's eyes), epistaxis, damage to cranial nerves I and II, and meningitis. Middle and posterior fossa injuries may damage cranial nerves VII and VIII and are associated with tinnitus, hemotympanum, and destruction of the cochlear vestibular apparatus. Ecchymosis of the mastoid process (Battle's sign) is common.

Compound depressed skull fracture: Neurologic changes are based on the extent of brain injury, but changes in LOC, pupillary changes, headache, cerebral edema, and IICP often accompany these injuries. Physical and diagnostic examination findings may include CSF leaks if the dura has been torn; tympanum rupture; and bruised, lacerated, or contused brain tissue.

Concussion: Headache, dizziness, vomiting, memory loss, and decreased attention and concentration skills. Moderate and severe injuries require close observation because cerebral edema and IICP can develop.

Contusion: Loss of consciousness common. Neurologic deficits may be generalized or focal, depending on the site and severity of injury. Cerebral edema often is a secondary complication.

Diffuse axonal injury: May occur with other injuries and is characterized by an immediate loss of consciousness, prolonged coma, and almost complete lack of recovery.

Subdural hematoma: With acute subdural hematoma, neurologic deterioration is seen within 24-72 h (or earlier) and is manifested by a changing LOC, ipsilateral dilated pupil, and contralateral extremity weakness. Subacute hematoma may present within 48 h to weeks after injury and manifests initially as a headache. Characteristically there is no clinical sign of improvement. LOC begins to deteriorate, and focal neurologic deficits ensue. Neurologic signs associated with a chronic subdural hematoma may occur weeks or months after injury. The progression of elusive fluctuating deficits, such as personality changes, memory loss, headache, extremity weakness, and incontinence, may signal chronic subdural hematoma, especially in high-risk groups such as elders or chronic alcohol users.

Subarachnoid hemorrhage (SAH): Highly associated with headache, changes in LOC, and meningeal signs such as nuchal rigidity, elevated temperature, and positive Kernig's sign (loss of ability to extend leg when thigh is flexed on abdomen).

Intracranial hematoma: Neurologic deficits based on the site and severity of injury.

Other physical assessment data: Baseline cardiovascular, pulmonary, gastrointestinal, genitourinary, and integumentary data should be completed, with reassessment on an ongoing basis.

COMPLICATIONS

Cardiac dysrhythmias: Commonly seen in brain-injured patients and probably related to autonomic (sympathetic and parasympathetic) derangement or compression of midbrain and brainstem structures. ECG changes seen with elevated ICP are prominent U waves, ST-segment changes, notched T waves, and prolongation of the QT interval. Bradycardic, supraventricular tachycardic, and ventricular dysrhythmias are seen as well. Cushing's syndrome, characterized by bradycardia, elevated systolic blood pressure (SBP), and a widening pulse pressure is a late sign indicating mechanical compression or severe metabolic dysfunction of the brainstem.

Aspiration with resultant pneumonia: Prevalent complication following brain injury. Aspiration may occur at the time of injury or as an iatrogenic complication of intubation, enteral feedings, or prolonged use of artificial airways. Whatever the cause, early detection reduces associated morbidity and mortality. Early detection methods that should be incorporated into the plan of care include checking tracheobronchial secretions for glucose (a sign that tube feedings have been aspirated inasmuch as sputum is negative for glucose), initiating enteral feeding protocols, and performing swallowing assessments. See "Nutritional Support" for **Risk for aspiration,** p. 16, and Table 1-4, p. 10, which discusses complications in the tube-fed patient.

Other complications: In addition, the patient with brain injury is predisposed to numerous complications that arise from injury to the central and autonomic nervous systems, concurrent injuries, hypoperfusion injury, and iatrogenic complications. These include adult respiratory distress syndrome (p. 247), pulmonary edema (p. 289), meningitis (p. 485), diabetes insipidus (p. 504), syndrome of inappropriate antidiuretic hormone (p. 511), gastrointestinal bleeding (p. 504), anemia (p. 587), and disseminated intravascular coagulation (p. 608).

DIAGNOSTIC TESTS

Skull x-ray: Detects structural deficits such as skull fractures and facial bone destruction, as well as air-fluid level in sinuses, abnormal intracranial calcification, pineal gland location (normally midline), and foreign bodies that are radiopaque.

Cervical spine x-ray: Demonstrates structural deficits of the spine and used to rule out associated cervical spine injuries, including fractures, dislocations, and subluxations. Cervical spine mobilization is mandatory in all trauma patients until the C-spine (cervical 1 through thoracic 1) is visualized completely and fractures are ruled out.

Computed tomography (CT) scan: Gray and white matter, blood, and CSF are detectable due to their different radiologic densities. Because CT scanning is capable of diagnosing cerebral hemorrhage, infarction, hydrocephalus, cerebral edema, and structural shifts, it continues to be the most important diagnostic tool for primary and secondary brain injury.

Magnetic resonance imaging (MRI):   Identifies type, location, and extent of injury. It provides spatial resolution, can follow metabolic processes, and detects structural changes.

Cerebral angiography: Invasive radiographic procedure that uses dye to examine the cerebral vasculature. It is used only as an adjunct study in diagnosing brain injury or if CT scan is unavailable.

Electroencephalography (EEG):   Measures spontaneous brain electrical activity *via* surface electrodes. It is useful in detecting areas of abnormal brain activity (irritability) associated with seizures and generalized brain activity related to drug overdose, coma, or suspected brain death. Drug therapy, especially anticonvulsants, alters brain activity, and therefore use of these drugs should be documented if the drug cannot be withheld 24-48 h before EEG testing.

Evoked responses: Evaluation of the electrical potentials (responses) of the brain to an external stimulus (i.e., auditory, visual, or somatosensory), thereby providing information related to lesions of the cortex or ascending pathways of the spinal cord, brainstem, or thalamus. Evoked potentials can be useful in determining the extent of injury in uncooperative, confused, or comatose patients and should be used when planning rehabilitation.

CSF analysis: Useful in determining infection in the brain-injured patient. Analysis of CSF should include color, turbidity/cloudiness, RBC and WBC counts, protein, glucose, electrolytes, Gram's stain, culture, and sensitivity.

Serum laboratory studies: To identify complications associated with injury. WBCs, Hgb, Hct, electrolytes, osmolality, albumin, and transferrin are monitored at least daily and more frequently during the acute phase.

COLLABORATIVE MANAGEMENT

Management focuses on treating the emergent pathology, controlling ICP, preventing complications, and initiating rehabilitation.

Surgical intervention: Performed to evacuate mass lesions (epidural, subdural, and intracranial hematomas), place ICP monitoring system, elevate depressed skull fractures, debride open wounds and brain tissue, and repair dural tears or scalp lacerations. Frontal lobectomies may be necessary to control severe increases in ICP.

Management of intracranial pressure dynamics: ICP monitoring is accomplished using a variety of techniques (Table 2-3). All monitoring systems provide a digital display of ICP, but CPP must be calculated (see p. 128). The goal is to maintain CPP between 60-80 mm Hg.

Reduction of ICP by CSF drainage: Accomplished only by using intraventricular or ventriculostomy systems. To prevent herniation when draining CSF, drainage collection bags must be maintained at the level of the tragus of the ear or higher, thereby preventing excessive CSF flow caused by a higher to lower pressure gradient.

Hyperventilation via mechanical ventilation: Used as an initial strategy to control ICP because it reduces $Paco_2$, thereby causing vasoconstriction of cerebral vessels and reduction of cerebral blood volume. Hyperventilation can be accomplished using control, assist control, intermittent mandatory ventilation (IMV), or spontaneous IMV techniques. $Paco_2$ should be maintained between 25-30 mm Hg and Pao_2 at levels >80 mm Hg to prevent hypoxia. See "Mechanical Ventilation," p. 19, for more information.

Diuresis therapy: Reduces cerebral brain volume by extracting fluid from the brain's intracellular compartment. Mannitol 20%, an osmotic diuretic, and furosemide (Lasix), a loop diuretic, are used most commonly. Mannitol may be given in 25-50 g doses as needed to reduce ICP or may be given q4-6h. Furosemide may be given in conjunction with mannitol at doses between 20-40 mg. Dehydration is a major complication with continued use of diuretics, and therefore strict attention must be paid to serum electrolyte and osmolality values. In addition to maintenance fluid therapy (75-100 ml/h), replacement of urine losses may be prescribed. Replacement therapy is based on the volume of urine collected 1 h after administration of the diuretic and is given either ml for ml or 0.5 ml for ml over a 3- to 4-h period.

Maintenance of blood pressure within an acceptable range: Imperative because both hypotension and hypertension can contribute to cerebral edema. Hypotension can result in decreased oxygen delivery to brain cells, thereby decreasing pH, elevating $Paco_2$, and causing cerebral vessels to vasodilate. Hypotension also reduces MAP and thus CPP. Dopamine HCl (Intropin), used at doses between 3-5 μg/kg/min, can effectively increase MAP and raise CPP.

The effects of hypertension (elevated CPP and increased cerebral edema) have not been well studied, but increased capillary permeability and petechial hemorrhage are seen with hypertension. Antihypertensive medications, such as labetalol HCl (Normodyne) or nitroprusside sodium (Nipride), may be necessary.

Reduction of metabolic demand: Important strategy when treating ICP problems, because cerebral blood supply must match demand in order to maintain cerebral function.

TABLE 2 - 3   Types of intracranial monitoring

System	Type	Placement	Advantages/uses	Disadvantages
Fluid-filled or fiberoptic	Intraventricular cannula	Lateral ventricle in nondominant hemisphere through burr hole	CSF measurement CSF drainage Drug administration Volume-pressure response testing	Rapid CSF drainage can result in collapsed ventricles or subdural hematoma Cannula tip may catch on ventricular wall Risk of intracerebral bleeding and infection May become plugged with debris Possible difficult insertion due to shifting or collapse of ventricle
Fluid-filled	Subarachnoid screw	Subarachnoid space through twist drill hole	Pressure monitoring Less risk of infection than cannula Useful with small ventricles Does not penetrate brain	Compliance testing may be unreliable No CSF drainage Some risk of infection Risk of hemorrhage or hematoma during insertion Brain may herniate into bolt, making recording unreliable
Electrical sensor	Epidural sensor	Epidural space Burr hole Fiberoptic sensor	Lowest risk of infection Easy to insert Dura not penetrated	No direct measurement of CSF No CSF drainage Inability to recalibrate to zero Cannot measure volume-pressure response
Fiberoptic	Intraparenchymal	Intraparenchymal *via* twist drill Fiberoptic sensor	Easy to insert Direct pressure Compliance testing One-time zero and calibration before insertion	Risk of intracerebral bleeding and infection No CSF drainage

- *Sedating agents:* Use of continuous drips of midazolam HCl (Versed) and narcotic analgesics, such as fentanyl citrate (Sublimaze) or morphine sulfate, is common. In addition, nondepolarizing agents, such as vecuronium bromide (Norcuron), are used to reduce metabolic demand. Sedation, analgesia, and paralysis may be used as combination therapy or as individual therapies. See "Sedating and Paralytic Agents," p. 40.

- *Seizure control:* Seizure activity may occur, especially in the presence of focal injuries such as depressed, comminuted, or compound skull fractures; contusions; and lacerations. Because seizure activity increases the metabolic demand of the brain, seizure prophylaxis using an anticonvulsant agent may be necessary. Phenytoin sodium (Dilantin) is most commonly used. A loading dose consisting of 500-1,000 mg IV is followed by a daily dose of 100 mg tid. Phenytoin must be administered slowly, 50 mg/min, and cannot be administered with a dextrose solution. Therapeutic levels should be maintained between 10-20 μg/ml.

- *Barbiturate coma:* Another method of reducing metabolic demand. High doses of barbiturates should never be used without continuous ICP and hemodynamic monitoring and controlled ventilation, because barbiturates induce profound cardiac and cerebral depression. Pentobarbital sodium (Nembutal) is the drug of choice. A loading dose between 5-10 mg/kg is given (discontinue if MAP falls <70 mm Hg), followed by a maintenance dose of 1-3 mg/kg/h to sustain a level of 3-5 mg/dl. Barbiturates are withdrawn gradually as the patient improves. Patients with barbiturate coma require intensive physical care and physiologic monitoring. When use of barbiturates does not improve the clinical condition, brain death criteria cannot be initiated until barbiturate levels return to zero.

- *Maintaining body temperature:* For every 1° C in temperature elevation, there is a 10%-13% increase in metabolic rate. Normal temperatures range from 35.8°-37.5° C (96.4°-99.5° F) with a diurnal variation of 1° C. Rectal temperatures are 0.2°-0.6° C higher than oral and can be 0.8° C higher than right atrial, esophageal, and oral temperatures during fever (Segatore, 1992). With brain injury, evaluation of the etiology of fever is important because it will influence treatment choice. Fever can be attributed to brain injury (central fever), an infectious process (peripheral fever), or drugs (drug fever). Central fever reflects a derangement in the hypothalamic thermoregulatory mechanism and is characterized by lack of sweating, no diurnal variation, plateaulike elevation patterns, elevations up to 41° C (105.8° F), absence of tachycardia, persistence for days or weeks, and temperature reduction with external cooling rather than with antipyretics. Peripheral fever is associated with wound infections, meningitis, sepsis, pneumonia, and other bacterial invasion. Sweating, diurnal variation, response to antipyretic agents, and tachycardia are characteristic of peripheral fever.

  Shivering, associated with hypothermia therapy, is the body's mechanism to increase heat production. Shivering not only increases metabolic demand, it also may increase ICP. Wrapping distal extremities in bath towels before initiating hypothermia is an effective measure for controlling shivering. Chlorpromazine (Thorazine) also may be used to control shivering, but it should be used with caution because it may have a hypotensive effect.

Modifying nursing care activities that raise ICP: Brief and rapid elevations in ICP are commonly seen during position changes or performance of other nursing care and cannot always be avoided. However, these elevations are transient and generally the ICP returns to resting baseline within a few minutes. Sustained increases (>5 min) should be avoided. All nursing care activities that increase ICP should be spaced to enable a return of ICP to baseline and maximizing of CPP. Clustering nursing care such as bathing, turning, and suctioning creates a stair-step rise in ICP, thereby promoting sustained increases.

- *Suctioning:* Causes a significant rise in ICP. To minimize adverse effects associated with suctioning, implement the guidelines found in Table 2-4.
- *Positioning:* Flexion, extension, and lateral movements can significantly raise ICP. Maintaining the neck in neutral position at all times is important. In patients with poor neck control, stabilize the neck with towel rolls or sandbags.
- *Elevating HOB:* Although HOB elevation at 30 degrees is believed to improve venous drainage and contribute to ICP reduction, ICP may be improved at higher or lower elevations. Adjust HOB elevation based on patient's clinical response.
- *Turning:* Turning the patient with IICP is not contraindicated but should be based on the patient's response to turning. Initially, turning from side to side will elevate pressure, but ICP should return to resting baseline after a few minutes. If the ICP does not return to resting baseline within 5 min, CPP may be compromised and the patient should be returned to a position that reduces ICP and maximizes CPP.
- *Bathing:* While bathing itself has not been documented as raising ICP, rapid turning from side to side associated with linen changes raises ICP because the length of the procedure does not allow sufficient time for the ICP to return to baseline. Evaluation of the patient's response may necessitate performing the linen change in stages or allowing adequate time for ICP to return to resting baseline.

T A B L E   2 - 4   Guidelines for suctioning patients at risk for increased intracranial pressure

- Suction only if the clinical status of the patient warrants.
- Precede suctioning with preoxygenation using 100% oxygen.
- Limit each suctioning pass to ≤10 sec.
- Limit suction passes to 2.
- Follow each pass with 60 sec of hyperventilation using 100% oxygen.
- Use negative suction pressure <120 mm Hg.
- Keep patient's head in a neutral position.
- Use a suction catheter with an outer-to-inner diameter ratio of 2:1.

- *Sensory stimulation:* This important rehabilitative technique for comatose patients has not been well studied in the unstable brain-injured patient with IICP. Therefore, assessment of the patient's response to conversation of any type should be ongoing, and conversation that is associated with sustained rises in ICP should be avoided. Aggressive tactile, olfactory, auditory, gustatory, and vestibular stimulation should be initiated in the comatose patient after ICP has returned to normal. Sensory stimulation should be discontinued but reattempted at a later time if adverse clinical effects are observed.

Nutritional support: Enteral nutrition is most physiologically compatible with gut function and should be initiated as early as possible after injury. When transpyloric (duodenum or jejunum) feeding tubes are used, enteral feedings can be initiated before bowel sounds return to normal. In some cases, gastric tubes for gastric decompression are used simultaneously with the transpyloric tubes. See "Nutritional Support," p. 16, for documentation of proper placement and checking of residual volumes. If enteral feedings are contraindicated or not tolerated by the patient, parenteral feedings are started.

Rehabilitation: Brain injury is highly associated with physical (paralysis, spasticity, and contractures) and cognitive impairments. Initiate early consultations with physical, occupational, and speech therapists to minimize the deficits and prepare the patient for an active rehabilitative program. Support also is available through the National Head Injury Foundation, 18A Vernon Street, Framingham, MA 01701; or the state chapter of the Head Injury Foundation.

NURSING DIAGNOSES AND INTERVENTIONS

Impaired gas exchange related to decreased oxygen supply and increased carbon dioxide production secondary to decreased ventilatory drive occurring with pressure on respiratory center, imposed inactivity, and possible neurologic pulmonary edema or chest injury

Desired outcomes: $Paco_2$ values remain between 25-30 mm Hg during hyperventilation, 35-40 mm Hg as ICP stabilizes, and 35-45 mm Hg by the time of discharge from ICU or transfer to rehabilitation unit. By the time of discharge from ICU or transfer to rehabilitation unit, patient has adequate gas exchange as evidenced by orientation to time, place, and person; Pao_2 ≥80 mm Hg; RR 12-20 breaths/min with normal depth and pattern (eupnea); and absence of adventitious breath sounds.

- Assess patient's respiratory rate, depth, and rhythm. Auscultate lung fields for breath sounds q1-2h and prn. Monitor for respiratory patterns described in Table 2-2. Be alert to IICP (see Table 6-3, p. 449).
- Assess patient for signs of hypoxia, including confusion, agitation, restlessness, and irritability. Remember that cyanosis is a late indicator of hypoxia.
- Ensure a patent airway *via* proper positioning of neck and frequent assessment of the need for suctioning. Ensure hyperoxygenation of patient before and after each suction attempt to prevent dangerous, suction-induced hypoxia.
- Monitor ABG values; consult physician for significant findings or

changes. Be alert to levels indicative of hypoxemia (Pa_{O_2} <80 mm Hg) and to Pa_{CO_2} ≥25-30 mm Hg, inasmuch as levels higher than this range may increase cerebral blood flow and thus ICP.
- Ensure that oxygen is delivered within prescribed limits.
- Assist with turning q2h, within limits of patient's injury, to promote lung drainage and expansion and alveolar perfusion. Unless contraindicated, raise HOB 30 degrees to enhance gas exchange.
- Encourage deep breathing at frequent intervals to promote oxygenation. Avoid coughing exercises for patients at risk for IICP.
- Perform chest physiotherapy as directed by physician or ICU protocol. Be aware that chest physiotherapy may increase ICP.
- Evaluate the need for an artificial airway in patients unable to maintain airway patency or adequate ventilatory effort.

Risk for infection (CNS) related to inadequate primary defenses secondary to direct access to the brain in the presence of skull fracture, penetrating wounds, craniotomy, intracranial monitoring, or bacterial invasion due to pneumonia or iatrogenic causes
Desired outcome: Patient is free of infection as evidenced by normothermia, WBC count ≤11,000/μl, negative culture results, HR ≤100 bpm, BP within patient's normal range, and absence of agitation, purulent drainage, and other clinical indicators of infection.
- Assess VS at frequent intervals for indicators of CNS infection. Be alert to elevated temperature and increased HR and BP.
- Monitor patient for signs of systemic infection, including discomfort, malaise, agitation, and restlessness.
- Inspect cranial wounds for the presence of erythema, tenderness, swelling, and purulent drainage. Obtain prescription for culture as indicated.
- Apply a loose sterile dressing (sling) to collect CSF drainage. Do not pack. Record amount, color, and character of drainage.
- Caution patient against coughing, sneezing, nose blowing, or other Valsalva-type maneuvers, because these activities can damage the dura further. Use orogastric tubes if basilar skull fractures or severe frontal sinus fractures are present.
- Ensure timely administration of prescribed antibiotics.
- Apply basic principles for care of invasive device used with ICP monitoring:
  □ Use good handwashing technique before caring for patient.
  □ If patient is not comatose, encourage him or her not to touch device; apply restraints *only* if necessary to keep patient from harm. Restraints can increase ICP by causing straining.
  □ Maintain aseptic technique during care of device, following agency protocol.

Decreased adaptive capacity: Intracranial, related to decreased cerebral perfusion pressure or infections that can occur with secondary head injury
Desired outcomes: Within 12-24 h of treatment/interventions, patient has adequate intracranial adaptive capacity as evidenced by equal and normoreactive pupils; RR 12-20 breaths/min with normal depth and pattern (eupnea); HR 60-100 bpm; ICP 0-15 mm Hg; cerebral perfusion pressure (CPP) 60-80 mm Hg; and absence of headache, vomit-

ing, and other clinical indicators of IICP. Optimally, by the time of discharge from ICU or transfer to rehabilitation unit, patient is oriented to time, place, and person and has bilaterally equal strength and tone in the extremities.

- Assess neurologic status at least hourly. Monitor pupils, LOC, and motor activity; also perform cranial nerve assessments (Appendix 4). A decrease in LOC is an early indicator of IICP and impending herniation. Changes in the size and reaction of the pupils, a decrease in motor function (e.g., hemiplegia, abnormal flexion posturing), and cranial nerve palsies all indicate impending herniation.
- Monitor VS at frequent intervals. Be alert to changes in respiratory pattern, fluctuations in BP and pulse, widening pulse pressure, and slow HR.
- Monitor patient for indicators of IICP (see Table 6-3, p. 449).
- Monitor hemodynamic status to evaluate CPP and ensure that it is 60-80 mm Hg. Be alert to decrease in mean systolic arterial blood pressure (<80 mm Hg) or increase in MAP. Perform ongoing assessment of ICP and CPP, recording pressures at least hourly until stable. Consult physician if pressure changes significantly (e.g., >15 mm Hg or other preestablished range). Perform ongoing calibration and zeroing of transducer to ensure accuracy of readings.
- Maintain a patent airway, and ensure precise delivery of oxygen to promote optimal cerebral perfusion.
- Facilitate cerebral venous drainage by maintaining neck in neutral position.
- To help prevent fluid volume excess, which could add to cerebral edema, ensure precise delivery of IV fluids at consistent rates.
- Ensure timely administration of medications that are prescribed for the prevention of sudden increase or decrease in BP, HR, RR.
- Treat elevations in ICP immediately (Table 2-5).

Ineffective thermoregulation related to trauma associated with injury to or pressure on the hypothalamus

---

T A B L E 2 - 5 Nursing interventions for patients with increased intracranial pressure

---

- Make sure HOB is elevated 30 degrees or to elevation known to decrease ICP.
- Loosen constrictive objects around neck that may be impeding blood flow.
- If patient has recently been repositioned, return patient to original position, since he or she might not be tolerating new position.
- Ensure that patient's head is maintained in a neutral position.
- Assess for factors that may be contributing to patient's IICP: distended bladder or abdomen, fear, anxiety.
- Evaluate activities (e.g., suctioning, bathing, dressing changes) that can increase pressure; reorganize care plan accordingly.
- Perform hyperoxygenation of patient before and after suctioning, according to ICU protocol.

Desired outcome: Patient becomes normothermic within 24 h of this diagnosis.

- Monitor for signs of hyperthermia: temperature >38.3° C (101° F), pallor, absence of perspiration, torso that is warm to the touch.
- As prescribed, obtain specimens for blood, urine, and sputum cultures to rule out underlying infection.
- Be alert to signs of meningitis: fever, chills, nuchal rigidity, Kernig's sign, Brudzinski's sign (see "Meningitis," p. 485).
- Assess wounds for evidence of infection, including erythema, tenderness, purulent drainage.
- If patient has hyperthermia, remove excess clothing and administer tepid baths, hypothermic blanket, or ice bags to axilla or groin.
- As prescribed, administer antipyretics such as acetaminophen.
- As prescribed, administer chlorpromazine to treat or prevent shivering, which can cause further increases in ICP.
- Keep environmental temperature at optimal range.
- Assess for possible drug fever reaction, which can occur with antimicrobial therapy.

Risk for disuse syndrome related to immobilization and prolonged inactivity secondary to brain injury, spasticity, or altered LOC
Desired outcome: Patient has baseline/optimal ROM without verbal or nonverbal indicators of pain.

- Begin performing passive ROM exercises q4h on all extremities immediately upon patient's admission. Monitor ICP during exercise, being alert to dangerous elevations outside of the established parameters. Consult with physical therapist accordingly.
- Teach passive ROM exercises to significant others. Encourage their participation in patient exercise as often as they are able.
- Reposition patient q2h within restrictions of the head and other injuries, using log-rolling technique as indicated.
- Ensure proper anatomic position and alignment. Support alignment with pillows, trochanter rolls, wrapped sandbags.
- For patient with spasticity, use foot cradles to keep linen off the feet. To maintain dorsiflexion, provide patient with shoes that are cut off at the toes, with the shoes ending just proximal to the head of the patient's metatarsal joints. Because there is no contact of the balls of the feet with a hard surface, the risk of spasticity will be minimized. Consult occupational therapist for use of splints or other supportive device.
- For patients without spasticity, use foot supports to prevent plantarflexion and external hip rotation.
- To maintain anatomic position of the hands, provide spastic patient with a splint or cone that is secured with an elastic band. Either device will limit spasticity by pressing on the muscles, while the elastic band will stimulate the extensor muscles, thereby promoting finger extension.

Impaired corneal tissue integrity (or risk for same) related to irritation associated with corneal drying and reduced lacrimal production secondary to altered consciousness or cranial nerve damage
Desired outcome: Patient's corneas are moist and intact.

- Assess for indicators of corneal irritation: red and itching eyes, ocu-

lar pain, sensation of a foreign object in the eye, scleral edema, and blurred vision.
- Avoid exposing patient's eyes to irritants such as baby powder or talc.
- Lubricate patient's eyes q2h with isotonic solution, either eye drops or ointment.
- Facilitate an ophthalmic consultation as indicated.

ADDITIONAL NURSING DIAGNOSES

See "Cerebral Aneurysm and Subarachnoid Hemorrhage" for **Decreased adaptive capacity:** Intracranial, p. 455. As appropriate, see nursing diagnoses and interventions under "Care of the Patient Following Intracranial Surgery," p. 463, and "Meningitis," p. 490. See "Status Epilepticus" for **Risk for trauma,** p. 467. Also see nursing diagnoses and interventions under "Nutritional Support" (particularly **Risk for aspiration,** p. 16); "Mechanical Ventilation," p. 24; "Hemodynamic monitoring," p. 37; "Prolonged Immobility," p. 78; "Psychosocial Support," p. 88; and "Psychosocial Support for the Patient's Family and Significant Others," p. 100. The patient with craniocerebral trauma is at risk for diabetes insipidus and syndrome of inappropriate antidiuretic hormone. See "Diabetes Insipidus" for **Fluid volume deficit,** p. 509, and "Syndrome of Inappropriate Antidiuretic Hormone" for **Risk for injury,** p. 513.

Chest trauma

PATHOPHYSIOLOGY

Chest trauma is a complex and multidimensional problem. It is usually categorized by cause.
Blunt injury: Occurs as a result of a direct, forceful blow to the chest. Usually the injury is "closed" in that there is no communication of the chest cavity with outside atmospheric pressure. A typical occurrence is a vehicular collision, during which there is impact of the thorax with the steering wheel. A crushing injury to the thorax also is considered blunt chest trauma.
Penetrating injury: Occurs as a result of stab or missile wounds to the thorax. This is an open chest injury because there is communication between the chest cavity and outside atmospheric pressure. Gunshots are the most common missile-type penetrating injuries, whereas knife wounds represent the most common stabbing chest injuries.

· · ·

Both blunt and penetrating chest wounds can lead to pneumothorax. In addition, thoracic injury can be severe enough to cause pulmonary or cardiac contusion or can lead to interference with the mechanical functions of the heart and lungs; therefore in-depth physical assessment is critical after the patient's injury.

ASSESSMENT

Subtle signs and symptoms and changes in the patient's condition can be clues to serious problems. Treat the patient as though a spinal cord injury has occurred until diagnostic tests have ruled it out. Be aware that subtle changes in mental status can signal a central nervous system insult as well as hypoxemia.

Blunt injury: Dyspnea, SOB, agitation, restlessness, anxiety, and severe chest pain during respirations that the patient can localize.

Potential complications: Pneumothorax, flail chest, hemothorax, pulmonary contusion, myocardial contusion, cardiac tamponade.

Inspection: RR >20 breaths/min; hyperpnea; ventilatory distress; use of accessory muscles of respiration; nasal flaring; decreased tidal volume; hemoptysis; asymmetric chest wall motion; paradoxic chest wall motion; inability to clear tracheobronchial secretions; splinting; jugular venous distention; cyanosis or pallor of the skin, lips, and nail beds; and ecchymosis, which can signal injury to underlying organs.

Palpation: Tracheal deviation; subcutaneous emphysema of the neck and upper portion of the chest; tenderness at fracture points; flail chest segment; weak pulse; cool, clammy skin; protrusion of bony fragments.

Percussion: Dullness over lung fields, which can signal hemothorax or atelectasis; hyperresonance over lung fields, signaling pneumothorax.

Auscultation: Diminished or absent breath sounds, respiratory stridor, bony crepitus over fracture sites, muffled heart tones, decreased BP, pericardial friction rub, paradoxic pulse, apical tachycardia. In addition, bowel sounds may be heard in the thorax as a result of rupture or tear of the diaphragm, allowing herniation of abdominal contents into the thorax.

Penetrating injury: Dyspnea, SOB, moderate chest pain, restlessness, anxiety.

Note: It is essential to perform a complete and rapid assessment with the patient's clothing removed. Entry sites may be deceptive, as the skin has an elastic quality and tends to close behind the penetrating object, thereby masking the size and extent of injury. Log roll the patient to visualize the exit wound, if present.

Potential complications: Hemothorax, pneumothorax, tension pneumothorax, hemorrhage, shock, and infection.

Inspection: RR >20 breaths/min; hyperpnea; respiratory distress; use of accessory muscles of respiration; nasal flaring; decreased tidal volume; asymmetric chest wall movement; inability to clear tracheobronchial secretions; splinting; and cyanosis or pallor of the skin, lips, and nail beds. During inspection, estimate blood loss on clothing and locate both entry and exit sites. Be alert to presence or severity of other wounds and to presence of ecchymosis, which can signal injury to underlying internal organs. Also note presence or absence of pulsations of the penetrating object, which may be imbedded in a major organ or blood vessel. Do not remove any penetrating object, because the object may have caused a sealing effect, and removing it could result in uncontrollable bleeding of the organ or vessel.

Palpation: Tracheal deviation, subcutaneous emphysema, weak or irregular pulse, cool and clammy skin.

Percussion: Dullness over lung fields as a result of hemothorax or atelectasis, hyperresonance over lung fields as a result of pneumothorax.

Auscultation: Sucking sound over point of entry during inspiratory phase; diminished breath sounds; respiratory stridor; muffled heart tones; apical tachycardia or bradycardia, depending on stage of shock; bowel sounds in thorax.

Flail chest: A severe complication of blunt chest trauma that occurs when three or more adjacent ribs fracture in two or more places (or the sternum is fractured, along with ribs adjacent to the sternum fracture). The fracture segment is free of the bony thorax and moves independently in response to intrathoracic pressure. Paradoxic chest wall motion is the hallmark symptom in diagnosing flail chest. Normally the chest expands on inspiration, creating a negative intrathoracic pressure; on expiration the chest wall retracts in response to positive pressure inside the chest. Because a flail chest segment is no longer attached to the bony thorax, it follows the pressure and retracts on inspiration (negative pressure is a pulling pressure) and bulges on expiration (positive pressure is a pushing pressure).

DIAGNOSTIC TESTS

Chest x-ray: Confirms presence of air or fluid in the pleural space; assists in determining extent of hemothorax or pneumothorax; and confirms presence or absence of fractures of the bony thorax, as well as mediastinal shift.

ABG analysis: Evaluates adequacy of oxygenation and presence or absence of acid-base abnormalities. Typical results will reflect hypoxemia (Pao_2 <80 mm Hg) and hypercapnia ($Paco_2$ >45 mm Hg) with concomitant respiratory acidosis (pH <7.35). Pulse oximetry may be used for continuous monitoring of oxygen saturation (see discussion, p. 230).

ECG: Reveals presence or absence of life-threatening dysrhythmias and provides a more thorough analysis of the heart's electrical activity. Although dysrhythmias are a common complication after chest trauma, this important test often is overlooked.

Hgb/Hct values: Levels determine the need for blood transfusion or fluid volume replacement.

WBC count: Baseline indicator of an infectious process.

COLLABORATIVE MANAGEMENT

Interventions are directed toward managing acute respiratory compromise while correcting the underlying pathophysiology or injuries that complicate or aggravate the patient's condition.

Oxygen therapy: Delivered by mask or cannula, depending on extent of hypoxemia.

Intubation: Maintains patent airway, decreases airway resistance and respiratory effort, provides route for easy removal of airway secretions, and allows for manual or mechanical ventilation, as necessary.

Mechanical ventilation: For cases of extreme respiratory distress or ventilatory collapse (see p. 19).

Blood replacement: A high priority in the trauma victim. Generally, blood loss is replaced with packed RBCs or whole fresh blood, when available. Blood replacement *via* a commercially prepared autotransfusion system is a widely accepted therapy. Use of colloid versus crystalloid fluids for volume replacement remains controversial. Many factors specific to the patient's condition and history dictate which fluid is the better volume expander. Volume usually is replaced with crystalloid fluids (e.g., normal saline, lactated Ringer's solution) rather than colloidal IV fluids (e.g., plasma, albumin) because colloids fail to provide significant benefits and carry with them the risk of development of ARDS and renal failure. Cost also is prohibitive. Two large-bore venous lines are inserted so that large volumes of fluid can be replaced rapidly.

Chest tube insertion: To remove accumulation of fluid or air from the chest cavity. A large-bore (26-30 Fr) thoracic catheter is inserted into the chest cavity through the second intercostal space, midclavicular line, or fifth lateral intercostal space, midaxillary line. Placement depends on the location and extent of the hemothorax or pneumothorax and on principles of gravity drainage. The catheter then is connected to a one-way flutter valve or to a closed chest-drainage system.

Analgesia: Manages pain, which can interfere with work of breathing. Generally, opioid analgesics are avoided or used cautiously because of respiratory depressive side effects. Intercostal nerve block may be performed to provide local pain relief.

Thoracentesis: Relieves life-threatening tension pneumothorax. A 14-gauge needle is inserted into the second intercostal space at the midclavicular line to ventilate the pressurized chest cavity or, in an emergency situation, to remove a massive hemothorax.

Stabilization and fixation of flail chest: Most flail chest injuries stabilize within 10-14 days without surgical intervention. Internal fixation involves the use of a volume-cycled ventilator to stabilize the fracture(s). In some cases the flail segment is fixated externally during a surgical procedure by wiring or otherwise attaching the segment to the intact bony structures.

Thoracotomy: Generally avoided unless complications develop after stabilization. Indications for thoracotomy include massive air leak in a functioning drainage system, continued or increased bleeding through a chest tube, refractory hypotension, acute deterioration, and cardiac tamponade.

NURSING DIAGNOSES AND INTERVENTIONS

Risk for fluid volume deficit related to active loss secondary to excessive bleeding occurring with chest trauma

Desired outcome: Patient is normovolemic as evidenced by BP and HR within patient's normal limits, stable weight, urine output ≥0.5 ml/kg/h, chest drainage ≤100 ml/h, and RR ≤20 breaths/min with normal depth and pattern (eupnea).

- Note condition of dressings at frequent intervals. Be sure to check sheets underneath patient. Report excessive drainage or bleeding (e.g., if dressings are saturated more frequently than q4h during the first 24-48 h). After the first 48 h bleeding should subside, and the dressing should not require changing more often than bid. At that time drainage should be serosanguineous or serous; however, any bright red bleeding should be reported promptly.

- Monitor drainage in closed chest-drainage system. Report significant increase in bright red blood or excessive drainage. Amounts >100 ml/h usually are considered excessive.
- Monitor functioning of autotransfusion equipment. Collaborate with physician for additional transfusion/fluid requirements based on the amount and rate of bleeding. Record accurate I&O status.
- Assess VS at frequent intervals. Be alert to decreased BP and to increased HR and RR, which can signal an impending shock state.
- Assess patient's hydration status by monitoring daily weight, as well as amounts of fluid intake and urinary output.
- Monitor patient's Hgb as an indicator of hemostasis. Be alert to a decrease in Hgb, which can occur with blood loss. Normal Hgb is ≥12 g/dl (female) or ≥14 g/dl (male).

ADDITIONAL NURSING DIAGNOSES

See "Major Trauma" for **Posttrauma response,** p. 123. See "Pneumothorax" for **Impaired gas exchange,** p. 261, and **Pain,** p. 263. For other nursing diagnoses and interventions, see "Psychosocial Support," p. 88, and "Psychosocial Support for the Patient's Family and Significant Others," p. 100.

Near drowning

PATHOPHYSIOLOGY

Near drowning can be defined as survival longer than 24 h after asphyxia related to submersion. Many adult drownings or near drownings are preceded by alcohol or drug ingestion, diving injuries, or medical catastrophes such as seizures or myocardial infarctions. Hypoxia, hypotension, pulmonary edema, and respiratory and metabolic acidosis are the most common problems after near drowning. Potential complications include neurologic deficits from cerebral anoxia, acute renal failure secondary to acute tubular necrosis, and disseminated intravascular coagulation (DIC). Near drowning can be categorized in two ways.

Near drowning with aspiration (wet): Occurs in 85%-90% of victims of near drowning. The aspirant is either the submersion fluid or gastric contents. Hypoxia results from a variety of mechanisms, including laryngospasm, bronchospasm, airway obstruction from aspirated contaminants, or pulmonary edema. *Freshwater* (hypotonic) *aspiration* results in loss of surfactant, which is caused by the presence of hypotonic solution in the lungs. This can lead to atelectasis because surface tension of the lung tissue increases, causing alveoli to collapse. A decrease in lung compliance also occurs. In turn the atelectasis and pulmonary edema lead to a ventilation-perfusion mismatch, which adds to the hypoxia and acidosis. *Saltwater* (hypertonic) *aspiration* results in a rapid shift of water and plasma proteins from the circulation into the alveoli. These fluid-filled alveoli are not ventilated, and the continued perfusion leads to ventilation-perfusion mismatch and hypoxia. Because the aspirated volume of either freshwater or saltwater is usually small, there is little effect on total blood volume. The intravascular depletion frequently seen is caused by increased capillary permeability (from anoxia) and loss of protein in the pulmonary edema fluid. Any contaminants that are aspirated (e.g., algae, chemicals, sand) can cause or contribute to obstruction and lead to asphyxiation. Bacterial pneumonia can develop, depending on the type of contaminant in the aspirant, and chemical pneumonitis can occur if gastric contents were aspirated.

Near drowning without aspiration (dry):   Represents 10%-15% of cases of near drowning. Death, if it occurs, results from asphyxiation secondary to laryngospasm. Laryngospasm usually is caused by water entering the airway, although it can be triggered by fear or pain.

Many deaths that have been attributed to near drowning may, in fact, be the result of one of two separate phenomena that can lead to aspiration: (1) *immersion syndrome,* which occurs with sudden immersion in cold water, resulting in hyperventilation; this increases the risk of swallowing or inhaling large amounts of cold water, which can lead to vagally stimulated bradycardia that results in loss of consciousness; and (2) *hyperventilation syndrome,* which occurs when divers hyperventilate to increase the duration time of breath-holding underwater. The normal impetus to breathe (increased $Paco_2$) is not present, and with exercise, oxygen stores continue to be used. Because breath-holding may not be terminated before oxygen supplies have reached dangerously low levels, dysrhythmias, seizure, or death from hypoxia can occur.

Hypothermia also is significant in near drowning. It is defined as a drop in core temperature to 33° C (91.4° F) or below. Its progression can cause muscle activity and vital functions to cease and ventricular fibrillation to occur (this happens at 28° C [83° F]). In some instances hypothermia protects the brain from permanent damage, depending on the victim's age and the degree of hypothermia, because of the decrease in cerebral metabolism that occurs when core body temperature reaches 25° C (77° F). This decrease in cerebral metabolism helps protect the brain from the effects of anoxia. Resuscitation should be continued until the victim is rewarmed to at least 32° C (90° F), because the heart may start beating at that temperature. Resuscitation is possible, even after 30 min of submersion. Resuscitation efforts frequently need to be continued for at least 1 h.

ASSESSMENT

The following criteria are based on postresuscitation findings:

CLINICAL PRESENTATION Depending on the severity and duration of the hypoxia, may include unconsciousness, seizures, nonspecific alterations in mental status (e.g., confusion, irritability, lethargy), neurologic deficits (motor, speech, visual), mild coughing, coughing up of pink and frothy sputum, vomiting, substernal chest pain, mottled and cold skin, cyanosis, fixed and dilated pupils, and abdominal distention.

PHYSICAL ASSESSMENT In the presence of pulmonary edema there may be resonance over lung fields and normal tactile fremitus. Auscultation of lung fields may reveal apnea, tachypnea (RR >20 breaths/min), shallow or gasping respirations, crackles, rhonchi, wheezes, supraventricular dysrhythmias, bradycardia (HR <60 bpm), tachycardia (HR >100 bpm), and ventricular fibrillation.

DIAGNOSTIC TESTS

ABG values: Initially may reflect hypoxemia (Pao_2 <80 mm Hg), hypercapnia ($Paco_2$ >45 mm Hg), and metabolic and respiratory acidosis (pH <7.35, serum bicarbonate <22 mEq/L). Often the $Paco_2$ will return to normal but the hypoxemia will persist. Pulse oximetry may be initiated for continuous monitoring of oxygen saturation (see p. 230).

Note: Initial ABG values may be within acceptable range, but because respiratory status can deteriorate quickly, serial monitoring is essential.

CBC count: To determine baseline hematologic status and presence of infection.

Serum electrolyte levels: Life-threatening changes in electrolyte levels are unusual after near drowning. Electrolyte disturbances are related to the quantity and tonicity of the water aspirated.

BUN and creatinine levels: To determine effects of hypoxia on renal tubular function. Creatinine is the most sensitive indicator of renal dysfunction. Acute tubular necrosis is a potential complication of near drowning.

Chest x-ray: Serial x-rays are necessary to determine presence or development of infiltrates, atelectasis, and pulmonary edema. The alveolar filling pattern, which is evaluated with pulmonary edema, is evidenced on x-ray by a soft, fluffy appearance with poorly demarcated lesions, often referred to as a ground-glass appearance.

Skull and spine x-rays: If CNS trauma has not been ruled out as a precipitating event, obtaining these x-rays is crucial. Until x-ray results are known, the patient's neck and spine must be immobilized.

COLLABORATIVE MANAGEMENT

Oxygen therapy: Oxygen (100%) is initiated immediately to treat hypoxia. High concentrations of oxygen are continued, even in alert patients with spontaneous ventilation, because of the risk of hypoxia and acidosis. Warmed oxygen 40°-43° C (104°-110° F) may be used as part of the rewarming process for patients with hypothermia.

Endotracheal intubation and positive end-expiratory pressure (PEEP):   Required when pulmonary edema or hypoxia is present and unresponsive to increasing levels of oxygen (Fio_2 ≥0.50 to maintain a Pao_2 ≥60 mm Hg). Intubation also assists in the maintenance of clear airways in patients who are unable to manage secretions independently. PEEP improves oxygenation by preventing the collapse of alveoli during expiration. It is especially useful after freshwater aspiration because it keeps alveoli open in the absence of adequate surfactant. PEEP should be removed cautiously because levels of surfactant can remain low for 48-72 h after freshwater aspiration.

Mechanical ventilation: Used in respiratory failure when lung compliance is decreased or when the patient is unable to maintain effective respiratory effort. PEEP is continued with mechanical ventilation when indicated. Patients with freshwater aspiration require 1½-2 times normal tidal volume at slower rates to allow optimal lung expansion and ventilation of alveoli. If neurologic involvement is present, decreased levels of $Paco_2$ can be achieved *via* mechanical hyperventilation.

Bronchoscopy: To remove aspirated contaminants, if necessary.

Rewarming for hypothermia: Warm, moist oxygen 40°-43° C (104°-110° F) may be used to elevate core temperature. Peritoneal lavage also is used for rewarming. Fluid for lavage is warmed to 37° C (98.6° F). The goal is quick rewarming to achieve a normal core temperature.

Pharmacotherapy: Metabolic acidosis is treated with sodium bicarbonate and careful monitoring of arterial pH. If bronchospasm is present, aerosolized bronchodilators may be used.

Note: Use of steroids and prophylactic antibiotics is controversial. Temperature elevation up to 38° C (101° F) during the first 24 h can be a normal response to injury. Antibiotics may be prescribed if fever ≥38° C (101° F) persists for longer than 24 h after the submersion.

Fluid and electrolyte management: Although uncommon, fluid and electrolyte abnormalities may occur. Usually no specific therapy is required for minor disturbances. Fluid volume may be replaced with crystalloid solutions (Ringer's lactate or normal saline).

Neurologic support: Depends on the severity of the neurologic impairment. Severe impairment may necessitate intracranial pressure monitoring, steroids, hyperosmolar diuretics (e.g., mannitol), mechanical ventilation to maintain $Paco_2$ <30 mm Hg or a barbiturate coma (see "Craniocerebral Trauma," p. 133), and deep hypothermia (core temperature <30° C [86° F]).

Management of event that precipitated the near drowning: Conditions such as alcohol or drug ingestion, seizure, myocardial infarction, or cervical spine fracture.

NURSING DIAGNOSES AND INTERVENTIONS

Impaired gas exchange related to alveolar-capillary membrane changes secondary to fluid accumulation in the lung or loss of surfactant

Desired outcome: Within 12 h of initiation of treatment, patient has adequate gas exchange as evidenced by the following ABG values: Pao_2 ≥60 mm Hg and $Paco_2$ ≤45 mm Hg. Within 3 days of treatment, RR is ≤20 breaths/min with normal depth and pattern (eupnea); breath sounds are clear and bilaterally equal; and patient is oriented to time, place, and person (depending on degree of permanent neurologic impairment).

- Auscultate lung fields at frequent intervals. Note the type and extent of adventitious breath sounds (e.g., crackles, rhonchi, friction rubs); document findings. Consult physician if acute changes occur.
- Monitor ABG values and/or oxygen saturation *via* pulse oximetry. Hypoxemia is common. Progressive hypoxemia may require in-

creased concentrations of oxygen or mechanical ventilation. Alert physician accordingly.

- Assess patient for indicators of increased respiratory effort: complaints of SOB, tachypnea (RR >20 breaths/min), change in the use of accessory muscles of respiration, nasal flaring, grunting, restlessness, and anxiety.
- Place patient in semi-Fowler's position to optimize lung expansion and decrease work of breathing.
- Assess patient's need for suctioning at frequent intervals. Document color, consistency, amount of sputum; frequency of suctioning to maintain clear airway; and patient's response to the procedure.
- If patient is receiving PEEP therapy, be aware that alveoli collapse when PEEP is removed. Oxygenation levels achieved before suctioning will not be attained immediately after PEEP is reinstituted because the effect PEEP exerts on alveoli is not instantaneous. To prevent dramatic decreases in Pao_2 with suctioning, use of a PEEP adapter or manual resuscitator is recommended for patients receiving high levels of PEEP. (See "Mechanical Ventilation," p. 20, for details.) An in-line suction device may prevent hypoxia associated with suctioning.
- Provide rest periods between activities to decrease oxygen demands.
- Explain all procedures to patient, and provide emotional support to decrease anxiety, which can contribute to oxygen consumption.

Hypothermia related to prolonged exposure to cold water during submersion

Desired outcomes: Within 24 h of initiating therapy, patient's core temperature increases to 35°-37° C (95°-98.6° F). BP, RR, and HR are within patient's normal limits.

- Use temperature probe to obtain a continuous measurement of patient's core temperature. If a pulmonary artery catheter is in place, the cardiac output thermodilution probe can be used to monitor core body temperature. The temperature of inspired gases may affect accuracy of this measurement. Other methods for measuring core temperature include bladder thermometry, rectal probe, or esophageal temperature probe, which is positioned in the lower third of the esophagus.
- Monitor patient's response to rewarming. Assess temperature and humidity level of inspired oxygen. Monitor temperature of instilled peritoneal lavage fluid. Do not attempt surface or external warming until core temperature is within acceptable limits (i.e., 35°-37° C [95°-98.6° F]). Premature surface rewarming can lead to the return of cold blood to the heart and precipitate an "after-drop" in core temperature.
- After core temperature has reached acceptable limits, monitor patient's response to active rewarming of body surface. Rewarming can be achieved by warm baths, heating pads, or lights. Cover patient's head to prevent heat loss from this exposed area. Use of blankets alone is an inadequate method of rewarming surface areas except in cases of mild hypothermia.
- Be aware of the likelihood of decreased drug metabolism during patient's hypothermic period.

Risk for infection related to increased environmental exposure secondary to aspiration of water and contaminants present in water

Desired outcome: Patient is free of infection as evidenced by body temperature ≤37.5° C (99.6° F) after the first 24 h, WBC count within normal limits for patient, clear sputum, and negative culture results.

- Monitor temperature q2h. Increases in temperature up to 38° C (100.4° F) are common during the first 24 h. After 24 h, an increased temperature may be indicative of infection.
- Monitor WBC count, being alert to increases from baseline values.
- Inspect sputum for changes in color, consistency, and amount.
- Use meticulous aseptic technique when suctioning patient's secretions.
- Collect sputum specimen for Gram's stain and culture and sensitivity as prescribed. These tests will identify the pathogen if infection is present.

ADDITIONAL NURSING DIAGNOSES

Also see "Major Trauma" for **Posttrauma response,** p. 123. See other nursing diagnoses and interventions in "Psychosocial Support," p. 88, and "Psychosocial Support for the Patient's Family and Significant Others," p. 100.

Cardiac trauma

PATHOPHYSIOLOGY

Cardiac trauma may be caused by blunt or penetrating injuries to the heart. *Blunt cardiac trauma* commonly is caused by acceleration-deceleration injuries in vehicular collision, during which the driver slams forward against the steering wheel. When this occurs, the heart muscle is injured by one or more of four mechanisms: compression of the heart between the sternum and vertebrae, bruising of heart tissue by bony structures, rupture or compression of coronary arteries by the blow, or cardiac rupture due to intrathoracic or intraabdominal pressure.

Blunt cardiac trauma can be classified as cardiac concussion or cardiac contusion. With cardiac concussion, the less severe injury, the patient will demonstrate many of the clinical signs and symptoms of cardiac trauma, without any evidence of cellular injury. Cardiac concussion leads to a transient myocardial dysfunction and some tissue edema but not to cellular damage or increase in serum CK-MB isoenzymes. The tissue damage, however, may lead to temporary cardiac dysrhythmias. In comparison, cardiac contusion involves demonstrable cellular damage. The patient has varying degrees of cellular injury and necrosis, ranging from small areas of bruising to full-thickness cellular necrosis and permanent myocardial scarring. The patient may exhibit signs and symptoms similar to those manifested by individuals with myocardial infarction. The walls of the right ventricle are those most often injured because they are located directly behind the sternum. Blunt trauma also may damage cardiac valves, particularly the aortic and mitral valves, the ventricular septum, and the papillary muscle attachment. Rupture of the left ventricle from blunt forces generally leads to death in a few minutes, whereas rupture of the right ventricle sometimes can be successfully managed. Ventricular rupture also may occur up to 2 wk after injury if the contused area of the heart fails to heal and instead softens and weakens.

Penetrating cardiac trauma is caused by gunshot wounds, stab wounds, or foreign bodies in the heart. The right ventricle, because of its anterior location, is the most common chamber involved in this type of injury. Penetrating injuries are the most common cause of intrapericardial hemorrhage (see "Acute Cardiac Tamponade," p. 152).

ASSESSMENT

HISTORY AND RISK FACTORS Motor vehicle collision, assault, sporting injuries, car-pedestrian collision.

CLINICAL PRESENTATION

Blunt injury: Precordial chest pain (difficult to distinguish from angina), bradycardia or tachycardia, SOB, guarded breathing.

Penetrating injury: Tachycardia, SOB, weakness, diaphoresis, acute anxiety, cool and clammy skin.

PHYSICAL ASSESSMENT

Blunt injury: Contusion marks on chest (may outline shape of steering wheel), flail chest (loss of continuity of bony thorax because of rib fracture) with resulting paradoxic respiratory movement of the chest wall, murmurs indicating valvular injury, atrial or ventricular gallops (if cardiac injury has decreased ventricular contractility).

Penetrating injury: Protrusion of penetrating instrument (e.g., knife, ice pick), external puncture wound, signs of cardiac tamponade (see "Acute Cardiac Tamponade," p. 152).

ECG AND HEMODYNAMIC MEASUREMENTS

Cardiac monitor: Sinus tachycardia, sinus bradycardia, ventricular tachycardia, ventricular fibrillation, asystole, and ST-segment and T-wave changes.

Arterial blood pressure: Decreased.

DIAGNOSTIC TESTS

There is no clear agreement on the diagnostic criteria for the medical diagnosis of cardiac contusion. Elevations of the CK-MB fraction and the results of echocardiography, electrocardiography, and myocardial scanning are considered useful aids in making the diagnosis, but no single test is widely accepted as the definitive diagnostic tool. In addition, these diagnostic methods lack sensitive and specific indicators of myocardial damage. The following diagnostic tests may demonstrate abnormal results with cardiac contusion.

Chest x-ray: Although heart muscle damage will not appear on routine chest x-ray, findings may reveal damage to bony structures of the chest.

Cardiac enzyme levels: CK and the MB subfraction may increase in the first 3-4 h after injury to levels >7%-8% of the total CK. In the patient with multiple trauma, however, the myocardium may not be the only source of CK-MB release. Injury to the liver, skeletal muscles, stomach, pancreas, and bowel also may lead to CK-MB elevations.

ECG: Cardiac injury may cause alterations in depolarization, repolarization, and muscle perfusion. The following abnormalities may occur: ST-segment changes, T-wave changes, prolongation of the QT interval, sinus tachycardia, heart block, and ventricular dysrhythmias. The ability of the ECG to determine myocardial contusion currently is being questioned. ECG changes are detected in <40% of all contusions, possibly because the right ventricle is the heart's most anterior structure and thus the area most likely to be damaged. The majority of ECG changes reflect changes in the large muscle mass of the left ventricle rather than the right.

Multiple-gated acquisition (MUGA) scan: In the presence of a contusion, detects decreased ability of the heart to pump efficiently.

Echocardiography: Detects abnormalities in wall motion and valvular function and presence of intracavity thrombi or pericardial effusion.

Transesophageal echocardiography (TEE):   A useful diagnostic tool when hemodynamic compromise occurs after chest trauma. It is particularly helpful in differentiating severe right ventricular contusion from acute cardiac tamponade. High-frequency sound waves are emitted from a transducer fitted to the end of a standard gastroscope approximately 9 mm in diameter. When the gastroscope is introduced into the esophagus, the transducer produces clear posterior images of the heart.

Technetium pyrophosphate myocardial scan: Identifies localized area(s) of radioisotope uptake by damaged myocardial cells, revealed as "hot spot(s)" on the scan.

COLLABORATIVE MANAGEMENT

For blunt injuries

Treatment of dysrhythmias: Antidysrhythmic agents (e.g., lidocaine for ventricular dysrhythmias and digitalis for pump failure or tachycardia) or temporary pacemakers for heart block. If rhythm disturbances do not appear in the first 5 days after trauma, they rarely occur later.

Relief of acute pain: Usually with IV morphine sulfate in small increments unless hypotension occurs.

Restriction of activity and institution of continuous observation

Immediate corrective surgical repair: For ruptured valve, torn papillary muscle, or torn intraventricular septum accompanied by hemodynamic instability.

Treatment of shock: With fluid resuscitation, pressor agents.

Treatment of myocardial failure: Oxygen, diuretics, positive inotropic agents, and monitoring with a pulmonary artery catheter for right- and left-sided heart pressures.

For penetrating injuries

Surgical intervention: Foreign bodies of reasonable size are localized by fluoroscopic examination and removed surgically.

Caution: Because of the potential for hemorrhage or pneumothorax, never remove a penetrating object until a surgeon is present.

Antimicrobial agents: To control infections that occur secondary to contamination by the penetrating instrument.

NURSING DIAGNOSES AND INTERVENTIONS

Altered peripheral, cardiopulmonary, renal, and cerebral tissue perfusion related to interruption of arterial and venous flow secondary to decreased cardiac contractility

Desired outcome: Within 12 h after injury, patient has adequate perfusion as evidenced by systolic BP ≥90 mm Hg (or within patient's normal range); HR ≤100 bpm; RR 12-20 breaths/min with normal depth and pattern (eupnea); ease of respiration; clear lung fields; urine output ≥0.5 ml/kg/h; brisk capillary refill (<2 sec); peripheral pulses >2+ on a 0-4+ scale; normal sinus rhythm; absence of neck vein distention with the HOB elevated to 30 degrees; and orientation to time, place, and person.

- Perform a complete cardiac assessment q4h, noting peripheral pulses, heart sounds, and capillary refill; assess heart rate and rhythm and BP hourly. For more assessment information, see **Decreased cardiac output,** p. 154, in "Acute Cardiac Tamponade" and **Impaired gas exchange,** p. 261, in "Pneumothorax."
- Perform a complete pulmonary assessment q4h, noting respiratory rate, depth, and effort. Auscultate lung fields q4h and as needed to evaluate for pulmonary congestion.
- Consult physician for changes in mental status, systolic BP <90 mm Hg or a drop of >20 mm Hg from trend, delayed capillary refill, or absent or thready peripheral pulses.
- Administer fluids as prescribed to maintain systolic BP at ≥90 mm Hg and urine output at ≥0.5 ml/kg/h.
- Maintain continuous cardiac monitoring for the first 3-4 days after cardiac trauma.
- If dysrhythmias occur, prepare to administer antidysrhythmic agents or assist with insertion of a transvenous temporary pacemaker.
- If hemodynamic instability occurs, place patient in supine position, if injuries allow, and prepare for initiation of pulmonary artery pressure monitoring.

Pain (acute precordial chest pain) related to biophysical injury secondary to myocardial damage and chest wall injury

Desired outcomes: Within 2 h after initiation of analgesic therapy, patient's subjective evaluation of discomfort improves, as documented by a pain scale. Nonverbal indicators, such as grimacing or diaphoresis, are absent or reduced.

- Assess and document location, type, severity, and duration of patient's discomfort. Devise a pain scale with patient, rating discomfort from 0 (no pain) to 10. Administer IV morphine or other analgesia as prescribed and record its effectiveness, using the pain scale. Pain may begin immediately after injury or after approximately 8 h. Usually, it is not affected by coronary vasodilators.
- Place patient in a position of comfort. Patients often prefer the HOB elevated at 30-45 degrees.
- If bony structures are damaged and pain limits coughing and deep breathing, assist patient with chest splinting during chest physio-

therapy. For some patients, intercostal nerve blocks may be necessary.
- Teach patient to recognize signs of posttraumatic pericarditis (i.e., fever, diaphoresis, and precordial chest pain) and to notify physician promptly if they occur.

ADDITIONAL NURSING DIAGNOSES

For other nursing diagnoses and interventions, see "Prolonged Immobility," p. 78; "Psychosocial Support," p. 88; and "Psychosocial Support of the Patient's Family and Significant Others," p. 100.

Acute cardiac tamponade

PATHOPHYSIOLOGY

Acute cardiac tamponade is the sudden accumulation of blood or fluid in the pericardial space, resulting in compression of the heart muscle and interference with cardiac filling during diastole and cardiac ejection during systole. Tamponade may occur as a result of blunt or penetrating cardiac trauma or as a complication after cardiac catheterization, anticoagulant therapy, myocardial infarction, or acute pericarditis.

The primary effect of sudden cardiac tamponade is hemodynamic compromise, with inadequate cardiac output and decreased tissue perfusion. Normally the pericardial sac contains 10-20 ml of fluid that protects the myocardium. Because the pericardial sac has minimal stretching ability, the sudden addition of as little as 50-100 ml of fluid can increase intrapericardial pressure markedly. As intrapericardial pressure increases and exceeds central venous pressure, the atria, ventricles, and coronary arteries become compressed. The compressed heart chambers, which no longer can hold their usual volume, cause a reduction in end-diastolic volume and end-diastolic fiber stretch and a decrease in stroke volume. Ultimately, decreased cardiac output and poor tissue perfusion occur.

ASSESSMENT

CLINICAL PRESENTATION Tachycardia, decreased BP, shock, pallor, confusion, restlessness, cold and clammy skin, dyspnea, oliguria, thready pulse.
Classic signs: Beck's triad (distended neck veins, hypotension, muffled heart tones). Distended neck veins usually are not present in acute traumatic tamponade (as compared with constrictive pericarditis) because of hypovolemia and an acceleration of blood into the right atrium during inspiration. Beck's triad occurs in <33% of patients with acute cardiac tamponade. Muffled heart tones may not be present if the patient is sitting upright because gravity pulls the blood toward the bottom of the pericardial sac.
PHYSICAL ASSESSMENT See Table 2-6.

Note: In severe hypovolemic states, physical signs may be masked.

T A B L E 2 - 6 Physical signs of acute cardiac tamponade

Physical sign	Explanation for findings
Muffled heart sounds	Accumulation of fluid surrounding the heart diminishes sounds of valve closure
CVP elevated to >12 mm Hg	Mean right atrial pressure is elevated because diastolic filling is impeded by atrial compression
Decreased BP	Compression by tamponade reduces ventricular filling, decreasing CO and BP
Jugular venous distention	As atria and ventricles become compressed, there is less space for diastolic filling, causing impairment of venous return
Pulsus paradoxus: a fall of ≥10 mm Hg in systolic BP during inspiration	Two possible explanations: (1) during each inspiration, blood pools in pulmonary veins, reducing left ventricular filling and output; (2) with inspiration, intraventricular septum shifts toward left ventricle, causing more volume to be drawn to right side rather than to left side of heart
Absence of Kussmaul's sign: Kussmaul's sign is a rise, rather than fall, in venous pressure during inspiration	On inspiration, blood is accelerated toward the right atrium because of septal shift toward left ventricle

ECG AND HEMODYNAMIC MEASUREMENTS

Cardiac monitor: May show evidence of sinus tachycardia or electrical alternans (see "ECG," below).

Pulmonary artery pressure: Elevation of right atrial pressure (early sign if severe hypotension does not occur); elevation of left ventricular end-diastolic pressure (late sign).

DIAGNOSTIC TESTS

ECG: May reveal ST-segment elevation, nonspecific ST and T-wave changes (representing myocardial ischemia), and electrical alternans (alternation of the QRS axis from beat to beat) caused by the heart's movement like a pendulum within the pericardial effusion. The underlying mechanism for this movement is not understood.

Chest x-ray: May reveal normal cardiac silhouette, clear lung fields, dilatation of the superior vena cava, and an enlarged mediastinum.

Echocardiography: May show echo-free space anterior to the right ventricular wall and posterior to the left ventricular wall, with a decrease in right ventricular chamber size. There will be right-to-left intraventricular septal shift during inspiration.

Transesophageal echocardiography (TEE): See discussion with "Cardiac Trauma," p. 150.

COLLABORATIVE MANAGEMENT

Pericardiocentesis: Needle aspiration of the pericardium by the subxiphoid or left parasternal approach to drain the pericardial space of the excess fluid. Often the blood removed from the pericardium will not clot due to breaking down of clotting factors (defibrination) within the pericardial sac by heart action. Evidence exists that pericardiocentesis alone does not manage acute pericardial tamponade; surgical exploration is recommended after this procedure because of the high incidence of recurrent bleeding if surgery is not performed.

Surgical procedures: Subxiphoid pericardiostomy involves a resection of the xiphoid process to drain the pericardial sac; it can be performed with the patient under local anesthesia. In addition, other more extensive surgical procedures such as a pericardiectomy can be used to decompress a pericardial tamponade. If the patient suddenly has signs of bradycardia (HR <50 bpm), severe hypotension (systolic BP <70 mm Hg), or cardiac arrest, an immediate thoracotomy is performed in the emergency department or ICU to allow for pericardial sac evacuation, hemorrhage control, and internal cardiac massage if needed.

Fluid resuscitation: To increase filling pressures during diastole, resulting in increased cardiac output and BP. Blood products, colloids, or crystalloids may be used.

Inotropic agents: To increase myocardial contractility and support cardiac output. Examples include dopamine, norepinephrine, phenylephrine, isoproterenol, and amrinone. For more information, see Appendix 7.

Oxygen, intubation, mechanical ventilation: Usually oxygen is administered *via* face mask; more aggressive therapy is used, as necessary, to correct hypoxia.

NURSING DIAGNOSES AND INTERVENTIONS

Decreased cardiac output related to decreased preload secondary to compression of ventricles by fluid in the pericardial sac

Desired outcome: Within 4-6 h after management with fluids or evacuation of tamponade, patient has adequate cardiac output as evidenced by mean RAP 4-6 mm Hg, mean PAWP 6-12 mm Hg, PAP 20-30/8-15 mm Hg, CO 4-7 L/min, systolic BP ≥90 mm Hg (or within patient's normal range), HR 60-100 bpm, normal sinus rhythm on ECG, and absence of new murmurs or gallops, distended neck veins, and pulsus paradoxus.

- Assess cardiovascular function by evaluating heart sounds and neck veins hourly. Consult physician for muffled heart sounds, new murmurs, new gallops, irregularities in rate and rhythm, and distended neck veins.
- Monitor all patients with blunt or penetrating trauma to the chest and abdomen for physical signs of acute cardiac tamponade (see Table 2-6), persistent hemodynamic instability, and shock out of proportion to the apparent blood loss.
- Evaluate patient for pulsus paradoxus: an abnormal decrease in ar-

T A B L E 2 - 7   Measuring paradoxic pulse

- After placing BP cuff on patient, inflate it above the known systolic BP. Instruct patient to breathe normally.
- While slowly deflating the cuff, auscultate BP.
- Listen for the first Korotkoff's sound, which will occur during expiration with cardiac tamponade.
- Note the manometer reading when the first sound occurs, and continue to deflate the cuff slowly until Korotkoff's sounds are audible throughout inspiration and expiration.
- Record the difference in millimeters of mercury between the first and second sounds. This is the pulsus paradoxus.

---

terial systolic BP during inspiration compared with that with expiration. See Table 2-7.

- Measure and record hemodynamic parameters. Consult physician for abnormalities or changes in trend. Early signs of tamponade include elevated RAP with normal BP. Later signs include elevated PAP in the presence of hypotension.
- Evaluate ECG for ST-segment changes, T-wave changes, rate, and rhythm. The optimal is sinus rhythm or sinus tachycardia. Maintain continuous cardiac monitoring.
- Administer blood products, colloids, or crystalloids through large-bore IV lines in the periphery, if possible. Compared with the longer and narrower central catheters, large-bore peripheral IV catheters provide less resistance to rapid infusion during fluid resuscitation. Use pressure infusers and rapid volume/warmer infusers for patients who require massive fluid resuscitation. Be prepared to administer pressor agents if fluid resuscitation does not support patient's BP.
- Have emergency equipment available for immediate pulmonary artery catheterization, central line insertion, pericardiocentesis, or thoracotomy.

Altered cardiopulmonary, peripheral, cerebral, and renal tissue perfusion related to interruption of arterial and venous flow secondary to compression of the myocardium by the collection of blood
Desired outcome: Within 4-6 h after management with fluids or evacuation of tamponade, patient has adequate perfusion as evidenced by orientation to time, place, and person; systolic BP $\geq$90 mm Hg (or within patient's normal range); RR 12-20 breaths/min with normal depth and pattern (eupnea) and ease of respirations; Sao_2 >95%; peripheral pulses >2+ on a 0-4+ scale; equal and normoreactive pupils; warm and dry skin; brisk capillary refill (<2 sec); and urine output $\geq$0.5 ml/kg/h.

- Assess tissue perfusion by evaluating the following at least hourly: LOC, BP, pulses, pupillary response, skin temperature, and capillary refill.
- Evaluate urine output hourly to ensure that it is at least 0.5 ml/kg/h. Assess urine specific gravity q4h; elevations (>1.030) may signal hypovolemia and inadequate renal perfusion.

- Maintain tissue perfusion by delivering prescribed blood products, colloids, or crystalloids.
- If hypotension occurs, be prepared to administer medication to maintain BP. Be familiar with dosage, side effects, and calculations necessary for administration. At frequent intervals, assess peripheral IV lines for evidence of infiltration. Pressor agents, which infiltrate subcutaneous tissues, jeopardize future tissue perfusion.

Note: When it is feasible, all pressor agents (e.g., norepinephrine, dopamine) should be infused through a central line.

- Have emergency equipment available for delivery of humidified oxygen, intubation, and mechanical ventilation.

ADDITIONAL NURSING DIAGNOSES

For other nursing diagnoses and interventions see "Prolonged Immobility," p. 78; "Psychosocial Support," p. 88; and "Psychosocial Support for the Patient's Family and Significant Others," p. 100.

Renal and lower urinary tract trauma

PATHOPHYSIOLOGY

Injuries to the kidneys and lower urinary tract (LUT), which includes the ureters, urinary bladder, and urethra, occur in <1% of all trauma patients but have the potential for lifelong complications or even death. These injuries often are overlooked in the initial trauma assessment because they frequently accompany life-threatening injuries that require aggressive and immediate management.

Blunt injuries are responsible for most renal and LUT trauma and are caused by vehicular collisions, falls, sports-related injuries, and assaults. Renal and LUT trauma also can occur after penetrating injuries, such as stab and gunshot wounds. The specific pathophysiology for each type of renal and LUT trauma is discussed in Table 2-8.

ASSESSMENT
Renal trauma

CLINICAL PRESENTATION Abdominal or flank pain, back tenderness, colicky pain with passage of blood clots, hemorrhage (pallor, diaphoresis, hypotension, tachycardia, restlessness, confusion), gross or microscopic hematuria.

Note: Gross hematuria is present in slightly more than half of patients with renal trauma and is considered an unreliable diagnostic sign.

PHYSICAL ASSESSMENT Hematoma over the flank of the eleventh or twelfth ribs; obvious wounds, contusions, or abrasions in the flank or abdomen; abdominal distention; Grey Turner's sign (bruising over the lower portion of the back and the flank due to a retroperitoneal hemorrhage); pain at the costovertebral angle; flank or abdominal mass.

T A B L E   2 - 8   Pathophysiology for renal and lower urinary tract trauma

Type of injury	Anatomic considerations	Pathophysiology and mechanism of injury	Result of injury
Renal trauma	Kidneys are well protected from injury posteriorly by muscles of the back, anteriorly by organs of the GI tract, and by a tough outer capsule and adipose tissue Kidneys are fixed in retroperitoneal space only by renal pedicle (vascular stem in renal hilum) and ureters Blunt renal injury is often due to compression of kidney by the twelfth rib, which rotates inwardly and squeezes kidney into lumbar spine	Renal trauma can be divided into three classifications: **Minor trauma: Incidence 85%** Bruising of renal parenchyma; superficial lacerations of renal cortex without rupture of renal capsule **Major trauma: Incidence 10%-15%** Major lacerations through cortex and medulla; continuation of laceration through renal capsule **Critical trauma: Incidence <5%** Renal vascular trauma in which kidney is shattered and renal pedicle is injured; fragmentation (renal fracture)	**Minor trauma:** Hematuria and flank tenderness that with rest and observation will usually result in a full recovery **Major trauma:** Hematuria, flank pain, and possible hypotension that may require surgical intervention **Critical injury:** Severe blood loss and shock requiring immediate surgical intervention
Ureteral trauma	Injury to upper part of ureter is uncommon because of its location deep in retroperitoneum Ureteral lacerations are most common at ureteropelvic junction, where upper ureter joins renal pelvis	Ureteral injury is most commonly associated with iatrogenic injuries during gynecologic, colonic, and vascular surgery Blunt injury may occur when ureter becomes crushed against spinal column When ureteral injury is not associated with iatrogenic injury, it usually occurs in the setting of severe abdominal compression or significant penetrating abdominal injury	Extravasation of urine or blood may lead to infection, abscess formation, hemorrhage, or shock; late complications include prolonged voiding time, ureteral strictures, and fistula formation

Continued.

T A B L E   2 - 8   Pathophysiology for renal and lower urinary tract trauma—cont'd

Bladder trauma	When bladder is distended, it extends above umbilicus and has less protection from trauma; the bladder ruptures at its point of least resistance (the dome), and blood and urine extravasate into the peritoneal cavity (intraperitoneal rupture) Extraperitoneal rupture occurs most often in conjunction with pelvic fractures; sharp bone fragments perforate bladder at its base, leading to extravasation of blood and urine into the space surrounding bladder base	Motor vehicle crashes are the most common cause of bladder rupture; bladder contusion often results from a direct blow or the cavitational effect of missiles (outward tissue acceleration away from the tract of the bullet); bladder rupture does not require extensive force, which may be a blunt blow to the lower abdomen	Bladder lacerations or rupture can lead to blood or urine extravasation outside of the peritoneal cavity (80%) and into the peritoneal cavity (20%); infection or hemorrhage can follow
Urethral trauma	Urethral injury is more common in males than females because the male urethra is 5 times longer; the male urethra is also rigidly fixed at the urogenital diaphragm (bulbous urethra), whereas the female urethra is short and mobile	Perineal trauma, straddle injuries, and pelvic fractures are often the causes of urethral injury; vehicular collisions with deceleration and shearing may also lead to injury of the posterior urethra	Urethral injury may lead to extravasation of blood and/or urine within penis; if disruption to Buck's fascia occurs, extravasation into upper thighs and peritoneum follows; hemorrhage or infection may also occur

Note: Physical signs may be masked because of the protection of the kidneys by abdominal organs, back muscles, and bony structures.

Ureteral trauma

CLINICAL PRESENTATION May be few early signs. Microscopic or gross hematuria may be present. If the ureter is completely transected, normal urine from the unaffected kidney may be voided. *Late signs* may include fever and flank or abdominal discomfort.

PHYSICAL ASSESSMENT Urine at the entrance or exit sites of penetrating wound, enlarging retroperitoneal mass.

Bladder trauma

CLINICAL PRESENTATION Suprapubic tenderness, inability to void spontaneously, gross hematuria (present in approximately 95% of patients). *Late signs* may include fever and abdominal discomfort.

PHYSICAL ASSESSMENT Perineal or scrotal edema and hematoma, abnormal position of prostate, abdominal distention, palpable suprapubic mass, palpable and overdistended bladder.

Urethral trauma

CLINICAL PRESENTATION Inability to void spontaneously, urethral bleeding, prostate tenderness, microscopic or gross hematuria, pain and tenderness of genitalia.

PHYSICAL ASSESSMENT Blood at urethral meatus, tracking of urine into tissues of the thighs or abdominal wall, bruised to discolored genitalia.

DIAGNOSTIC TESTS

Retrograde urethrogram: A small urinary catheter is inserted and the balloon inflated to 2 ml in the distal anterior urethra, 2 cm from the urinary meatus. Contrast material, 5-10 ml, is injected and a single x-ray is taken to outline the inner size and shape of the urethra. In urethral rupture, extravasation of the contrast material occurs, usually near the membranous urethra.

Cystogram: If no urethral tear is found on retrograde urethrogram, a catheter is inserted into the bladder. The bladder is filled with 300 ml of contrast material. After x-rays are obtained to determine if intraperitoneal or extraperitoneal extravasation of contrast material occurs, the bladder is drained and repeat x-rays are taken to check for small posterior ruptures.

Excretory urogram/intravenous pyelogram: Contrast material is administered intravenously and is filtered by the kidneys before excretion through the urinary tract. X-rays provide visualization of the normal or injured structures of the kidneys, ureters, or bladder.

Caution: Check patient for a history of allergy to iodine, iodine-containing foods, or contrast material. Adequate hydration and sometimes diuretics are needed to rid the body of contrast material after this test.

Renal ultrasound: A transducer transmits high-frequency sound waves through the urinary tract. The resultant echoes are amplified and converted into electrical impulses that are displayed on an oscilloscope.

The sound waves demonstrate the presence or absence of fluid accumulation, blood clots, and LUT structural damage.

Radionuclide imaging: After IV injection of a radionuclide, a radioactivity-detecting device scans and records the radioactive uptake to evaluate for injured LUT structures and alterations in renal blood flow. It takes 6-24 h for the substance to be excreted from the patient's body.

Blood urea nitrogen values: Measurement of the nitrogen fraction of urea, the end product of protein metabolism. Renal dysfunction causes insufficient excretion of urea, elevating nitrogenous wastes in the blood. In renal trauma, BUN level also may increase because of body catabolism or dehydration. Normal value is 10-20 mg/dl.

Serum creatinine levels: Measurement of a nonprotein end product of creatinine metabolism. Creatinine level measures renal damage more accurately than does the BUN level because renal impairment is virtually the only cause of elevated serum creatinine. Creatinine production is fairly constant day to day because production is proportional to muscle mass. Creatinine is freely filtered at the glomerulus and minimally reabsorbed, causing creatinine excretion to be roughly proportional to glomerular filtration rate. Normal value is 0.7-1.5 mg/dl.

Clearance tests: Clearance is the volume of plasma that can be cleared of a specific substance during a specified period of time. Clearance tests evaluate the extent of injury by assessing renal filtration, reabsorption, secretion, and renal plasma flow. Creatinine, inulin (a plant starch), and urea are the substances usually tested.

Kidney-ureter-bladder (KUB) radiography: Evaluates position, size, structure, and defects of kidney and LUT structures. Abnormal findings include retroperitoneal hematoma, fracture of the lower ribs or pelvis, foreign bodies, organ displacement, or fluid accumulation.

CT scan: Imaging of the kidneys *via* a series of cross-sectional slices that are then interpreted by computer. CT scanning after renal trauma may reveal hematomas, renal lacerations, renal infarcts, or extravasation of urine.

Renal angiography: Arterial injection of a contrast medium, permitting identification on x-ray of renal vasculature and functional tissue. After renal trauma, angiography permits identification of renal pedicle injury, renal infarct, intrarenal hematoma, lacerations, and shattered kidney.

Note: Assess patient for allergy to contrast medium, and maintain adequate hydration during and after the procedure.

MRI: Clarifies the surgical approach necessary for trauma such as traumatic posterior urethral injury and enables estimation of the length of injury.

COLLABORATIVE MANAGEMENT

Pharmacotherapy

Antibiotics: For positive urine culture results, penetrating injuries, or peritonitis.

Analgesics: IV morphine sulfate usually relieves the pain and can be readily reversed with naloxone if complications, such as hypotension or bradypnea, occur.

Management of complications

Hemorrhage shock: Rapid volume resuscitation.

Infections: Blood and urine cultures, antibiotics.

Renal dysfunction: Evaluation of need for fluid restriction; dietary restrictions of protein, sodium, or potassium; peritoneal dialysis; continuous arteriovenous hemofiltration (CAVH); continuous venovenous hemofiltration (CVVH); or hemodialysis. See "Renal Replacement Therapies," p. 410, for more information.

Catheterization: If patient is unable to void. Catheter should be passed only as far as it will progress without undue force. If any resistance is met during catheterization, a urethrogram is indicated. If blood is present at the urethral meatus, the patient should not be catheterized under any circumstances before the urethrogram is obtained inasmuch as the blood may signal urethral injury. In the presence of urethral injury, an improperly placed catheter can cause subsequent incontinence, impotence, and urethral strictures. In renal trauma, diversion of urine may be required by nephrostomy tube, depending on location of injury or in cases of coexisting pancreatic and duodenal injury. A suprapubic catheter may be used to manage severe urethral lacerations and urethral disruption. Internal ureteral catheters (ureteral stents) may be indicated for ureteral trauma, particularly for gunshot wounds, to maintain ureteral alignment, ensure urinary drainage, and provide support during anastomosis.

Surgical correction: Indicated for transected ureter, partial ureteral tears of more than a third of the circumference of the ureter, bladder perforation with associated abdominal injuries or intraperitoneal rupture, and injuries accompanied by rapidly expanding, pulsating hematomas. See Table 2-9 for examples of procedures for the various types of renal and LUT injuries.

NURSING DIAGNOSES AND INTERVENTIONS

Altered urinary elimination related to mechanical trauma secondary to injury to the kidney and LUT structures

Desired outcome: Within 6 h after immediate trauma management, patient has a urinary output of ≥0.5 ml/kg/h with no evidence of bladder distention.

- Ensure adequate urinary outflow by encouraging patient to void. If patient is unable to void, assess the need for urinary catheterization or suprapubic drainage by palpating gently for a full bladder. As indicated, discuss the need for a urinary catheter with physician. Monitor for the following signs of kidney or LUT trauma:
  □ Urge but inability to void spontaneously in spite of adequate volume replacement
  □ Blood at the urethral meatus
  □ Difficult or unsuccessful urinary catheterization
  □ Anuria after urinary catheterization
  □ Hematuria
- Do not catheterize patient if there is blood at the urethral meatus unless a urethrogram has indicated that catheterization can be per-

T A B L E   2 - 9   **Surgical procedures for renal and lower urinary tract trauma**

Type of injury	Surgical indications/surgical management
Minor renal trauma	None needed. Rest and observation with careful follow-up to prevent progressive deformity and to evaluate BP.
Major renal trauma	Surgical intervention if hypotension and hemodynamic instability occur.
Critical renal trauma	Immediate surgical exploration; low rates of renal salvage.
Proximal ureteral injury	Primary ureterostomy with end-to-end anastomosis.
Distal ureteral injury	Ureteral stenting or percutaneous nephrostomy, depending on location and extent of injury.
Bladder injury	Use of suprapubic drainage versus indwelling urethral catheter drainage is controversial. Use of suprapubic catheter avoids complications of prolonged urethral catheterization, particularly in males who are prone to the development of urethral strictures.
Urethral injury	Suprapubic cystotomy and drainage for temporary urinary evacuation. Urethral splinting and surgical reconstruction usually are delayed for 3-6 mo to allow reduction in bruising and swelling, which could delay healing of urinary structures.

formed safely. Do not force a catheter if resistance is felt. Call physician for consultation if urethral injury is suspected.
- Monitor serum BUN and creatinine. Elevations reflect ineffective removal of waste products. Normal values are as follows: serum BUN ≤20 mg/dl; serum creatinine ≤1.5 mg/dl.
- Document I&O hourly. Assess patency of urinary collection system hourly to determine if clots are occluding the system. If indicated, obtain prescription for catheter irrigation or call physician to irrigate catheter, according to agency policy.
- Sudden cessation of urine flow through the collection system (particularly if past output was >50 ml/h) indicates possible catheter obstruction. If catheter irrigation does not resume urine drainage, consider changing the urinary catheter after discussion with physician.
- Ensure that the nephrostomy tube is not occluded by patient's weight or external pressure. Irrigate the nephrostomy tube *only* if prescribed, and with ≤5 ml of fluid, because the renal pelvis can hold no more than 10 ml fluid.
- Assess entrance site of the nephrostomy tube for bleeding or leakage of urine. Catheter blockage with clots or catheter dislodging can cause a sudden decrease in urine output. Consult physician if urine output is <0.5 ml/kg/h.
- Assess urine for color and presence or absence or clots. Expect he-

maturia for the first 24-48 h after nephrostomy tube insertion. Consult physician if gross bleeding (with or without clots) occurs.

- Ensure adequate hydration to allow for clearing of contrast material from patient's system after diagnostic testing.

Risk for infection related to inadequate primary defenses and tissue destruction secondary to bacterial contamination of the urinary tract system occurring with penetrating trauma, rupture of the bladder into the perineum, or instrumentation

Desired outcome: Patient is free of infection as evidenced by normothermia, WBC count ≤11,000 μl, and negative results of urine and wound drainage testing for infective organisms.

- Use aseptic technique when caring for urinary drainage systems. Maintain catheters and collection container at a level lower than the bladder to prevent reflux; keep drainage tubing unkinked.
- Record the color, odor, and specific gravity of urine each shift. Culture urine specimen when infection is suspected.
- Monitor patient's WBC count daily and temperature q4h for elevations.
- Assess patient each shift for signs of peritonitis: abdominal pain, abdominal distention with rigidity, nausea, vomiting, fever, malaise, and weakness.
- Assess catheter exit site each shift for the presence of erythema, swelling, or drainage.
- Assess thigh, groin, and lower portion of abdomen for indicators of urinary extravasation: swelling, pain, mass(es), erythema, tracking of urine along fascial planes.
- Assess surgical incision for approximation of suture line and evidence of wound healing, noting presence of erythema, swelling, and drainage. Note and record color, odor, and consistency of wound drainage. As prescribed, culture any drainage that appears purulent or is foul smelling; notify physician of results.
- At least q8h assess skin at all catheter entrance sites for indicators of irritation: erythema, drainage, and swelling.
- Cleanse insertion site q8h with antimicrobial solution. Apply sterile gauze pad(s) over suprapubic catheter exit site and tape securely with paper tape. Change dressings q24h or as soon as they become wet. If erythema and swelling occur as a result of maceration from contact with urine, consider use of a pectin wafer skin barrier for extra protection.

Pain (acute tenderness in lower abdomen) related to physical injury associated with LUT structural injury, procedures for urinary diversion, or surgical incisions

Desired outcomes: Within 2 h after giving analgesia, patient's subjective evaluation of discomfort improves, as documented by a pain scale. Nonverbal indicators of discomfort, such as grimacing, are absent.

- Assess patient for pain at least q4h. Devise a pain scale with patient, rating discomfort from 0 (no pain) to 10. Be alert to shallow breathing in the presence of abdominal pain, which can cause inadequate pulmonary excursion. Medicate promptly and document patient's response to analgesia, using the pain scale. IV narcotics may be indicated if the injury is severe.

- Explain the cause of the pain to the patient.
- Assist patient into a position of comfort. Often knee flexion will relax lower abdominal muscles and help reduce discomfort.
- Implement nonpharmacologic measures for coping with pain: diversion, touch, conversation. Also see discussion of pain, p. 66.

Pelvic fractures

PATHOPHYSIOLOGY

The pelvis is composed of three bones: two innominate bones and the sacrum. The innominate bones are each composed of three bones (ilium, pubis, and ischium) that fuse after childhood. The two innominate bones are joined by the symphysis pubis, a fibrous cartilage joint that connects the two pubic bones anteriorly, and attached posteriorly to a third bone, the sacrum, by a system of ligaments termed the posterior osseous ligamentous structures.

Motor vehicle collisions and auto-pedestrian trauma cause approximately two thirds of all pelvic fractures, which have mortality rates of up to 50% in some studies. For a pelvic fracture to occur, a large force is needed because these bones are stabilized by a strong network of ligaments. Pelvic fractures have been classified by several systems, but perhaps the most helpful are the systems that classify fractures by their stability and mechanism of injury (see Table 2-10). Pelvic fractures are considered stable fractures when the posterior osseous ligamentous structures are intact. An unstable pelvic fracture occurs when the osseous ligamentous structures are disrupted posteriorly and portions of the pelvis can move in any direction.

The most serious complications from a pelvic fracture are hemorrhage and exsanguination, which cause up to 60% of the deaths from pelvic injuries. The pelvis receives a rich supply of blood from a complex system of interconnected collateral arteries and the venous plexus of the iliac system, often called the "vascular sink." The aorta and internal iliac artery have close proximity to the pelvis as well. This complex vascular network easily can be damaged or disrupted by the same forces that injure the pelvis, or pelvic fragments can damage vascular structures. Because the retroperitoneal space can hold as much as 4 L of blood before spontaneous tamponade occurs, acute blood loss is difficult to identify until systemic symptoms, such as those with shock, appear. In addition, damage to the sciatic and sacral nerves may occur with sacral and sacroiliac disruption.

ASSESSMENT

HISTORY AND RISK FACTORS Motor vehicle or motorcycle crash, auto-pedestrian collision, fall, industrial accident, crush injury, sports injury.

CLINICAL PRESENTATION Suprapubic tenderness; pain over the iliac spines; signs and symptoms of hemorrhagic shock (tachycardia, delayed capillary refill, decreased urinary output, decreased extremity temperature, pallor, hypotension); signs and symptoms of urinary in-

T A B L E 2 - 1 0   Classification of pelvic fractures

Classification of injury	Mechanism of injury	Description
Anteroposterior compression	External rotation is caused by a crushing force on the posterior superior iliac spines.	"Open book injury;" The force causes the symphysis pubis to spring open. Rupture of anterior sacroiliac and sacrospinous ligaments occurs, but posterior ligaments are intact. Stable vertically but can rotate externally. May be associated with ruptured bladder (intraperitoneal) if injury occurs when bladder is full.
Lateral compression	Internal rotation from a high-energy injury that causes direct pressure to crush anterior sacrum. Pressure on the greater trochanter causes the femoral head to displace the anterior pubic rami.	Most common type of injury. Often does not affect posterior ligamentous complex. Partially unstable fracture that is rotationally unstable but vertically stable. May have extensive soft tissue injury. May be associated with ruptured bladder (extraperitoneal).
Vertical shear (Malgaigne's fracture)	Excessive force from trauma such as falls and crush injuries in a vertical plane leads to unstable disruption of the anterior and posterior ring.	Most severe injury with the highest mortality rates. Very unstable. Complete disruption of the posterior osseous ligamentous system. Often accompanied by injuries of the skin and subcutaneous tissues or injuries to the gastrointestinal, genitourinary, vascular, and neurologic systems.
Complex fracture	Excessive and powerful forces from many directions.	Pelvic ring disruptions resulting in bizarre fractures or dislocations in a combination of injury patterns. Usually very unstable.

juries (up to 15% of trauma victims with a pelvic fracture have associated renal and lower urinary tract injuries; see p. 156).

Note: Initial evaluation of a patient with multiple trauma and a pelvic fracture may reveal no obvious evidence of pelvic injury.

PHYSICAL ASSESSMENT Groin, genitalia, and suprapubic swelling or ecchymosis; swelling and ecchymosis of medial thigh or lumbosacral area; pelvic instability (asymmetry or abnormal movement on downward pressure of the iliac crests); crepitus; lower extremity shortening; abnormal lower extremity internal rotation; "frog-leg positioning" of the lower extremities; hematuria or urethral bleeding; vaginal bleeding; blood in the rectum; lower extremity paresis or hypoesthesia; absence of plantar flexion and ankle jerk reflexes; unequal or weak peripheral pulses.

Note: Lacerations of the perineum, groin, or buttocks are assumed to be caused by compound open pelvic fractures until proven otherwise.

DIAGNOSTIC TESTS
Pelvic x-ray
Anteroposterior view: Differentiates between a stable and unstable fracture; shows overall alignment, hip assessment, and location of fractures.
Inlet view: Determines rotational displacement, posterior displacement, sacral fractures.
Outlet view: Demonstrates superior rotation, vertical migration, sacral fractures.
CT scan: Ascertains pattern of pelvic injury. This is the most reliable method for determining injury to the posterior portion of the pelvis and is particularly successful in identifying sacral and sacroiliac joint injury.
Angiography: Identifies the site of bleeding, which often occurs at multiple points in the pelvic circulation. Two groups of patients have angiograms: those who undergo full laparotomy and are discovered to have an expanding pelvic retroperitoneal hematoma, and those with a pure pelvic injury who bleed internally.
Hematocrit: A value that fails to stabilize, falls, or fails to rise with transfusion is an indication of ongoing bleeding. A falling Hct is a late sign of hemorrhage and occurs only after significant blood loss.
Excretory urography (intravenous pyelogram), cystography, and urography: Used to determine associated injuries (see "Renal and Lower Urinary Tract Trauma," p. 159).

COLLABORATIVE MANAGEMENT
Pelvic stabilization
External immobilization: Defined as any device that is applied to immobilize the pelvis either externally or percutaneously through the skin into the bone. External fixation can be accomplished at the scene of injury to preserve function and prevent further orthopedic and neurovascular injury. Pneumatic antishock garments (PASG) sometimes are used to immobilize bony injuries as well as provide a tamponade

effect, but their use is controversial (see below). If abnormal shortening or rotation has occurred with the injury, the lower extremities should be supported and stabilized in the position in which they were found with a wooden backboard and supported by pillows, towels, or blankets taped in place with cloth tape. Most patients are managed with bed rest, spica casts, or sling traction. Emergency external fixation devices, consisting of one pin in each iliac wing connected by a bar, can be inserted to provide pelvic stability. If an emergency laparotomy is needed, a more complex external fixation device may be applied.

Note: Use of an external fixation device is not sufficient for maintaining reduction in the posterior pelvis or for stabilizing the pelvic posterior elements. As long as the patient is on bed rest or in traction, it will, however, sufficiently manage the patient's fracture in the acute phase.

Internal immobilization: Surgical open reduction and immobilization of unstable pelvic ring disruptions with plates, screws, or other devices that are surgically implanted internally. Permanent fixation requires close anatomic reduction because it will be the final form of pelvic stabilization.

Surgical exploration: May occur along with ligation or vessel repair when the patient is hemorrhaging. The surgeon can limit blood inflow to the pelvic circulation by ligation of the internal iliac artery to control pelvic bleeding. Because many collateral vessels exist in the pelvic circulation, infarction is unusual after this procedure. Surgical exploration, however, is not always recommended. When the peritoneal space is entered, the tamponade is released and bleeding can increase. In addition, the extensive vascular sink makes identification of bleeding vessels difficult. Instead of surgical exploration, some patients undergo angiography and selective embolization of bleeding points with either an autologous blood clot or particulate gel foam.

Massive fluid resuscitation: Rapid fluid replacement with blood, colloids, or crystalloids. If >2 L of blood are required in the 8 h following the initial resuscitation, additional measures to manage bleeding are indicated.

Pneumatic antishock garment (PASG, also known as military antishock trousers [MAST]):   Device composed of three compartments: two leg and one abdominal. When inflated the compartments result in immobilization and compression of pelvic injuries. Leg compartments may be inflated to 40 mm Hg and the abdominal compartment to 30 mm Hg after endotracheal intubation to maintain the patient's airway. Failure of bleeding to cease within 3-6 h of placement may signal a major vascular laceration. Use of PASG is controversial. Some studies show that when used, prehospital mortality increases because of increased prehospital time. In addition, PASG increases afterload and can cause hemodynamic dysfunction.

Pharmacotherapy

Antibiotics: For open fractures (controversial) and for positive cultures of wounds, blood, and urine.

Analgesics: IV morphine sulfate usually relieves pain and readily can be reversed with naloxone if complications, such as hypotension or bradypnea, occur.

Vasopressors: For hypotension **only** after sufficient volume replacement has occurred (see Appendix 7).

Tetanus immunization: Booster is given if history is unknown or if a booster is needed.

NURSING DIAGNOSES AND INTERVENTIONS

Fluid volume deficit related to active blood loss secondary to injury to the pelvis and pelvic sink

Desired outcomes: Within 12 h after injury, patient's fluid status is adequate as evidenced by regular HR ≤100 bpm, bilaterally strong and equal peripheral pulses, warm and dry extremities, brisk (<2 sec) capillary refill, systolic BP ≥90 mm Hg (or within 10% of patient's normal range), and urine output ≥0.5 ml/kg/h. If hemodynamic monitoring is present, PAWP is ≥6 mm Hg and CI is ≥2.5 L/min/m². Patient is awake, alert, and oriented to time, place, and person without restlessness or confusion.

- Perform a complete assessment of fluid balance qh until patient is stable, noting all cardiac, hemodynamic, urinary, and CNS parameters. Consult physician for early signs of hemorrhage: delayed capillary refill, tachycardia, decreased urinary output, and changes in mental status.
- Administer blood products, colloids, or crystalloids as prescribed through a large-bore peripheral IV or trauma catheter. Unless peripheral access is unavailable, avoid using standard central lines or triple-lumen catheters for fluid resuscitation inasmuch as their length and narrow gauge increase resistance to flow and slow fluid administration.
- Use pressure infusers and rapid warmer/infusers for patients who require massive fluid/blood resuscitation. Be prepared to administer pressor agents only after fluid replacement is in progress. Vasopressors never should be used to maintain BP in the patient without adequate fluid volume replacement.
- Prepare to move the patient to the operating room rapidly if necessary for repair of pelvic vasculature.
- Place the patient flat until fluid volume status is stabilized if other injuries do not preclude position and if the patient has adequate airway and breathing in that position. Avoid Trendelenburg position because of the risk of aspiration, negative hemodynamic consequences, and decreased pulmonary excursion.
- If recommended by physician, assist with placement of PASG to tamponade pelvic bleeding. If the patient is placed in PASG, wrap extremities in towels before application, maintain compartment pressures as prescribed, and check peripheral pulses and neurovascular status q2h. Deflate PASG slowly (e.g., q6h in increments of 5 mm Hg) when prescribed. Deflate the abdominal compartment before the leg compartments.

Risk for infection related to inadequate primary defenses secondary to open pelvic fractures, percutaneous external fixation devices, or surgical procedure

Desired outcome: Within 24 h after injury, soft tissues begin to heal without purulent drainage or erythema; WBC count is ≤11,000 µl; cultures of blood and wounds are negative; pin insertion site is free of erythema, edema, or purulent drainage; and surgical wounds are well approximated and without erythema, edema, or purulent drainage.

- For initial wound care, remove any gross contamination from the wound and cover any exposed soft tissue and bone with wet sterile dressings. Avoid dressings soaked in povidone-iodine to minimize iodine absorption and local tissue irritation. Prevent reentry of a portion of dirty bone or soft tissue into a wound. See "Infection Prevention and Control," Appendix 8, for indications for use of sterile gloves, mask, and eye protection when managing large wounds.
- Monitor all wounds, incisions, and pin insertion sites on external fixation devices q4h for presence of erythema, drainage, and edema.
- Perform pin care as prescribed (e.g., q4-6h). Pin care is controversial and may include removing dried exudate to allow the pin holes to drain freely. In contrast, some experts believe that exudate is a part of the normal healing process and provides a tight interface between the skin and pin, thereby limiting bacterial invasion into the wounds. Unless contraindicated, wrap a loose, open gauze dressing around the insertion site of the pin.

Impaired physical mobility related to pelvic immobilization secondary to pelvic ring instability

Desired outcomes: Immediately after pelvic immobilization, patient maintains appropriate body alignment; external fixation devices and traction remain in place. At the time of hospital discharge, patient exhibits full ROM in uninjured extremities.

- Position patient in proper body alignment.
- Apply compression boots if appropriate to limit the effects of venous stasis. Remove boots at least every shift to provide skin care. Consider using compression boots on upper extremities if appropriate to aid in venous return.
- Provide active and passive ROM to uninjured extremities every shift as appropriate.
- Maintain traction by keeping it free hanging. Do not remove weights even when repositioning.
- Use caution when turning and positioning to maintain body alignment. If patient has an unstable fracture that has not yet been reduced, consult orthopedic surgeon before moving patient. Some patients can be turned from side to side until internal fixation is accomplished. Also consult physician regarding the appropriate HOB elevation and write this information on Kardex or computer care plan.
- Do not hold onto external fixation device when turning patient.

Impaired skin integrity related to initial injury, physical immobility, and placement of external fixation or PASG secondary to pelvic injury

Desired outcomes: Within 12 h of injury and throughout hospitalization, patient has timely wound healing. Patient does not develop pressure ulcers nor experience tissue injury from the external fixation device.

- Cover the ends of all wires on the external fixation device with cork or gauze to protect the patient from injury.
- Apply padding to any traction slings.
- Apply alternating air mattress or other specialty mattresses.

- If patient can be positioned laterally, pad the external fixation device to prevent damage to the patient's skin. Provide padding over bony prominences and any body area that comes in contact with a rigid surface.
- Keep all skin areas clean and dry to minimize the risk of pressure ulcers.
- If PASG is used, place towels under the device to protect patient's skin. After PASG is deflated, assess the skin on the anterior and posterior body surfaces carefully and initiate appropriate skin care regimen.
- See "Wound and Skin Care," p. 57, for more interventions.

Note: Also see "Pain," p. 66, for management of discomfort.

Compartment syndrome (ischemic myositis)

PATHOPHYSIOLOGY

Compartment syndrome is defined as increased pressure within an anatomic compartment that compromises the circulation, viability, and function of tissues within the compartment. Failure to diagnose compartment syndrome is the most common cause of litigation against the medical profession in North America. It is a surgical emergency that requires rapid intervention to prevent permanent cosmetic or functional deformity or loss of limb. Although compartment syndrome most commonly follows fractures, especially those of the tibia and fibula, it can occur from a variety of conditions (Table 2-11). Although compartment syndrome may be acute or chronic (exercise-related forms), this discussion focuses on acute forms.

As compartmental tissue pressure increases, it compromises capillary blood flow. Unremitting pressure results in tissue injury, which causes the release of histamine, producing vasodilatation and increased capillary permeability. Dilated blood vessels and loss of fluids and proteins through the more permeable capillaries contribute to higher tissue pressures. These higher pressures eventually exceed capillary pressure and, ultimately, venous pressure, which in turn promotes further tissue ischemia. Tissue ischemia results in the release of additional histamine, which exacerbates the problem. As a result of impaired venous return, anaerobic metabolism creates more lactic acid, which stimulates vasodilatation, increases BP, and elevates tissue pressure even further. Finally, as compartmental pressure continues to increase, arteriolar spasm occurs from arteriolar compression, further contributing to lower capillary hydrostatic pressure. As this cycle continues, ischemic tissue begins to necrose, resulting in permanent tissue changes.

Sustained hypotension and shock have been associated with a greater incidence of compartment syndrome. As systemic BP decreases, the likelihood of tissue ischemia increases, because it then takes less compartmental pressure to result in arteriolar spasm. Therefore periods of hypotension may result in increased tissue injury at lower compartmental pressure, and persons in shock are more susceptible to compartment syndromes.

The average interval between the initial injury to the compartment and the beginning symptoms of compartment syndrome is 2 h. Compartmental tissue ischemia that lasts longer than 6 h results in tissue necrosis and irreversible tissue changes. Neurologic injury begins within 30 min of inadequate blood supply and may become functionally irreversible after 4 to 6 h.

ASSESSMENT

HISTORY AND RISK FACTORS Any patient with a peripheral injury listed in Table 2-11 is at risk. Patients undergoing IV therapy and those with

TABLE 2-11 Causes of compartment syndrome

Localized compartmental trauma	Tissue reaction/edema formation	Coagulation defects	Other
Fractures	Prolonged use of operative tourniquets	Hemophilia	Compression during obtundation (anesthesia, drug overdose)
Surgery		Anticoagulant therapy	
Hematoma			
Venomous bites (snake, spider)	Arterial or venous obstruction		Infiltrated IV therapy
Vascular injury	Limb reimplantation		Muscle hypertrophy (e.g., shin splints)
Postischemic swelling	Burns (especially when circumferential)		Constrictive dressings, inflatable splints or casts
Crush injuries			
Electrical injuries	Excessive exercise (e.g., march gangrene)		Closure of fascial defects
	Nephrotic syndrome		Hypothermia or hyperthermia
			Clostridium perfringens infections
			Rocky Mountain spotted fever
			Legionnaires' disease
			Use of PASG (pneumatic antishock garment) or MAST (military antishock trousers) on injured *and* uninjured extremities

Modified from Callahan J: *Orthop Nurs* 4(4):11-15, 1985.

circumferential casts or dressings are at risk for iatrogenic compartment syndrome.

CLINICAL PRESENTATION

Early indicators: Pain out of proportion to the injury is the cardinal symptom. Passive motion of the involved muscle group (*via* passive extension of the digits) significantly increases the pain. Palpation of the compartment reveals a tense compartment and slowed capillary refill. Tissue pressures vary with the method of measurement; in general, normal tissue pressures vary from 0-10 mm Hg and sustained pressures >30 mm Hg result in tissue necrosis. Pressures >16 mm Hg are sufficient to collapse thin-walled lower extremity veins, further contributing to the pathogenesis.

Late indicators: If compartment syndrome is left untreated, the necrosed muscle becomes fibrosed and contracted, resulting in a functionally useless compartment (e.g., Volkmann's ischemic contracture), which drastically affects function of the involved limb. The importance of early recognition and treatment of compartment syndrome is reinforced by the fact that decompression fasciotomy seldom restores lost myoneural function. Complications of fasciotomy include wound infection, the potential for osteomyelitis, and large scars.

PHYSICAL ASSESSMENT

Muscle involvement: Inability to control pain with usual amounts of opiates in any patient at risk for compartment syndrome requires closer physical assessment. Pain on passive extension or flexion of the digits is an early finding indicative of muscle tissue involvement.

Neurovascular involvement: Increasing extremity circumference, decrease in or loss of two-point discrimination, sluggish capillary refill, and tautness and tenderness over tissue compartments are signs of early neurovascular involvement. Eventually, all neurovascular structures traversing the involved compartment will show deficit. *Late findings* include the *six P's:* *p*ain (increased with pressure applied over the compartment and passive movement of the digits), *p*allor, *p*olar (coolness), *p*ulselessness, *p*aresthesia, and *p*aralysis.

DIAGNOSTIC TESTS

Intracompartmental pressure monitoring: Although simple needle manometers may be used to measure compartment tissue pressures, they are subject to obstruction from muscle tissue and are inappropriate for continuous monitoring. Wick or slit catheters allow continuous pressure monitoring *via* fluid-filled catheters and pressure monitors. Pressures that indicate the need for fasciotomy vary with clinical indicators, the patient's systemic condition, and the measurement technique. Methods of measuring compartment pressure and associated critical values include *needle* (pressure within 10-30 mm Hg of diastolic BP), *continuous infusion* (pressure >45 mm Hg), and *wick* or *slit catheter* (>30-35 mm Hg). In the presence of factors favorable to the development of compartment syndrome (see Table 2-11) and low systemic BP, the delta pressure should be determined (delta pressure equals mean arterial pressure minus compartmental pressure). Delta pressures of ≤30 mm Hg for 6 h or ≤40 for 8 h require prompt consultation with the physician.

Arteriograms and venograms: Radiologic examination of blood vessels may be performed when embolus, thrombus, or other vascular injury is suspected.

Transcutaneous Doppler venous flow and/or duplex imaging: Enable noninvasive determination of impaired venous flow as an adjunct to the clinical signs for diagnosing compartment syndrome.

MRI spectroscopy: May be used to determine presence of muscle ischemia.

Pulse oximetry: May be used to assess perfusion of distal tissues. Readings should be compared to readings from a contralateral, uninvolved extremity.

COLLABORATIVE MANAGEMENT

Release of external pressure: Loosening or removing circumferential casts and padding or dressings; escharotomy for circumferential burns or frostbite.

Analgesia: Parenteral opiates often with sedative adjuncts (e.g., hydroxyzine HCl, promethazine HCl).

Ice and extremity elevation: Recommended with fractures to promote vasoconstriction when there is no evidence of impaired microcirculation (i.e., decreased capillary refill, pallor, pulselessness, or coolness of the extremity). Once microcirculation has been impaired, however, use of ice and extremity elevation is **contraindicated** inasmuch as further impairment of circulation is likely to result.

Fasciotomy of myofascial compartment: Imperative for strongly suspected compartment syndrome to permit unrestricted swelling. After a few days, the fasciotomy is closed primarily; skin grafting may be needed to ensure complete coverage of the exposed compartments.

Compartment syndrome caused by vascular injury: Requires exploration of the involved vessel to facilitate application of papaverine (e.g., a smooth muscle relaxant that causes local vasodilatation), injection of a bolus of fluid to regain normal internal artery dynamics, and repair of lacerations or resection of involved vessels.

NURSING DIAGNOSES AND INTERVENTIONS

Altered peripheral (compartment) tissue perfusion (or risk for same) related to interruption of capillary blood flow secondary to increased pressure within the anatomic compartment

Desired outcomes: Throughout duration of the hospitalization, patient has adequate perfusion to compartment tissues as evidenced by brisk (<2 sec) capillary refill; peripheral pulses >2+ on a 0-4+ scale; normal tissue pressures (0-10 mm Hg); and absence of edema, tautness, and the six P's for the involved compartment. Within 2 h of admission patient verbalizes understanding of the importance of reporting symptoms indicative of impaired neurovascular status.

- Monitor neurovascular status of injured extremity with each VS check (at least q2h). Assess for increased pain on passive extension or flexion of the digits. Monitor for sluggish capillary refill, decrease in or loss of two-point discrimination, increasing limb edema, and tautness over individual compartments. As available, use pulse oximetry to assess distal tissue perfusion and report significant differences from oximetry readings taken from the uninvolved contralateral extremity. Also assess for the six P's: *p*ain (especially on passive digi-

tal movement and with pressure over the compartment), *p*allor, *p*olar (coolness), *p*ulselessness, *p*aresthesia, and *p*aralysis.
- Report deficits in neurovascular status promptly. Loosen circumferential dressings as indicated. Apply ice when appropriate (see above).
- Teach patient the symptoms that necessitate prompt reporting: increasing pain, paresthesia (diminished sensation, hyperesthesia, or anesthesia), paralysis, coolness, sluggish capillary refill, or pulselessness.
- Monitor tissue pressures on a continuous basis if an intracompartmental pressure device is present. Consult physician if pressures exceed normal or preestablished levels. Be aware that pressures >10 mm Hg may be significantly elevated above normal.
- Be alert to increased susceptibility to tissue injury with slightly increased compartmental tissue pressures in hypotensive states.

Pain related to physical factors (tissue ischemia) secondary to compartment syndrome
Desired outcomes: Throughout duration of the hospitalization, patient's subjective evaluation of discomfort improves as documented by a pain scale. Nonverbal indicators of discomfort, such as grimacing, are absent or diminished. Within 2 h of admission, patient verbalizes understanding of the need to report uncontrolled or increasing pain.
- Assess the patient's complaints of pain for onset, duration, progression, and intensity. Devise a pain scale with patient, rating discomfort "0" for no pain to "10" for unbearable. Patients with impaired ability to communicate may require a visual scale.
- Determine if passive stretching of digits and pressure over limb compartments increase the pain, inasmuch as both are likely to occur with compartment syndrome.
- Adjust the medication regimen to the patient's needs; document medication effectiveness. Promptly report uncontrolled pain.
- Prevent pressure on involved compartment and neurovascular structures.
- If patient has had a fasciotomy, be aware that if the pain does not subside after this procedure, it could indicate an incomplete fasciotomy. Pain that increases several days after a fasciotomy may signal compartmental infection.
- Continue to monitor neurovascular function with each VS check to assess for recurring compartment syndrome or infection.

Risk for infection related to inadequate primary defenses secondary to necrotic tissue, wide compartmental fasciotomy, and open wound
Desired outcomes: Throughout duration of the hospitalization, patient is free of infection as evidenced by normothermia, WBC count ≤11,000 μl, erythrocyte sedimentation rate (ESR) ≤20 mm/h (women) or ≤15 mm/h (men), and absence of wound erythema and other clinical indicators of infection. Within 24 h of admission patient verbalizes understanding of the need to report promptly any indicators of infection.
- Monitor patient for fever, increasing pain, and laboratory data indicative of infection (e.g., increased WBC count, increased ESR).
- Assess exposed wounds and dressings for erythema, increasing wound drainage, purulent wound drainage, increasing wound circumference, edema, and localized tenderness.

- Assess neurovascular structures for deficit, which can signal infection or pressure from adjacent inflamed tissues.
- After primary closure or grafting of wound, continue to assess wound for signs of infection.
- Be aware of and assess for chronic infection and osteomyelitis as potential complications after compartment syndrome.
- Caution patient about the need to report the following indicators of infection: fever, localized warmth, increasing pain, increasing wound drainage (especially if purulent), swelling, and redness.
- Consult with physician promptly regarding significant findings.

Body image disturbance related to physical changes secondary to large, irregular fasciotomy wound and skin grafted scar; loss of function and cosmesis of an extremity; or amputation

Desired outcomes: Within the 24 h period before discharge from ICU, patient acknowledges body changes and demonstrates movement toward incorporating changes into self-concept. Patient does not exhibit maladaptive response (e.g., severe depression) to wound or functional loss.

- Encourage questions about compartment syndrome, therapeutic interventions, and long-term effects.
- Provide time for verbalization of feelings regarding change in appearance and function. Encourage discussion of these feelings with patient's significant other.
- Identify and emphasize patient's strengths to facilitate adaptation to cosmetic and functional loss. Help patient set realistic goals for recovery.
- Facilitate patient's progression through the grieving process, as appropriate.
- Recognize individuality in adjustment; enable patient to determine when to view or discuss the injury.
- If the extremity will be amputated (and it is feasible within the time frame), collaborate with physician regarding visit by an amputee who has successfully adapted, and who can serve as patient's role model.
- Begin to encourage maximum self-care. Provide necessary adjunctive aids (e.g., built-up utensils, button hooks, orthotics) to facilitate independence.
- For patients with functional loss or amputation, introduce the ability for compensation *via* use of orthotics and adjunctive devices to facilitate self-care.

Acute spinal cord injury

PATHOPHYSIOLOGY

In general, a spinal cord injury (SCI) results from concussion, contusion, laceration, hemorrhage, or impairment of blood supply to the spinal cord. This trauma to the spinal cord may be secondarily increased by the ischemia and subsequent edema that occur. Most often, SCI is caused by a vehicular collision, a sports-related incident, or an act of violence. Of the 7,000-10,000 new SCIs per year, half of the involved population have complete injuries of the spinal cord with loss of voluntary motor and sensory function below the level of the lesion. Approximately two thirds have injuries to the cervical area of the spinal cord. Although life expectancy is good after injury, morbidity and mortality most often are the result of infection. Pulmonary complications (atelectasis, pneumonia), renal complications (infection, calculi, septicemia), and pulmonary disease account for 30%-40% of all deaths. A higher incidence of left lower lobe pneumonia and atelectasis is associated with high-level injuries, possibly due to changes in respiratory patterns, ineffective cough, positioning problems, and the anatomy of the left mainstem bronchus, which branches at an oblique angle, making it more difficult to access for suctioning.

SCI is classified in several ways: according to *type and cause,* such as open (gunshot or stab wound) or closed (motor vehicle accident, falls, sports-related incident); *site* (level of the spinal cord involved); *mechanism,* such as flexion (e.g., occurring as a result of sudden deceleration in a head-on collision, backward fall down a flight of stairs, or diving into a swimming pool) or extension (e.g., whiplash or fall involving hyperextension of the neck); *stability* (integrity of the supporting structures such as ligaments or bony facets); and whether the injury is *complete* or *incomplete* ("complete" meaning the absence of all voluntary motor, sensory, and vasomotor function below the level of injury, and "incomplete" meaning the presence of some percentage of voluntary motor or sensory function below the level of injury).

Fractures involving the vertebral bodies: These fractures may or may not cause SCI. Conversely, severe SCI can occur without evidence of damage to the vertebrae. With more severe fractures, such as the "burst" fracture (fragmentation of a vertebral body with penetration of the spinal cord), there is almost always paralysis. Penetration of the spinal cord with bony fragments may cause hemorrhage, infection, and leakage of CSF.

Spinal shock: Immediately after SCI most patients experience a period of spinal shock, which is the loss of all reflex activity below the level of injury. It may last minutes or be prolonged for days or weeks. Generally the duration is 1-6 wk, although periods of 6 mo to 1 yr have been reported. Generally, the more quickly the individual shows signs of return to function, the better the prognosis.

Neurogenic shock: Patients with injuries to the upper thoracic and cervical regions may experience cardiovascular instability due to interruption of the descending sympathetic pathways. This interruption results in loss of vasomotor tone and sympathetic innervation to the heart. The loss of sympathetic innervation causes venous pooling in the extremities and splanchnic vasculature, which decreases venous return to the heart, resulting in low cardiac output and low tissue perfusion pressure. This causes bradycardia and hypotension.

ASSESSMENT

CLINICAL PRESENTATION

Spinal shock: Flaccid paralysis of all skeletal muscles; absence of DTRs, cutaneous sensation, proprioception (position sense), visceral and somatic sensation, and penile reflex; urinary and fecal retention; anhidrosis (absence of sweating).

Neurogenic shock: Vasodilatation, bradycardia, hypotension.

Note: Although spinal shock is seen in SCIs at *any* level, the loss of central control of peripheral vascular tone (neurogenic shock) occurs most dramatically in high cervical spine injuries, with interruption of the sympathetic nervous system. Profound bradycardia and hypotension are possible. With spinal cord injuries lower than the midthoracic area, the patient will experience a phase of neurogenic shock, with loss of sympathetic innervation to vasculature below the level of the lesion; however, the effects of that loss are not as dramatic. The patient will be susceptible to bradycardia and hypotension in relation to position change, but this will not be as serious a problem.

Recovery phase of spinal shock: As spinal shock subsides, the patient may experience the following: (1) flexor spasms evoked by cutaneous stimulation, (2) reflex emptying of the bowel and bladder, (3) extensor or flexor rigidity, (4) hyperreflexic DTRs, and (5) reflex priapism or ejaculation in the male, evoked by cutaneous stimulation.

Levels of cord injury

C4 and above: Loss of all muscle function, including muscles of respiration. With complete cord transection the patient will die, probably at the scene of the injury, unless immediate ventilation is initiated.

C4-C5: Same as preceding but with possible sparing of the phrenic nerve. This means that the patient probably will require assisted ventilation because of weak or absent intercostal muscle function. Patient will be tetraplegic/quadriplegic.

C6-C8: Quadriplegia will occur, but patient will retain function of diaphragm and accessory muscles of respiration and may have some movement of neck, shoulders, chest, and upper portion of arms.

T1-T3: Will have neck, shoulder, chest, arm, hand, and respiratory function; will experience difficulty maintaining a sitting position.

T4-T10: Same as preceding but with more stability of trunk muscles. The lower the lesion, the greater the independence. The patient will be paraplegic.

Note: 80% of persons with lesions at or above T6 (tetraplegics/quadriplegics/high paraplegics) will have episodes of autonomic dysreflexia (AD). See discussion that follows.

T11-L2: Will have use of upper extremities, neck, and shoulders. Chest and trunk muscles will provide stability, and patient will have some muscle function of upper portion of thigh. At this level there may be loss of voluntary bowel and bladder control, but the patient will have reflex emptying of the bowel. Men may experience difficulty achieving and maintaining an erection and may have decreased seminal emission.

L3-S1: Will have muscle function of all muscle groups in the upper portion of the body and most of the muscle function in the lower extremities. There will be loss of voluntary bowel and bladder function, with reflex emptying. Men may experience decreased ability or lack of ability to have an erection, with decreased seminal emission.

S2-S4: Will have function of all muscle groups but may have some lower extremity weakness. There may be flaccidity of bowel and bladder, as well as loss of the ability to have a reflex erection.

Cord syndromes

Anterior cord syndrome: This syndrome involves injury to the anterior portion of the spinal cord supplied by the anterior spinal artery and may be associated with acute traumatic herniation of an intervertebral disk. Surgical decompression is necessary, and the prognosis varies with each patient and depends on the degree of structural damage and edema.

- *Clinical presentation:* Varying degrees of paralysis occur below the level of the injury, along with diminution of pain and temperature sensations. Patient will retain senses of touch, motion, position, and vibration.

Central cord syndrome: Generally seen with hyperextension injuries or interruption of blood supply to the cervical spinal cord. Usually it is seen in older adults, with some evidence of vertebral injury noted on radiography. In this syndrome, motor and sensory deficits are less severe in the lower extremities than in the upper extremities due to the central arrangement of cervical fibers in the spinal cord. Incomplete injuries carry a relatively good prognosis. Steroids are used to decrease edema, and many patients are able to ambulate with an assistive device and may regain bowel and bladder function. Regaining useful function in the hands carries a less favorable prognosis.

- *Clinical presentation:* Motor and sensory deficits usually are severe in the upper extremities and profound in the hands and fingers. With sparing of sacral and some lumbar fibers there will be some motor and sensory function in the perineum, genitalia, and lower extremities.

Lateral cord (Brown-Séquard) syndrome: Results from a horizontal hemisection of the spinal cord (e.g., from a gunshot or stab wound). Patients usually have bilateral motor and sensory impairment, with a relative difference in function from one side to the other. Prognosis usually is good for recovery of upper and lower extremity function.

- *Clinical presentation:* Ipsilateral weakness and decrease in light touch, vibratory, and position senses, with contralateral hypalgesia. Usually there are bilateral motor and sensory deficits, but motor activity will be better on one side and sensory activity will be better on the other.

Horner's syndrome: Seen after an incomplete (partial transection) injury in the cervical region of the spinal cord. The lesion affects either the preganglionic sympathetic trunk or the postganglionic sympathetic neurons of the superior cervical ganglion. It usually affects the ipsilateral side of the face.

- *Clinical presentation:* Ipsilateral miosis, enophthalmos (backward displacement of the eye in its socket), ptosis, and anhidrosis.

Autonomic dysreflexia (AD): Life-threatening response of the autonomic nervous system to a stimulus, creating an exaggerated sympathetic nervous system response. This response can occur during the acute phase of SCI or it may not appear until several years after injury. It affects individuals with lesions at or above T6. If AD is not identified promptly, treated, and reversed, the potential consequences include seizures, subarachnoid hemorrhage, and fatal cerebrovascular accident.

- *Causes:* Stimuli to the *bladder* (most common) such as distention, infection, calculi, cystoscopy; *bowel* such as fecal impaction, rectal examination, suppository insertion; or *skin* such as tight clothing or sheets, temperature extremes, sores, or areas of broken skin.
- *Clinical presentation:* Classic triad includes a throbbing headache, cutaneous vasodilatation, and sweating, which occur above the level of the lesion. The patient also may exhibit the following: hypertension (BP >250-300/150 mm Hg), nasal congestion, flushed skin (above the level of the lesion), blurred vision, nausea, and bradycardia. Below the level of the lesion there will be pilomotor erection (goose bumps), pallor, chills, and vasoconstriction.

DIAGNOSTIC TESTS

Spinal x-rays: AP and lateral films are obtained to detect fractures or dislocations of vertebral bodies, narrowing of the spinal canal, and hematomas. Additional views (odontoid [open-mouth], bilateral oblique, flexion-extension) or tomograms may be necessary to view some levels of the spinal cord, particularly in obese and heavily muscled patients.

Caution: This stage in the evaluation of the patient with a possible SCI is extremely dangerous, because any sudden or incorrect movement of the injured area could cause further trauma to the spinal cord.

CT scan: Same purpose as preceding; may reveal soft tissue injury.
Magnetic resonance imaging: Same purpose as preceding; will define internal organ structures, detect tissue changes such as edema or infarction, and evaluate blood flow patterns and blood vessel integrity.
Myelography: To identify site of spinal canal blockage, which can occur as a result of fractures, dislocations, or herniation or protrusion of an intervertebral disk. Radiopaque dye is injected into the spinal subarachnoid space through a lumbar or cervical puncture.
Pretest: Have patient or family member sign a consent form. Question patient or significant others regarding patient's sensitivity to iodine, shellfish, or contrast material. Ensure that NPO status is maintained for 4-6 h.
Posttest: If a water-soluble dye was used (e.g., metrizamide), elevate HOB for at least 8 h to prevent dye from irritating cerebral meninges. Seizures are a complication of this dye substance. If an oil-based dye (e.g., Pantopaque) was used, it will be removed *via* the puncture site immediately after the test or during surgery if it is scheduled after the test. Keep patient flat for 6-8 h after dye removal.
Pulmonary fluoroscopy: To evaluate the degree of diaphragmatic movement in a person with a high cervical injury. If the injury is at C5 or below, the diaphragm will move up and down with inspiration; however, if the injury is at a slightly higher level, the innervation of the diaphragm may be partial, causing paradoxic respiratory movements that will lead to an ineffective breathing pattern. If this occurs, the patient will require assisted ventilation.

Hgb and Hct values: To detect blood loss due to hemorrhage caused by internal injury.
Urinalysis: To detect the presence of bacteria or blood, which indicates contused kidneys or ruptured bladder.
ABG values and pulmonary function studies: To assess effectiveness of respirations and to detect the need for oxygen, tracheostomy, and mechanical ventilation.
Sputum cultures: Periodic screening to detect onset of respiratory infection and select appropriate antibiotic therapy.

COLLABORATIVE MANAGEMENT

Immobilization of the injured site: With or without surgical intervention.
Cervical spine injury: Skeletal traction is used to immobilize and reduce the fracture or dislocation. Traction may be achieved *via* Vinke, Gardner-Wells, Trippi-Wells, or Crutchfield tongs, which are inserted through the outer table of the skull. These tongs are attached to ropes and pulleys with weights to achieve bony reduction and proper alignment. The patient may be placed on a special frame or bed (e.g., Roto-Rest kinetic treatment table). The patient also may be immobilized with a halo device and a plaster or fiberglass jacket for skeletal fixation of the head and neck. This device allows for earlier mobilization and rehabilitation.

Surgical intervention during the immediate postinjury phase is controversial. Surgery may be performed if (1) the neurologic deficit is progressing, (2) there are compound fractures, (3) the injury involves a penetrating wound of the spine, (4) there are bone fragments in the spinal canal, or (5) there is acute anterior spinal cord trauma. Surgeries may include decompression laminectomy, closed or open reduction of the fracture, or spinal fusion for stabilization.
Thoracic spine injury: May require surgical stabilization *via* Harrington rods or laminectomy with spinal fusion, using bone taken from the iliac crest.
Lumbar spine injury: May necessitate surgical stabilization with laminectomy and spinal fusion. If the injury is stable, it may be treated with closed reduction. Some patients with lumbar spine injury may be immobilized with a halo device with femoral distraction. This device may be connected to traction with weights for reduction and stabilization before surgery.
Respiratory management: The need for assisted ventilation is based on level of injury, ABG values, and the results of pulmonary function tests, pulmonary fluoroscopy, and physical assessment data. In addition, the need for ventilatory assistance is considered likely with injuries at C4 and above, patients >40 yr of age, smokers, associated chest trauma, and immersion injuries. Initially, the patient may require intubation, and later, tracheotomy. Persons with high cervical injury who survive the initial injury but have paralysis of the muscles of respiration may require permanent tracheostomy with mechanical ventilation. Some of these individuals may be candidates for phrenic nerve stimulation, which if successful can give the patient periodic independence from the ventilator. Phrenic nerve stimulation is performed only at specialized spinal cord trauma centers.

Aggressive pulmonary care: To prevent, detect, and treat atelectasis, pulmonary infection, and respiratory failure inasmuch as pulmonary problems are a major source of morbidity and mortality in the patient with SCI. Chest physiotherapy, intubation, and ventilation are instituted as indicated.

Fluid management: In patients with neurogenic shock, blood volume is normal but the vascular space is enlarged, causing peripheral pooling, decreased venous return, and decreased cardiac output. Careful fluid repletion, usually with crystalloids, is indicated. Pressor therapy is initiated for patients unresponsive to fluid volume replacement (see discussion under "Pharmacotherapy," below). For fluid management in patients with multisystem trauma, see "Major Trauma," p. 115.

Gastric tube placement: To decompress the stomach, prevent aspiration of gastric contents, and decrease the risk of paralytic ileus (often seen within 72 h of injury in patients with lesions higher than T6).

Urinary catheterization: Insertion of an indwelling or intermittent catheter to decompress an atonic bladder in the immediate postinjury phase (spinal shock). With the return of the reflex arc after spinal shock subsides, a reflex neurogenic bladder that fills and empties automatically will develop in patients with lesions above T12. Patients with lesions at or below T12 generally will have an atonic, areflexic neurogenic bladder that overfills, distending the bladder and causing overflow incontinence. Intermittent catheterization may be necessary.

Pharmacotherapy

Methylprednisolone: Because neuromembranes are 40% fat (compared with 5%-10% fat for other body cell membranes), administration of this adrenal steroid within 8 h of injury inhibits lipid peroxidation, which in turn protects the neuromembrane from further destruction. In addition, it improves blood flow to the injury site, facilitating tissue repair. A large dose (30 mg/kg) is administered by IV bolus over a 15-min period. After a 45-min wait, 5.4 mg/kg/h is then administered in a continuous IV infusion over a 23-h period and then stopped. If the infusion is interrupted for any reason, it must be recalibrated so that the entire dose can be completed within the original 23 h.

Osmotic diuretics (e.g., mannitol, urea): To decrease edema at the site of injury.

Antacids: To prevent gastric ulceration, which may occur post-SCI due to hyperacidity of gastric secretions and increased production of gastric acid. The risk of ulceration with hemorrhage is further increased if steroids are used.

Histamine H_2-receptor antagonists (e.g., cimetidine, ranitidine): To suppress secretion of gastric acid and to prevent or treat ulcers in the patient with increased production of gastric acid and an increased susceptibility to gastric ulceration and perforation (see Table 8-13, p. 555).

Stool softeners (e.g., docusate sodium): To begin bowel retraining program and prevent fecal impaction with distention of the bowel, which could stimulate an episode of AD.

Hyperosmolar laxatives (e.g., glycerin suppository): To prevent fecal impaction and facilitate movement of the bowels on a regular basis (part of a bowel program).

Irritant or stimulant laxatives (e.g., bisacodyl):   To stimulate bowel movements as part of a bowel training program.

Analgesics (e.g., acetaminophen or acetaminophen with codeine):   To decrease pain associated with the injury or surgery.

Sedatives: To decrease anxiety due to the injury, hospitalization, or fear of the prognosis.

Antihypertensives (e.g., hydralazine hydrochloride, methyldopa, nitroprusside sodium):   To treat the severe hypertension that occurs in AD.

Vasopressors (e.g., epinephrine):   To treat the hypotension that may occur in the immediate postinjury stage due to loss of vasomotor control below the level of injury, with resultant vasodilatation and a relative hypovolemia (see Appendix 7).

Note: Orthostatic hypotension may become a permanent problem, especially in patients with cervical and high thoracic injuries. Care givers must be taught to move the patient slowly into the upright position to avoid a sudden drop in BP, which can cause cerebral hypoxia and loss of consciousness. Abdominal binders and Ace bandages or thigh-high antiembolic stockings also may aid in preventing orthostatic hypotension.

Bronchodilators (theophylline):   To dilate bronchioles and facilitate removal of secretions. Early use of theophylline is recommended in patients with a history of COPD, smoking, and evidence of difficulty moving secretions. Some research indicates that theophylline may increase diaphragmatic contractility and reduce respiratory fatigue.

Mucolytic agents (guaifenesin, acetylcysteine):   To reduce tenacity and viscosity of purulent and nonpurulent secretions.

Antibiotics: To prevent or treat wound, respiratory, or urinary tract infection.

Anticoagulants (heparin):   To prevent thrombophlebitis, deep vein thrombosis, and pulmonary emboli.

Note: Patients with SCI are at high risk for development of vascular complications because they are immobilized, have lost vasoconstrictive capabilities below the level of injury, and cannot constrict the muscles in the lower extremities to facilitate venous flow. Patients who are not candidates for anticoagulation may have an inferior vena cava umbrella or Greenfield filter inserted to trap emboli traveling from the lower extremities to the lungs.

NURSING DIAGNOSES AND INTERVENTIONS

Impaired gas exchange related to altered oxygen supply associated with hypoventilation secondary to paresis or paralysis of the muscles of respiration (diaphragm, intercostals) occurring with high cervical spine injury or ascending cord edema

Desired outcomes: Within 24 h of this diagnosis and throughout remaining hospitalization, patient has adequate gas exchange as evidenced by orientation to time, place, and person; $Pao_2 \geq 80$ mm Hg; and $Paco_2 \leq 45$ mm Hg. RR is 12-20 breaths/min with normal depth and pattern (eupnea), HR is 60-100 bpm, BP is stable and within patient's normal range, and vital capacity is ≥ 1 L. Motor and sensory losses remain at the same spinal cord level as the initial findings.

Note: Patients with cervical injuries usually arrive in the ICU with intubation already in place. However, with some high thoracic or low cervical lesions, patients who ventilate independently in the emergency department may arrive in the ICU without assisted ventilation. Such a patient may be at risk for an increasingly higher level of cord damage because of hemorrhage and edema, which can result in a higher level of dysfunction and a change in respiratory status that requires assisted ventilation.

- Assess for signs of respiratory dysfunction: shallow, slow, or rapid respirations; vital capacity <1 L; changes in sensorium; anxiety; restlessness; tachycardia; pallor; and inability to move secretions.
- Monitor ABG studies; report abnormalities. Be particularly alert to Pao_2 <60 mm Hg, $Paco_2$ >50 mm Hg, and decreasing pH inasmuch as these findings indicate the need for assisted ventilation, possibly due to atelectasis, pneumonia, or respiratory fatigue.
- Monitor vital capacity at least q8h. If it is <1 L, Pao_2/PAo_2 ratio is ≤ 0.75, or copious secretions are present, intubation is recommended.
- Monitor chest x-rays and consult physician for abnormalities.
- Monitor patient for evidence of ascending cord edema: increasing difficulty with swallowing secretions or coughing, presence of respiratory stridor with retraction of accessory muscles of respiration, bradycardia, fluctuating BP, and increased motor and sensory loss at a higher level than the initial findings.
- Before attempting oral intubation with neck flexion, ensure that cervical x-rays have confirmed the absence of cervical involvement. If patient exhibits evidence of respiratory distress and cervical involvement has not been ruled out, do not hyperextend the neck for resuscitation; instead, use either nasal intubation or orotracheal intubation with manual cervical spine immobilization.
- If patient has undergone immobilization *via* placement of cranial tongs or traction with a halo apparatus, monitor patient's respiratory status q1-2h for the first 24-48 h and then q4h if patient's condition is stable. Be alert to absent or adventitious breath sounds, and inspect chest movement to ensure that the plaster or fiberglass vest is not restricting diaphragmatic movement.
- If intubation *via* ET tube or tracheostomy becomes necessary, explain the procedure to patient and significant others.
- See "Mechanical Ventilation," p. 19, for interventions related to mechanical ventilation.

Ineffective airway clearance (or risk for same) related to decreased or absent cough reflex secondary to cervical or high thoracic spine injury

Desired outcome: Within 24-48 h of this diagnosis, patient has a clear airway as evidenced by absence of adventitious breath sounds.

- Monitor patient's respiratory status and be alert to the following indicators of ineffective airway clearance: adventitious breath sounds (i.e., crackles, rhonchi), decreased or absent breath sounds (bronchial, bronchovesicular, vesicular), increased HR (>100 bpm) and BP (>10 mm Hg over patient's normal), decreased tidal volume ($<75\%-85\%$ of predicted value) or vital capacity (<1 L), shallow or rapid respirations (>20 breaths/min), pallor, cyanosis, increased restlessness, and anxiety.

- Monitor and report abnormal ABG values (i.e., decreased Pao_2 or increased $Paco_2$) and chest x-ray results.
- Suction secretions as often as needed, as indicated by auscultation findings. Always hyperoxygenate before suctioning.

Note: Be alert for bradycardia associated with tracheal suctioning. Some authorities suggest giving atropine before suctioning.

- If indicated by the assessment findings, prepare patient for intubation or tracheostomy with mechanical ventilation. See "Mechanical Ventilation," p. 19, for more information.
- If patient does not require intubation with mechanical ventilation, implement the following measures to improve airway clearance:
  - □ Place patient in semi-Fowler's position unless it is contraindicated (e.g., patient is in cervical tongs with traction).
  - □ Turn patient from side to side at least q2h to help mobilize secretions.
  - □ Keep room humidified to help loosen secretions.
  - □ Unless contraindicated, keep patient hydrated with at least 2-3 L/day of fluid.
  - □ If patient has respiratory muscle control, teach coughing and deep-breathing exercises, which should be performed at least q2h.
  - □ If patient's cough is ineffective, implement the following method, known as "quad coughing": Place palm of hand under patient's diaphragm and push up on the abdominal muscles as patient exhales.

Note: Be aware that using the "quad cough" maneuver in patients with intracaval filters to prevent pulmonary emboli has been reported to have significant complications, including bowel perforation and filter migration and deformation.

Dysreflexia (AD) (or risk for same) related to abnormal response of the autonomic nervous system to a stimulus
Desired outcomes: Patient has no symptoms of AD as evidenced by dry skin above the level of injury, BP within patient's normal range, HR ≥60 bpm, and absence of headache and other clinical indicators of AD. ECG demonstrates normal sinus rhythm.
- Assess for the classic triad of AD: throbbing headache, cutaneous vasodilatation, and sweating above the level of injury. In addition, extremely elevated BP (e.g., ≥250-300/150 mm Hg), nasal stuffiness, flushed skin (above the level of the injury), blurred vision, nausea, and bradycardia can occur. Be alert to the following signs of AD that occur below the level of injury: pilomotor erection, pallor, chills, and vasoconstriction.
- Assess for cardiac dysrhythmias, optimally *via* cardiac monitor during initial postinjury stage (2 wk).
- Be aware of and implement measures to prevent factors that may precipitate AD: *bladder stimuli* (i.e., distention, calculi, infection, cystoscopy); *bowel stimuli* (i.e., fecal impaction, rectal examination, suppository insertion); *skin stimuli* (i.e., pressure from tight clothing or sheets, temperature extremes, sores, or areas of broken skin).
- If indicators of AD are present, implement the following measures:

- □ Elevate HOB or place patient in a sitting position. This will decrease BP by promoting cerebral venous return.
- □ Monitor BP and HR q3-5min until patient stabilizes.
- □ Determine and remove offending stimulus.
  - —If, for example, the patient's bladder is distended, catheterize cautiously, using a sufficient amount of a lubricant that contains a local anesthetic.
  - —If patient has an indwelling urinary catheter, check for obstruction, such as granulation in catheter or kinking of tubing. As indicated, irrigate catheter, using no more than 30 ml normal saline.
  - —If urinary tract infection is suspected, obtain a urine specimen for culture and sensitivity once the crisis stage has passed.
  - —Check for fecal impaction. Perform the rectal examination gently, using an ointment containing a local anesthetic (e.g., Nupercaine).
  - —Check for sensory stimuli, and loosen clothing, bed covers, or other constricting fabric as indicated.
- Consult physician for severe or prolonged hypertension or other symptoms that do not abate. Severe or prolonged elevations of BP may result in life-threatening consequences: seizures, subarachnoid or intracerebral hemorrhage, fatal cerebrovascular accident.
- As prescribed, administer antihypertensive agent and monitor its effectiveness.
- Remain calm and supportive of patient and significant others during these episodes.
- Upon resolution of the immediate crisis, answer patient's and significant others' questions regarding cause of the AD. Provide patient and family teaching regarding signs and symptoms and methods of treatment of AD. This is particularly critical for the patient with SCI who has sustained injury above T6, because these patients are at risk for AD for life.

Decreased cardiac output related to relative hypovolemia secondary to enlarged vascular space occurring with neurogenic shock

Desired outcome: Within 24 h of this diagnosis, patient has adequate cardiac output as evidenced by orientation to time, place, and person; systolic BP ≥90 mm Hg (or within patient's normal range); HR 60-100 bpm; RAP 4-6 mm Hg; PAP 20-30/8-15 mm Hg; PAWP 6-12 mm Hg; SVR 900-1,200 dynes/sec/cm^{-5}; normal amplitude of peripheral pulses (>2+ on a 0-4+ scale); urinary output ≥0.5 ml/kg/h; and normal sinus rhythm on ECG.

- Monitor patient for indicators of decreased cardiac output: drop in systolic BP >20 mm Hg, systolic BP <90 mm Hg, or a continuous drop of 5-10 mm Hg with each assessment; HR >100 bpm, irregular HR, lightheadedness, fainting, confusion, dizziness, flushed skin; diminished amplitude of peripheral pulses; change in BP, HR, mental status, and color associated with a change in position. Monitor I&O, and be alert to urine output <0.5 ml/kg/h for 2 consecutive hours. Also assess hemodynamic measurements. In the presence of neurogenic shock, anticipate decreased RAP, PAP, PAWP, and SVR. (See Table 1-13, p. 32.)

- Continuously assess cardiac rate and rhythm per cardiac monitor; report changes in rate and rhythm.
- Implement measures to prevent episodes of decreased cardiac output due to orthostatic hypotension:
  - Change patient's position slowly.
  - Perform ROM exercises q2h to prevent venous pooling.
  - Apply elastic antiembolic hose as prescribed to promote venous return.
  - Avoid placing pillows under patient's knees, "gatching" the bed, or allowing patient to cross the legs or sit with legs in a dependent position.
  - Collaborate with physical therapy personnel in progressing patient from a supine to upright position, using a tilt table.
- As prescribed, administer fluids to control *mild* hypotension.
- Administer and monitor for therapeutic effects of vasopressors (see Appendix 7).
- Ensure adequate volume repletion before or concurrent with pressor therapy.

Risk for injury related to risk of development of gastric ulcer (Cushing's) or gastritis secondary to increased gastric acid production

Desired outcome: Result of patient's gastric pH test is >5, and patient has no symptoms of gastric ulcer as evidenced by gastric aspirate and stool culture that are negative for blood, BP within patient's normal range, HR ≤100 bpm, and absence of midepigastric or referred shoulder pain.

Note: Patients sustaining major trauma are at high risk for development of gastritis/gastric ulcers due to increased production of gastric acid. Although ulceration can occur at any time in the patient with SCI, it is most likely to occur within 3 wk of the injury.

- Assess for indicators of GI ulceration or hemorrhage: midepigastric pain (dull, gnawing, burning ache) if patient has sensation; and hematemesis, melena, constipation, anemia, pallor, decreased BP, increased HR, and complaints of shoulder pain.
- Test gastric aspirate and stools for blood q8h. Promptly consult physician if blood is present.
- Monitor CBC for signs of anemia: decreases in Hct, Hgb, and RBCs. Normal values are as follows: Hct 40%-54% (male) or 37%-47% (female), Hgb 14-18 g/dl (male) or 12-16 g/dl (female), and RBCs 45-60 million/μl (male) or 40-55 million/μl (female).
- As prescribed, implement measures to treat or prevent ulceration and hemorrhage:
  - Monitor gastric pH q2h; administer antacids q2-4h or as prescribed to maintain gastric pH >5.
  - Administer histamine H_2-receptor antagonists to suppress secretion of gastric acids, decrease irritating effects of gastric secretions, and facilitate healing.
  - Insert gastric tube and attach to low intermittent suction to remove gastric contents.
  - Prepare patient for surgery as indicated.
- For the patient with GI ulceration and hemorrhage, bowel perfora-

tion is an added risk. Be alert to the following indicators: pallor, shock state, abdominal distention, vomiting of material that resembles coffee grounds, absent bowel sounds, elevated WBC count ($>11,000/\mu l$), and presence of air on abdominal x-ray. In some cases the only indicators are tachycardia and shoulder pain. Bowel perforation is an emergency situation, requiring immediate surgical intervention.

Altered peripheral and cardiopulmonary tissue perfusion (or risk for same) related to interruption of blood flow associated with thrombophlebitis, deep vein thrombosis (DVT), and pulmonary emboli (PE) secondary to venous stasis, vascular intimal injury, and hypercoagulability occurring as a result of decreased vasomotor tone and immobility

Desired outcome: Patient is free of symptoms of thrombophlebitis, DVT, and pulmonary emboli within 48 h of initiation of therapy, as evidenced by absence of heat, swelling, discomfort, and erythema in the calves and thighs; HR $\leq$100 bpm; RR $\leq$20 breaths/min with normal pattern and depth (eupnea); BP within patient's normal range; Pao_2 $\geq$80 mm Hg; and absence of chest or shoulder pain.

- The high-risk interval for this diagnosis is the 6-12 wk period after injury. Assess for indicators of thrombophlebitis and DVT: unusual heat and erythema of calf or thigh, increased circumference of calf or thigh, tenderness or pain in extremity (depending on patient's level of injury and whether injury is complete or incomplete), pain in the calf area with dorsiflexion (positive reaction for Homans' sign).
- Assess for indicators of pulmonary emboli: sudden chest or shoulder pain, tachycardia, dyspnea, tachypnea, hypotension, pallor, cyanosis, cough with hemoptysis, restlessness, increasing anxiety, low Pao_2.
- Implement measures to prevent development of thrombophlebitis, DVT, and pulmonary emboli:
  - Change patient's position at least q2h to prevent venous pooling.
  - Perform ROM exercises on all extremities q1-2h to promote venous return and prevent venous stasis.
  - Avoid use of knee gatch or pillows under the knees, which can compromise circulation.
  - If patient is out of bed and in a chair, do not allow patient to cross legs at the knee or sit with legs dependent for longer than ½-1 h. For the patient experiencing some return of spinal reflex arcs below the level of the injury with spasticity of lower extremities, caution patient to alert nurse should legs become crossed.
  - Apply sequential compression devices or antiembolic hose as prescribed.
  - Maintain adequate hydration of at least 2-3 L/day, unless contraindicated, to prevent dehydration and concomitant increase in blood viscosity, which can promote thrombus formation.
  - Administer prophylactic low-dose heparin as prescribed.
- If the patient exhibits signs of thrombophlebitis or DVT, implement the following:
  - Consult physician.
  - Maintain bed rest unless otherwise directed.

□ Maintain rest of affected extremity, keeping extremity in a neutral or elevated position, as prescribed.

□ Discourage activities that promote vasoconstriction, such as smoking.

□ Administer anticoagulants and antiplatelet aggregating agents as prescribed.

Note: Patients with SCI who are not candidates for anticoagulation may require surgical intervention (intracaval filter) to prevent pulmonary emboli due to thrombophlebitis or DVT.

□ Apply warm, moist heat as prescribed. Use of heat is controversial, however, due to concern that heat causes vasodilatation, which may mobilize a thrombus.

• If patient exhibits evidence of pulmonary emboli, perform the following, in addition to the aforementioned interventions for thrombophlebitis and DVT:

□ Elevate HOB if not contraindicated.

□ Administer oxygen.

□ As prescribed, administer vasopressors (for hypotension) and analgesics (for pain).

□ Prepare patient for diagnostic procedure (i.e., perfusion lung scan) or surgical intervention (e.g., insertion of intracaval filter).

□ Remain calm and provide support and reassurance to patient and significant others.

• See "Pulmonary Emboli," p. 251, for more information.

Risk for impaired skin integrity related to prolonged immobility secondary to immobilization device or paralysis

Desired outcome: Patient's skin remains intact during hospital course.

• Perform a complete skin assessment at least q8h. Pay close attention to skin that is particularly susceptible to breakdown (i.e., skin over bony prominences and around halo vest edges). Be alert to erythema, warmth, open or macerated tissue, and foul odors (indicative of infection with tissue necrosis).

• Turn and reposition patient, and massage susceptible skin at least q2h. Post a turning schedule, and include patient in the planning and initiating of this schedule.

Caution: Do not turn patient without a written prescription until the injured area of the spinal cord has been stabilized. If turning is allowed before immobilization with tongs, halo, or surgery, use log-rolling technique only, using at least three people to turn patient: *one to support the head and neck and keep them in alignment during the procedure, and two to turn the patient.*

• Keep skin clean and dry.

• Pad halo jacket edges (e.g., with sheepskin) to minimize irritation and friction.

• Provide pressure-relief mattress most appropriate for patient's injury.

• For more information related to the maintenance of skin and tissue integrity, see "Wound and Skin Care," p. 57.

Altered nutrition (or risk for same): Less than body requirements related to decreased oral intake secondary to anorexia, difficulty eating in prone position, fear of choking and aspiration, and inability to feed self due to paralysis of upper extremities; and decreased GI motility secondary to autonomic nervous system dysfunction

Desired outcome: Within 24-72 h of this diagnosis, patient has adequate nutrition as evidenced by balanced nitrogen state per nitrogen balance studies, serum albumin 3.5-5.5 g/dl, thyroxine-binding prealbumin 20-30 mg/dl, and retinol-binding protein 4-5 mg/dl.

- Perform a complete baseline assessment of patient's nutritional status. See "Nutritional Support," p. 1.
- Assess patient's readiness for oral intake: presence of bowel sounds, passing of flatus, or bowel movement.

Note: Next to fecal impaction, paralytic ileus is the second most common GI disorder of patients with SCI. It usually occurs within 72 h of the injury and is associated with gastric distention. (See **Constipation,** p. 193.)

- When the patient begins an oral diet, progress slowly from liquids to solids as tolerated.
- Monitor and record percentage of each meal eaten by patient.
- Implement measures to maintain or improve patient's intake.
  - Obtain dietary consultation to provide patient with his or her favorite foods, as well as those that are of high nutritious value.
  - Make mealtime pleasant: provide oral hygiene before and after meals, and decrease external stimuli (which also will help patient concentrate on chewing and swallowing and thus minimize the risk of aspiration).
  - Provide small, frequent feedings inasmuch as they may be more readily digested; less likely to cause abdominal distention, which may compromise respiratory movement; and less fatiguing.
  - If patient is in a Stryker wedge frame or Foster bed, feed in a prone position to minimize the risk of aspiration. If patient is in a halo device or has been stabilized, feed in high Fowler's position.
  - Feed patient slowly, providing small, bite-size pieces, which facilitate digestion and help prevent choking.
  - Provide straws for liquids; teach patient to sip slowly.
- Once patient's condition has been stabilized, consult with occupational therapy personnel for selection of assistive devices that will enable patient to feed self.

Urinary retention related to inhibition of the spinal reflex arc secondary to spinal shock after SCI

Desired outcome: Within 24 h of this diagnosis, patient has urinary output of $\geq$0.5 ml/kg/h with output comparable to intake.

Caution: Urinary retention with stretching of the bladder muscle may trigger AD. Therefore it is critical to assess for retention and to treat it promptly.

- Assess for indicators of urinary retention: suprapubic distention and intake greater than output.
- Catheterize patient on admission as prescribed. Patients usually have

an indwelling catheter for the first 48-96 h after injury, followed by intermittent catheterization in an attempt to retrain the bladder.
- Ensure continuous patency of the drainage system to prevent reflux of urine into the bladder or blockage of flow, which could cause urinary retention or UTI, which may precipitate AD.
- Maintain a fluid intake of at least 2.5-3 L/day to prevent early stone formation due to mobilization of calcium.
- Tape the catheter over the pubis in both the male and female patient to prevent traction on the catheter, which can lead to ulcer formation in the urethra and erosion of the urethral meatus.
- If the patient remains catheterized for >14 days, a culture and sensitivity is recommended with possible administration of a sulfonamide to prevent bacteremia.
- If an episode of AD is triggered by a distended bladder, obstructed catheter, kinked tubing, or UTI, implement the following:
  □ Have someone notify physician.
  □ If patient is not already catheterized, catheterize patient, using an anesthetic jelly.
  □ If the catheter is obstructed, gently instill no more than 30 ml normal saline in an attempt to open the catheter.
  □ If the catheter remains obstructed, remove it and insert another, using an anesthetic lubricating agent.
  □ If a UTI is the suspected triggering factor, obtain a specimen of urine for culture and sensitivity testing.
  □ For other treatment interventions, see **Dysreflexia,** p. 184.

Reflex incontinence related to uninhibited activity of the spinal reflex arc secondary to recovery phase from spinal shock in patients with cord lesions above T12

Desired outcome: Patient does not experience urinary incontinence.
- As prescribed, catheterize patient on a regularly scheduled basis (e.g., q3-4h).
- If episodes of urinary incontinence occur, catheterize more frequently. If >400 ml of urine is obtained, catheterize more often and reduce fluid intake.
- Measure the amount of residual urine, and attempt to increase the length of time between catheterizations as indicated by decreased amounts (e.g., <50-100 ml urine).

Note: Recent studies recommend continuing 3-4 h intermittent catheterizations to prevent >300-400 ml of urine from accumulating in the bladder. Amounts of urine >400 ml are associated with a significant increase in the rate of infection.

- Monitor and record I&O. Encourage a consistent intake of fluids, evenly distributed throughout the day, to prevent overdistention, which can cause incontinence and increase the risk for AD.
- Decrease fluid intake before bedtime to prevent nighttime incontinence.
- Discourage intake of caffeine-containing beverages and foods (e.g., colas, chocolate, coffee, tea) because they have a diuretic effect and may stimulate increased urine production, bladder spasms, and reflex incontinence.

- Teach patient and significant others the procedure for intermittent catheterization. Alert them to the indicators of UTI (restlessness, incontinence, malaise, anorexia, fever, cloudy or foul-smelling urine) and the importance of adequate fluid intake, regular urine cultures, good handwashing technique, and cleansing of the urinary catheter before catheterization. (The patient with a lesion above T12 whose bladder indicates a neurogenic reflex eventually may be able to empty the bladder automatically and may not require catheterization.)

Caution: UTI is one of the leading causes of morbidity and mortality in the patient with SCI. This patient may not be aware of the presence of UTI until he or she is severely ill due to a pyelonephritis (calculi, infection, septicemia).

Urinary retention (with overflow incontinence) related to loss of reflex activity for micturition and bladder flaccidity secondary to cord lesion at or below T12
Desired outcome: Patient has urinary output without incontinence.
- As prescribed, either insert an indwelling urinary catheter or catheterize patient intermittently on a regularly scheduled basis (e.g., q3-4h).
- If intermittent catheterization is used and episodes of urinary incontinence occur, catheterize more frequently. If >400 ml of urine is obtained, catheterize more often and reduce fluid intake.
- Measure the amount of residual urine, and attempt to increase the length of time between catheterizations, as indicated by decreased amounts (i.e., <50-100 ml urine).

Note: Recent studies recommend continuing 3- to 4-h intermittent catheterizations to prevent >300-400 ml of urine from accumulating in the bladder. Amounts of urine >400 ml are associated with a significant increase in the rate of infection.

- Monitor and record I&O. Distribute fluids evenly throughout the day to prevent overdistention, which can cause incontinence and increase the risk for AD.
- Decrease fluid intake before bedtime to prevent nighttime incontinence.
- Discourage intake of caffeine-containing beverages and foods (e.g., colas, chocolate, coffee, tea) because they have a diuretic effect and may stimulate increased urine production.
- When patient or significant other is ready, teach bladder-emptying techniques such as straining or Credé method.

Note: Even with these techniques, patients may experience dribbling of urine, which will necessitate catheterization or incontinence undergarments.

- Teach patient and significant others the procedure for intermittent catheterization. Alert them to the indicators of UTI (restlessness, incontinence, malaise, anorexia, fever, cloudy or foul-smelling urine) and the importance of adequate fluid intake, regular urine cultures, good handwashing technique, and cleansing of the urinary catheter before catheterization.

Caution: UTI is one of the leading causes of morbidity and mortality in the patient with SCI. This patient may not be aware of the presence of UTI until he or she is severely ill as a result of pyelonephritis (calculi, infection, septicemia).

Ineffective thermoregulation related to inability of the body to adapt to environmental temperature changes secondary to poikilothermic reaction occurring with SCI

Desired outcome: Within 2-4 h of this diagnosis patient becomes normothermic.

Note: With SCI the patient may become poikilothermic, meaning that the patient adapts his or her own body temperature to that of the environment and is unable to control core body temperature *via* vasodilatation to lose heat or vasoconstriction to conserve heat.

- Monitor patient's temperature at least q4h, and assess patient for signs of ineffective thermoregulation: complaints of being too warm, excessive diaphoresis, warmth of skin above level of injury, complaints of being too cold, pilomotor erection (goose bumps), or cool skin above the level of injury.
- Implement measures to attain normothermia:
  - Regulate room temperature.
  - Provide extra blankets to prevent chills.
  - Protect patient from drafts.
  - Provide warm food and drink if patient is chilled; provide cool drinks if patient is warm.
  - Use fans or air conditioners to prevent overheating.
  - Remove excess bedding to facilitate heat loss.
  - Provide a tepid bath or cooling blanket to facilitate cooling.

Risk for injury related to potential of paralytic ileus with concomitant risk of AD secondary to SCI

Desired outcome: Patient remains free of symptoms of paralytic ileus, as evidenced by auscultation of normal bowel sounds, and free of symptoms of AD, as evidenced by BP within patient's normal range; vision normal for patient; dry skin above the level of injury; HR ≥60 bpm; and absence of headache, nasal congestion, flushed skin above the level of injury, and nausea; as well as absence of the following findings below the level of injury: pilomotor erection (goose bumps), pallor, chills.

Note: Paralytic ileus occurs most often in patients with SCI at T6 and above and usually within the first 72 h after the injury.

- Assess for indicators of paralytic ileus: decreased or absent bowel sounds, abdominal distention, anorexia, vomiting, and altered respirations as a result of pressure on the diaphragm. Report significant findings promptly.
- Observe closely for signs of AD, which can be triggered by disten-

tion of the abdomen (for assessment and treatment of AD, see interventions with **Dysreflexia,** p. 184).
- If indicators of paralytic ileus appear, implement the following, as prescribed:
  □ Restrict oral or enteral intake.
  □ Insert gastric tube to decompress the stomach; attach to suction.
  □ Insert a rectal tube if prescribed.

Caution: Stimulation of the rectum by a rectal tube may precipitate an episode of AD; therefore application of anesthetic ointment before insertion is recommended.

- If patient has a rectal tube in place, he or she may not have sensation in the rectal area. Therefore special care is necessary to prevent damage to the rectal mucosa and anal sphincter. Remove the tube as soon as possible.

Constipation or fecal impaction related to neuromuscular impairment secondary to spinal shock
Desired outcome: Within 24-48 h of this diagnosis and subsequently q2-3 days (or within patient's preinjury pattern) patient has bowel elimination of soft and formed stools.
- Monitor patient for indicators of constipation (nausea, abdominal distention, malaise) and fecal impaction (nausea, vomiting, increasing abdominal distention, palpable colonic mass, or presence of hard fecal mass on digital examination).
- Until bowel sounds are present and paralytic ileus has resolved, maintain patient on NPO status, with gastric suction.
- Perform a gentle digital examination to determine presence of fecal impaction and check for rectal reflexes.
- Before the return of rectal reflex arc, it may be necessary to remove feces from the rectum manually. If a fecal impaction is present in an atonic bowel, a small-volume enema may be necessary.

Caution: Be aware that overdistention of the bowel or stimulation of the anal sphincter due to impaction, rectal examination, or enema may precipitate AD. Use generous amounts of anesthetic lubricant when performing rectal examination or administering an enema.

Constipation related to lack of voluntary control of the anal sphincter and lack of sensation of a fecal mass after return of reflex arc associated with neuromuscular impairment
Desired outcome: Within 24-48 h of this diagnosis and subsequently q2-3 days (or within patient's preinjury pattern) patient has bowel elimination of soft and formed stools.
- Obtain history of patient's preinjury bowel elimination pattern.
- Assist patient with selection of menu items that are high in fiber.
- Unless contraindicated, maintain a minimum fluid intake of 2-3 L/day.
- Administer stool softeners (e.g., docusate sodium) daily.
- If possible, avoid enemas for long-term bowel management, as the patient with SCI cannot retain the enema solution. If, however, impaction occurs, a gentle small-volume cleansing enema, followed by manual removal of fecal material, may be necessary.

- Assess patient's readiness for bowel retraining program, including neurologic status and current bowel patterns, noting frequency, amount, and consistency. Usually bowel retraining is initiated when the patient is neurologically stable and can resume a sitting position.
- Because use of a bed pan may impair the patient's ability to evacuate the bowel, provide a bedside commode, if allowed.
  - Provide ample time each day for bowel elimination. One-half hour after mealtime coincides with the gastrocolic reflex.
  - Ensure patient's privacy.
  - Stimulate the rectal sphincter with digital stimulation or insert suppository (i.e., bisacodyl) to initiate reflex peristalsis with reflex evacuation.

Caution: See precautions with **Dysreflexia**, p. 184.

  - If patient has upper extremity function, teach him or her how to perform digital rectal stimulation, insertion of suppository, and abdominal massage to facilitate bowel movement.

Risk for infection related to inadequate primary defenses (broken skin) secondary to presence of invasive immobilization devices

Desired outcome: Patient is free of infection at insertion site for tongs or halo device as evidenced by normothermia, negative culture results, and absence of erythema, swelling, warmth, purulent drainage, or tenderness at insertion site.

- Assess insertion sites q8h for indicators of infection: erythema, swelling, warmth, purulent drainage, and increased or new tenderness. Also be alert to pin migration. If the pin appears to be loose, consult physician and instruct patient to remain still until the pin can be secured.
- Perform pin care as prescribed. One regimen involves cleansing the site with povidone-iodine or half-strength normal saline and hydrogen peroxide, leaving any superficial crust intact, followed by application of an antibiotic ointment. An alternative regimen involves cleansing with povidone-iodine or hydrogen peroxide and no antibiotic ointment. Sterile dressings may be applied around the pins, or the area may be left open to air according to physician or agency policy. Collaborate with physician to develop an effective pin care regimen for the patient. Use sterile applicators, and follow aseptic technique during all pin care procedures.

Sensory/perceptual alterations (visual) related to presence of immobilization device or use of therapeutic bed

Desired outcome: Following intervention(s), patient expresses satisfaction with visual capabilities.

- Assess for factors that limit the patient's visual capabilities: presence of tongs, cervical traction, halo device; and use of Stryker wedge frame or Foster bed, or Roto-Rest kinetic treatment table.
- Provide for increased visualization of patient's surroundings:
  - Obtain prism glasses for patient who must remain supine or is unable to turn his or her head because of halo traction device. If prism glasses are unavailable, provide a hand mirror for patient with upper extremity function.

- Position mirrors to increase the amount of area that can be visualized from patient's position.
- Approach patient and converse within patient's visual field.
- Keep clocks, calendars, and other personal objects within patient's visual field.

Sexual dysfunction or altered sexuality pattern related to trauma associated with SCI

Desired outcome: Patient verbalizes sexual concerns before discharge from ICU.

- Assess patient's level of sexual function or loss from a neurologic and psychologic perspective. The general rule for men is that the higher the lesion, the greater the chance of maintaining the ability to have an erection, but with less chance for ejaculation. For women, ovulation may stop for several months due to stress after the injury. Ovulation usually returns, however, and the woman can become pregnant and have a normal pregnancy. Both men and women with high lesions may experience feelings of excitement similar to a pre-injury orgasm.
- Evaluate your own feelings about sexuality. If you are uncomfortable discussing this subject with the patient, arrange for a knowledgeable staff member to speak with patient about his or her concerns.
- Elicit patient's knowledge, concerns, and questions about his or her sexual function after the SCI.
- It is normal for men to experience a reflex erection upon resolution of the spinal shock, particularly for individuals with lesions in the cervical and thoracic areas. Reassure patient that this is normal and therefore nothing to be embarrassed about.
- Expect acting-out behavior related to the patient's sexuality. This is a normal response to the patient's concern regarding his or her sexual prognosis.
- Provide accurate information regarding expected sexual function in an open, interested manner, based on your assessment of the patient's readiness for information.
- Facilitate communication between the patient and his or her partner.
- Refer patient and his or her partner to a sex therapist or other knowledgeable rehabilitation professional upon resolution of the critical stages of SCI.
- Also provide patient with the following addresses and phone numbers:
  - National Spinal Cord Injury Association, 369 Elliot St., Newton Upper Falls, MA 02164.
  - Spinal Cord Injury Hot Line: 800-638-1733.
  - American Spinal Injury Association, 250 East Superior St., Room 619, Chicago, IL 60611.

ADDITIONAL NURSING DIAGNOSES

For other nursing diagnoses and interventions, see the following as appropriate: "Nutritional Support," p. 12; "Mechanical Ventilation," p. 24; "Prolonged Immobility," p. 78; "Psychosocial Support," p. 88; and "Psychosocial Support for the Patient's Family and Significant Others," p. 100.

Abdominal trauma

PATHOPHYSIOLOGY

The degree of injury to abdominal contents is related to the nature of the force applied and the consistency of the affected structures. Forces involved may be blunt or penetrating, and organs are categorized as solid (e.g., liver, spleen, pancreas) or hollow (e.g., stomach, intestine). Penetrating abdominal trauma typically results in injury to organs in the direct path of the instrument or missile, but high-velocity weapons (e.g., rifles) cause injury not only to tissue in the direct path of the missile but to adjacent organs as well because of energy shock waves that surround the missile path. Injury inflicted by stab wounds follows a predictable pattern and involves less tissue destruction than does injury from gunshot wounds, although stab wounds to major vascular structures (e.g., aorta) and organs (e.g., liver) can be fatal. Blunt abdominal trauma typically results in injury to solid viscera because hollow viscera tend to be more compressible. Hollow organs, however, may rupture, especially when full, if there is a sudden increase in intraluminal pressure. The rate of complications and death increases greatly if injury to multiple abdominal organs is sustained.

Abdominal trauma results in direct injury to organs, blood vessels, and supporting structures. Other pathophysiologic changes associated with abdominal trauma include (1) massive fluid shifts related to tissue damage, blood loss, and shock, (2) systemic inflammation and metabolic changes associated with stress and catecholamine release, (3) coagulation problems associated with massive hemorrhage and multiple transfusions, (4) inflammation, infection, and abscess formation due to release of GI secretions and bacteria into the peritoneum, and (5) nutritional and electrolyte alterations that develop as a consequence of disruption of GI tract integrity. Prolonged hypovolemia and shock result in organ ischemia and ultimately failure (see "Major Trauma," "Adult Respiratory Distress Syndrome," "Cardiogenic Shock," "Acute Renal Failure," "Hepatic Failure," and "Disseminated Intravascular Coagulation"). The following brief overview summarizes common injuries.

Spleen: The organ most frequently injured after blunt trauma. Massive hemorrhage from splenic injury is common. Splenic injury often is associated with hepatic or pancreatic injury. All efforts are made to repair the spleen, because total splenectomy increases the long-term risk of infection, especially in children and young adults.

Liver: Because of its large size and location, it is the organ most frequently involved in penetrating trauma and often is affected by blunt injury as well. Control of bleeding and bile drainage are major concerns with hepatic injury.

Lower portion of esophagus and stomach: Occasionally, the lower portion of the esophagus is involved in penetrating trauma. Because the stomach is flexible and readily displaced, it usually is not injured with blunt trauma, but it may be injured by direct penetration. Injury to either one results in the escape of irritating gastric fluids and the release of free air below the level of the diaphragm. Esophageal injuries often are associated with thoracic injuries.

Pancreas and duodenum: Although traumatic pancreatic or duodenal injury occurs relatively infrequently, it is associated with high morbidity and mortality rates because of the difficulty of detecting these injuries and the likelihood of massive injury to nearby organs. Because these organs are retroperitoneal, clinical indicators of injury often are not obvious for several hours.

Small intestine and mesentery: These injuries are common and may be caused by penetrating or nonpenetrating forces. Compromised intestinal blood flow with eventual infarction is the consequence of undetected mesenteric damage. Perforations or contusions can result in release of bacteria and intestinal contents into the abdominal cavity, causing serious infection.

Colon: Injury most frequently caused by penetrating forces, although lap belts, direct blows, and other blunt forces cause a small percentage of colonic injuries. Because of the high bacterial content, infection is even more a concern than it is with small bowel injury. Most patients with significant colon injuries require temporary colostomy.

Pelvis: See "Renal and Lower Urinary Tract Trauma," p. 156.

Major vessels: Injuries to the abdominal aorta and inferior vena cava most often are caused by penetrating trauma, but they also occur with deceleration injury. Hepatic vein injuries frequently are associated with juxtahepatic vena caval injury and result in rapid hemorrhage. Blood loss after major vascular injury is massive, and survival depends on rapid transport to a trauma center and immediate surgical intervention.

Retroperitoneal vessels: Tears in retroperitoneal vessels associated with pelvic fractures or damage to retroperitoneal organs (pancreas, duodenum, kidney) can cause bleeding into the retroperitoneum. Even though the retroperitoneal space can accommodate up to 4 L of blood, detection of retroperitoneal hematomas is difficult and sophisticated diagnostic techniques may be required.

ASSESSMENT

HISTORY Details regarding circumstances of the accident and mechanism of injury are invaluable in detecting the presence of specific injuries. In addition, the time of the patient's last meal, previous abdominal surgeries, and use of safety restraints (if appropriate) should be ascertained. If possible, information concerning current medications and allergies, particularly to contrast material, antibiotics, and tetanus toxoid, should be obtained. The history may be difficult to obtain due to alcohol or drug intoxication, head injury, breathing difficulties, or impaired cerebral perfusion. In such cases, family members and emergency personnel may be valuable sources of information.

CLINICAL PRESENTATION A wide variation can occur. Mild tenderness to severe abdominal pain may be present, with the pain either localized to the site of injury or diffuse. Blood or fluid collection within the peritoneum causes irritation that results in involuntary guarding, rigidity, and rebound tenderness. Fluid or air under the diaphragm may cause referred shoulder pain. Kehr's sign (left shoulder pain caused by splenic bleeding) also may be noted, especially when the patient is recumbent. Nausea and vomiting may occur, and the conscious patient who has sustained blood loss often complains of thirst, an early sign of hemorrhagic shock. Symptoms of abdominal injury may be minimal or absent in the patient who is intoxicated or has sustained head or spinal cord injury.

Note: The absence of signs and symptoms does not exclude the presence of major abdominal injury. Outward signs of injury are absent in up to 36% of patients with abdominal trauma (Beachley, 1993).

PHYSICAL ASSESSMENT Abdominal assessment is highly subjective, and serial evaluations by the same examiner are strongly recommended to detect subtle changes.

Inspection: Abrasions and ecchymoses may indicate underlying injury. Ecchymosis over the LUQ suggests splenic rupture, and erythema and ecchymosis across the lower portion of the abdomen suggest intestinal injury caused by lap belts. *Grey Turner's sign,* a bluish discoloration of the flank, may indicate retroperitoneal bleeding from the pancreas, duodenum, vena cava, aorta, or kidneys. *Cullen's sign,* a bluish discoloration around the umbilicus, may be present with intraperitoneal bleeding from the liver or spleen. Ecchymoses may take hours to days to develop, depending on the rate of blood loss. The absence of ecchymosis does not exclude major abdominal trauma and massive internal bleeding. In the event of gunshot wounds, entrance and exit (if present) wounds should be identified.

Auscultation: It is important to auscultate before palpation and percussion, because these maneuvers can stimulate the bowel and confound assessment findings. Bowel sounds are likely to be decreased or absent with abdominal organ injury or intraperitoneal bleeding. The presence of bowel sounds, however, does not exclude significant abdominal injury. Immediately after injury, bowel sounds may be present, even with major organ injury. Bowel sounds should be auscultated in each quadrant q1-2h in patients with suspected abdominal injury. Absence of bowel sounds is expected immediately after surgery. Failure to auscultate bowel sounds within 24-48 h after surgery suggests ileus, possibly caused by continued bleeding, peritonitis, or bowel infarction.

Palpation: Tenderness to light palpation suggests pain from superficial or abdominal wall lesions, such as that occurring with seat-belt contusions. Deep palpation may reveal a mass in the area of hematoma. Internal injury with bleeding or release of GI contents into the peritoneum results in peritoneal irritation and certain assessment findings. Table 2-12 describes signs and symptoms that suggest peritoneal irritation. Subcutaneous emphysema of the abdominal wall usually is caused by thoracic injury but also may be produced by bowel rupture. Measurements of abdominal girth may be helpful in identifying increases in girth attributable to gas, blood, or fluid. Visual evaluation of abdominal distention is a late and unreliable sign of bleeding.

Percussion: Unusually large areas of dullness may be percussed over ruptured blood-filled organs. For example, a fixed area of dullness in the LUQ suggests a ruptured spleen. An absence (or decrease in the size) of liver dullness may be caused by free air below the diaphragm, a consequence of hollow viscus perforation, or, in unusual cases, displacement of the liver through a ruptured diaphragm. The presence of

---

T A B L E 2 - 1 2   Signs and symptoms that suggest peritoneal irritation

---

· Generalized abdominal pain or tenderness
· Involuntary guarding of the abdomen
· Abdominal wall rigidity
· Rebound tenderness
· Abdominal pain with movement or coughing
· Decreased or absent bowel sounds

---

tympany suggests gas; dullness suggests that the enlargement is caused by blood or fluid.

VITAL SIGNS AND HEMODYNAMIC MEASUREMENTS Ventilatory excursion often is diminished because of pain, thoracic injury, or diaphragmatic elevation due to abdominal distention. With initial compensatory tachycardia and vasoconstriction caused by blood loss, a normal BP usually is maintained until blood loss becomes major. At that point BP deteriorates to an MAP <70 mm Hg. Vascular resistance remains high. A diminished CVP and PAP reflect hypovolemic shock; CO decreases because of hypovolemia but will normalize with correction. Initial hypothermia is common. See "Major Trauma," p. 114, for hemodynamic findings associated with hyperdynamic and MODS responses to injury.

DIAGNOSTIC TESTS

Hct level: Serial levels reflect the amount of blood lost. If measured immediately after the injury, the Hct level may be normal, but serial levels will reveal dramatic decreases during resuscitation and as extravascular fluid mobilizes during the recovery phase. Major blood loss is common with intraabdominal injury.

WBC count: Leukocytosis is expected immediately after injury. Splenic injuries in particular result in the rapid development of a moderate to high WBC count. A later increase in WBCs or a shift to the left reflects an increase in the number of neutrophils, which signals an inflammatory response and possible intraabdominal infection. In the patient with abdominal trauma, ruptured abdominal viscera must be considered as a potential source of infection.

Platelet count: Mild thrombocytosis occurs immediately after traumatic injury. Spontaneous bleeding and a very low platelet count (<20,000-30,000 μl) signal the need for platelet transfusion.

Glucose levels: Initially elevated due to catecholamine release and insulin resistance associated with major trauma. Glucose metabolism is abnormal after major hepatic resection, and patients with significant hepatic injury should be monitored at frequent intervals to prevent severe hypoglycemic episodes.

Electrolytes: Sodium, potassium, and chloride levels may drop due to gastric suctioning or vomiting.

BUN: Elevations are associated with shock, dehydration, GI bleeding, infection, and impaired kidney function.

Amylase levels: Elevated serum levels are associated with pancreatic or upper small bowel injury, but values may be normal even with severe injury to these organs. Delayed elevation suggests traumatic pancreatitis.

Liver enzymes: Elevations of AST, ALT, and ALP reflect hepatic dysfunction due to liver ischemia during prolonged hypotensive episodes or direct traumatic damage. Fluctuations in these enzyme levels during the postoperative period can be used to detect evidence of liver necrosis.

Bilirubin: Elevated direct (conjugated) indicates the liver's inability to excrete bilirubin. Elevated indirect (unconjugated) indicates rapid destruction of RBCs or possible retroperitoneal hematoma.

X-rays: Flat and upright chest x-rays exclude chest injuries (frequently associated with abdominal trauma) and establish a baseline, inasmuch as surgery is likely. In addition, chest, abdominal, and pelvic x-rays may reveal fractures, missiles, free intraperitoneal air, hematoma, or hemorrhage.

Occult blood: Gastric contents and stool should be tested for blood in the initial and recovery periods because GI bleeding can occur both as a result of direct injury and of later complications, including gastric erosion.

Diagnostic peritoneal lavage (DPL):   Involves insertion of a peritoneal dialysis catheter into the peritoneum to check for intraabdominal bleeding. DPL is indicated for confirmed or suspected blunt abdominal trauma for the following patients: (1) those in whom signs and symptoms of abdominal injury are obscured by intoxication, head or spinal cord trauma, opiate administration, or unconsciousness, (2) those about to undergo general anesthesia for repair of other injuries (e.g., orthopedic, facial), and (3) any patient with equivocal assessment findings. DPL is unnecessary for patients with obvious intraabdominal bleeding or other indications for immediate laparotomy (see "Surgical Considerations" in the following section).

If gross blood is recovered when the catheter is inserted, immediate laparotomy is indicated. If blood is not recovered, 1 L of normal saline or Ringer's lactate is infused rapidly through the catheter and then drained into a sterile bedside drainage device. If possible, the patient is moved from side to side after fluid instillation in order to distribute the lavage fluid evenly. If the drained lavage is grossly bloody, intraperitoneal bleeding is confirmed. Other indicators of positive lavage results are $>100,000$ RBC/μl, >500 WBC μl, amylase >175 U/dl, presence of bile or bacteria, or obvious intestinal contents in the drainage.

Note: An indwelling urinary catheter is inserted before DPL to prevent inadvertent puncture of a full bladder. The stomach is decompressed with a gastric tube in order to check for bleeding and avoid pressure on a full stomach, vomiting, and aspiration.

CT scan: Can detect intraperitoneal and retroperitoneal bleeding and free air (associated with rupture of hollow viscera). It is most useful in assessing injury to solid abdominal organs.

Angiography: Performed selectively to evaluate injury to spleen, liver, pancreas, duodenum, and retroperitoneal vessels when other diagnostic findings are equivocal.

Caution: Because of the large amount of contrast material used during this procedure, monitor urine output closely for several hours for a decrease and ensure adequate hydration.

ADDITIONAL DIAGNOSTIC TESTS

Abdominal injuries often are associated with multisystem trauma. Also see diagnostic test discussions in "Major Trauma," p. 114, "Craniocerebral Trauma," p. 130, "Chest Trauma," p. 141, "Cardiac Trauma," p. 149, "Renal and Lower Urinary Tract Trauma," p. 159, and "Acute Spinal Cord Injury," p. 179.

COLLABORATIVE MANAGEMENT

Oxygen: Abdominal injury may result in poor ventilatory efforts due to pain or compression of thoracic structures. High-flow supplemental oxygen is indicated initially and then titrated according to ABG values.

Fluid management: Because massive blood loss is associated with most abdominal injuries, immediate volume resuscitation is critical. Initially, Ringer's lactate or a similar balanced salt solution is given. Colloid solutions such as albumin are helpful in the postoperative period if hypoalbuminemia occurs as a result of hepatic injury or ischemia or if there are low filling pressures and evidence of decreased plasma oncotic pressure. Typed and cross-matched fresh blood is the optimal fluid for replacement of large blood losses. However, inasmuch as fresh whole blood is rarely available, a combination of packed cells and fresh frozen plasma often is used. See "Major Trauma," p. 115, for more information.

Pneumatic antishock garment (PASG, MAST):   Can be used as a temporary means to elevate BP in patients with severe abdominal trauma and marked hypovolemia. See "Major Trauma," p. 116, for more information.

Gastric intubation: Gastric tube permits gastric decompression, aids in removal of gastric contents, and prevents accumulation of gas or air in the GI tract. Aspirated contents can be checked for blood to aid in the diagnosis of lower esophageal, gastric, or duodenal injury. The tube usually remains in place until bowel function returns.

Pharmacotherapy

Antibiotics: Abdominal trauma is associated with a high incidence of intraabdominal abscess, sepsis, and wound infection, particularly with injury to the terminal ileum and colon. Persons with penetrating or blunt trauma and suspected intestinal injury are started on parenteral antibiotic therapy immediately. Broad-spectrum antibiotics are continued postoperatively and stopped after several days unless there is evidence of infection.

Analgesics: Because opiates alter the sensorium, making evaluation of the patient's condition difficult, they seldom are used in the early stages of trauma. Analgesics are used in the immediate postoperative period to relieve pain and promote ventilatory excursion.

Tetanus prophylaxis: Tetanus immunoglobulin and tetanus toxoid are considered on the basis of CDC recommendations (see Table 2-1). **Nutrition:**   Patients with abdominal trauma have complex nutritional needs because of the hypermetabolic state associated with major trauma and traumatic or surgical disruption of normal GI function. Often infection and sepsis contribute to a negative nitrogen state and increased metabolic needs. Prompt initiation of parenteral feedings in patients unable to accept enteric feedings and the administration of supplemental calories, proteins, vitamins, and minerals are essential for healing. For additional information, see "Nutritional Support," p. 1.

Surgical considerations for penetrating abdominal injuries: Removing penetrating objects can result in additional injury; thus attempts at removal should be made only under controlled situations with a surgeon and operating room immediately available. The issue of mandatory surgical exploration versus observation and selective surgery, especially with stab wounds, remains controversial. There is a trend toward observation of patients without obvious injury or peritoneal signs. Indications for laparotomy include one or more of the following: (1) penetrating injury suspected of invading the peritoneum, (2) positive peritoneal signs (e.g., tenderness, rebound tenderness, and involuntary guarding), (3) shock, (4) GI hemorrhage, (5) free air in the peritoneal cavity as seen on x-ray, (6) evisceration, (7) massive hematuria, and (8) positive findings on diagnostic peritoneal lavage.

Note: The patient should be evaluated for peritoneal signs at least hourly by the same examiner. Consult surgeon immediately if the patient shows peritoneal signs, evidence of shock, gastric or rectal bleeding, or gross hematuria.

Surgical considerations for nonpenetrating abdominal injuries: Physical examination usually is reliable in determining the necessity for surgery in alert, cooperative, unintoxicated patients. Additional diagnostic tests such as DPL or CT scan are necessary to evaluate the need for surgery in the patient who is intoxicated or unconscious, or who has sustained head or spinal cord trauma. Immediate laparotomy for blunt abdominal trauma is indicated under the following circumstances: (1) clear signs of peritoneal irritation (see Table 6-16), (2) free air in the peritoneum, (3) hypotension due to suspected abdominal injury or persistent and unexplained hypotension, (4) positive DPL findings, (5) GI aspirate or rectal smear positive for blood, or (6) other positive findings in diagnostic tests such as CT scan or arteriogram. Carefully evaluated, stable patients with blunt abdominal trauma may be admitted to critical care for observation. These patients should be evaluated in the same manner as that described in "Surgical Considerations for Penetrating Abdominal Injuries," above. It is important to note that damage to retroperitoneal organs such as the pancreas and duodenum may not cause significant signs and symptoms for 6-12 h or longer. Relatively slow bleeding from abdominal viscera may not be clinically apparent for 12 h or longer after the initial injury. In addition, the nurse should be aware that complications such as bowel obstruction due to adhesions or narrowing of the bowel wall from localized ischemia, inflammation, or hematoma may develop days or weeks after the traumatic event. The need for vigilant observation in the care of these patients cannot be overemphasized.

NURSING DIAGNOSES AND INTERVENTIONS

Fluid volume deficit related to active loss secondary to physical injury

Desired outcomes: Within 12 h of this diagnosis, patient becomes normovolemic as evidenced by MAP ≥70 mm Hg, HR 60-100 bpm, normal sinus rhythm on ECG, CVP 2-6 mm Hg, PAWP 6-12 mm Hg, CI ≥2.5 L/min/m^2, SVR 900-1,200 dynes/sec/cm^{-5}, urinary output ≥0.5 ml/kg/h, warm extremities, brisk capillary refill (<2 sec), and distal pulses >2+ on a 0-4+ scale.

- Monitor BP q15min, or more frequently in the presence of obvious bleeding or unstable VS. Be alert to changes in MAP of >10 mm Hg. Even a small but sudden decrease in BP signals the need to consult the physician, especially with the trauma patient in whom the extent of injury is unknown.
- Monitor HR, ECG, and cardiovascular status q15min until volume is restored and VS are stable. Check ECG to note HR elevations and myocardial ischemic changes (i.e., ventricular dysrhythmias and ST-segment changes), which can occur because of dilutional anemia in susceptible individuals.
- In the patient with evidence of volume depletion or active blood loss, administer pressurized fluids rapidly through several large-caliber (16-gauge or larger) catheters. Use short, large-bore IV tubing (trauma tubing) to maximize flow rate. Avoid use of stopcocks, because they slow the infusion rate. Fluids should be warmed to prevent hypothermia.

Caution: Evaluate patency of IV catheters continuously during rapid-volume resuscitation.

- Measure central pressures and thermodilution CO q1-2h or more frequently if there is ongoing blood loss. Calculate SVR and PVR q4-8h or more often in unstable patients. Be alert to low or decreasing CVP and PAWP. An elevated HR, along with decreased PAWP, decreased CO/CI, and increased SVR, suggests hypovolemia (see Table 4-17, p. 364, for hemodynamic profile of hypovolemic shock). Anticipate slightly elevated HR and CO due to hyperdynamic cardiovascular state in some patients who have undergone volume resuscitation, particularly during the preoperative phase. Also anticipate mild to moderate pulmonary hypertension, especially in patients with concurrent thoracic injury, such as pulmonary contusion, smoke inhalation, or early adult respiratory distress syndrome (ARDS). ARDS is a concern in patients who have sustained major abdominal injury, inasmuch as there are many potential sources of infection and sepsis that make the development of ARDS more likely (see "Adult Respiratory Distress Syndrome," p. 247).
- Measure urinary output q1-2h. Be alert to output <0.5 ml/kg/h for 2 consecutive hours. Low urine output usually reflects inadequate intravascular volume in the patient with abdominal trauma.

- Monitor for physical indicators of hypovolemia, including cool extremities, capillary refill >2 sec, and absent or decreased amplitude of distal pulses.
- Estimate ongoing blood loss. Measure all bloody drainage from tubes or catheters, noting drainage color (e.g., coffee ground, burgundy, bright red [see Table 2-13]). Note the frequency of dressing changes due to saturation with blood to estimate amount of blood loss *via* wound site.

Pain related to physical injury secondary to external trauma or surgery

Desired outcomes: Within 2 h of this diagnosis, patient's subjective evaluation of discomfort improves, as documented by a pain scale. Nonverbal indicators of discomfort, such as grimacing, are absent.

- Evaluate patient using a pain scale for presence of preoperative and postoperative pain. Preoperative pain is anticipated and is a vital diagnostic aid. The nature of postoperative pain also can be important. Incisional and some visceral pain can be anticipated, but intense pain or prolonged pain, especially when accompanied by other peritoneal signs, can signal bleeding, bowel infarction, infection, or other complications.

T A B L E 2 - 1 3   Characteristics of gastrointestinal drainage

Source	Composition and usual character
Mouth and oropharynx	Saliva; thin, clear, watery; pH 7
Stomach	Hydrochloric acid, gastrin, pepsin, mucus; thin, brownish to greenish; acidic
Pancreas	Enzymes and bicarbonate; thin, watery, yellowish brown; alkaline
Biliary tract	Bile, including bile salts and electrolytes; bright yellow to brownish green
Duodenum	Digestive enzymes, mucus, products of digestion; thin, bright yellow to light brown, may be greenish; alkaline
Jejunum	Enzymes, mucus, products of digestion; brown, watery with particles
Ileum	Enzymes, mucus, digestive products, greater amounts of bacteria; brown, liquid, feculent
Colon	Digestive products, mucus, large amounts of bacteria; brown to dark brown, semiformed to firm stool
Postoperative (GI surgery)	Initially, drainage expected to contain small amounts of fresh blood appearing bright to dark; later, drainage mixed with old blood appearing dark brown (coffee-ground); and then approaches normal composition
Infection present	Drainage cloudy, may be thicker than usual; strong or unusual odor, drain site often erythematous and warm

- Recognize that opiate analgesics can decrease GI motility, causing nausea, vomiting, and delay of bowel activity. These factors are especially significant if the patient has had a recent laparotomy.
- See this diagnosis in "Major Trauma," p. 119, and in Chapter 1, p. 74, for additional pain interventions.

Risk for infection related to inadequate primary defenses secondary to physical trauma or surgery; related to inadequate secondary defenses due to decreased hemoglobin or inadequate immune response; related to tissue destruction and environmental exposure (especially to intestinal contents); and related to multiple invasive procedures

Desired outcome: Patient is free of infection as evidenced by core or rectal temperature $<37.8°$ C ($100°$ F); HR ≤100 bpm; CI ≤4 L/min/m^2; SVR ≥900 dynes/sec/cm^{-5}; orientation to time, place, and person; and absence of unusual redness, warmth, or drainage at surgical incisions and drain sites.

- Note color, character, and odor of all drainage. Report the presence of foul-smelling or abnormal drainage. See Table 2-13 for a description of the *usual* character of GI drainage.
- As prescribed, administer pneumococcal vaccine in patients with total splenectomy to minimize the risk of postsplenectomy sepsis.
- If evisceration occurs initially or develops later, do not reinsert tissue or organs. Place a saline-soaked gauze over the evisceration, and cover with a sterile towel until the evisceration can be evaluated by the surgeon.
- For more interventions, see this diagnosis in "Major Trauma," p. 119.

Altered gastrointestinal tract tissue perfusion related to interruption of arterial or venous blood flow or hypovolemia secondary to physical injury

Desired outcome: By the time of hospital discharge, patient has adequate GI tract tissue perfusion as evidenced by normoactive bowel sounds; soft, nondistended abdomen; and return of bowel elimination.

- Auscultate for bowel sounds hourly during the acute phase of abdominal trauma and q4-8h during the recovery phase. Report prolonged or sudden absence of bowel sounds during the postoperative period, because these signs may signal bowel ischemia or mesenteric infarction.
- Evaluate patient for peritoneal signs (see Table 2-12), which may occur initially as a result of injury or may not develop until days or weeks later if complications due to slow bleeding or other mechanisms occur.
- Ensure adequate intravascular volume (see **Fluid volume deficit,** p. 203).
- Evaluate laboratory data for evidence of bleeding (e.g., serial Hct) or organ ischemia (e.g., AST, ALT, LDH). Desired values are as follows: Hct $>28\%$-30%, AST 5-40 IU/L, ALT 5-35 IU/L, and LDH 90-200 ImU/ml.
- Document amount and character of GI secretions, drainage, and excretions. Note changes that suggest bleeding (presence of frank or occult blood), infection (e.g., increased or purulent drainage), or obstruction (e.g., failure to eliminate flatus or stool within 3-4 days of surgery).
- Stress the importance of seeking medical attention if indicators of

infection or bowel obstruction occur (e.g., fever, severe or unusual abdominal pain, nausea and vomiting, unusual drainage from wounds or incisions, or a change in bowel habits).

Impaired tissue integrity related to mechanical factors (including physical injury); increased metabolic needs secondary to trauma/stress response; altered circulation secondary to hemorrhage or direct vascular injury; and exposure to irritants (gastric secretions)

Desired outcome: Patient has adequate tissue integrity by the time of hospital discharge as evidenced by wound healing within an acceptable time frame (according to extent of injury) and absence of skin breakdown due to GI drainage.

- Protect the skin surrounding tubes, drains, or fistulas, keeping the areas clean and free from drainage. Gastric and intestinal secretions and drainage are highly irritating and can lead to skin excoriation. If necessary, apply ointments, skin barriers, or drainage pouches to protect the surrounding skin. If available, consult ostomy nurse for complex or involved cases.
- For other interventions, see this diagnosis in "Major Trauma," p. 120.

Altered nutrition: Less than body requirements related to decreased intake secondary to disruption of GI tract integrity (traumatic or surgical) and increased need secondary to hypermetabolic posttrauma state

Desired outcome: Within 5 days of this diagnosis, patient has adequate nutrition as evidenced by maintenance of baseline body weight and state of nitrogen balance on nitrogen studies.

- Collaborate with physician, dietitian, and pharmacist to estimate patient's metabolic needs on the basis of type of injury, activity level, and nutritional status before injury.
- Consider patient's specific injuries when planning nutrition. For example, expect patients with hepatic or pancreatic injury to have difficulty with blood sugar regulation. Patients with trauma to the upper GI tract may be fed enterally, but feeding tube must be placed distal to the injury. Disruption of the GI tract may require a feeding gastrostomy or jejunostomy. Patients with major hepatic trauma may have difficulty with protein tolerance.
- Ensure patency of gastric or intestinal tubes to maintain decompression and encourage healing and return of bowel function. Avoid occlusion of the vent side of sump suction tubes, because this may result in vacuum occlusion of the tube. Use caution when irrigating gastric or other tubes that have been placed in or near recently sutured organs.
- For additional information, see this diagnosis in "Major Trauma," p. 121.

Body image disturbance related to creation of stoma (often without the patient's prior knowledge) or mutilating physical injury

Desired outcome: By the time of hospital discharge, patient acknowledges body changes, views and touches affected body part, and demonstrates movement toward incorporating changes into self-concept.

- Evaluate the patient's reaction to the stoma or missing/mutilated body part by observing and noting evidence of body image disturbance (see Table 1-41, p. 97).

- Anticipate feelings of shock and disbelief initially. Be aware that trauma patients usually do not receive the emotional preparation for ostomy, amputation, and other disfiguring surgery that the patient undergoing elective surgery receives.
- Anticipate and acknowledge normalcy of feelings of rejection and isolation (and uncleanliness in the case of fecal diversion).
- Offer patient opportunity to view stoma/altered body part. Use mirrors if necessary.
- Encourage patient and significant others to verbalize feelings regarding altered/missing body part.
- Offer patient the opportunity to participate in care of ostomy, wound, or incision.
- Confer with surgeon regarding advisability of a visit by an ostomate or a patient with similar alteration in body part.
- Be aware that most colostomies are temporary in persons with colonic trauma. This fact can be reassuring to the patient, but it is important to verify the type of colostomy with the surgeon before explaining this to the patient.

ADDITIONAL NURSING DIAGNOSES

Also see "Major Trauma" for **Hypothermia,** p. 121 and **Posttrauma response,** p. 123. For additional information, see other diagnoses under "Major Trauma," as well as nursing diagnoses and interventions in the following sections, as appropriate: "Hemodynamic Monitoring," p. 37; "Prolonged Immobility," p. 78; "Psychosocial Support," p. 88; "Psychosocial Support for the Patient's Family and Significant Others," p. 100; "Peritonitis," p. 565; "Enterocutaneous Fistula," p. 580; and "Shock," p. 635.

Burns

PATHOPHYSIOLOGY

Burns usually involve damage to the skin, an organ that protects against infection, controls body temperature, and prevents loss of body fluids, as well as affecting external appearance and influencing body image. Burns also may involve other major organs (e.g., cardiac due to electrical burn or pulmonary caused by smoke inhalation). The causative agent in burn injury may be thermal (scalding hot liquid or steam, hot metal, flame), electrical, chemical, or radiation. The burn agent, the patient's age, the intensity and duration of exposure to the offending agent, the burn's location and depth, and the percentage of body exposure determine outcome.

Burns are categorized based on depth or magnitude. The longer and more intense the exposure to the burn agent, the greater the severity of burn depth and magnitude. A burn injury may be described as partial or full thickness relative to the layer(s) of skin and tissues involved. Partial-thickness injuries are further differentiated into superficial and deep partial-thickness categories. *Superficial partial-thickness injury,* commonly referred to as "first-degree" burn (e.g., sunburn), damages the epidermis. The epidermis is composed of keratinized fiber, which is replenished continuously from underlying desquamated cells that migrate to the superficial layer and form a protective barrier between the host and the environment. These burns heal within 24-72 h. *Deep partial-thickness injury,* called a "second-degree" burn, involves varying levels of the dermis, which contains structures essential to skin function (e.g., sweat and sebaceous glands, hair follicles, sensory and motor nerves, and capillary network). These burns heal within 3-35 days, depending on depth, because epidermal elements germinate and migrate until the epidermal surface is restored. *Full-thickness injury,* a "third-degree" burn, exposes the poorly vascularized fat layer, which contains adipose tissue, roots of sweat glands, and hair follicles; these burns destroy all epidermal elements. Wounds <4 cm in diameter are allowed to heal by granulation and migration of healthy epithelium from wound margins; larger wounds are closed *via* skin grafting.

Electrical burn injuries often reveal only superficial injury on initial inspection, but extensive damage may occur to deep and underlying tissues, nerves, blood vessels, and muscles along the conduction path and at the electrical current exit site. Careful assessment is needed to determine the full extent of the injury.

The American Burn Association (ABA) has developed an injury severity grading system that categorizes burns as minor, moderate, and major (Table 2-14). The ABA advocates that major burns be treated in a burn center or facility with expertise in burn care. Moderate burns usually require hospitalization, although not necessarily in a burn unit, and minor burns often are treated in the emergency department or on an outpatient basis.

Care for the patient with burn injury is provided in three stages, based on the pathologic changes that occur. The first stage, the emergency period, lasts from the time of injury to 48 h postburn. The second stage, the acute phase, begins with resolution of the fluid shift and continues until all wounds are closed or, in some agencies, when open wound areas are <10% of the total body surface area (TBSA). This stage can last from 3 days to a month or several months. The last stage, the rehabilitative stage, can continue for many years and seldom is a focus for critical care nurses, although patient and family teaching may begin in earlier stages of care.

T A B L E 2 - 1 4   ABA classification system

Magnitude of burn injury	Partial thickness		Full thickness adults and children (%BSA)	Special location*	Complications (poor risk, fractures, other trauma)
	Adult (%BSA)	Children (%BSA)			
Major	>25%	>20%	>10%	+	+
Moderate	15%-25%	10%-20%	<10%	—	—
Minor	<15%	<10%	<2%	—	—

BSA, Body surface area.
*Hands, face, eyes, ears, feet, and/or genitalia.

ASSESSMENT

General clinical presentation:　Before focusing on burn size and depth, assess the basic ABCs of patient care: airway, breathing, and circulation. To determine the severity of the burn injury, consider the percentage of body surface area burned, burn depth, location(s) (including inhalation injury), patient's age, and patient's past medical history.

The extent of the burn wound is estimated quickly by means of the Berkow formula, commonly known as the "rule of nines" (Figure 2-1). For adults each body part is assigned a percentage of surface area to establish the degree of involvement: head and neck 9%, each arm 9%, anterior portion of chest 18%, posterior portion of chest 18%, each leg 18%, and the genitalia 1%. For odd-shaped burns the surface area of the patient's palm usually equals 1% of the total BSA. A more accurate assessment tool is the Lund and Browder chart (Figure 2-2), which is more detailed and accounts for the changes in body parts according to age.

Respiratory system:　First, determine airway patency. The patient is at high risk for airway obstruction owing to swelling caused by the heat, smoke, or chemically traumatized mucous membranes of the nasopharyngeal passage or by constriction around the neck or chest caused by eschar formation. Note, in particular, the presence of singed

Multisystem Stressors

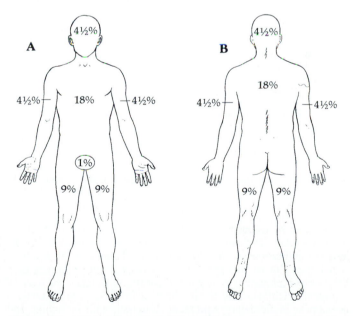

Figure 2-1:　Estimation of adult burn injury: rule of nines. **A,** Anterior view. **B,** Posterior view. (From Thompson JM et al: *Mosby's manual of clinical nursing,* ed 3, St Louis, 1993, Mosby.)

BURNS

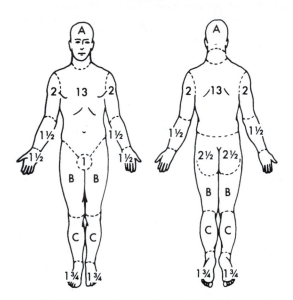

Relative percentages of areas affected by growth
(age in years)

	0	1	5	10	15	Adult
A: half of head	9½	8½	6½	5½	4½	3½
B: half of thigh	2¾	3¼	4	4¼	4½	4¾
C: half of leg	2½	2½	2¾	3	3¼	3½

Second degree _____ and
Third degree   _____ =
Total percent burned ____

Figure 2-2:   Estimation of burn injury: Lund and Browder chart. Areas designated by letters *(A, B,* and *C)* represent percentages of body surface area that vary according to age. The accompanying table indicates the relative percentages of these areas in various stages of life. (From Thompson JM et al: *Mosby's manual of clinical nursing,* ed 3, St Louis, 1993, Mosby.)

nasal hairs, burns in the perioral area, change in voice, or coughing up of soot. Gas exchange may be further compromised by smoke inhalation and carbon monoxide poisoning. Tissues in the lower respiratory tract can be damaged by direct contact with products of combustion and inhalation of vaporized caustic substances, such as sulfur, nitrogen, aldehydes, and hydrochloric acid. Respiratory damage may not appear immediately. Epithelial sloughing with bronchitis and respiratory distress occur 6-72 h postburn. Carbon monoxide (CO) has an affinity for hemoglobin that is 200 times that of oxygen, resulting in hypoxia owing to the prevention of hemoglobin from binding with oxygen and being transported to the tissues. Tissue oxygenation is inadequate and physiologic effects worsen as the level of CO increases. Symptoms range from headache and decreased visual acuity to coma and death.

Risk factors: History of having been burned in a confined area. Patients with a preexisting cardiac or respiratory condition and those who are heavy smokers are most susceptible to respiratory complications associated with smoke inhalation.

Clinical indicators: Include crackles, rhonchi, stridor, severe hoarseness, hacking cough, labored breathing, dyspnea, tachypnea, and possible altered LOC due to hypoxia. Cherry red skin coloring, headache, tinnitus, vertigo, and convulsions may be signs of CO poisoning.

Note: Physical evidence of respiratory compromise may be absent initially, despite pulmonary injury. Progression to airway obstruction and acute respiratory distress can occur rapidly.

Cardiovascular system: Circulatory compromise secondary to burn injury results from fluid shifts, direct damage to the heart or blood vessels, obstruction of microcirculation, compression of blood vessels, and hemorrhage caused by clotting disorders. Extent of injury determines the degree of circulatory compromise. Increased capillary permeability due to the inflammatory response at the site(s) of the burn injury results in a shift of intravascular fluid into the interstitial spaces. This fluid shift causes a decrease in circulating volume and increased viscosity of the remaining intravascular fluid. In response to the burn injury, there is an increase in catecholamine, cortisol, renin-angiotensin, ADH, and aldosterone production as the body struggles to retain sodium and water to replenish intravascular fluid. Patients may complain of thirst, dry mucous membranes, and tingling or numbness in their extremities.

Risk factors: Patients with renal disease, diabetes, or preexisting cardiac, vascular, or respiratory conditions may have complications associated with fluid resuscitation therapy.

Clinical indicators: Signs of shock, such as decreased LOC, pallor, dry mucous membranes, and cool skin temperature; tachycardia, hypotension, and decreased filling pressures (CVP, PAP, PAWP); decreased or absent peripheral pulses and delayed capillary refill; hemoconcentration and thrombus formation; impaired peripheral perfusion with possible obstruction due to circumferential burns of the extremities; cardiac dysrhythmias due to direct cardiac damage (electrical burns) and electrolyte imbalance, such as hyperkalemia caused by cellular hemolysis during the first 24-36 h postburn; and peripheral edema due to fluid shifts and hypoproteinemia. Muscle weakness caused by elevated fat mobilization from fatty acids and triglycerides, as well as by electrolyte imbalances, may occur with major burns.

Gastrointestinal system: Blood flow is shunted away from the GI tract, and peristalsis is slowed or may be stopped completely, causing paralytic ileus (usually resolves within 72 h after burn injury). There is also high risk for development of life-threatening stomach and intestinal ulceration with hemorrhage (associated with a gastric pH of <5). This condition is referred to as Curling's ulcer or stress ulcer.

Nutritional deficits are a common concern due to a dramatically elevated basal metabolic rate with high protein and fat catabolism, resulting in high caloric needs and electrolyte imbalances due to fluid shifts and cell hemolysis. The increased metabolic rate is proportional to the burn size. Inability to meet nutritional needs through oral or enteral feedings may necessitate use of parenteral nutritional therapy.

Risk factors: History of peptic ulcer or duodenal ulcer disease, steroid use, preexisting malnourishment, or alcohol abuse.

Clinical indicators: Absence of bowel sounds, stools, and flatus and presence of nausea and vomiting, possibly with occult blood (hematemesis), and abdominal distention due to accumulated flatus.

Renal system: Hemoconcentration and reduced circulatory volumes result in decreased renal flood flow and low urinary output. A high myoglobin or hemoglobin load may be reflected by dark, concentrated urine. Continued poor renal perfusion can result in acute tubular necrosis and renal failure with buildup of metabolic waste products and electrolyte imbalances (see "Acute Renal Failure," p. 385).

Risk factors: History of renal disease, previously compromised renal function, chronic cardiovascular disease, diabetes mellitus, and collagen-vascular disease.

Clinical indicators: Urine output <0.5 ml/kg/h; dark, amber, "thick" urine; high urine specific gravity; elevated urine nitrogen and proteinuria, and decreased creatinine clearance; glycosuria secondary to a decreased glucose tolerance and decreased insulin effectiveness.

Integumentary system: Loss of skin integrity results in fluid loss through evaporation, hypothermia, and increased risk of infection. Hypertrophic scar formation can result in contractures with limitations in extremity ROM. Keloids, an overgrowth of scar tissue most commonly found in individuals of dark pigmentation, may present a challenge to normal healing and require special treatment. Circumferential burns can cause constriction of underlying tissue, blood vessels, and muscles (compartment syndrome, see p. 170) with tissue necrosis secondary to circulatory compromise to underlying muscle.

Clinical indicators: Deep partial-thickness and full-thickness burn wounds of varied magnitude (Tables 2-15 and 2-16).

Wound sepsis: Ongoing evaluation for wound sepsis is imperative, because sepsis is the primary cause of death in burn injury. The larger the wound, the higher the risk for infection.

Risk factors: Concomitant injuries (e.g., fractures), long-term steroid therapy, immunosuppression, diabetes mellitus, invasive procedures, history of cardiopulmonary or vascular disease, and delayed antimicrobial therapy.

Clinical indicators: Increased rapidity of eschar separation, increased amount of exudate, and isolated pockets that contain purulent material all suggest burn wound sepsis. Disappearance of well-defined burn margins and presence of edema, discoloration, and superficial ulceration of burned skin at wound margin/skin interface are other indicators. Granulation tissue may become pale and boggy; focal black, dark brown, or violet areas of discoloration may appear in the wound; partial-thickness burn may change from pink or mottled red to full-thickness necrosis (i.e., sloughing of subcutaneous fat layer); vesicular lesions may appear in healing or healed partial-thickness injury;

TABLE 2-15   Characteristics of burn wound depth

Criterion	Partial thickness	Full thickness
Cause	Flash, flame, ultraviolet (sunburn), hot liquid or solid, chemicals, radiation	Extended contact with flame, hot liquid or solid, steam, chemical, electrical, radiation
Surface appearance	*Superficial:* Dry, no blisters or edema *Deep:* Moist blebs, blisters, edema, oozing of plasmalike fluid	Dry, leathery, eschar; thrombosed blood vessels may be visible
Color	Cherry red to mottled white; will blanch and refill	Ranges in color from red to khaki; waxy; charred; does not blanch
Sensation	*Superficial:* Very painful to the touch *Deep:* Extremely sensitive to touch, temperature, and air currents	Anesthetized to touch and temperature because of destruction of sensory nerve endings
Healing	3-35 days	Grafting required for wounds $\geq$4 cm

TABLE 2-16   Factors determining burn severity

Criterion	Factors
Extent	Severity depends on intensity and duration of exposure
Depth	Severity depends on intensity and duration of exposure
Age	Patients <2 yr and >60 yr
Medical history	Preexisting conditions such as heart disease, chronic renal failure
Body part	Special burn areas: hands, face, eyes, ears, feet, and genitalia
Complications	Burns with concomitant trauma (e.g., fractures)

and erythematous, nodular lesions may be present in unburned skin. In addition, there may be hemorrhagic discoloration of subeschar fat, with remaining eschar spongy and poorly demarcated; cellulitis of unburned skin (common with gram-positive invasion); turquoise-colored, sweet-smelling exudate (with *Pseudomonas* infection).

Signs of systemic/septic shock: Include changes in LOC (confusion, disorientation, agitation); labile temperature ranging from 35°-40.5° C (95°-105° F), gastric distention, and paralytic ileus. Other indicators include tachycardia, tachypnea, decreased BP with low SVR, malaise, nausea and anorexia, hyperglycemia, and glycosuria.

DIAGNOSTIC TESTS

Serial ABG values: Will demonstrate hypoxemia and acid-base abnormalities.

Carboxyhemoglobin level: Determines presence of carbon monoxide in the blood secondary to smoke inhalation.

Serial chest x-rays: Usually normal on patient's admission; however, changes 24-48 h after injury may reflect atelectasis, pulmonary edema, or acute respiratory distress.

Culture and sensitivity studies: To evaluate sputum, blood, urine, and wound tissue for evidence of infection. Burn wound sepsis is defined as microorganisms 10^5/g of burn wound tissue with active invasion of adjacent, viable, unburned skin. Examples of gram-negative organisms that may be found include *Pseudomonas aeruginosa, Klebsiella, Serratia, Escherichia coli,* and *Enterobacter cloacae.* Less frequently, gram-positive organisms *(Staphylococcus* and *Streptococcus)* and fungal organisms *(Candida* and *Aspergillus)* may be present.

Note: If a burn wound culture is positive for group A *Streptococcus* sp., this may signal the need for an epidemiologic investigation. Contact your facility's infection control nurse or epidemiology department for assistance in evaluating such a culture, especially if more than one patient's culture is positive at approximately the same time.

Laryngoscopy and bronchoscopy: Although not routine, may be helpful in determining presence of extramucosal carbonaceous material and the state of the mucosa (e.g., edema, denudation, erythema, blistering) in inhalation injuries.

Vital capacity, tidal volume, and inspiratory force measurements: Performed q2-4h to evaluate respiratory status. They will demonstrate falling values with inhalation injury associated with the development of respiratory distress or failure.

Urine specimen: Culture and sensitivity studies performed for early detection and treatment of urinary tract infection. Urinalysis and 24-h urine collection for total nitrogen, urea nitrogen, creatinine, and amino acid nitrogen values may indicate return of capillary integrity (3-5 days postburn) and mobilization of third-space fluids, the degree of catabolism present, and the onset or resolution of acute renal failure. Myoglobin, a muscle pigment, may be found in the urine (myoglobinuria) after muscle injury.

Note: Continued elevation of BUN and creatinine levels may signal inadequate fluid intake or acute renal failure (see "Intrarenal" section of "Acute Renal Failure," p. 394).

Baseline blood work
Hematocrit: Increased secondary to fluid shifts from intravascular space.
Hemoglobin: Decreased secondary to hemolysis.
Serum sodium: Decreased secondary to massive fluid shifts into interstitial spaces.
Serum potassium: Elevated due to cell lysis and fluid shifts into interstitial spaces.

BUN: Elevated secondary to hypovolemic status, increased protein catabolism, and possible development of acute renal failure.

Total protein: Decreased secondary to leakage of plasma proteins into interstitial spaces.

Creatinine kinase (CK): Evaluated as an index of muscle damage; thus it is particularly important in electrical injuries. The higher the CK, the more extensive the muscle damage.

ECG: Myocardial damage secondary to electrical burn injury may be evident.

COLLABORATIVE MANAGEMENT

Humidified oxygen therapy: Treats hypoxemia and prevents drying and sloughing of the mucosal lining of the tracheobronchial tree.

Intubation and mechanical ventilation: As indicated for respiratory distress. Because laryngeal edema resolves in 3-5 days, tracheostomy is avoided for upper airway distress.

Bronchodilators and mucolytic agents: Aid in the removal of secretions.

Escharotomy (surgical incision through the eschar or fascia): Relieves respiratory distress secondary to circumferential, full-thickness burns of neck and trunk, or in extremities to lessen pressure from underlying edema and to restore adequate perfusion. It may be performed at the bedside or in the emergency room. Indications for escharotomy include cyanosis of distal unburned skin, delayed capillary filling, progressive neurologic changes (may mimic compartment syndrome), burns of thorax that restrict respiratory motion, and weak or absent peripheral pulses. See "Compartment Syndrome," p. 170, for more information.

Fluid resuscitation therapy: Fluid replacement protocols are based on body weight and percentage of body surface area burned and are designed to replenish lost body fluids and maintain organ perfusion without circulatory overload. Various formulas are used to estimate fluid requirements for burn patients during the acute phase of injury (Table 2-17). Colloids generally are avoided during the first 24 h after burn injury because increased capillary permeability causes leakage of protein into the interstitial tissues, resulting in edema formation. In the most commonly used formulas, crystalloid fluids are used in the first 24 h, with small amounts of colloid fluids added during the second 24 h postinjury. The Parkland formula, which is most commonly used, recommends administration of 4 ml fluid/kg body weight/percentage body area burned. The first half of the calculated volume is infused over the first 8 h when fluid shifts are greatest. For example, if the patient was injured 2 h before arrival at the hospital and initial infusion of fluid, the first half of the calculated 24-h fluid need is infused over the next 6 h. The second half is then infused over the following 16 h.

Note: Calculate fluid infusion time from the time of injury, not the time of hospital admission. Fluid formulas provide guidelines but should be modified, based on individual patient responses and needs. Patients with electrical injuries may have greater fluid needs than suggested by cutaneous injury. The presence of inhalation injury, ethanol intoxication, or crushing injuries also affects acute fluid requirements.

T A B L E 2 - 1 7 **Formulas used in estimating fluid requirements for adults during the acute phase of burn injury**

Formula	First 24 h			Second 24 h		
	Crystalloid/electrolyte solution	Colloid-containing fluid/plasma equivalent	Dextrose in water	Crystalloid/electrolyte solution	Colloid-containing fluid/plasma equivalent	Dextrose in water
Parkland	Lactated Ringer's 4 ml/kg/% TBSA burned				20%-60% of calculated plasma volume	As necessary for maintaining urinary output
Brooke	Lactated Ringer's 1.5 ml/kg/% TBSA burned	0.5 ml/kg/% TBSA burned	2 L	½-¾ of first 24-h requirement	½-¾ of first 24-h requirement	2 L
Modified Brooke	Lactated Ringer's 2 ml/kg/% TBSA burned				0.3-0.5 ml/kg/% TBSA burn	As necessary for maintaining urinary output
Evans	Normal saline 1 ml/kg/% TBSA burned	1 ml/kg/% TBSA burned; dextran 70 in normal saline or whole blood	2 L	½ of first 24-h requirement	½ of first 24-h requirement	2 L

Indwelling urinary catheter: Enables accurate measurement of urine output.

Gastric suction: Allows aspiration of gastric contents, a necessary procedure because of the potential for paralytic ileus in patients with a ≥30% BSA burn or alcohol intoxication.

Tetanus-toxoid prophylaxis: Given intramuscularly to combat *Clostridium tetani,* an anaerobic infection. See Table 2-1.

IV morphine sulfate: The drug of choice for pain management. It usually is initiated as a large dose and then given in small increments as needed for comfort.

Note: All medications, except for tetanus toxoid, are administered intravenously to avoid sequestration of medication, which then would "flood" the vascular system with the return of capillary integrity and the diuresis of third-spaced fluids.

Antacids/histamine H_2-receptor antagonists: Maintain gastric pH >5 and prevent development of Curling's ulcer. Many burn centers are finding that early initiation of gastric tube feedings is effective in preventing Curling's ulcer.

Dietary regimen: High metabolic activity and increased protein catabolism related to burn injury result in a significant increase in energy requirements and nutritional needs. Energy requirements may be estimated using one of several formulas based on body size and extent of burn with adjustment for age. Additional injury or poor preburn nutritional status may increase nutritional needs. The appropriate mix of protein, fat, and carbohydrates is controversial, but a positive nitrogen state has been achieved with patients who are administered high-protein, high-carbohydrate diets. Use of high-fat, low-carbohydrate diets has been suggested to facilitate weaning of patients from the ventilator, since increased CO_2 production results from high-carbohydrate loads. The method of delivery for nutritional support may vary based on patient tolerance. The oral route may be inadequate or contraindicated due to injury or anorexia. Enteral feedings are an inexpensive method of delivery, which, if tolerated, may decrease GI acidity and ulcer formation. Central parenteral nutrition may be initiated for the patient with paralytic ileus or one who is unable to tolerate an adequate amount of enteral feedings.

Multivitamin and mineral supplements: Vitamins A and C and zinc are especially important for promoting wound healing.

IV antibiotics: As indicated for specific culture and sensitivity findings.

Wound care: Cleansing, débridement (manual, enzymatic, or surgical), and antimicrobial therapy (i.e., topical agents: silver sulfadiazine [Silvadene], povidone-iodine, mafenide, silver nitrate) control bacterial proliferation and provide a wound capable of producing granulation tissue and a capillary network.

Split-thickness skin grafting: Provides closure for full-thickness injuries. Biologic dressings such as cadaver skin or porcine or amniotic membranes may be used for temporary closure before autografting.

NURSING DIAGNOSES AND INTERVENTIONS

Impaired gas exchange (or risk for same) related to smoke inhalation with tracheobronchial swelling and carbonaceous debris; related to competition of CO with O_2 for hemoglobin; and related to hypoventilation associated with circumferential burns to neck and thorax

Desired outcome: Within 1 h of treatment/intervention, patient exhibits adequate gas exchange as evidenced by Pao_2 ≥80 mm Hg; oxygen saturation ≥95%; RR 12-20 breaths/min with a normal pattern and depth (eupnea); absence of adventitious breath sounds and other clinical indicators of respiratory dysfunction; and orientation to time, place, and person.

- Assess and document respiratory status hourly, noting rate and depth, breath sounds, and LOC. Be alert to a declining respiratory status as evidenced by crackles, rhonchi, stridor, severe hoarseness, hacking cough, labored breathing, dyspnea, tachypnea, restlessness, and decreasing LOC. Consult physician promptly for all significant findings.
- Monitor serial ABG values for decreasing Pao_2 and oxygen saturation and increasing $Paco_2$ as evidence of worsening hypoxemia. Also be alert to gradually declining values in vital capacity, tidal volume, and inspiratory force (see Table 3-1, p. 231).
- Place patient in high Fowler's position to enhance respiratory excursion.
- Teach patient the necessity of coughing and deep-breathing exercises q2h, including incentive spirometry.
- Monitor for indicators of upper airway distress (e.g., severe hoarseness, stridor, dyspnea and, less frequently, CNS depression) and lower airway distress (e.g., crackles, rhonchi, hacking cough, and labored or rapid breathing). Report significant findings promptly.
- Administer oxygen therapy, mechanical ventilation, or bronchodilator treatment (i.e., theophylline, sympathomimetics) as prescribed.

Ineffective airway clearance (or risk for same) related to increased secretions and inflammation and swelling of nasopharyngeal mucous membranes secondary to smoke irritation and impaired cough; related to compression of neck and chest cavity and decreased expansion of alveoli secondary to circumferential burns

Desired outcome: Patient has a clear airway within 10-30 min of treatment/intervention as evidenced by auscultation of normal breath sounds over the lung fields; a state of eupnea; and orientation to time, place, and person.

- Assess and document respiratory status hourly, noting breath sounds, rate and depth of respirations, and LOC. Be alert to a declining respiratory status as evidenced by crackles, rhonchi, stridor, labored breathing, dyspnea, tachypnea, restlessness, and decreasing LOC. Consult physician promptly for all significant findings.
- Assess and document character and amount of secretions after each coughing and deep-breathing exercise.
- Reposition patient from side to side q1-2h to help mobilize secretions.
- As prescribed, administer percussion and postural drainage to facilitate airway clearance (this is contraindicated with fresh skin grafts).
- Perform oropharyngeal or ET suctioning as indicated by the pres-

ence of adventitious breath sounds and the patient's inability to clear the airway effectively by coughing.

Fluid volume deficit related to active loss through the burn wound and leakage of fluid, plasma proteins, and other cellular elements into the interstitial space

Desired outcome: Within 24-48 h of this diagnosis, patient becomes normovolemic as evidenced by BP 110-120/70-80 mm Hg (or within patient's normal range), peripheral pulses >2+ on a 0-4+ scale, urine output ≥0.5 ml/kg/h, and urine specific gravity 1.010-1.030.

- Monitor patient for evidence of fluid volume deficit, including tachycardia, decreased BP, decreased amplitude of peripheral pulses, urine output <0.5 ml/kg/h, thirst, and dry mucous membranes.
- Monitor I&O; administer fluid therapy as prescribed, titrating hourly infusion to maintain urine output at a minimum of 30-50 ml/h.
- Monitor weight daily; report significant gains or losses. For example a 2 kg acute weight loss may signal a 2 L fluid loss. However, weight loss also may be due to catabolism and an increased metabolic rate as the body attempts to heal itself.
- Monitor urine specific gravity. As fluid resuscitation occurs, urine specific gravity will become normal, reflecting a normovolemic status; conversely, an elevated value occurs with a dehydrated state and a decreased value reflects an overhydrated state.
- Monitor serial Hct, Hgb, serum sodium, and serum potassium values. As the circulating volume is restored, the Hct decreases to within normal limits. Hgb values may decrease secondary to hemolysis within the first 1-2 h after burn injury. Transfusions with packed RBCs generally are required by day 5 after burn injury. Usually potassium is elevated during the first 24-36 h postburn due to hemolysis and the lysis of cells. After 72-96 h, hypokalemia may occur as cell membranes regain their integrity and the patient experiences diuresis. At this point it may be necessary to add potassium to the IV solutions. Consult physician for significant anemia or electrolyte imbalance.
- Monitor patient for evidence of fluid volume excess secondary to rapid fluid resuscitation, especially in patients with preexisting respiratory or cardiac disease. Be alert to excessive urine output, crackles, SOB, and tachypnea.
- Confer with physician regarding use of mannitol to promote osmotic diuresis and prevent renal tubular sludging due to myoglobinuria. Other diuretics are avoided because they further deplete an already compromised intravascular volume.
- With the onset of spontaneous diuresis, decrease infusion rates by 25% for 1 h as prescribed if the urine output is 30-50 ml/h for 2 consecutive hours. Continue to reduce rates gradually according to intake/output ratio and clinical status.

Pain related to burn injury

Desired outcomes: Within 1 h of treatment/intervention, patient's subjective evaluation of discomfort improves as documented by a pain scale. Nonverbal indicators of discomfort are absent or diminished.

- Assess patient's level of discomfort at frequent intervals. Devise a pain scale with patient, rating discomfort from 0 (no pain) to 10. Patients with partial-thickness burns may experience severe pain because of exposure of sensory nerve endings. Pain tolerance decreases with prolonged hospitalization and sleep deprivation.

- Monitor patient for clinical indicators of pain: increased BP, tachypnea, dilated pupils (unless patient has received narcotic analgesia), shivering, rigid muscle tone, or guarded position.
- Administer narcotic analgesia and tranquilizers as prescribed and, if they are given orally, at least 30-45 min before painful procedures.
- Provide a full explanation of procedures and honest feedback, using a calm, organized, and firm manner.
- Employ nonpharmacologic interventions as indicated: relaxation breathing, guided imagery, soft music.
- Ensure that patient receives periods of uninterrupted sleep (optimally 90 min at a time) by grouping care procedures when possible and limiting visitors.
- See p. 66 for additional information about pain management.

Impaired tissue integrity/Altered peripheral tissue perfusion related to thermal injury, circumferential burns, edema, and hypovolemia

Desired outcomes: Patient's wound exhibits evidence of granulation and healing by primary intention or split-thickness skin grafting within an acceptable time frame.

Note: Healing time varies with the extent of injury. Tissue perfusion in burned extremities is adequate as evidenced by peripheral pulses >2+ on a scale of 0-4+, brisk capillary refill (<2 sec), and skin temperature warm to the touch. Tissue healing occurs without overgrowth (keloid) formation.

- Assess and document time and circumstances of burn injury, as well as extent and depth of burn wound (see Tables 2-15 and 2-16).
- In burned extremities, evaluate tissue perfusion by hourly monitoring of capillary refill, temperature, and peripheral pulses. Be alert to signs of decreased peripheral perfusion, including coolness of the extremity, weak or absent peripheral pulses, and delayed capillary refill. Consult physician for significant findings.
- Cleanse and débride wound as prescribed. Control ambient temperature carefully to prevent hypothermia.
- Apply topical antimicrobial treatments as prescribed, using aseptic technique.
- Elevate burned extremities at or above heart level to promote venous return and to prevent excessive dependent edema formation.
- To prevent pooling of fluid or seroma formation, which contributes to graft loss, express fluid between graft and recipient bed as prescribed by using a rolling motion with sterile applicators. Always roll the applicator in the same direction over the graft to prevent disruption of graft "take." If prescribed, aspirate hematomas or seromas with a tuberculin syringe and a 26-gauge needle. This also is performed to prevent pooling of fluids.
- Monitor type and amount of drainage from wounds. Promptly report the presence of bright red bleeding, which would inhibit graft "take," and purulent exudate, which indicates infection.
- Maintain immobility of grafted site for 3 days or as prescribed. This

is achieved with a combination of positioning, splinting, or light pressure and sedation. In some instances, restraints, stents, bulky dressings, or occlusive dressings may be required to maintain immobilization and promote hemostasis of graft.

- Elevate grafted extremity at or above heart level to promote venous return and decrease pooling of blood and plasma.
- Apply elastic wraps to grafted legs to promote venous return.
- Use bed cradle to prevent bedding from coming in contact with open grafted area.
- Provide donor site care as prescribed, and be alert to signs of donor site infection (see **Risk for infection,** p. 223.)
- Apply compression netting to graft and incision sites. Teach patient about need for extended compression to prevent skin overgrowth.

Altered gastrointestinal tissue perfusion related to hypovolemia and interruption in blood flow associated with splanchnic vasoconstriction secondary to fluid shifts and catecholamine release

Desired outcome: Patient has adequate GI tissue perfusion as evidenced by auscultation of 5-34 bowel sounds/min within 48-72 h after burn injury and bowel elimination within patient's normal pattern.

Note: Be aware that prolonged impaired perfusion to GI organs increases the likelihood of such complications as decreased bowel sounds, adynamic ileus, and the development of gastritis and Curling's ulcer.

- Monitor bowel sounds q2h. Be alert to decreasing or absent bowel sounds, which occur with adynamic ileus.
- During period of absent bowel sounds, maintain gastric tube to intermittent low suction as prescribed. Ensure patency and position of the tube.
- Maintain NPO status until return of bowel sounds.
- Monitor gastric pH level q2h. Administer antacids as prescribed to maintain pH ≥ 5. If prescribed, start gastric tube feedings immediately to protect the patient's gastric mucosa from irritation.
- Administer histamine H_2-receptor antagonists as prescribed to prevent formation of gastric acids (see Table 8-13, p. 555).
- Test gastric aspirate for blood q8h. Promptly report presence of blood to physician.

Altered nutrition: Less than body requirements of protein, vitamins, and calories related to hypermetabolic state secondary to burn wound healing

Desired outcome: By the time of discharge from the critical care unit, patient has adequate nutrition as evidenced by stable weight, balanced nitrogen state per nitrogen studies, serum albumin ≥ 3.5 g/dl, thyroxine-binding prealbumin 20-30 mg/dl, retinol-binding protein 4-5 mg/dl, and evidence of burn wound healing and graft "take" within an acceptable time frame.

- Record all intake for daily calorie counts. Measure weight daily, and evaluate on the basis of patient's preburn weight.
- Monitor serum albumin, thyroxine-binding prealbumin, retinol-binding protein, and urine nitrogen measurements. Burn patients undergo long periods of catabolism, with large amounts of nitrogen excreted in the urine. Serum values will be decreased from normal.

Be alert to continuing deficiencies, weight loss, and poor graft "take," all of which are signals that nutritional needs are not being met.

- Provide high-protein, high-calorie diet as prescribed. When patient can take foods orally, promote supplemental feedings of snacks such as milkshakes and ice cream between meals.
- Confer with physician regarding need for enteral feedings in patients with burns >10% BSA, preinjury illness, or associated injuries, inasmuch as they have calorie requirements that cannot be met orally. Patients with ileus that persists for more than 4 days or those unable to meet caloric needs enterally will require TPN as prescribed by physician.
- Assess patient preferences relative to foods high in protein and carbohydrates. Encourage family members to provide desired foods.
- For additional information, see "Nutritional Support," p. 1.

Sensory/perceptual alterations (tactile and visual) related to altered reception secondary to medications, sleep pattern disturbance, pain, and altered dermal status

Desired outcome: Within 24-48 h of this diagnosis, patient verbalizes orientation to time, place, and person and describes rationale for necessary treatments.

- Assess patient's orientation to time, place, and person.
- Answer patient's questions simply and succinctly, providing information regarding immediate surroundings, procedures, and treatments. During the emergent phase of the burn injury, anticipate the necessity of having to repeat information at frequent intervals.
- For patient with full-thickness injury, explain why tactile sensation is decreased or absent and that it will return with eschar separation and débridement.
- If patient's eyelids are swollen shut due to facial edema, reassure patient that he or she is not blind and that swelling will resolve within 3-5 days.
- Touch patient often on unburned skin to provide nonpainful tactile stimulation.
- For additional information, see this nursing diagnosis in "Psychosocial Support," p. 90.

Body image disturbance related to biophysical changes secondary to burn injury

Desired outcomes: Within 72 h of this diagnosis, patient acknowledges body changes and demonstrates movement toward incorporating changes into self-concept. Patient does not exhibit maladaptive responses such as severe depression.

- Assess patient's perceptions and feelings about the burn injury and changes in life-style and relationships, especially those with significant other.
- Involve significant other in as much care as possible to maintain bond with patient.
- Respect patient's need to express anger over body changes.
- Provide information about cosmetic aids and use of clothing to help conceal burns.
- Praise patient's attempts to enhance appearance. Praise and encour-

age patient's expressed desires regarding public excursions after hospital discharge.

- Provide names and telephone numbers of support groups for burn patients.
- For additional information, see this nursing diagnosis, p. 97, and Table 1-41, p. 97.

Risk for disuse syndrome related to immobilization from pain, splints, or scar formation

Desired outcome: Patient displays complete ROM without verbal or nonverbal indicators of discomfort.

- Provide ROM exercises q4h. When possible, combine with hydrotherapy in a Hubbard tank.
- Apply splints as recommended by physical therapy personnel to maintain body parts in functional positions and to prevent contracture formation.
- For graft patient, institute ROM exercises and ambulation on fifth postgraft day, or as prescribed. Premedicate with prescribed analgesic to aid in patient's mobility.

Risk for infection related to inadequate primary and secondary defenses secondary to traumatized tissue, bacterial proliferation in burn wounds, presence of invasive lines or urinary catheter, and immunocompromised status

Desired outcome: Patient is free of infection as evidenced by normothermia, WBC count $\leq$11,000 μl, negative culture results, well-defined burn wound margin, and absence of pockets that contain purulent matter and other clinical indicators of burn wound infection.

- Except for eyebrows, shave all hair within 5 cm of wound margin to prevent contamination of wound.
- Monitor temperature q2h. Report temperatures >38.9° C (102° F).
- Assess burn wound daily for status of eschar separation and granulation tissue formation, color, vascularity, sensation, and odor. Be alert to signs of infection, including fever, elevated WBC count, rapid eschar separation, increased amount of exudate, pockets that contain purulent material, disappearance of a well-defined burn margin with edema formation, wound discoloration (e.g., black or dark brown), change in color of partial-thickness burn from pink or mottled red to full-thickness necrosis, superficial ulceration of burned skin at wound margins, pale and boggy granulation tissue, hemorrhagic discoloration of subeschar fat, and spongy and poorly demarcated eschar. Consult physician for significant changes.
- Assess appearance of grafted site, including adherence to recipient bed, appearance, and color. Be alert to erythema, hyperthermia, increasing tenderness, purulent drainage, and swelling around the grafted site.
- Observe for clinical indicators of sepsis: tachypnea, hypothermia, hyperthermia, ileus, subtle disorientation, unexplained metabolic acidosis, and glucose intolerance, as evidenced by glycosuria and elevated blood sugar levels (see "Shock," p. 608).
- As prescribed, obtain wound, blood, sputum, and urine culture specimens in the presence of a temperature >38.9° C (102° F).
- Administer systemic antibiotics and antipyretics as prescribed.

- Ensure aseptic technique when administering care to burned areas and performing invasive techniques.
- Place patients 18-60 yr of age with burns >30% BSA and patients >60 yr of age with burns >20% BSA in protective isolation.
- For patients with skin grafts, monitor donor site for evidence of infection, including purulent drainage, undefined borders, and foul odor.

Knowledge deficit: Self-care during the rehabilitative stage

Desired outcome: Within the 24-h period before discharge from the critical care unit, patient and significant others verbalize knowledge about prescribed medications and demonstrate and verbalize knowledge about techniques that facilitate continued wound healing and limb mobility.

- Review the splinting and exercise program for contracture prevention, as directed by physical therapist. Teach patient and significant others to monitor for pain or pressure due to improperly applied splint and to assess splinted extremity for coolness, pallor, cyanosis, decreased pulses, and impaired function.
- Discuss skin care, emphasizing the following:
  □ Explain that a lubricating cream without alcohol (e.g., Nivea) should be applied several times a day and after bathing to promote soft and pliant skin and assist with control of pruritus.
  □ Explain that dressings or padding should be applied to areas that may be traumatized by pressure.
  □ Teach patient to avoid exposure to sun, because healed skin is highly sensitive to ultraviolet rays for up to 1 year.
  □ Explain to a darker-skinned patient that permanent pigmentation changes are likely to occur due to destruction of melanocytes and that burned areas usually will stay pink.
  □ Review wound care. Provide simplified dressing change procedure; explain indicators of infection and importance of notifying physician should they appear.
  □ Teach patient the importance of wearing pressure garment as prescribed to prevent excessive or hypertrophic scarring.
- Review nutrition needs: Explain the importance of maintaining an adequate intake of protein and calories for optimal wound healing.
- Provide a list of medications, including drug name, purpose, dosage, schedule, precautions, and potential side effects.
- Discuss home care and the importance of counseling to provide support for adjustment to life outside the hospital environment after disfiguring injury.
- Provide addresses and telephone numbers of local support groups for burn patients.
- Stress the importance of follow-up care; confirm date and time of first appointment if it has been established.

ADDITIONAL NURSING DIAGNOSES

For other nursing diagnoses and interventions, see the following, as appropriate: "Nutritional Support," p. 12; "Mechanical Ventilation," p. 24; "Wound and Skin Care," p. 58; "Pain," p. 74; "Prolonged Immobility," p. 78; "Psychosocial Support," p. 88; "Psychosocial Support for the Patient's Family and Significant Others," p. 100; and "Infection Prevention and Control," Appendix 8.

Selected Bibliography

American College of Chest Physicians–Society for Critical Care Medicine Consensus Conference Committee: Definitions for sepsis and organ failure and guidelines for the use of innovative therapies in sepsis, *Chest* 101(6):1644-1655, 1992.

Apple S, Thurkauf GE: Preparing for and understanding transesophageal echocardiography, *Crit Care Nurse* 12(6):29-34, 1992.

Balski JD, Cantelmo NL, Menzoian JO: Complications of caval interruption by Greenfield filter in quadraplegics, *J Vasc Surg* 9(4):558-562, 1989.

Bastnagel Mason P: Neurodiagnostic testing in critically injured adults, *Crit Care Nurse* 1(4):64-75, 1992.

Batlle FJ, Northrup BE: Pathophysiology of acute spinal cord injury, *Trauma Quarterly* 9(2):29-37, 1993.

Bayley EW: Wound healing in the patient with burns, *Nurs Clin North Am* 25(1):205-222, 1990.

Beachly M, Farrar J: Abdominal trauma: putting the pieces together, *Am J Nurs* 93(11):26-34, 1993.

Bishop MH: Relationship between supranormal circulatory values, time delays, and outcome in severely traumatized patients, *Crit Care Med* 21(1):56-63, 1993.

Bolton P, Von Rotz N: Management of an open abdominal wound with a synthetic covering, *Crit Care Nurse* 14(2):44-51, 1993.

Bracken MB et al: A randomized clinical trial of methylprednisolone and naloxone used in the treatment of acute spinal cord injuries, *N Engl J Med* 322:1405-1411, 1990.

Buckman RF et al: Penetrating cardiac wounds: prospective study of factors influencing initial resuscitation, *J Trauma* 34(5):717-725, 1993.

Burgess MC: Initial management of a patient with extensive burn injury, *Crit Care Nurs Clin North Am* 3(2):165-179, 1991.

Calistro AM: Burn care basics and beyond, *RN* 56(3):26-31, 1993.

Cammermyer M, Appledorn C: *Core curriculum for neuroscience nursing,* Chicago, 1993, American Association of Neuroscience Nurses.

Cardona VC et al: *Trauma nursing: from resuscitation through rehabilitation,* ed 2, Philadelphia, 1994, Saunders.

Carlson DE, Jordan BS: Implementing nutritional therapy in the thermally injured patient, *Crit Care Nurs Clin North Am* 3(2):221-235, 1991.

Carter CT, Shafer N: Incidence of urethral disruption in females with traumatic pelvic fractures, *Am J Emerg Med* 11(3):218-220, 1993.

Cohen JR: Pulmonary management of the patient with spinal cord injury, *Trauma Quarterly* 9(2):38-43, 1993.

Crosby L, Parsons C: Cerebrovascular response of closed head-injured patients to a standardized endotracheal tube suctioning and manual hyperventilation procedure, *J Neurosci Nurs* 24(1):40-49, 1992.

Dalton JR: Urologic management of the patient with spinal cord injury, *Trauma Quarterly* 9(2):72-81, 1993.

Ditunno JF, Marino RJ, Crozier KS: Neurologic and functional assessments in acute spinal cord injury: uses in prognosis and management, *Trauma Quarterly* 9(2):44-52, 1993.

Duncan DJ, Driscoll DM: Burn wound management, *Crit Care Nurs Clin North Am* 3(2):199-221, 1991.

Dyer C, Roberts D: Thermal trauma, *Nurs Clin North Am* 25(1):85-117, 1990.

Edwards KP: Orthopedic trauma: pelvic fractures, *Today's OR Nurse* 15(4):24-28, 1993.

Fishburn MJ, Marino RN, Ditunno JF: Atelectasis and pneumonia in acute spinal cord injury, *Arch Phys Med Rehabil* 71(3):197-200, 1990.

Fontaine DK: The cutting edge in trauma, *Crit Care Nurse* (June suppl):14-15,21, 1993.

Fuhrman GM et al: The single indication for cystography in blunt trauma, *J Trauma* 59(6):335-337, 1993.

Gennarelli T et al: Influence of the type of intracranial lesion on outcome from severe head injury, *J Neurosurg* 56(1):26-32, 1982.

Goldberg SP, Karalis DG, Ross JJ: Severe right ventricular contusion mimicking cardiac tamponade: the value of transesophageal echocardiography in blunt chest trauma, *Ann Emerg Med* 22(4):745-747, 1993.

Hammond SG: Chest injuries in the trauma patient, *Nurs Clin North Am* 25(1):35-43, 1990.

Hilton G, Frei J: High-dose methylprednisolone in the treatment of spinal cord injury, *Heart Lung* 20(6):675-680, 1991.

Hilton G, Frei J: Methylprednisolone for acute spinal cord injury, *J Neurosci Nurs* 24(4):234-237, 1992.

Hughes MC: Critical care nursing for the patient with spinal cord injury, *Crit Care Nurs Clin North Am* 2(1):33-40, 1990.

Interqual: The ISD-A review system with adult ISD criteria, August 1992, North Hampton, NH and Marlboro, MA, Interqual, Inc.

Jordan K: Chest trauma: how to detect—and to react to—serious trouble, *Nursing* 20(9):34-42, 1990.

Kaplan AJ, Norcross ED, Crawford FA: Predictors of mortality in penetrating cardiac trauma, *Am Surg* 59(6):338-341, 1993.

Keller C, Williams A: Cardiac dysrhythmias associated with central nervous system dysfunction, *J Neurosci Nurs* 25(6):349-355, 1993.

Kerr M et al: Head-injured adults: recommendations for endotracheal suctioning, *J Neurosci Nurs* 25(2):86-91, 1993.

Kim MJ, McFarland GK, McLane AM: *Pocket guide to nursing diagnoses,* ed 6, St Louis, 1995, Mosby.

Lawrence DM: Gastrointestinal trauma, *Crit Care Nurs Clin North Am* 5(1):127-140, 1993.

Lekander B, Cerra F: The syndrome of multiple organ failure, *Crit Care Nurs Clin North Am* 2(2):331-342, 1990.

McAnich JW et al: Renal gunshot wounds: methods of salvage and reconstruction, *J Trauma* 35(2):279-284, 1993.

McGee D, Dalsey W: The mangled extremity: compartment syndrome and amputations, *Emerg Med Clin North Am* 10(4):783-800, 1992.

McMurtry RY, McLellan BA: *Management of blunt trauma,* Baltimore, 1990, Williams & Wilkins.

Mubarak S: Compartment syndromes. In Chapman MW, editor: *Operative orthopedics,* Philadelphia, 1993, Lippincott.

Narumi Y et al: MR imaging of traumatic posterior urethral injury, *Radiology* 188(2):439-443, 1993.

Neff JA, Kidd PS: *Trauma nursing: the art and science,* St Louis, 1993, Mosby.

Paone RF, Reacock JB, Smith DL: Diagnosis of myocardial contusion, *South Med J* 86(8):867-870, 1993.

Park PK, Ziring BS, Merli GJ: Prophylaxis of deep venous thrombosis in patients with acute spinal cord injury, *Trauma Quarterly* 9(2):93-99, 1993.

Reich SM, Cotler JM: Mechanisms and patterns of spine and spinal cord injuries, *Trauma Quarterly* 9(2):7-28, 1993.

Reilly E, Yucha C: Multiple organ failure syndrome, *Crit Care Nurs* 14(2):25-31, 1993.

Robins EV: Burn shock, *Crit Care Nurs Clin North Am* 2(2):299-307, 1990.

Ross D: Acute compartment syndrome, *Orthop Nurs* 10(2):33-38, 1991.

Ross D: Ischemic myositis (compartment syndrome). In Swearingen PL, editor: *Manual of medical-surgical nursing care,* ed 3, St Louis, 1994, Mosby.

Rudy E et al: Endotracheal suctioning in adults with head injury, *Heart Lung* 20(6):667-674, 1991.

Rue III LW, Cioffi Jr WG: Resuscitation of thermally injured patients, *Crit Care Nurs Clin North Am* 3(2):181-198, 1991.

Segatore M: Fever after traumatic brain injury, *J Neurosci Nurs* 24(2):104-109, 1992.

Slye D: Orthopedic complications: compartment syndrome, fat embolism syndrome, and venous thromboembolism, *Nurs Clin North Am* 26(1):113-132, 1991.

Smith A, Fitzpatrick E: Penetrating cardiac trauma: surgical and nursing management, *J Cardiovasc Nurs* 7(2):52-70, 1993.

Sommers MS: Alcohol and trauma: the critical link, *Crit Care Nurse* 14(2):82-93, 1993.

Summers TM: Psychosocial support of the burned patient, *Crit Care Nurs Clin North Am* 3(2):237-243, 1991.

Vos H: Making headway with intracranial hypertension, *Am J Nurs* 93(2):28-39, 1993.

Williams A, Coyne S: Effects of neck position on intracranial pressure, *Am J Crit Care* 2(1):68-71, 1993.

Worthington P, Crowe MA, Armenti VT: Nutritional support for patients with SCI, *Trauma Quarterly* 9(2).82-92, 1993.

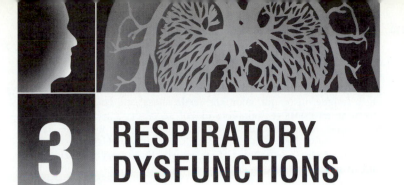

3 RESPIRATORY DYSFUNCTIONS

Status asthmaticus

PATHOPHYSIOLOGY

Status asthmaticus (SA) is a severe, life-threatening bronchospasm that critically diminishes the diameter of the patient's airway. The hyperreactive bronchial airways respond to a variety of irritants with diffuse narrowing as a result of bronchospasm and bronchial inflammation, causing mucosal edema, increased mucus production, and plugging. When an episode of bronchospasm is not reversed after 24 h of maximum doses of traditional beta-agonist and theophylline therapy, the patient is diagnosed with SA. Precipitating factors include allergens (airborne or ingested), respiratory infection, chemical irritants (e.g., smoke, air pollution), physical irritants (e.g., cold air, exercise) and, in some individuals, emotional stress. Although the attack can happen suddenly, there usually is a more gradual onset, with symptoms of increased sputum production, coughing, wheezing, and dyspnea occurring over several days. The patient experiences increased work of breathing, which increases insensible water loss through exhaled water vapor and diaphoresis. Oral intake may be decreased, which contributes further to the hypovolemia. Mucus becomes thick and begins to plug the airways. Terminal bronchioles become occluded completely from mucosal edema and tenacious secretions. Ventilation-perfusion mismatch occurs as poorly ventilated alveoli continue to be perfused. Shunting of blood from nonventilated alveoli to other alveoli cannot compensate for the diminished ventilation, and hypoxia occurs. Tachypnea and tachycardia evolve as compensatory mechanisms. As a result, oxygen requirements and work of breathing increase. If the patient is not treated promptly, respiratory collapse can occur, and death by asphyxiation is possible.

ASSESSMENT

CLINICAL PRESENTATION Coughing, chest tightness, increased sputum production, increased RR (>20 breaths/min), labored breathing, dyspnea, fatigue, insomnia, anorexia, restlessness, and confusion.

PHYSICAL ASSESSMENT Agitation, use of accessory muscles of respiration, chest retractions, nasal flaring, diaphoresis, decreased tactile fremitus and hyperresonance over lung areas in which there is air trapping, and dullness over areas of atelectasis. Expiratory wheezing, prolonged expiratory phase, and coarse rhonchi may be auscultated. In addition, the patient may have hypotension, pulsus paradoxus >10 mm Hg, and apical tachycardia (HR >100 bpm). Cyanosis of the lips and nail beds is a late sign of respiratory compromise.

Note: An absence of wheezing in the presence of other signs and symptoms of respiratory distress may be a result of severe bronchial constriction, which dangerously narrows airways during both inspiratory and expiratory phases. The volume of air moved through the airways is so minimal that it does not cause a sound. If this occurs, respiratory collapse may be imminent.

DIAGNOSTIC TESTS

ABG analysis: Evaluates status of oxygenation and acid-base balance. Initially, Pao_2 is normal and then decreases as the ventilation-perfusion mismatch becomes more severe. Usually, $Paco_2$ is decreased in early stages of SA due to hyperventilation. When $Paco_2$ is normal or greater than normal, respiratory failure may be imminent due to relative hypoventilation.

Pulse oximetry (Spo_2): Safe, noninvasive technology that measures the oxygen saturation of arterial blood, which then can be displayed continuously. Pulse oximetry uses red and infrared wavelengths of light to calculate arterial saturation based on the difference between light transmitted and light absorbed by the RBCs. Correlation of peripheral oxygen saturation values measured by oximetry with arterial saturation (Sao_2) is within 2% when Sao_2 is >50%. Factors that may affect the oxyhemoglobin dissociation curve (temperature, pH, $Paco_2$, anemia, hemodynamic status) may adversely affect the accuracy of pulse oximetry measurements. Also, the presence of other forms of Hgb in the blood (carboxyhemoglobin, a byproduct of smoking and smoke, or methemoglobin, which is formed by the use of drugs such as lidocaine and nitroglycerin) can produce falsely high readings. Normal reading is $\geq 90\%$. When initiating pulse oximetry, it is helpful to obtain ABG values to compare and evaluate $Paco_2$ and pH.

Pulmonary function testing: Forced expiratory volume (FEV) is decreased during acute episodes because of severely narrowed airways that prevent forceful exhalation of inspired volume (Table 3-1).

Chest x-ray: Useful in ruling out other causes of respiratory failure (e.g., foreign body aspiration, pulmonary edema, pulmonary embolism, pneumonia). The x-ray usually shows lung hyperinflation due to air trapping and a flat diaphragm related to increased intrathoracic volume.

T A B L E 3 - 1　Pulmonary function tests in status asthmaticus

Test	Description	Normal values	Parameters in SA
FVC	Total amount of gas exhaled as forcefully and rapidly as possible after maximal inspiration	≥80% of predicted normal	Normal or slightly decreased due to air trapping
FEV_1	Volume of gas exhaled over first second of FVC	≥75% of predicted normal	Decreased due to obstruction; may return to normal after inhalation of aerosolized bronchodilator
FEF	Average rate of flow during middle half of FEV; an accurate estimate of airway resistance	≥80% of predicted normal	Decreased due to small airways obstruction; may return to normal after inhalation of aerosolized bronchodilator

FEF, Forced expiratory flow; *FEV_1*, forced expiratory volume in 1 sec; *FVC*, forced vital capacity.

Sputum:　Gross examination may show increased viscosity or actual mucous plugs. Culture and sensitivity may show microorganisms if infection is the precipitating event.

CBC count:　Differential will show increased eosinophils in patients not receiving corticosteroids, which is indicative of allergic response. The hematocrit (Hct) may be increased due to hypovolemia.

Serum theophylline level:　Important baseline indicator for patients who are on this therapy regimen. Acceptable therapeutic range is 10-20 mg/ml. The therapeutic level is close to the toxic level, and the patient must be monitored for side effects (e.g., nausea, nervousness, dysrhythmias). Serial levels are drawn at frequent intervals.

ECG:　Presence of sinus tachycardia is an important baseline indicator, because the use of some bronchodilators (e.g., metaproterenol) may produce cardiac stimulant effects and dysrhythmias.

Urine specific gravity:　An important indicator of hydration. Values higher than normal (1.010-1.020) occur with dehydration.

COLLABORATIVE MANAGEMENT

Respiratory failure in SA is relative to the increased work of breathing and increased minute ventilation requirements. Primarily, management is directed toward decreasing bronchospasm and increasing pulmonary ventilation. Other interventions are directed toward treatment of sequelae.

Oxygen therapy:　Generally, patients with SA have profound hypoxia and can tolerate high doses of oxygen (4-8 L). However, if the patient has chronic CO_2 retention, he or she may not tolerate >2-3 L oxygen, inasmuch as higher doses might impair the drive to breathe, which is a hypoxic drive. Oxygen therapy is begun immediately to correct hypoxemia, and the Pao_2 is kept above normal to compensate for the increased oxygen demands imposed by the increased work of breathing. The oxygen is humidified to help liquefy secretions. The degree of hypoxemia and patient response determine the method of oxygen delivery. The patient may prefer a nasal cannula, but a high-flow system delivers more precise and higher Fio_2. Comfort, however, is important, especially if the patient will not wear a mask because of feelings of suffocation.

Intubation and mechanical ventilation: Elected if $Paco_2$ continues to rise, if Pao_2 falls to <60 mm Hg, or if patient experiences intolerable respiratory distress. Therapy ensures adequate alveolar ventilation and provides a pathway for clearing airway secretions *via* suctioning. See discussion, p. 19

Pharmacotherapy: Vigorous therapy is initiated to improve bronchospasm. Treatment is continued until wheezing is eliminated and pulmonary function tests return to baseline.

Bronchodilators: Dilate smooth muscles of the airways (Table 3-2).

Corticosteroids: Given intravenously during the acute phase of SA to decrease the inflammatory response. Dosage varies according to severity of episode and whether patient currently is taking steroids.

Note: Acute adrenal insufficiency can develop in patients who take steroids routinely at home if these drugs are not given to the patient during hospitalization.

Sedatives and tranquilizers: Generally avoided unless patient is extremely agitated and unable to cooperate with therapy, inasmuch as these agents depress the CNS response to hypoxia, hypercapnia, and airway obstruction.

Buffers: Metabolic acidosis may develop as a compensatory mechanism for early respiratory alkalosis during which patient is hyperventilating and exhaling greater than normal amounts of CO_2. Sodium bicarbonate may be given to correct severe metabolic acidosis. The physiologic response to bronchodilators improves with correction of metabolic acidosis.

Antibiotics: Given if infectious pulmonary process is suspected, as evidenced by fever, purulent sputum, or leukocytosis.

Fluid replacement: To liquefy secretions and replace insensible losses. Generally, crystalloid fluids (i.e., D_5W or D_5NS) are used.

Chest physiotherapy: Generally contraindicated in acute phases of SA because of acute respiratory embarrassment and hyperreactive state of airways. Once the crisis is over, the patient may benefit from percussion and postural drainage q2-4h to help mobilize secretions.

NURSING DIAGNOSES AND INTERVENTIONS

Impaired gas exchange related to altered oxygen supply secondary to decreased alveolar ventilation present with narrowed airways

Desired outcome: Within 2-4 h of initiation of treatment, patient has adequate gas exchange as evidenced by Pao_2 >60 mm Hg, $Paco_2$ 35-45 mm Hg, and pH 7.35-7.45 (or ABG values within 10% of patient's baseline). Within 24-48 h of initiation of treatment, RR is 12-20

T A B L E   3 - 2   Bronchodilators used in status asthmaticus

Medication	Usual dosage	Action	Side effects
epinephrine	0.2-0.5 ml of 1:1,000 solution given SC q15-30min	Immediate adrenergic effects; activates adrenergic sympathomimetic receptors; acts on alpha-, $beta_1$-, and $beta_2$-receptors; relieves bronchospasm	Cardiac stimulation, palpitations, anxiety
terbutaline (Brethine)	0.2-0.3 ml given SC q30min × 3 doses	Selective beta-adrenergic; relaxes bronchial smooth muscle	Fewer than with epinephrine and usually transient; increased HR (>120 bpm), nervousness, tremor, palpitations, nausea, vomiting, headache
methylxanthines (theophylline, aminophylline)	*Loading dosage:* 6 mg/kg given as IV bolus. **Note:** Loading dose may be omitted if the patient is already taking oral methylxanthine and serum level is therapeutic *Maintenance dosage:* 0.1-0.5 μg/kg/h given *via* continuous IV infusion	Short-acting nonadrenergic; directly relaxes smooth muscle of bronchial airways and pulmonary vasculature	Nausea, vomiting, GI bleeding, gastric distress, HR >120 bpm, decreased BP, restlessness. **Note:** Toxic levels are close to therapeutic loads; serum levels should be monitored closely to ensure correct dosage adjustment; dysrhythmias may result from theophylline toxicity

Note: Isoproterenol and isoetharine are two inhalants usually avoided during acute SA because the patient's gas flow may be too minimal to provide adequate distribution of medication. Aerosolized drugs may be used once other routes achieve bronchodilatation.

breaths/min with normal depth and pattern (eupnea), and breath sounds are clear and bilaterally equal.

- Observe for signs and symptoms of hypoxia (e.g., restlessness, agitation, changes in LOC). Remember that cyanosis of the lips and nail beds is a late indicator of hypoxia.
- Position patient for comfort and to promote optimal gas exchange. Usually this is accomplished by high Fowler's position, with the patient leaning forward and elbows propped on the over-the-bed table to promote maximal chest excursion. Record patient's response to positioning.
- Auscultate breath sounds at frequent intervals. Monitor for decreased or adventitious sounds (e.g., wheezes, rhonchi).
- Encourage patient to breathe slowly and deeply. Teach pursed-lip breathing technique to assist patient with controlling his or her respirations:
  1. Inhale through the nose.
  2. Form lips in an "O" shape as if whistling.
  3. Exhale slowly through pursed lips.
- Record patient's response to breathing technique. Educate significant others in coaching.
- Deliver oxygen as prescribed; monitor Fio_2 to ensure that oxygen is within prescribed concentrations.
- Monitor ABG or pulse oximetry values. Be alert to decreasing Pao_2 and increasing $Paco_2$ with ABG analysis or decreasing saturation levels with pulse oximetry, which are signals of respiratory failure.

Ineffective airway clearance related to presence of increased tracheobronchial secretions; and related to decreased ability to expectorate secondary to fatigue.

Desired outcome: Within 24-48 h of initiating treatment, patient's airway is free of excess secretions as evidenced by eupnea and absence of adventitious breath sounds and excessive coughing.

- At frequent intervals, assess patient's ability to clear tracheobronchial secretions. Keep emergency suction equipment at the bedside.
- Encourage oral fluid intake within patient's prescribed limits to help decrease viscosity of the secretions.
- Encourage patient to cough effectively at frequent intervals to clear secretions:
  1. Instruct patient to take several deep breaths. Instruct significant others in coaching this technique.
  2. After the last inhalation, teach patient to perform a succession of coughs (usually three to four) on the same exhalation until most of the air has been expelled.
  3. Explain that patient may need to repeat this technique several times before the cough becomes productive.
- After crisis phase of SA has been resolved, ensure that patient receives chest physiotherapy as prescribed; document patient's response to treatment. If appropriate, teach significant others to perform chest physiotherapy.
- Ensure that oxygen is humidified to aid in liquefying tracheobronchial secretions.

Activity intolerance related to imbalance between oxygen supply and demand secondary to decreased alveolar oxygen supply and greater metabolic oxygen demands due to increased work of breathing

Desired outcome: Within 24-48 h of initiation of treatment, patient verbalizes a decrease in fatigue and associated symptoms.

- Organize and group assessment procedures and activities to provide patient with frequent rest periods (optimally, at least 90-120 min).
- Teach patient progressive muscle relaxation technique (see **Health-seeking behavior,** p. 323). Teach significant others how to coach patient in using relaxation techniques.
- Decrease metabolic demands for oxygen by limiting or pacing patient's activities and procedures.
- If patient is restless, which increases oxygen demand, ascertain the cause of the restlessness (e.g., if restlessness is related to anxiety, help reduce anxiety by providing reassurance, enabling family members to stay with patient, and offering distractions such as soft music or television.)
- Explain all procedures and offer support to minimize fear and anxiety, which can increase oxygen demands.
- Schedule rest times after meals to avoid competition for oxygen supply during digestion.
- Monitor Spo_2 by pulse oximetry during activity to evaluate limits of activity and recommend optimal positions for oxygenation.
- Assess temperature q2-4h. Consult physician for increases, and provide treatment as prescribed to decrease temperature and thus oxygen demands.

ADDITIONAL NURSING DIAGNOSES

See "Acute Pneumonia," for **Risk for infection** (nosocomial pneumonia), p. 242. For other nursing diagnoses and interventions, see "Psychosocial Support," p. 88, and "Psychosocial Support for the Patient's Family and Significant Others," p. 100.

Acute pneumonia

PATHOPHYSIOLOGY

Pneumonia is an acute infection that causes inflammation of the parenchyma (alveolar spaces and interstitial tissue) of the lung. As a result of the inflammation, the involved lung tissue becomes swollen and the air spaces fill with liquid. Pneumonias can be classified into two groups: community acquired and hospital associated (nosocomial). Pneumonias that occur in the immunocompromised host can be acquired in the community or can be associated with hospitalization. The infecting organisms are often distinctive in this population and will be described separately. (See Table 3-3 for a detailed discussion by pneumonia type.)

Community acquired: Persons with this type of pneumonia seldom require hospitalization and are seen in intensive care areas only when

Text continued on p. 240.

T A B L E 3 - 3   Assessment guidelines by pneumonia type

Type/pathogen	Risk groups	Onset	Defining characteristics	Complications/comments
Community acquired				
Pneumococcal (*Pneumococcus pneumoniae, Streptococcus pneumoniae*)	Persons >40 yr, especially males. Risk increases with alcoholism and debilitating diseases (e.g., COPD, CHF, multiple myeloma, sickle cell disease). Viral upper respiratory tract infections often precede this pneumonia.	Abrupt	Single shaking chill, fever, pleuritic chest pain, severe cough, SOB, rust-colored sputum, and diaphoresis. Many patients also have herpes labialis, abdominal pain and distention, and paralytic ileus.	Pleural effusions, empyema, impaired liver function, bacteremia, and meningitis. Incidence of pneumococcal pneumonia peaks in winter and early spring. Mortality rate increases if more than one lobe is involved.
Mycoplasma (*Mycoplasma pneumoniae*)	School-aged children to young adult (5-30 yr). Intrafamilial spread is common.	Gradual	Cough, sore throat, fever, headache, chills, malaise, anorexia, nausea, vomiting, diarrhea. In children arthralgia involving the large joints is common.	Rare. Persistent cough and sinusitis are possible. Pulse-temperature dissociation is common.
Legionnaires' (*Legionella pneumophila*)	Middle-aged, elderly (males at increased risk) populations; smokers; individuals with malignancy, immunosuppression, or chronic renal failure; exposure to contaminated construction site.	Abrupt	Malaise, headache within 24 h, fever with normal HR, shaking chills, progressive dyspnea, cough that may become productive; GI symptoms, including anorexia, vomiting, diarrhea; arthralgia, myalgia.	Respiratory failure, hypotension, shock, acute renal failure.

Viral influenza A	Elderly persons with chronic diseases (e.g., COPD, diabetes mellitus, CHF); pregnancy.	1 wk after onset of influenza symptoms	Severe dyspnea, cyanosis, scant sputum occasionally with blood, fever, persistent and dry cough.	Rapid course leading frequently to acute respiratory failure; secondary bacterial pneumonia.
Haemophilus influenzae	Adults (especially ≥50 yr of age) with chronic diseases (e.g., diabetes mellitus, COPD, chronic alcohol ingestion).	2-6 wk after URI	Fever, chills, dyspnea, cough, nausea, vomiting, pain.	Fever may be minimal or absent; HR and RR may be normal.
Nosocomial				
Klebsiella* (*Klebsiella pneumoniae*) (also may be acquired in the community)	Males >40 yr, alcoholics; patients with diabetes mellitus, COPD, heart disease; those previously treated with antibiotics or ET intubation.	Abrupt	Chills, fever, productive cough (copious purulent green or "currant jelly" sputum). Severe pleuritic chest pain, dyspnea, cyanosis, jaundice, vomiting, and diarrhea.	Lung abscess and empyema, necrotizing pneumonitis with cavitation, acute respiratory failure. High mortality rate (~50%). Aspiration of oropharyngeal flora is responsible for nosocomial and community-acquired cases.

Enterobacter and *Serratia* are enteric organisms that cause pneumonia with the same clinical pattern as *Klebsiella* organisms.

Continued.

T A B L E 3 - 3 Assessment guidelines by pneumonia type—cont'd

Type/pathogen	Risk groups	Onset	Defining characteristics	Complications/comments
Pseudomonas (also may be acquired in the community)	Patients neutropenic from chemotherapy or immunosuppressed secondary to cortisone therapy or other illnesses.	Gradual	Fever, chills, confusion, delirium, bradycardia, purulent sputum (green, foul smelling).	Rarely occurs in previously healthy adults; high mortality rate.
Proteus	Older adults with debilitating underlying diseases.	Abrupt	High fever, chills, pleuritic chest pain.	Rare. Localizes to areas that already are damaged. Occurs as a mixed infection; has four pathogenic species with differing antibiotic susceptibilities.
Staphylococcus aureus	Patients with debilitating diseases (e.g., diabetes mellitus, renal failure, liver disease, COPD); those with a prior viral or influenza infection; IV drug abusers.	Abrupt with community acquired; insidious with hospital associated.	Cough, chills, high fever, pleuritic pain, progressive dyspnea, cyanosis, bloody sputum.	Pulmonary abscesses, empyema, pleural effusions; slow response to antibiotics.
Aspiration of gastric contents	Patients with impaired gag/cough reflexes; general anesthesia; presence of NG/ET tube.	Gradual: latent period between aspiration and onset of symptoms.	Fever, wheezes, crackles (rales), rhonchi, dyspnea, cyanosis.	Physiologic response depends on pH of material aspirated: ≥ 2.5, little necrosis occurs; < 2.5, atelectasis, pulmonary edema, hemorrhage, and necrosis can occur.

Immunocompromised patient

Pneumocystis (*Pneumocystis carinii*)	Patients with AIDS or organ transplants.	Insidious	Several weeks of fever, nonproductive cough, night sweats, dyspnea; hypoxemia with few auscultatory signs.	Bronchoscopy with transbronchial biopsy usually required for diagnosis.
Aspergillosis (*Aspergillus*)	Patients with AIDS, COPD, and transplants (especially autogolous bone marrow transplant); also those receiving cytotoxic agents or steroids.	Abrupt with immunosuppression; insidious with COPD.	High fever; fungal ball within lung cyst or cavity; nonproductive cough; pleuritic chest pain.	Cavitation frequently occurs; hematogenous spread common in immunocompromised patients.

CHF, Congestive heart failure; *URI,* upper respiratory infection.

an underlying medical condition such as chronic obstructive pulmonary disease (COPD), cardiac disease, diabetes mellitus, or an immunocompromised state necessitates special care.

Hospital associated (nosocomial):   These pneumonias usually occur after aspiration of oropharyngeal flora in an individual whose resistance is altered or whose coughing mechanisms are impaired (e.g., a patient who has undergone thoracoabdominal surgery). Bacteria invade the lower respiratory tract *via* three routes: aspiration of oropharyngeal organisms (most common route), inhalation of aerosols that contain bacteria, or hematogenous spread to the lung from another site of infection (rare). Alteration of oropharyngeal flora frequently occurs in debilitated hospitalized patients, especially those receiving antibiotics. Gram-negative pneumonias result in a high mortality rate, even with appropriate antibiotic therapy. *Aspiration pneumonia* is a nonbacterial cause of hospital-associated pneumonia that occurs when gastric contents are aspirated. If the alveolar-capillary membrane is affected, adult respiratory distress syndrome (ARDS) may be seen.

Immunocompromised patient: Immunosuppression and neutropenia are predisposing factors in the development of nosocomial and community-acquired pneumonias, from both common and unusual pathogens. The patient's underlying disease state is a determining factor in susceptibility to specific pathogens. Usually, patients with neutropenia resulting from acute leukemia or cytotoxic agents have gram-negative bacilli as the source of pneumonia. Severely immunocompromised patients are affected not only by bacteria but also by fungi *(Candida, Aspergillus* spp.*),* viruses (cytomegalovirus), and protozoa *(Pneumocystis carinii).* Most commonly, *Pneumocystis carinii* is seen in patients with HIV disease or in those who have received organ transplants.

ASSESSMENT

Findings are influenced by the patient's age, extent of the disease process, underlying medical condition, and pathogen involved.

RISK FACTORS In addition to the risk factors listed in Table 1-3, any factor that alters the integrity of the lower airways, thereby inhibiting ciliary activity, increases the likelihood of pneumonia. These factors may include hypoventilation, hyperoxia (increased Fio_2), hypoxia, and chemical irritants such as smoke.

CLINICAL PRESENTATION Cough (productive and nonproductive), sputum (rust colored, purulent, bloody, or mucoid), fever, pleuritic chest pain (more common in community-acquired bacterial pneumonias), dyspnea, chills, headache, myalgia. The older adult may be confused or disoriented and run low-grade fevers but initially may have few other signs and symptoms.

PHYSICAL ASSESSMENT Presence of nasal flaring and expiratory grunt; use of accessory muscles of respiration (scalene, sternocleidomastoid, external intercostals); decreased chest expansion caused by pleuritic pain; dullness on percussion over affected areas; tachypnea (RR >20 breaths/min), tachycardia (HR >100 bpm), decreased or bronchial breath sounds (absent if severe), high-pitched and inspiratory crackles (increased by or heard only after coughing), and low-pitched inspiratory crackles caused by airway secretions.

Note: Findings may be normal, even with an abnormal chest x-ray and vice versa.

DIAGNOSTIC TESTS

ABG analysis: Hypoxemia (Pao_2 <80 mm Hg) and hypocapnia ($Paco_2$ <35 mm Hg), with a resultant respiratory alkalosis (pH >7.45), will be seen in the absence of an underlying pulmonary disease. In severe cases the $Paco_2$ can be <35 mm Hg because CO_2 elimination may be affected.

Pulse oximetry (Spo_2): See description, p. 230.

CBC count: WBC count will be increased (>11,000 μl) in the presence of bacterial pneumonias. Normal or low WBC count will be seen with viral or mycoplasma pneumonias.

Sputum for Gram's stain and culture and sensitivity tests: If a sputum culture is prescribed, it should be obtained from the lower respiratory tract before initiation of antibiotic therapy. It can be obtained *via* expectoration, suctioning, transtracheal aspiration, bronchoscopy, or open-lung biopsy.

Blood culture and sensitivity: To determine presence of bacteremia and aid in identification of the causative organism.

Culture and sensitivity of pleural effusion fluid: Especially useful in identifying pathogen involved in nosocomial pneumonias.

Serologic studies: Acute and convalescent titers are drawn to diagnose viral pneumonia. Rises in antibody titers are a positive sign for viral infection.

Acid-fast stain: To rule out tuberculosis.

Chest x-ray: To identify anatomic involvement, extent of disease, and presence of consolidation, pleural effusions, and cavitation:

Lobar: Entire lobe involved.

Segmental (lobular): Only parts of a lobe involved.

Bronchopneumonia: Affects alveoli contiguous to the involved bronchi.

COLLABORATIVE MANAGEMENT

Oxygen therapy: Administered when ABG values demonstrate presence of hypoxemia. Special care must be taken not to abolish the drive to breathe if patient has a chronic lung disorder and is known to retain CO_2. Initially, in patients with chronic CO_2 retention, oxygen is delivered in low concentrations while closely monitoring ABG levels. If Pao_2 does not rise to acceptable levels (e.g., >60 mm Hg), Fio_2 is increased in small increments, with concomitant ABG checks or monitoring *via* pulse oximetry.

Intubation and mechanical ventilation: Intubation may be necessary if patient is unable to maintain a patent airway because of tenacious or copious secretions, ineffective cough, or fatigue. Mechanical ventilation is required if patient is unable to maintain adequate ABG values (Pao_2 >60 mm Hg) with supplemental oxygen. High concentrations of oxygen and positive end-expiratory pressure (PEEP) may be necessary in severe cases of pneumonia that lead to acute respiratory failure.

Pharmacotherapy

Antibiotics: Prescribed empirically on the basis of presenting signs and symptoms, clinical findings, and chest x-ray results until sputum or blood culture results are available. Erythromycin is the most commonly used antibiotic in community-acquired pneumonia. Antimicrobial therapy in critically ill patients usually is parenteral and guided by sensitivity of the causative organism. Many of the organisms responsible for nosocomial pneumonias are resistant to multiple antibiotics. Proper identification of the organism, determination of sensitivity, and attainment of therapeutic drug levels are critical for effective therapy.

Antipyretics and analgesics: To reduce temperature and provide relief for pleuritic pain. Patients with pneumonia may have significant pleuritic pain that requires administration of narcotics for relief. When narcotics (e.g., codeine, morphine sulfate, meperidine) are given, varying degrees of depression occur. Careful and frequent monitoring of the patient's respiratory rate and depth, as well as oxygen saturation, *via* pulse oximetry is necessary.

Hydration: IV fluids may be necessary to replace fluids lost from insensible sources (e.g., tachypnea, diaphoresis with fever).

Isolation: Some patients with pneumonia may require isolation and Transmission-based Precautions (see "Infection Prevention and Control," Appendix 8).

Percussion and postural drainage: Indicated if deep breathing, coughing, and moving about in bed or ambulation are ineffective in raising and expectorating sputum.

NURSING DIAGNOSES AND INTERVENTIONS

Risk for infection (nosocomial pneumonia) related to inadequate primary defenses (e.g., decreased ciliary action), invasive procedures (e.g., intubation), and/or chronic disease

Desired outcome: Patient is free of infection as evidenced by normothermia, WBC count within normal limits for patient, and sputum clear to whitish in color.

- Perform good handwashing procedure before and after contact with respiratory secretions (even though gloves were worn) and before and after contact with patient with tracheostomy or intubation. Inform visitors of effective precautions or pertinent isolation procedures.
- Identify presurgical candidate who is at increased risk for nosocomial pneumonia: individuals who are >70 yr old or obese; who have COPD or a history of smoking, abnormal results of pulmonary function tests (especially decreased forced expiratory flow rate), or tracheostomy; who anticipate a prolonged period of intubation; or who will have upper abdominal or thoracic operations.
    - Before surgery, provide patient and significant others with verbal and written instructions and demonstrations of turning, coughing, and deep-breathing exercises to perform after surgery to prevent respiratory tract infection. Make sure the patient verbalizes knowledge of the exercises and their rationale and *returns* the demonstrations appropriately.
    - Be aware that most patients can expand their lungs effectively after surgery but will not do so unless they are encouraged. At

frequent intervals, encourage lung expansion: deep breathing, coughing if secretions are present, turning in bed, and walking (may not be possible in critical care). In addition, use of incentive spirometry promotes periodic, voluntary lung expansion greater than tidal volume. Educate significant others to encourage these activities.

- ☐ If pain interferes with lung expansion, control it by administering prn analgesics ½ h before deep-breathing exercises and providing support of wound areas with hands or pillows placed firmly across site of incision.
- ☐ For patients who cannot remove secretions effectively by coughing, perform procedures that stimulate coughing such as chest physiotherapy, which includes breathing exercises, postural drainage, and percussion.
- ☐ If the patient has an endotracheal or tracheostomy tube, provide a fast, deep breath with a manual resuscitator to stimulate the cough receptors.
- Identify patients who are at high risk for aspiration: individuals who have a depressed LOC or dysphagia, or a gastric tube in place.
- For patient with depressed LOC, consult physician regarding need for a method of feeding in which risk of aspiration is minimal (e.g., small-bore weighted feeding tube that migrates to the duodenum, total parenteral nutrition [TPN], or gastrostomy).
- For patient with a gastric tube in place, turn onto right side rather than back during feeding and provide continuous, rather than bolus, feedings. Elevate HOB to at least 30 degrees during feedings and for 1 h after any feeding or medication.
- Recognize the following ways in which nebulizer reservoirs can contaminate patient: introduction of nonsterile fluids or air, manipulation of nebulizer cup, or backflow of condensate from delivery tubing into reservoir or into patient when tubing is manipulated.
- Use only sterile fluids and dispense them aseptically.
  - ☐ Replace (rather than replenish) solutions and equipment at frequent intervals (e.g., empty reservoir completely and refill with sterile solution q8-24h, according to agency protocol).
  - ☐ Change breathing circuits q48h; if used for multiple patients, replace breathing circuit with sterilized or disinfected breathing circuit between patients.
  - ☐ Fill fluid reservoirs immediately before use.
  - ☐ Discard any fluid that has condensed in tubing; do not allow it to drain back into reservoir or into patient.
- Recognize risk factors for patients with tracheostomy or ET tubes: presence of underlying lung disease or other serious illness, increased colonization of oropharynx or trachea by aerobic gram-negative bacteria, greater access of bacteria to lower respiratory tract, and cross-contamination due to manipulation of these tubes.
  - ☐ Employ "no-touch" technique or use sterile gloves on both hands until tracheostomy wound has healed or formed granulation tissue around the tube.
- Suction on an "as needed" rather than a routine basis, inasmuch as frequent suctioning increases the risk of trauma and cross-contamination.

- Always wear gloves on both hands when suctioning to protect against transmission of the herpes simplex virus (HSV) from the patient's oral secretions; transmission of HSV into openings in the skin (e.g., a hangnail) can cause herpetic whitlow.
- Consider use of an in-line suction device to reduce the risk of infection or contamination.

Risk for fluid volume deficit related to increased insensible loss secondary to hyperventilation, fever, and use of supplemental oxygen; and related to reduced fluid intake

Desired outcome: Patient is normovolemic as evidenced by urinary output $\geq$0.5 ml/kg/h, specific gravity 1.010-1.020, no clinical evidence of hypovolemia (such as furrowed tongue), stable weight, BP within patient's normal range, CVP 2-6 mm Hg, PAP 20-30/8-15 mm Hg, CO 4-7 L/min, MAP 70-105 mm Hg, HR 60-100 bpm, and SVR 900-1,200 dynes/sec/cm^{-5}.

- Monitor I&O hourly. Initially intake should exceed output during volume replacement therapy. Consult physician for urine output <0.5 ml/kg/h for 2 consecutive hours. Measure urine specific gravity q8h; expect it to decrease with therapy.
- Monitor VS and hemodynamic pressures for signs of continued hypovolemia. Be alert to decreased values in BP, CVP, PAP, CO, and MAP, as well as increased HR and SVR.
- Weigh patient daily, at the same time of day (preferably before breakfast) on a balanced scale, with the patient wearing the same type of clothing. Document the type of scale used (e.g., standing, bed, chair).
- Administer PO and IV fluids as prescribed. Document patient's response to replacement therapy.
- Monitor for signs and symptoms of fluid overload or too-rapid fluid administration: crackles (rales), SOB, tachypnea, tachycardia, increased CVP, increased pulmonary artery (PA) pressures, neck vein distention, and edema.

ADDITIONAL NURSING DIAGNOSES

See "Near Drowning" for **Impaired gas exchange,** p. 146. See "Status Asthmaticus" for **Ineffective airway clearance,** p. 234 and **Activity intolerance,** p. 235. As appropriate, see nursing diagnoses and interventions in "Nutritional Support," p. 12; "Mechanical Ventilation," p. 24; "Prolonged Immobility," p. 78; "Psychosocial Support," p. 88; and "Psychosocial Support for the Patient's Family and Significant Others," p. 100.

Pulmonary hypertension

PATHOPHYSIOLOGY

Pulmonary hypertension is defined as a mean pulmonary artery pressure (MPAP) >20 mm Hg. Primary pulmonary hypertension, which is rare, is a process for which a cause cannot be described. With secondary pulmonary hypertension the cause can be identified (see Table 3-4 for a discussion of etiologic factors).

T A B L E 3 - 4 **Etiologic factors in the development of pulmonary hypertension**

Cause	Clinical examples
Congenital heart disease with left-to-right shunt	Ventricular septal defect, atrial septal defect, patent ductus arteriosus
Congenital heart disease with diminished pulmonary blood flow	Tetralogy of Fallot, transposition of the great vessels
Obstruction to pulmonary venous outflow (congenital and acquired)	Mitral valve disease, left ventricular failure, stenosis of large pulmonary veins, portal hypertension
Pulmonary embolism and thrombosis	
Chronic alveolar hypoxia	High-altitude hypoxia, COPD, obstructive sleep apnea, obesity (hypoventilation syndrome), neuromuscular disease processes
Diffuse pulmonary fibrosis	Lupus erythematosus, systemic sclerosis, sarcoidosis, idiopathic interstitial fibrosis

Rising pulmonary artery pressure (PAP) increases pulmonary vascular resistance (PVR), which in turn causes two responses in the vasculature: standby vessels open to increase the surface area available for perfusion, and the capillaries distend to accommodate the increased blood flow. Although these responses reduce PVR initially, the system eventually fails if the increased pressure becomes chronic due to vasoconstriction that occurs in response to chronic alveolar hypoxia. Whereas most of the vascular system responds to hypoxia by dilating in an effort to increase blood flow to vital organs, the pulmonary vasculature responds to alveolar hypoxia by vasoconstriction, a beneficial mechanism that shunts blood away from underventilated areas in the lungs to better ventilated areas, thereby improving oxygenation. This regional mechanism is not strong enough to correct the ventilation/perfusion imbalance, however. Generally, Pao_2 decreases to ≤ 60 mm Hg before vasoconstriction occurs; the lower the Pao_2, the more severe the vasoconstriction.

The rise in PAP and the resulting increase in PVR from acute hypoxia are completely reversible after the hypoxia has been resolved. In the presence of chronic hypoxia, however, the pulmonary vasculature undergoes permanent changes (i.e., hypertrophy and hyperplasia), causing thickening of the vessel and narrowing of the lumen. In addition, polycythemia develops as a compensatory mechanism to increase oxygen transport; this condition increases blood viscosity, which in turn increases PVR.

The functions of the heart and lungs are interdependent. Increased PVR stimulates the right ventricle to increase the pumping force in order to maintain adequate cardiac output. The right ventricle dilates and hypertrophies under the constant strain and workload. Eventually, the right side of the heart weakens and is unable to accommodate venous blood returning to the heart. As a result, pressure in the systemic venous circulation increases, causing cor pulmonale or right-sided heart failure. See "Congestive Heart Failure/Pulmonary Edema," p. 289, for further discussion of right-sided heart failure.

ASSESSMENT

Because the low-resistance pulmonary vascular bed is clinically silent until late in the disease process, onset is insidious.

CLINICAL PRESENTATION
Early indicators: Hyperventilation, vague chest discomfort.
Late indicators: Tachypnea, dyspnea, orthopnea, chest congestion.
PHYSICAL ASSESSMENT Cyanosis of the lips and nail beds, edema of the hands and feet, anasarca (generalized, massive edema), distended jugular veins, right ventricular heave (visible left parasternal systolic lift), accentuated pulmonary component of the second heart sound, right ventricular diastolic gallop, pulmonary ejection click, distant breath sounds, basilar crackles.
HEMODYNAMIC MEASUREMENTS MPAP will be >20 mm Hg. Normally, pulmonary artery pressures (PAP) range from 8-15 mm Hg during diastole to 20-30 mm Hg during systole, with an MPAP of 15 mm Hg.

DIAGNOSTIC TESTS

ABG values: Will vary but are important to the differential diagnosis of the cause of pulmonary hypertension. Generally, Pao_2 will be <60 mm Hg, whereas $Paco_2$ will be within normal limits (35-45 mm Hg) unless COPD is the cause of the pulmonary hypertension, at which time it may be elevated.
Chest x-ray: Will confirm anatomic abnormalities associated with chronic right ventricular failure (right ventricular dilatation or hypertrophy), enlarged pulmonary artery secondary to increased pressure, and diminished diaphragmatic excursion.
ECG: May show right-axis deviation, right bundle-branch block, and enlarged P waves.
Echocardiography: May reveal enlarged right atrium and right ventricle, diminished wall motion, pulmonic valve malfunction (midsystolic closure or delayed opening).
Pulmonary function tests: Also important for the differential diagnosis of the underlying pathologic condition; will vary according to cause. For normal values, see Table 3-1.
Pulmonary angiography and perfusion scans: To rule out an embolic event as the underlying cause.
Hemodynamic monitoring: Pressures in the pulmonary vasculature are measured by way of the flow-directed pulmonary artery (e.g., Swan-Ganz) catheter. Data will differentiate or quantify the contribution of the left or right ventricular failure and measure the response to pharmacotherapy.
Open-lung biopsy: Usually avoided unless the cause of pulmonary hypertension cannot be diagnosed by less invasive studies. Data obtained from biopsy specimen may establish the type of pulmonary vascular disease and assess extent of the disease process.
RBC/Hct values: May be increased above normal.

COLLABORATIVE MANAGEMENT

The goal of medical management is to diagnose and treat the underlying disorder or process causing the pulmonary hypertension. Treatment is directed primarily toward increasing myocardial contractility or reducing right ventricular afterload caused by the high pulmonary vascular resistance.

Oxygen therapy: By eliminating hypoxia, pulmonary vascular vasoconstriction is reduced, which in turn may reduce right ventricular afterload.

Pharmacotherapy

Diuretics: Reduce circulating volume *via* loss of sodium and water, which may decrease PAP and right ventricular workload. In turn, this reduces leftward septal bulging seen with right ventricular overload.

Digitalis: Generally used only in cor pulmonale with biventricular failure. Otherwise, the inotropic effects of digitalis can increase cardiac output and pulmonary resistance, which are deleterious in the presence of right ventricular failure.

Bronchodilators (e.g., aminophylline, isoproterenol, terbutaline): Act as afterload reducers by decreasing pulmonary vascular resistance and increasing right ventricular ejection fraction. By improving gas exchange, bronchodilators may decrease hypoxic vasoconstriction of the pulmonary vascular bed.

Vasodilators (e.g., nitrates, hydralazine, calcium channel blockers, prostaglandins E_1 and I_2): Reverse pulmonary vasoconstriction, which will reduce right ventricular afterload and enhance pulmonary blood flow.

NURSING DIAGNOSES AND INTERVENTIONS

Note: As appropriate, see nursing diagnoses and interventions in "Nutritional Support," p. 12; "Prolonged Immobility," p. 78; "Psychosocial Support," p. 88; and "Psychosocial Support for the Patient's Family and Significant Others," p. 100. See "Near Drowning" for **Impaired gas exchange,** p. 146. See "Status Asthmaticus" for **Activity intolerance,** p. 235. Refer to "Congestive Heart Failure/Pulmonary Edema," p. 293, for nursing diagnoses and interventions related to the care of patients with heart failure.

Adult respiratory distress syndrome

PATHOPHYSIOLOGY

Adult respiratory distress syndrome (ARDS) is an often fatal condition, with a mortality rate approaching 60%. Although ARDS often is a result of a direct injury to the lung resulting from trauma or infection, it is more likely to occur as a sequela to an indirect insult to the lung. In either case, the hallmark of ARDS is multisystem organ failure and sepsis. Although the cause of ARDS is not understood completely, the site of injury is the alveolar-capillary membrane. Normally this membrane is permeable only to smaller molecules, such as water and electrolytes. The balance of the forces of hydrostatic pressure (pushing) and osmotic pressure (pulling) keeps fluids in their proper place and maintains the interstitium and alveoli in a relatively dry state. All of the etiologic factors that lead to the development of ARDS (see "History and Risk Factors" in the next section) cause an increase in the permeability of the alveolar-capillary membrane, either by altering hydrostatic or osmotic pressure or by injuring the alveolar epithelium or capillary endothelium. This enables the passing of larger molecules (e.g., albumin and globulin) across the membrane. Essentially, this altered permeability leads to a leaky membrane and an accumulation of protein-rich fluid in the interstitial and intraalveolar spaces, interfering with gas exchange at this critical level. As the leak grows larger, the interstitium, alveoli, and terminal airways become filled with fluid, blood, and protein. Surfactant activity is reduced, either because the cell producing the surfactant is destroyed or because the surfactant is inactivated. The alveoli tend to collapse and resist reexpansion in the absence of surfactant. Gas exchange no longer can occur, and these areas become a mass of interstitial and alveolar edema, hemorrhage, and focal atelectasis. Ventilation-perfusion mismatching, with resultant hypoxia, occurs as areas of the lung are perfused but not ventilated. Arterial oxygen tension (Pao_2) begins to fall, there is an increase in the shunt fraction (the amount of blood returning to the arterial system without passing through ventilated regions of the lung), and physiologic dead space increases. The patient becomes fatigued as the work of breathing increases in response to ever-stiffening lungs, and respiratory failure is possible.

ASSESSMENT

HISTORY AND RISK FACTORS Trauma, hemorrhagic shock, gram-negative sepsis, sepsis with disseminated intravascular coagulation (DIC), inhalation of toxic substances, severe pneumonitis, aspiration of gastric contents, near drowning, air or fat embolus, acute pancreatitis, postperfusion cardiopulmonary bypass, oxygen toxicity, drug overdose, neurologic injury, immunosuppression, and massive blood transfusion.

CLINICAL PRESENTATION Will vary, depending on the pathophysiology contributing to the ARDS. The following are general early and late indicators. The goals are to diagnose ARDS in the early stages when treatment is much less complex and the patient is less critically ill and to reduce additional insults to the respiratory and other organ systems.
Early indicators: Dyspnea, restlessness, hyperventilation, cough, increased work of breathing, chest clear on auscultation.
Late indicators: Cyanosis, pallor, grunting respirations, adventitious breath sounds, rapid and shallow breathing, intercostal-suprasternal retractions, tachypnea, tachycardia, diaphoresis, mental obtundation.

DIAGNOSTIC TESTS

ABG analysis: Essential to the diagnosis of ARDS. Refractory hypoxemia is a key indicator (decreasing Pao_2 that is unresponsive to increasing Fio_2). Initially, the pH is above normal (>7.45) because the patient hyperventilates and exhales greater-than-normal levels of CO_2. As ARDS worsens, the pH falls below 7.35 due to respiratory acidosis, which may be further complicated by metabolic acidosis resulting from the anaerobic metabolism induced by hypoxia.

Pulse oximetry: Used for continuous monitoring of oxygenation (see discussion, p. 230).

Mixed venous oxygen saturation (Svo$_2$):   Svo$_2$ is a more sensitive indicator of oxygen available for tissue oxygenation. Normal values range from 60%-80%. A value <50% is associated with impaired tissue oxygenation.

Serial chest x-rays: May be normal in the early stages. As ARDS progresses, the lung shows bilateral diffuse infiltrates. In later stages there may be few air spaces left in the lung, a condition that gives the lung a completely white appearance on x-ray.

Pulmonary function tests: Static and dynamic lung compliance will be decreased. Lung volumes also will be decreased, particularly functional residual capacity (FRC).

Hemodynamic monitoring: Measurements of PAWP are important to the differential diagnosis. PAWP is normal in ARDS, but high (>12 mm Hg) in cardiogenic pulmonary edema. PAWP is a more sensitive indicator of fluid balance than is CVP and is obtained at frequent intervals in conjunction with fluid therapy.

Tracheal protein/plasma protein ratio: A relatively new diagnostic tool used to differentiate between cardiogenic and noncardiogenic pulmonary edema (ARDS). It compares total protein in tracheal aspirate with total protein in plasma. Ratio in cardiogenic pulmonary edema is <0.5, whereas the ratio in ARDS generally is >0.7.

Lactic acid level: Lactic acid is a byproduct of anaerobic metabolism and will accumulate in the serum in the presence of hypoxemia. The presence of arterial lactate contributes to acidosis.

P(A-a)o$_2$:   Alveolar-arterial oxygen tension difference. Normally, it increases approximately 4 mm Hg with each decade of life. The value increases above normal in ARDS and reflects the intrapulmonary shunting that occurs secondary to alveolar flooding.

QS/QT: Ratio of shunt to cardiac output. Measures intrapulmonary shunting. Normal physiologic shunt is 3%-4%; may increase to 15%-20% with ARDS.

COLLABORATIVE MANAGEMENT

The goals for management are twofold: first, maintenance of adequate arterial oxygenation and pulmonary ventilation, and second, treatment of the underlying pathophysiologic condition that caused the ARDS.

Oxygen therapy: To provide acceptable Pao$_2$ levels (>60 mm Hg) with Fio$_2$ ≤0.50.

Mechanical ventilation: Indicated if the patient cannot receive adequate oxygen with acceptable concentrations of Fio$_2$ (≤0.50). Mechanical ventilation is indicated for nearly all patients with ARDS because decreased lung compliance significantly increases work of breathing and the increase in physiologic dead space causes a compensatory increase in ventilatory requirements.

Positive end-expiratory pressure (PEEP):   Used in conjunction with mechanical ventilation, PEEP allows for better arterial oxygenation (Pao$_2$) with administration of lower levels of inspired oxygen tension (Fio$_2$). It also increases functional residual capacity by recruiting or maintaining open alveoli that are otherwise collapsed. High pressures (5-20 cm H$_2$O) are mechanically maintained at the end of the expiratory cycle, allowing alveoli to remain open and thus participate in gas exchange. For a more complete discussion of PEEP, see p. 20 in "Mechanical Ventilation."

Corticosteroids: Although use of steroids is controversial and their efficacy is not well established, short-term, high-dose corticosteroids may be useful in stabilizing the alveolar-capillary membrane to prevent further deterioration. Corticosteroids also may be useful in the chronic phases of ARDS.

Fluid therapy: Primary goal is to maintain a minimum pulmonary artery wedge pressure (PAWP) to provide adequate cardiac output. Usually, the patient's fluid volume is kept slightly depleted due to leakage of excess fluids into the interstitium through damaged capillary membrane. The use of crystalloid versus colloid fluids is controversial. Both types of fluid have been shown to leak across the alveolar-capillary membrane. Generally, colloids are reserved for those patients with hypoalbuminemia, and crystalloids are used for all other patients.

Sedation: Extremely agitated patients may receive medication such as morphine sulfate. Those patients too combative to cooperate with mechanical ventilation procedure may be placed under heavy sedation with agents such as propofol (Diprivan) or paralyzed with a neuro-blocking agent, such as vecuronium bromide (Norcuron). It is imperative that the care giver recognize that although the paralyzed patient may appear comatose, he or she may be alert and extremely anxious because of the total lack of muscle control. These patients must receive appropriate sedation (e.g., lorazepam [Ativan]) and analgesia (e.g., morphine), and they will require expert psychosocial nursing interventions. See "Sedating and Paralytic Agents," p. 40.

Nutritional support: Energy outlay with respiratory failure is high, in part because of the increased work of breathing. If the patient is unable to consume adequate calories with enteral feedings, TPN *via* peripheral or central access is instituted.

NURSING DIAGNOSES AND INTERVENTIONS

Impaired gas exchange related to alveolar-capillary membrane changes secondary to increased permeability with alveolar injury and collapse

Desired outcome: Within 12-24 h of initiation of therapy, patient has adequate gas exchange as evidenced by the following ABG values: $Pa_{O_2} > 60$ mm Hg, $Pa_{CO_2} < 45$ mm Hg, and pH 7.35-7.45. Within 4-6 days of initiation of therapy, patient's RR is 12-20 breaths/min with a normal pattern and depth (eupnea) and absence of adventitious breath sounds.

- Assess and document character of respiratory effort: rate, depth, rhythm, and use of accessory muscles of respiration.
- Assess patient for signs and symptoms of respiratory distress: restlessness, anxiety, confusion, tachypnea (RR >20 breaths/min).
- Assess breath sounds with each VS check to ascertain their presence and character. Adventitious sounds, which usually are present in the later stages of ARDS, are not as likely to occur during the early stage.
- Monitor serial ABG values and consult physician for significant

changes. Explain need for frequent analysis to patient and significant others.

- Compare ABG saturation with pulse oximetry saturation for accuracy. Consult physician for pulse oximetry values <90%.
- Administer oxygen and monitor Fio_2 as prescribed.
- Monitor and record pulmonary function tests as prescribed, especially tidal volume and minute ventilation. Expect decreased tidal volume and increased minute ventilation with respiratory distress.
- Encourage patient to slow the rate of respirations by using pursed-lip breathing technique.
- Position patient for comfort and to promote adequate gas exchange. Usually, semi-Fowler's to high Fowler's position is therapeutic.
- Keep oral airway and self-inflating manual ventilating bag at the bedside for emergency use. Keep emergency intubation equipment at the bedside for use should patient's condition deteriorate.

ADDITIONAL NURSING DIAGNOSES

Also see "Status Asthmaticus" for **Activity intolerance,** p. 235. As indicated, see nursing diagnoses and interventions in "Nutritional Support," p. 12; "Mechanical Ventilation," p. 24; "Prolonged Immobility," p. 78; "Psychosocial Support," p. 88; and "Psychosocial Support for the Patient's Family and Significant Others," p. 100.

Pulmonary emboli

PATHOPHYSIOLOGY

Pulmonary perfusion disorders are the result of any obstruction of blood flow in the pulmonary vasculature. The two most common abnormalities of pulmonary perfusion are thrombotic emboli and fat emboli. Venous air emboli are also discussed.

Thrombotic emboli (TE): The most common pulmonary perfusion abnormality, TEs are caused by a dislodged blood clot from the systemic circulation, typically the deep veins of the legs or pelvis. Most often, the iliofemoral venous system is implicated. Thrombus formation is the result of one or more of the following factors: blood stasis, alterations in clotting factors, and injury to vessel walls. Many patients with TE do not exhibit signs and symptoms of deep vein thrombosis (DVT). The formed thrombus becomes dislodged and travels to the pulmonary circulation, where it obstructs one or both branches of the pulmonary artery or a subdivision. Total obstruction leading to pulmonary infarction is rare, because the pulmonary circulation has multiple sources of blood supply. Early diagnosis and appropriate treatment reduce mortality to less than 10%. Although most thrombotic emboli resolve completely, leaving no residual deficits, some patients may be left with chronic pulmonary hypertension.

Fat emboli: The most common nonthrombotic cause of pulmonary perfusion disorders, fat emboli are the result of two events: the release of free fatty acids that cause a toxic vasculitis, followed by thrombosis and obstruction of small pulmonary arteries by fat.

Venous air emboli: Almost always an iatrogenic complication with multiple causes, including surgical procedures, insertion of pulmonary artery catheters and central venous catheters, hemodialysis, endoscopy, and injection of contrast media. Small amounts of air may be completely asymptomatic secondary to rapid reabsorption. A larger bolus of air into the right ventricle may completely obstruct pulmonary blood flow, leading to cardiac arrest. In severe cases, venous air embolus may have a mortality rate >50%. Rapid diagnosis and treatment are essential.

ASSESSMENT
Thrombotic emboli
HISTORY AND RISK FACTORS
Prolonged immobilization: Especially significant when it coexists with surgical or nonsurgical trauma, carcinoma, or cardiopulmonary disease. Risk increases as length of immobilization increases.
Cardiac disorders: Atrial fibrillation, congestive heart failure, myocardial infarction, rheumatic heart disease, or any low cardiac output state.
Surgical intervention: Risk increases in postoperative period, especially for patients with pelvic, thoracic, and abdominal surgery and for those with extensive burns or musculoskeletal injuries of the hip or knee.
Pregnancy: Especially during the postpartum period.
Trauma: Especially fractures of the lower extremities, hip fractures in the older adult, burns, and acute head and spinal cord injuries. The degree of risk is related to the severity, site, and extent of trauma.
Carcinoma: Particularly neoplasms involving the breast, lung, pancreas, and genitourinary and alimentary tracts.
Obesity: Patients with a ≥20% increase in ideal body weight have an increased incidence of TE.
Varicose veins or prior thromboembolic disease
Age: Risk of thromboembolism is greatest between 55-65 yr of age.

Note: Low-dose heparin prophylaxis (e.g., 5,000 U subcutaneously q8-12h) frequently is initiated in high-risk groups (except for neurosurgical patients). Low molecular weight (LMW) heparins, e.g., dalteparin (Fragmin) and enoxaparin (Lovenox), may be used for DVT prophylaxis in certain high-risk surgical patients, such as with abdominal surgery and hip replacements.

CLINICAL PRESENTATION Often nonspecific but may involve sudden onset of dyspnea, tachypnea, restlessness, and anxiety. The patient also may have a nonproductive cough, palpitations, nausea, and syncope. With a large embolism, oppressive substernal chest discomfort will be present. Fever, pleuritic chest pain, and hemoptysis are present with pulmonary infarction.
PHYSICAL ASSESSMENT RR >20 breaths/min, HR >100 bpm, crackles, decreased chest wall excursion secondary to splinting, S_3 and S_4 gallop rhythms, diaphoresis, edema, and cyanosis. Temperature may be elevated if pulmonary infarction has occurred, and transient pleural friction rub may be present.

Fat emboli

HISTORY AND RISK FACTORS

Multiple long bone fractures: Especially fractures of the femur and pelvis (see p. 164).

Trauma to adipose tissue or liver.

Burns (see p. 207).

Osteomyelitis.

Sickle cell crisis (see p. 588).

CLINICAL PRESENTATION Typically, patient is without symptoms for a period lasting 12-24 h after embolization; this period ends with sudden cardiopulmonary and neurologic deterioration: dyspnea, restlessness, confusion, delirium, and coma.

PHYSICAL ASSESSMENT RR >20 breaths/min; HR >100 bpm; increased BP; elevated temperature; petechiae, especially of the upper torso and axillae; inspiratory crowing; and expiratory wheezes.

Venous air emboli

HISTORY AND RISK FACTORS

Recent surgical procedure.

Pulmonary artery/central venous catheter insertion.

Misuse of closed-wound suction unit.

Cardiopulmonary bypass.

Hemodialysis.

Endoscopy.

CLINICAL PRESENTATION Dependent on severity of the bolus. Agitation, confusion, cough, dyspnea, and chest pain.

PHYSICAL ASSESSMENT RR >20 breaths/min, HR >100 bpm, wheezing, hypotension, mill wheel murmur.

DIAGNOSTIC TESTS

Thrombotic emboli

ABG values: Hypoxemia (Pao_2 <80 mm Hg), hypocapnia ($Paco_2$ <35 mm Hg), and respiratory alkalosis (pH >7.45) usually are present. A normal Pao_2 does not rule out the presence of TE. Pulse oximetry is used for continuous monitoring of oxygen saturation (see p. 230).

Alveolar-arterial oxygen pressure difference: $P(A-a)o_2$ usually will be >10 mm Hg, depending on the severity of the perfusion disorder and the degree of ventilation-perfusion mismatch.

Chest x-ray: Initially, the chest x-ray shows normal findings or an elevated hemidiaphragm will be present. After 24 h the x-ray may reveal small infiltrates secondary to atelectasis from decrease in surfactant. More specific findings are abnormal blood vessel diameters (i.e., obstruction of right pulmonary artery would cause dilatation of left pulmonary artery) and shapes (i.e., the affected blood vessel may taper to a sharp point and disappear). If pulmonary infarction is present, infiltrates and pleural effusions may be seen within 12-36 h.

ECG: If TEs are extensive, signs of acute pulmonary hypertension may be present: right-shift QRS axes, tall and peaked P waves, ST-segment changes, and T-wave inversion in leads V_1-V_4.

Pulmonary ventilation-perfusion scan: A scan is used to detect the presence of abnormalities of ventilation or perfusion in the pulmonary system. The patient inhales radioactive-tagged gases, and radioactive particles are injected peripherally. If there is a mismatch of ventilation and perfusion (e.g., normal ventilation with decreased perfusion), vascular obstruction is likely.

Pulmonary angiography: This is the definitive study for TEs. It is an invasive procedure involving catheterization of the right ventricle and injection of dye into the pulmonary artery (PA) to visualize pulmonary vessels. An abrupt vessel "cut off" may be seen at the site of embolization. Usually, filling defects are seen.

Hemodynamic studies: If TEs lead to increased pulmonary vascular resistance, PA pressure will be elevated. PA pressures increase significantly (>20 mm Hg) if 30%-50% of the pulmonary arterial tree is affected. If massive TEs are present and PA pressure increases to >40 mm Hg, right ventricular failure can develop, leading to a decrease in cardiac output and hypotension.

Fat emboli

ABG values: Hypoxemia (Pao_2 <80 mm Hg) and hypercapnia ($Paco_2$ >45 mm Hg) will be present with a respiratory acidosis (pH <7.35).

Chest x-ray: A pattern similar to ARDS is seen: diffuse, extensive bilateral interstitial and alveolar infiltrates.

CBC count: May reveal decreased hemoglobin (Hgb) and Hct secondary to hemorrhage into the lung, in addition to thrombocytopenia.

Venous air emboli

ABG values: Hypoxemia (Pao_2 <80 mm Hg), hypercapnia ($Paco_2$ >45 mm Hg), and respiratory acidosis (pH <7.35) generally are present in severe cases.

Chest x-ray: Reveals changes consistent with pulmonary edema or air-fluid levels in the main pulmonary artery system.

Pulmonary artery pressure: Acutely elevated without elevation of PAWP.

COLLABORATIVE MANAGEMENT

Thrombotic emboli

Oxygen therapy: Delivered at appropriate concentration to maintain a Pao_2 of >60 mm Hg.

IV heparin therapy: Treatment of choice. It is started immediately in patients without bleeding or clotting disorders and in whom TE is strongly suspected.

Initial dose: IV bolus of 5,000-10,000 U.

Maintenance dose: 2-4 h after initial dose, either a continuous IV infusion of 1,000 U/h or 5,000-7,500 U q4h. Maintenance continues for 7-14 days, during which time the patient is placed on bed rest to ensure that the thrombus is firmly attached to the vessel wall before ambulation is attempted.

Goals of therapy: To inhibit thrombus growth, promote resolution of the formed thrombus, and prevent further embolus formation. These goals are achieved by keeping partial thromboplastin time (PTT) at 1½-2½ times the normal. This test should be done just before the next intermittent dose of heparin. In addition, platelet counts should be obtained q3days, because thrombocytopenia and paradoxic arterial thrombosis can occur as a result of heparin therapy.

Protamine sulfate: Heparin antidote, which should be readily available during heparin therapy. Fatal hemorrhage occurs in 1%-2% of patients undergoing heparin therapy. Risk of bleeding is greatest in women >60 yr of age.

Oral anticoagulants (warfarin sodium): Started 48-72 h after initiation of heparin therapy. The two are given simultaneously for 6-7 days to allow time for warfarin to inhibit vitamin K–dependent clotting factors before heparin is discontinued.

Prothrombin time (PT): Monitored daily, with a goal of 1¼-1½ times normal. Once the patient's condition has stabilized and the heparin is discontinued, weekly monitoring of PT is acceptable. After hospital discharge the PT should be monitored q2wk for as long as the patient continues to take warfarin.

Maintenance: Usually 10 mg/day, continued for 3-6 months and based on the continued presence of risk factors. Certain tumors (e.g., Trousseau's syndrome) necessitate lifetime therapy.

Note: Subcutaneous heparin therapy is an effective alternative to warfarin, with less risk of bleeding. The dose of heparin must be adjusted while the patient is hospitalized to ensure a PTT of 1½ times that of normal.

Vitamin K: Reverses the effects of warfarin in 24-36 hours. Fresh frozen plasma may be required in cases of serious bleeding.

Caution: Warfarin crosses the placental barrier and can cause spontaneous abortion and birth defects.

Thrombolytic therapy: These drugs lyse clots *via* conversion of plasminogen to plasma and may be given in the first 24-72 h after TE to speed the process of clot lysis, especially when severe cardiopulmonary compromise has occurred. After the first 24-72 h of thrombolytic therapy, heparin therapy is initiated. Thrombolytic therapy may be preferred for initial treatment of TE in patients with hemodynamic compromise; in those with >30% occlusion of pulmonary vasculature; and in patients for whom therapy was initiated no later than 3 days after onset of TE.

Note: Up to 33% of patients who receive thrombolytic therapy have hemorrhagic complications. Discontinuing the drug and administering fresh-frozen plasma are the appropriate treatments.

Streptokinase: Loading dose of 250,000 IU in normal saline or D_5W given IV over a 30-min period. Maintenance dose is 100,000 IU/h given IV for 24-72 h.

Urokinase: Loading dose of 4,400 IU/kg body weight in 5 ml of solution given IV over 10 min. Maintenance dose is 4,400 IU/kg/h for 12 h.

Tissue plasminogen activator: Given 50 mg/h for 2 h.

Thrombin time: Monitors therapy for all three drugs. The test is repeated q4h during therapy to ensure adequate response, which should be 2-5 times normal. A PTT can be used instead of thrombin time and should be 2-5 times control. Once thrombolytic therapy is stopped, thrombin time or PTT should be checked frequently until values fall below 2 times normal. When the values are below 2 times normal, heparin is started and continued as described in the second entry of the preceding list.

Contraindications: Active internal bleeding, cerebrovascular accident, or intracranial bleeding within 2 months of TE. Other contraindications include trauma or surgery within 15 days of TE, diastolic hypertension >100 mm Hg, recent cardiopulmonary resuscitation, pregnancy, and <10 days postpartum.

Surgical interventions: Inferior vena caval interruption and pulmonary embolectomy may be indicated in select cases. Inferior vena caval interruption most often involves the transvenous insertion of an umbrella filter (e.g., Greenfield filter) that prevents the passage of major emboli from deep venous thrombi in the lower extremities.

Fat emboli

Oxygen: Concentration of oxygen is based on clinical picture, ABG results, and patient's prior respiratory status. Intubation and mechanical ventilation may be required.

Steroids: Cortisone, 100 mg, or methylprednisolone, 30 mg/kg, is used to decrease local injury to pulmonary tissue and pulmonary edema.

Diuretics: Pulmonary edema develops in approximately 30% of patients with fat emboli, necessitating use of diuretics.

Venous air emboli

Emphasis is on prevention. Ensure that central venous catheter is inserted with the patient in Trendelenburg position. Use Luer-Lok connectors on all IV tubing to prevent a disconnection. Should venous air embolus occur despite precautions, the following are anticipated.

Oxygen therapy: 100% Fio_2 is initiated immediately.

Trendelenburg position with a left decubitus tilt: To minimize further movement of air bolus through the heart and into the pulmonary vasculature and beyond.

Aspiration of air: If a central venous catheter is in place near the right atrium, an attempt is made to aspirate the air.

NURSING DIAGNOSES AND INTERVENTIONS

Impaired gas exchange related to altered blood flow secondary to presence of pulmonary emboli

Desired outcome: Within 12 h of initiation of therapy, patient has adequate gas exchange as evidenced by the following ABG values: Pao_2 ≥60 mm Hg, $Paco_2$ 35-45 mm Hg, and pH 7.35-7.45. Within 2-4 days of initiating therapy, patient's RR is 12-20 breaths/min with normal depth and pattern (eupnea).

- Monitor serial ABG values, assessing for the desired response to treatment: increased Pao_2 (≥60 mm Hg) and correction of respiratory alkalosis ($Paco_2$ ≥35 mm Hg and pH <7.45). Report lack of response to treatment or worsening ABG values. If pulse oximetry is present, monitor oxygen saturation.
- Monitor patient for signs and symptoms of increasing respiratory dis-

tress, and consult physician for significant findings: RR increased from baseline, increasing dyspnea, anxiety, cyanosis.
- Ensure delivery of prescribed concentrations of oxygen.
- Position patient for comfort and optimal gas exchange. Ensure that the area of the lung affected by the emboli is not dependent when patient is in the lateral decubitus position. Position patient with the unaffected side down and elevate HOB 30 degrees. This will ensure a better ventilation-perfusion match, thereby improving Pao_2.
- Avoid positioning patient with knees bent (i.e., "gatching" the bed), because this impedes venous return from the legs and can increase the risk of TE.
- Ensure that patient performs deep-breathing exercises 3-5 times q2h.
- Decrease metabolic demands for oxygen by limiting or pacing patient's activities and procedures.
- Explain all procedures and offer support to minimize fear and anxiety, which can increase oxygen demands.
- Schedule rest times after meals to avoid competition for oxygen supply during digestion.

Altered protection related to risk of clotting anomalies secondary to anticoagulation or thrombolytic therapy

Desired outcomes: Patient is free of bleeding signs or, if bleeding occurs, it is not prolonged.
- Monitor serial PTT or thrombin times. Report values outside the desired therapeutic ranges. Optimal range for PTT is 1½-2½ times that of control value and for thrombin time 2-5 times that of normal.
- Ensure easy access to antidotes for prescribed treatment:
  - *Protamine sulfate:* 1 mg counteracts 100 U of heparin. Usually, the initial dose is 50 mg.
  - *Vitamin K:* 20 mg given subcutaneously.
  - *Epsilon-aminocaproic acid* (e.g., Amicar): Reverses the fibrinolytic condition related to thrombolytic therapy.

Note: Although use of epsilon-aminocaproic acid as an antidote has not been approved, it has been used in some emergency situations.

- Inspect the following sites for evidence of bleeding: any entry site of an invasive procedure, oral mucous membranes, wounds, and nares; inspect the torso and extremities for evidence of petechiae or ecchymoses. Also check stool, urine, sputum, and vomitus for occult blood, using agency-approved method for testing. Be alert to complaints of back pain or other site-specific pain (e.g., headache), which may signal occult bleeding.
- Apply pressure over puncture sites until bleeding stops, usually 5-10 min for venous site and 10-20 min for arterial site. Apply pressure dressing over arterial puncture sites to stop oozing of blood.
- To prevent hematoma formation, avoid giving IM injections.
- Monitor Hgb and Hct. Consult physician for significant findings, including decreases in values or failure to see appropriate increases after transfusion.
- To avoid negative interactions with anticoagulants or thrombolytic therapy, establish compatibility of all drugs before administering them:

- □ *Heparin:* Digitalis, tetracyclines, nicotine, and antihistamines decrease the effect of heparin therapy. Establish compatibility before infusing other IV drugs through heparin IV line.
- □ *Warfarin sodium:* Numerous drugs result in a decrease or an increase in response to treatment with warfarin. Consult with pharmacist to obtain specific information about patient's medication profile.
- □ *Thrombolytic therapy:* No specific drug interactions are noted. However, do not infuse other medications through the same IV line.
- Because aspirin and nonsteroidal antiinflammatory drugs (e.g., ibuprofen) are platelet-aggregation inhibitors and can prolong episodes of bleeding, avoid use of *any* drug that contains these agents.
- Discuss with patient and significant others the importance of reporting promptly the presence of bleeding from any source.
- Teach patient the necessity of using sponge-tipped applicators and mouthwash for oral care to minimize the risk of gum bleeding during hospitalization when anticoagulant therapy is most intensive. Instruct patient to shave with an electric razor rather than a safety razor.
- If patient is restless and combative, provide a safe environment: pad the side rails, restrain patient as necessary to prevent falls, and use extreme care when moving patient to avoid bumping extremities into side rails.

Knowledge deficit: Oral anticoagulant therapy, potential side effects and complications, and foods and medications to avoid during therapy
Desired outcome: Within 24 h of initiation of oral anticoagulant therapy, patient and/or significant others verbalize knowledge of patient's prescribed anticoagulant drug, the potential side effects, and foods and medications to avoid during oral anticoagulant therapy.

- Determine patient's knowledge of oral anticoagulant therapy. As appropriate, discuss the drug name, purpose, dosage, schedule, potential side effects, and complications of therapy.
- Inform patient of the potential side effects and complications of anticoagulant therapy: easy bruising, prolonged bleeding from cuts, spontaneous nose bleeds, black and tarry stools, and blood in urine and sputum.
- Teach the rationale and application procedure for antiembolism stockings. Explain that patient should put them on in the morning before getting out of bed.
- Stress the importance of preventing impairment of venous return from the lower extremities by avoiding prolonged sitting, crossing of the legs, and constrictive clothing.
- Teach patient about foods high in vitamin K (e.g., fish, bananas, dark green vegetables, tomatoes, and cauliflower), which can interfere with anticoagulation.
- Caution patient that a soft-bristled toothbrush, rather than a hard-bristled one, and an electric razor, rather than a safety razor, should be used during anticoagulant therapy while at home.
- Instruct patient to consult with physician before taking any new OTC or prescribed drugs. The following are among many drugs that enhance the response to warfarin: aspirin, ibuprofen, cimetidine, and

trimethoprim. Drugs that decrease the response include antacids, diuretics, oral contraceptives, and barbiturates, among others.

ADDITIONAL NURSING DIAGNOSIS

See "Status Asthmaticus" for **Activity intolerance,** p. 235.

Pneumothorax

PATHOPHYSIOLOGY

Pneumothorax is an accumulation of air between the parietal and visceral pleura. There are three types of pneumothorax.

Spontaneous: A type of closed pneumothorax in which the chest wall remains intact with no leak to the atmosphere. It results from the rupture of a bleb or bulla on the visceral pleural surface, usually near the apex. In a *primary* spontaneous pneumothorax the cause of the rupture is unknown, although it may result from a weakness related to a respiratory infection. The affected individual is usually a young male (20-40 yr of age), previously healthy, and a smoker. Generally, onset of symptoms occurs at rest rather than with vigorous exercise or coughing. The potential for recurrence is great, with the second pneumothorax occurring an average of 2-3 yr after the first. A primary spontaneous pneumothorax is rarely life threatening. A *secondary* spontaneous pneumothorax is related to an underlying lung disease (COPD, cystic fibrosis, tuberculosis, malignant neoplasm). The symptoms are more severe than with the primary spontaneous pneumothorax, and this disorder may be life threatening because of the underlying lung disease. In addition, recurrence rates are high in this population.

Traumatic: Can be open or closed. An open pneumothorax occurs when air enters the pleural space from the atmosphere through an opening in the chest wall, such as with a penetrating injury or an invasive medical procedure (e.g., lung biopsy, thoracentesis, or placement of a central line into a subclavian vein). A closed pneumothorax occurs when the visceral pleura is penetrated but the chest wall remains intact, with no atmospheric leak. This usually occurs with blunt trauma that results in a fracture and dislocation of the ribs. It also may occur from the use of PEEP or after CPR. For more information about blunt chest injuries, see "Chest Trauma," p. 139.

Tension: Occurs when air enters the pleural space through a pleural tear during inspiration. Air continues to accumulate but cannot escape during expiration because of intrapleural pressure, which is greater than alveolar pressure. This leads to a one-way or flap-valve effect. As the pressure increases, it is transmitted to the mediastinum. This results in a mediastinal shift toward the unaffected side, which further impairs ventilatory efforts. The increase in pressure also compresses the vena cava, which impedes venous return, leading to a decrease in cardiac output and, ultimately, to circulatory collapse if it is not diagnosed and treated quickly. Tension pneumothorax is a life-threatening medical emergency. Although it can occur with a spontaneous pneumothorax, it most often is associated with trauma or infection, or it can occur during mechanical ventilation in patients who require positive-pressure ventilation.

ASSESSMENT

The clinical presentation will vary in degree, depending on the type and size of pneumothorax.

Spontaneous or traumatic: Sudden onset of sharp, stabbing chest pain on the affected side, which may radiate to the shoulder; moderate to severe dyspnea; anxiety.

Inspection: Decreased chest wall movement on affected side.

Palpation: Tracheal shift toward unaffected side, subcutaneous emphysema (crepitus), tactile and vocal fremitus decreased or absent on affected side.

Percussion: Hyperresonance on affected side.

Auscultation: Absent or decreased breath sounds on affected side; increased RR. Moderate tachycardia (HR >140 bpm) may be present.

Tension: Severe dyspnea; chest pain on affected side; cool, clammy, mottled skin; anxiety and restlessness.

Inspection: Decreased chest wall movement on affected side, expansion of affected side throughout respiratory cycle, jugular vein distention.

Palpation: Tracheal shift toward unaffected side, subcutaneous emphysema in neck and chest.

Percussion: Hyperresonance on affected side.

Auscultation: Absent or decreased breath sounds on affected side, distant heart sounds, increased RR (>20 breaths/min), decreased BP, increased HR (may be >140 bpm).

Caution: Tension pneumothorax is life threatening. Immediate medical intervention is critical.

DIAGNOSTIC TESTS

Chest x-ray: Will show size of the pneumothorax and any tracheal shift. The affected side will show air in the pleural space, expansion of the chest wall, lowering of the diaphragm, and partial to total collapse of the lung.

ABG analysis: Hypoxemia (Pao_2 <80 mm Hg) will be evident immediately after a moderate to large pneumothorax that occupies ≥15% of the hemithorax. As the pneumothorax resolves, arterial oxygen saturation returns to normal. Hypoxemia may be accompanied by respiratory acidosis (pH <7.35) and hypercapnia ($Paco_2$ >45 mm Hg).

ECG: May reveal decrease in QRS amplitude, precordial T-wave inversion, rightward shift of frontal QRS axis, and small precordial R voltage.

COLLABORATIVE MANAGEMENT

Oxygen therapy: Administered when ABG values demonstrate the presence of hypoxemia, which usually occurs with a large pneumothorax.

Analgesia: Provides relief of pain of pneumothorax or its treatment.

Thoracentesis: Performed immediately in tension pneumothorax to remove air from the chest cavity. A large-bore needle is inserted into the second intercostal space, midclavicular line, which correlates to the superior portion of the anterior axillary lobe. A sudden rushing out of air confirms the diagnosis of tension pneumothorax. To decrease the risk of further pleural laceration as the chest reexpands, a stylet introducer needle with a plastic sheath may be used. The needle is removed after penetration, and the plastic catheter sheath is left in place to allow decompression of the chest cavity. After air aspiration, chest tubes are inserted.

Chest tube placement: A chest tube may be inserted in a patient who has symptoms of a pneumothorax, depending on the severity of collapse. Chest tubes produce inflammation and, ultimately, scarring of the pleura and may help prevent recurrent spontaneous pneumothoraces. Patients with recurrent pneumothoraces require chest tubes because their visceral pleurae do not seal promptly. Chest tubes (26-30 Fr) are inserted in the second or third lateral intercostal space, midclavicular line. During insertion, the patient should be in an upright position so that the lung falls away from the chest wall. A small, 1-2 cm incision is made, and the chest tube is placed, sutured in place, and connected to an underwater-seal drainage system. Usually simple underwater-seal drainage is all that is necessary for 6-24 h. Suction may be used, depending on the size of the pneumothorax, the patient's condition, and the amount of drainage. A one-way flutter valve may be used with the chest tube instead of the underwater-seal drainage system. The flutter valve allows air to escape but prevents its reentry. The flutter valve is placed on the end of the chest tube. Suction can be applied with the flutter valve in place. After chest tube insertion and removal of air from the pleural space, the lung begins to reexpand. A chest tube may produce inflammation of the pleura, causing pleuritic pain, slight temperature elevation, and pleuritic friction rub.

Thoracotomy: Often indicated because of the risk of continuous recurrence if patient has had two or more spontaneous pneumothoraces on one side, or if resolution of the pneumothorax does not occur within 7 days. Thoracotomy may involve mechanical abrasion of the pleural surfaces with a dry sterile sponge or chemical abrasion *via* an agent such as tetracycline solution or talc, both of which result in pleural adhesions to prevent recurrence. A partial pleurectomy may be performed instead of mechanical or chemical abrasion.

NURSING DIAGNOSES AND INTERVENTIONS

Impaired gas exchange related to decreased alveolar blood flow and decreased oxygen supply secondary to increased pleural pressure

Desired outcome: Within 2-6 h of initiation of treatment, patient exhibits adequate gas exchange as evidenced by Pao_2 $\geq$60 mm Hg and $Paco_2$ $\leq$45 mm Hg (or values within 10% of patient's baseline values, which depend on underlying pathophysiology), RR $\leq$20 breaths/min with normal depth and pattern (eupnea), and orientation to time, place, and person.

- Monitor serial ABG results to detect continued presence of hypercapnia or hypoxemia. Monitor O_2 saturation *via* pulse oximetry as indicated. Consult physician for new or persistent hypoxemia or hypercapnia.

- Observe for indicators of hypoxia, including increased restlessness, anxiety, and changes in mental status.
- Assess patient for increasing respiratory distress: increased RR, diminished or absent movement of chest wall on affected side, complaints of increased dyspnea, and cyanosis.
- Position patient to allow for full expansion of unaffected lung. Semi-Fowler's position usually provides comfort and allows adequate expansion of chest wall. The patient also can be turned unaffected side down with the HOB elevated to ensure a better ventilation-perfusion match.
- Change patient's position q2h to promote drainage and lung reexpansion and to facilitate alveolar perfusion.
- Encourage patient to take deep breaths, providing necessary analgesia to decrease discomfort during deep-breathing exercises. Deep breathing will promote full lung expansion and may decrease the risk of atelectasis.
- Ensure delivery of prescribed concentrations of oxygen.
- Assess and maintain closed chest-drainage system:
  □ Tape all connections and secure chest tube to thorax with tape.
  □ Avoid all kinks in the tubing, and ensure that the bed and equipment are not compressing any component of the system.
  □ Maintain fluid in underwater-seal chamber, and suction chamber at appropriate levels.
  □ Be aware that the suction apparatus does not regulate the amount of suction applied to the closed drainage system. The amount of suction is determined by the water level in the suction control chamber. Minimal bubbling is optimal. Excessive bubbling causes rapid evaporative loss.

Note: Suction aids in the reexpansion of the lung, but removing suction for short periods of time, such as for transporting, will not be detrimental or disrupt the closed drainage system.

  □ Be aware that fluctuations in the long tube of the underwater-seal chamber indicate a patent chest tube. Fluctuations stop when either the lung has reexpanded or there is a kink or obstruction in the chest tube.
  □ Bubbling in the underwater-seal chamber occurs on expiration and is a sign that air is leaving the pleural space.
  □ Continuous bubbling on both inspiration and expiration in the underwater-seal chamber is a signal that air is leaking into the drainage system. Locate and seal the system's air leak, if possible.
- Keep necessary emergency supplies at the bedside: (1) petrolatum gauze pad to apply over insertion site if the chest tube becomes dislodged and (2) sterile water in which to submerge the chest tube if it becomes disconnected from the underwater-seal system. *Never* clamp a chest tube without a specific directive from the physician, inasmuch as clamping may lead to tension pneumothorax because the air can no longer escape.

Caution: Follow your agency's policy regarding chest tube stripping. Be aware that this mechanism for maintaining chest tube patency is controversial and has been associated with high negative pressures in the pleural space, which can damage fragile lung tissue. Chest tube stripping may be indicated when bloody drainage or clots are visible in the tubing. Squeezing alternately hand-over-hand along the drainage tube may generate sufficient pressure to move fluid along the tube.

Pain related to biophysical injury as a result of chest tube placement and pleural irritation
Desired outcomes: Within 1-2 h of initiating analgesic therapy, patient's subjective evaluation of discomfort improves as documented by a pain scale. Nonverbal indicators of discomfort, such as grimacing and splinting on inspiration, are absent.
- Give patient and significant others appropriate information regarding chest tube placement and maintenance.
- At frequent intervals, assess patient's degree of discomfort, using patient's verbal and nonverbal cues. Devise a pain scale with patient, rating discomfort on a scale of 0 (no pain) to 10 (worst pain). Medicate with analgesics as prescribed, evaluating and documenting the effectiveness of the medication on the basis of the pain scale.
- Position patient on unaffected side to minimize discomfort from chest tube insertion site. Administer medication 30 min before initiating movement.
- Teach patient to splint affected side during coughing, moving, or repositioning. Move patient as a unit to enhance stability and comfort.
- Schedule activities to provide for periods of rest, which may increase patient's pain threshold.
- Stabilize chest tube to reduce pull or drag on latex connector tubing. Tape chest tube securely to thorax, and loop latex tubing on bed beside patient.
- Teach patient to maintain active ROM on the involved side to prevent development of a stiff shoulder from the immobility.

ADDITIONAL NURSING DIAGNOSES
See "Status Asthmaticus" for **Activity intolerance,** p. 235. Also see appropriate nursing diagnoses and interventions in "Psychosocial Support," p. 88; and in "Psychosocial Support for the Patient's Family and Significant Others," p. 100.

Acute respiratory failure

PATHOPHYSIOLOGY

Acute respiratory failure is a clinical event in which there is impairment of either alveolar ventilation or pulmonary vascular perfusion or both. The accompanying increased work of breathing places demands on the cardiopulmonary system that exceed functional reserves. The result can be detrimental to respiratory homeostasis. Clinically, respiratory failure exists when Pao_2 is <50 mm Hg with the patient at rest and breathing room air. $Paco_2$ ≥50 mm Hg or pH <7.35 is significant for acute respiratory acidemia. Although a variety of disease processes can lead to respiratory failure, three basic mechanisms are involved.

Alveolar hypoventilation: Occurs as a result of reduction in alveolar minute ventilation. Because differential indicators (cyanosis and somnolence) occur late in the process, the condition may go unnoticed until hypoxia is severe.

Ventilation-perfusion mismatch: Considered the most common cause of hypoxia. Normal alveolar ventilation occurs at a rate of 4 L/min, with normal pulmonary vascular blood flow occurring at a rate of 5 L/min. The normal ventilation/perfusion ratio is 0.8:1. Any disease process that interferes with either side of the equation upsets the physiologic balance and can lead to respiratory failure as a result of reduction in arterial oxygen levels.

Diffusion disturbances: Processes that physically impair gas exchange across the alveolar-capillary membrane. Diffusion is impaired because of the increase in anatomic distance the gas must travel from the alveoli to the capillaries and from the capillaries to the alveoli.

Right-to-left shunting (intrapulmonary shunt):   Occurs when the aforementioned processes go untreated. Large amounts of blood pass from the right side of the heart to the left and out into the general circulation without adequate ventilation; therefore blood is poorly oxygenated. This process occurs when alveoli are atelectatic or fluid filled, inasmuch as these conditions interfere with gas exchange. Unlike the first three responses, hypoxia secondary to right-to-left shunting does not improve with the administration of oxygen, because the additional Fio_2 is unable to cross the alveolar-capillary membrane.

Note: See Table 3-5 for a description of some of the disease processes that can lead to acute respiratory failure.

ASSESSMENT

CLINICAL PRESENTATION Indicators of acute respiratory failure vary according to the underlying disease process and severity of the failure. Acute respiratory failure is one of the most common causes of impaired LOC. Often it is misdiagnosed as congestive heart failure (CHF), pneumonia, or cerebrovascular accident (CVA). Sometimes the onset of acute respiratory failure is so insidious that it is missed because staff members do not want to disturb the patient who appears to be sleeping.

Early indicators: Dyspnea, restlessness, anxiety, headache, fatigue, cool and dry skin, increased BP, tachycardia, and cardiac dysrhythmias.

Intermediate indicators: Confusion, lethargy, tachypnea, hypotension caused by vasodilatation, cardiac dysrhythmias.

Late indicators: Cyanosis, diaphoresis, coma, respiratory arrest.

DIAGNOSTIC TESTS

ABG analysis: Assesses adequacy of oxygenation and effectiveness of ventilation. Typical results are Pao_2 <60 mm Hg, $Paco_2$ ≥45 mm

T A B L E 3 - 5   Disease processes leading to the development of respiratory failure

Impaired alveolar ventilation	*Ventilation or perfusion disturbances*
COPD (emphysema, bronchitis, asthma, cystic fibrosis)	Pulmonary emboli
Restrictive pulmonary disease (interstitial fibrosis, pleural effusion, pneumothorax, kyphoscoliosis, obesity, diaphragmatic paralysis)	Atelectasis
	Pneumonia
	Emphysema
	Chronic bronchitis
	Bronchiolitis
	Adult respiratory distress syndrome
Neuromuscular defects (Guillain-Barré syndrome, myasthenia gravis, multiple sclerosis, muscular dystrophy)	*Diffusion disturbances*
	Pulmonary/interstitial fibrosis
	Pulmonary edema
	Adult respiratory distress syndrome
Depression of respiratory control centers (drug-induced cerebral infarction, inappropriate use of high-dose oxygen therapy)	Anatomic loss of functioning lung tissue (tumor pneumonectomy)

Hg, and pH <7.35, which are consistent with severe respiratory acidosis. Pulse oximetry is used for continuous monitoring of oxygen saturation (see p. 230).

Mixed venous oxygen saturation (Svo₂):   Mixed venous blood gases are drawn intermittently or measured continuously from the distal tip of the pulmonary artery catheter. A blood sample taken from this site ensures complete mixing of the blood returned from all parts of the body. Changes in Svo₂ provide an early indication of perfusion failure or increased tissue demands for oxygen. Svo₂ is a more sensitive indicator of oxygen available for tissue oxygenation than Spo₂. Normal values are 60%-80%. A value <50% is associated with impaired tissue oxygenation.

Chest x-ray: Ascertains presence of underlying pathophysiology or disease process that may be contributing to the failure.

COLLABORATIVE MANAGEMENT

Correction of hypoxemia: First treatment priority. Pao₂ levels <30 mm Hg for longer than 3-4 min may cause permanent brain damage or death. Oxygen therapy and chest physiotherapy, in conjunction with pharmacotherapy (e.g., bronchodilators, steroids, antibiotics), often improve ABG levels sufficiently to remove the patient from danger.

Correction of abnormal pH level: Second treatment priority. Adequate cellular and metabolic functioning is hindered when pH level remains outside the normal range of 7.35-7.45. When the pH is <7.25, IV sodium bicarbonate may be used conservatively and usually only when the patient is mechanically ventilated. A pH >7.45 may be managed by placing a rebreathing mask on the patient or increasing dead space on mechanical ventilator circuitry.

Intubation and mechanical ventilation: The purposes of intubation and mechanical ventilation are to restore alveolar ventilation, restore pH level within normal limits, and decrease work of breathing. Early intubation can prevent further airway collapse and tissue injury. In most cases the patient will require intubation and mechanical ventilation to provide adequate respiratory function and stabilize ABG levels. Mechanical support is used until the underlying cause of the failure can be corrected and the patient can resume ventilatory efforts independently. Mechanical ventilation is discussed in greater depth in Chapter 1.

NURSING DIAGNOSES AND INTERVENTIONS

See sections relating to patient's underlying pathologic condition (e.g., "Mechanical Ventilation," p. 24, and "Chest Trauma," p. 142).

Selected Bibliography

Atkins P: Respiratory consequences of multi-system crisis: the adult respiratory distress syndrome, *Crit Care Nurs Quart* 16(4):27-38, 1994.

Carden D, Smith K: Pneumonia, *Emerg Med Clin North Am* 7(2):255-278, 1989.

Centers for Disease Control: Guideline for prevention of nosocomial pneumonia, *Am J Infect Control* 22:247-292, 1994.

Civetta J, Taylor R, Kirby R: *Critical care,* ed 2, Philadelphia, 1992, Lippincott.

Currie D: Pulmonary embolism: diagnosis and management, *Crit Care Nurs Quart* 13(2):41-49, 1990.

Dettenmeier P: *Pulmonary nursing care,* St Louis, 1992, Mosby.

Ellstrom K: What's causing your patient's respiratory distress, *Nursing* 20(11):57-61, 1990.

Epstein CD, Henning RJ: Oxygen transport variables in the identification and treatment of tissue hypoxia, *Heart Lung* 22(4):328-348, 1993.

Gillepsie D, Rehder K: Body position and ventilation perfusion relationships in unilateral pulmonary disease, *Chest* 91(1):75-79, 1987.

Horne M, Swearingen PL: *Pocket guide to fluids, electrolytes, and acid-base balance,* ed 2, St Louis, 1993, Mosby.

Howard C: Respiratory disorders. In Swearingen PL, editor: *Manual of medical-surgical nursing care: nursing interventions and collaborative management,* ed 3, St Louis, 1994, Mosby.

Interqual: *The ISD-A review system with adult ISD criteria,* August 1992, North Hampton, NH, and Marlboro, MA, Interqual.

Kim MJ, McFarland GK, McLane AM: *Pocket guide to nursing diagnosis,* ed 6, St Louis, 1995, Mosby.

Niederman M et al: Pneumonia in the critically ill hospitalized patient, *Chest* 97(1):170-181, 1990.

Reischman R: Review of ventilation and perfusion physiology, *Crit Care Nurse* 8(7):24-28, 1988.

Roberts S: Pulmonary tissue perfusion, altered: emboli, *Heart Lung* 16(2):128-137, 1987.

Schmitz T: The semi-prone position in ARDS: five case studies, *Crit Care Nurse* 11(5):22-33, 1991.

Shapiro B: *Clinical application of respiratory care,* ed 4, Chicago, 1991, Mosby.

Siskind M: A standard for care of the nursing diagnosis of ineffective airway clearance, *Heart Lung* 18(5):444-451, 1989.

Sonnesso G: Are you ready to use pulse oximetry? *Nursing* 21(8):60-64, 1991.

Szaflarski NL: Use of pulse oximetry in critically ill adults, *Heart Lung* 18(5):444-452, 1989.

Teplitz L: Responding to an air embolism, *Nursing* 22(7):33, 1992.

Thompson B, Hales C: Hypoxic pulmonary hypertension: acute and chronic, *Heart Lung* 15(5):457-465, 1986.

Traver G, Flodquist-Priestly G: Management problems in unilateral lung disease with emphasis on differential lung ventilation, *Crit Care Nurse* 6(4):40-50, 1986.

Wollschlager C, Khan FA: Secondary pulmonary hypertension: clinical features, *Heart Lung* 15(4):336-340, 1986.

Young N, Gorzeman J: Managing pneumothorax and hemothorax, *Nursing* 21(4):56-57, 1991.

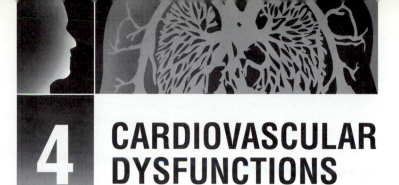

4 CARDIOVASCULAR DYSFUNCTIONS

Acute chest pain

PATHOPHYSIOLOGY

Chest discomfort or pain associated with myocardial ischemia is called angina pectoris. It can occur at rest or with exercise and may result from a sudden decrease in coronary blood flow due to coronary thrombosis or spasm or from the inability to increase coronary blood flow sufficiently to meet myocardial oxygen demands (e.g., during exercise). Acute chest pain due to ischemia may occur when coronary perfusion pressure is low, as in sudden hypotension, or when oxygen demands are greatly elevated, as in aortic stenosis. Pathogenic mechanisms that can cause acute chest pain due to ischemia include the following: atherosclerosis, platelet aggregation in diseased vessels, transient coronary artery thrombosis, hemorrhage into atheromatous plaque, abnormal vasoconstriction (spasm) of a coronary artery, and extracardiac factors such as anemia or thyrotoxicosis.

ASSESSMENT

HISTORY AND RISK FACTORS Familial history of coronary artery disease (CAD), age >65 yr, male sex (risk for females increases after menopause), cigarette smoking, hypercholesterolemia, hyperlipidemia, hypertension, diabetes, obesity, increased stress, sedentary life-style.

CLINICAL PRESENTATION Pain that usually is precipitated by exertion or emotional upset; subsides with rest; lasts for 1-4 min but not longer than 30 min; subsides gradually when precipitating factor is removed; is relieved by nitroglycerin, usually within 45-90 sec.

Chest pain with myocardial ischemia: Abrupt or gradual onset of substernal discomfort described as deep, visceral, squeezing, choking, burning, heavy, tight, or aching. Many patients will deny the presence of chest "pain" but will admit to severe chest "discomfort" or "pressure."

Chest pain with transmural infarction: More severe, of longer duration (i.e., >30 min), unrelieved by nitroglycerin.

Forms of angina

Stable: Has not increased in frequency or severity over a period of several months.

Unstable: A broad category that includes several types. Usually the quality of pain has changed or increased in frequency, duration, or severity; can occur with lessened exertion or at rest.

□ Wellen syndrome: Unstable angina, usually associated with left anterior descending (LAD) coronary artery lesions.

□ Rest angina.

□ New onset angina.

□ Preinfarction or crescendo: Unstable angina with the potential for progression to infarction.

Prinzmetal's (variant):   May occur at rest, long after exercise, and during sleep; usually caused by coronary vasospasm.

PHYSICAL ASSESSMENT BP may be elevated related to the sympathetic response to chest pain. BP may decrease if pain is caused by ischemia, which can result in decreased myocardial contractile strength and decreased cardiac output. HR may increase in response to hypoxia and enhanced sympathetic tone. S_4 heart sound may be audible during ischemic episodes.

DIAGNOSTIC TESTS

Also see "Acute Myocardial Infarction," p. 279, for a description of other diagnostic tests that may be performed, such as multiple-gated acquisition (MUGA) scanning, positron emission tomography (PET), and technetium pyrophosphate.

ECG: May establish diagnosis of ischemic heart disease if characteristic changes are present, although the absence of abnormality does not rule out this disease. In the absence of pain and with the patient at rest, the 12/18-lead ECG may be normal; therefore this test must be obtained during an episode of chest pain. ST-segment and T-wave changes, which occur during spontaneous chest pain and disappear with relief of the pain, are significant. The most characteristic change is depression of the ST segment with or without T-wave inversion. In variant or Prinzmetal's angina, the ST segments may be elevated during the chest pain episode.

   With Wellen syndrome, characteristic changes include inverted symmetric T waves with little or no ST elevation.

Cardiac catheterization: To determine presence and extent of coronary artery disease as the cause of the chest pain.

Stress test: Patient exercises while being monitored by electrocardiography. Its purpose is to elicit chest pain and document any associated ECG changes. Positive stress test results elicit at least 1 mm horizontal depression or downsloping ST segment in one or more leads that lasts 0.08 sec. In addition, frequent PVCs or runs of ventricular tachycardia are suggestive of ischemia.

Thallium treadmill: Normal myocardial tissue will accumulate thallium, whereas infarcted or ischemic areas will have decreased uptake, appearing as "cold spots" on the scan. To identify areas of decreased uptake, the patient exercises after an injection of thallium. A scan is obtained both immediately after exercise and 4 h later to determine if areas with decreased uptake fill in after 4 h. Ischemic areas that fill in are considered to have viable tissue and reversible damage, whereas areas that remain as "cold spots" are diagnosed as infarcted.

Serum enzyme levels: To rule out the occurrence of myocardial infarction (see "Acute Myocardial Infarction," p. 279).

Chest x-ray: May reveal cardiac enlargement. In patients with ischemic heart disease, cardiomegaly signals the presence of myocardial ischemia and decreased myocardial contractility.

COLLABORATIVE MANAGEMENT

Relief of acute pain: Drugs are administered and titrated to reduce or eliminate chest pain.

Oral, sublingual, and other forms of nitroglycerin (NTG): Can be used for short-term therapy or longer-lasting prophylactic effects.

IV nitroglycerin: For unstable angina, it is titrated until relief is obtained.

IV morphine sulfate: Given in small increments (i.e., 2 mg) until relief is obtained. This medication is usually not necessary unless a myocardial infarction (MI) is occurring.

Calcium channel blockers (e.g., nifedipine): Block the movement of calcium into the cells, causing vasodilatation of the coronary and peripheral arteries to relieve chest pain caused by coronary artery spasm. In addition, they decrease contraction and oxygen demand. Nifedipine may be given sublingually for rapid onset of action.

Reduction of cardiac workload to decrease oxygen demand

Beta-adrenergic blocking agents (e.g., propranolol): To decrease HR, BP, and myocardial contractility.

Limit activities: Restrictions based on patient's activity tolerance.

Oxygen: Usually 2-4 L/min by nasal cannula, or mode and rate as directed by ABG values.

Management of unstable angina: May include administration of an anticoagulant and antiplatelet drug (ASA) to prevent thrombus formation.

Percutaneous transluminal coronary angioplasty (PTCA): Invasive procedure for improving blood flow through stenotic coronary arteries. A balloon-tipped catheter is inserted into the coronary arterial lesion, and the balloon is inflated to compress the plaque material against the vessel wall, thereby opening the narrowed lumen. PTCA is indicated for the surgical candidate whose angina is refractory to medical treatment. It also is performed in individuals with postinfarction angina, postbypass angina, and chronic stable angina. The ideal candidate has single-vessel disease with a discrete, proximal, noncalcified lesion.

During the procedure the patient is sedated lightly; given a local anesthetic at the insertion site, usually the femoral artery; and ECG electrodes are placed on the chest. A pulmonary artery catheter is passed through the vena cava and right atrium into the heart in order to measure heart pressure. A pacing wire may be inserted as well. An introducer sheath is inserted into the femoral artery, a guidewire is passed into the aorta and coronary artery, and the balloon catheter is passed over the guidewire to the stenotic site. The patient may be asked to take deep breaths and cough to facilitate passage of the catheter. Heparin is given to prevent clot formation, and intracoronary NTG and sublingual nifedipine are administered to dilate coronary vessels and prevent spasm. The balloon is inflated repeatedly for 60-90 sec at a pressure of 4-11 atm. Subsequently, radiopaque dye is injected to determine whether the stenosis has been reduced to less than 50% of the vessel diameter, which is the goal of the procedure. The introducer sheath is left in the femoral artery for up to 12 h after PTCA for heparin infusion or in the event of the need for repeat angiography.

Complications after PTCA include acute coronary artery occlusion, acute myocardial infarction (AMI), coronary artery spasm, bleeding, circulatory insufficiency, renal hypersensitivity to contrast material, hypokalemia, vasovagal reaction, dysrhythmias, and hypotension. Restenosis can occur 6 weeks to 6 months after PTCA, although the patient may not experience angina.

Excimer laser coronary angioplasty (ELCA):   Enables treatment of distal coronary lesions in tortuous arteries. The laser ablates only the tissue it contacts.

Intracoronary stent procedure: Stents are metal-mesh tubes used to keep arteries open. Balloon-expanded stents are most commonly used in the United States and are inserted during a procedure similar to PTCA.

Percutaneous balloon valvuloplasty: Used to dilate stenotic aortic valves in patients who are not candidates for surgery because of advanced age (>80 yr) or who refuse surgery. These patients may have chest pain due to critical stenosis of the aortic valve with decreased blood flow through coronary arteries (see p. 328).

NURSING DIAGNOSES AND INTERVENTIONS

Pain (chest) related to biophysiologic injury secondary to decreased oxygen supply to the myocardium

Desired outcomes: Within 1 h of intervention, patient's subjective evaluation of discomfort improves, as documented by a pain scale. Nonverbal indicators, such as grimacing, are absent.

- Assess and document the character of the patient's chest pain, including location, duration, quality, intensity, precipitating and alleviating factors, presence or absence of radiation, and associated symptoms. Devise a pain scale with patient, rating discomfort from 0 (no pain) to 10.
- Measure BP and HR with each episode of chest pain. BP and HR may increase because of sympathetic stimulation as a result of pain. If the chest pain is caused by ischemia, the heart muscle may not be functioning normally and cardiac output may decrease, resulting in

a low BP. In addition, dysrhythmias such as bradycardia and ventricular ectopy may be noted with ischemia.

- Obtain a 12- or 18-lead ECG during patient's episode of chest pain. During angina, ischemia usually is demonstrated on the ECG by ST-segment depression and T-wave inversion.
- Administer nitrates as prescribed, titrating IV nitroglycerin so that chest pain is relieved, yet systolic BP remains >90 mm Hg. NTG drip is usually 100 mg nitroglycerin in 250 ml D_5W. Begin with 3 ml/min, which is 19.8 μg/min. Titrate by increments of 3 ml q5min (or 19.8 μg q5min) up to a maximum dosage determined by agency protocol or physician.
- After each titration of intravenous NTG, evaluate patient's BP and the effects of therapy in relieving patient's chest pain. If slight hypotension occurs (80-90 mm Hg systolic), reduce the flow rate to ½ or less of the infusing dose. If severe hypotension (<80 mm Hg systolic) occurs, stop the infusion and contact the physician for further directions. In either situation the physician may prescribe a low-dose positive inotropic agent (e.g., dopamine or dobutamine) to enhance cardiac contractility. For additional information, see "Inotropic and Vasoactive Agents," Appendix 7.
- Monitor for side effects of NTG, including headache, hypotension, syncope, facial flushing, and nausea. If side effects occur, place patient in a supine position and consult physician for further interventions.
- As prescribed, administer beta-blockers and calcium channel blockers, which relieve chest pain by diminishing coronary artery spasm, causing coronary and peripheral vasodilatation, and decreasing myocardial contractility and oxygen demand. Monitor for side effects, including bradycardia and hypotension. Be alert to indicators of heart failure, including fatigue, SOB, weight gain, and edema, and to indicators of heart block such as syncope and dizziness.
- Administer heparin and ASA as prescribed. Heparin usually is administered in a 500 U IV bolus, followed by 1,000 U/h, which is titrated according to PTT results.
- Administer oxygen per nasal cannula at 2-4 L/min, as prescribed.
- Position patient according to his or her comfort level.
- Provide care in a calm and efficient manner; reassure and support patient during chest pain episodes.
- Maintain a quiet environment and group patient care activities to allow for periods of uninterrupted rest.
- Ensure that activity restrictions and bed rest are maintained; teach patient the importance of activity limitation and its rationale: to minimize oxygen requirements and thus decrease chest pain.
- Instruct patient to report any further episodes of chest pain.
- For more information about pain, see p. 66 in Chapter 1.

Activity intolerance related to imbalance between oxygen supply and demand secondary to decreased cardiac output associated with coronary artery disease

Desired outcome: Within the 12-24 h period before discharge from CCU, patient exhibits cardiac tolerance to increasing levels of activity as evidenced by RR <24 breaths/min, normal sinus rhythm on ECG, BP within 20 mm Hg of patient's normal range, HR <120 bpm (or

T A B L E 4 - 1   **Activity level progression for hospitalized patients***

Level		Activity
I	Bed rest	Flexion and extension of extremities qid, 15 times each extremity; deep breathing qid, 15 breaths; position change from side to side q2h
II	OOB to chair	As tolerated, tid for 20-30 min
III	Ambulate in room	As tolerated, tid for 20-30 min
IV	Ambulate in hall	Initially, 50-200 ft bid; progressing to 50-200 ft qid

*__Signs of activity intolerance:__ Decrease in BP >20 mm Hg; increase in HR to >120 bpm (or >20 bpm above resting HR in patients receiving beta-blocker therapy).

within 20 bpm of resting HR for patients on beta-blocker therapy), and absence of chest pain.

- Assist patient with identifying activities that precipitate chest pain and teach patient to use NTG prophylactically before the activity.
- Assist patient as needed in progressive activity program, beginning with level I and progressing to level IV, as tolerated (Table 4-1).
- Assess patient's response to activity progression. Be alert to presence of chest pain, SOB, excessive fatigue, and dysrhythmias. Monitor for a decrease in BP >20 mm Hg and an increase in HR to >120 bpm (>20 bpm above resting HR in patients receiving beta-blocker therapy).
- Teach patient about measures that prevent complications of decreased mobility, such as active ROM exercises. (For additional details, see "Prolonged Immobility," p. 78.)

Knowledge deficit: Disease process and its life-style implications

Desired outcome: Within the 24-h period before discharge from the step-down unit, patient verbalizes understanding of his or her disease, as well as the necessary life-style changes that may modify risk factors.

- Teach patient about ischemia and its resultant chest pain, referred to as "angina pectoris."
- Discuss the pathophysiologic process underlying patient's angina, using drawings or heart models as indicated.
- Assist patient in identifying his or her own risk factors (e.g., cigarette smoking, high-stress life-style).
- Teach patient about risk-factor modification:
  □ *Diet low in cholesterol and saturated fat:* Provide sample diet plan for meals that are low in cholesterol and saturated fat. Teach patient about foods that are high and low in cholesterol and saturated fat (Tables 4-3 and 4-4). Stress the importance of reading food labels.
  □ *Smoking cessation:* Teach patient that smoking causes the coronary arteries to constrict, thus decreasing blood flow to the heart.
  □ *Stress management:* Discuss the role that stress plays in angina. Explain that stress increases sympathetic tone, which can cause the BP and HR to increase, resulting in increased oxygen demand.

T A B L E   4 - 2   **Guidelines for a progressive at-home walking program**

Week	Distance	Time
1	100-200 ft	2 ×/day
2	200-400 ft	2 ×/day
3	¼ mi	8-10 min
4	½ mi	15 min
5	1 mi	30 min
6	1¾ mi	30 min
7	2 mi	40 min

By employing relaxation techniques such as imagery, meditation, or biofeedback, one can decrease the effects of stress on the heart. For a sample relaxation technique, see **Health-seeking behavior,** p. 323.

- Teach patient about the prescribed medications, including name, purpose, dosage, action, schedule, precautions, and potential side effects.
- Teach patient the actions that should be taken if chest pain is unrelieved or increases in intensity. If chest pain occurs:
  1. Stop and rest.
  2. Take one NTG; wait 5 min. If pain is not relieved, take a second NTG; wait 5 min. If pain is not relieved, take a third NTG.
  3. Lie down if headache occurs. Explain that the vasodilatation effect of NTG causes a decrease in BP, which may result in orthostatic hypotension and transient headache.
  4. If the pain is not relieved after three NTGs taken over a 15-min period, call physician or dial 911 or local emergency number.
- Explain to patient that it is no more beneficial to be in the emergency department than it is to be at home during episodes of chest pain due to angina and therefore traveling to a hospital at the first sign of chest pain usually is unnecessary.
- Review activity limitations and prescribed progressions. (Tables 4-1 and 4-2). Provide the following information:

When you are discharged from the hospital, it is important that you continue your walking program. The following guidelines [in Table 4-2] are to help you plan a program that is right for you. Don't overestimate your ability; rather, start off slowly and build up. Depending on how you feel, you may only be able to stay at one level or you may progress to 2 mi quickly. Remember to warm up and cool down with stretches for 5-7 min and to walk 3-5 times each week. In addition:

- Avoid sudden energetic activities.
- Plan for regular rest periods in the afternoon.
- Let your body guide you regarding whether to increase or decrease activity.
- Inform your physician of any changes in activity tolerance, such as the development of new symptoms with the same activity.

- □ Avoid exercising outdoors in very cold, hot, or humid weather. Extreme weather places an additional stress on the heart. If you do exercise in extremes of weather, decrease the pace and monitor your response carefully.
- Pulse monitoring: Teach patient how to take pulse, including parameters for target heart rates and limits.
- Sexual activity guidelines: Because sexual activity is a physical activity, certain guidelines can help the patient and his or her partner enjoy a satisfying sexual relationship while minimizing the workload of the heart:
  - □ Rest is beneficial before engaging in intercourse.
  - □ Find a position that is comfortable for you and your partner. Assuming a different position that is uncomfortable to both may increase the workload of the heart.
  - □ Medications such as NTG may be taken prophylactically by the patient before intercourse to prevent chest pain.
  - □ Postpone intercourse for 1-1½ h after eating a heavy meal.
  - □ Report the following symptoms to your physician if they are experienced after sexual relations: SOB, increased HR that persists for more than 15 min, unrelieved chest pain.

For patients undergoing percutaneous transluminal coronary angioplasty

Knowledge deficit:　Angioplasty procedure and postprocedural care
Desired outcomes:　Within the 24-h period before the procedure, patient describes the rationale for the procedure, how it is performed, and postprocedural care. Patient relates discharge instructions within the 24-h period before discharge from the CCU.

- Assess patient's understanding of CAD and the purpose of angioplasty. Evaluate patient's style of coping and degree of information desired.
- As appropriate for coping style, discuss the following with patient and significant others:
  - □ Location of patient's CAD, using heart drawing.
  - □ Use of local anesthesia and sedation during procedure.
  - □ Insertion site of catheter: groin or arm.
  - □ Sensations that may occur: mild chest discomfort; a feeling of heat as the dye is injected.
  - □ Use of fluoroscopy during procedure. Determine patient's history of sensitivity to contrast material.
  - □ Ongoing observations made by nurse after procedure: BP, HR, ECG, leg or arm pulses, blood tests.
  - □ Importance of lying flat in bed 6-12 h after procedure.
  - □ Necessity for nursing assistance with eating, drinking, and toileting needs after procedure.
  - □ Need for increased fluid intake after procedure to wash dye out of system.
  - □ Discharge instructions: Importance of taking antiplatelet drugs to prevent restenosis, avoidance of strenuous activity during first few weeks at home, follow-up visit with cardiologist 1 week after hospital discharge, signs and symptoms to report to physician (i.e., GI upset, repeat of angina, fainting).

- If patient and significant others express or exhibit evidence of anxiety regarding the upcoming procedure, try to arrange for them to meet with another patient who has had a successful angioplasty.

Decreased cardiac output (or risk for same) related to negative inotropic changes secondary to vessel occlusion, infarction, coronary artery spasm, and cardiac tamponade; and related to electrical factors secondary to angioplasty-induced dysrhythmias

Desired outcomes: Within 24 h of this diagnosis, patient exhibits adequate cardiac output, as evidenced by BP within normal limits for patient; HR 60-100 bpm; normal sinus rhythm on ECG; peripheral pulses >2+ on a 0-4+ scale; warm and dry skin; hourly urine output ≥0.5 ml/kg; measured CO 4-7 L/min; RAP 4-6 mm Hg, PAP 20-30/8-15 mm Hg, PAWP 6-12 mm Hg; and patient awake, alert, oriented, and free from anginal pain.

- Monitor BP, RAP, and PAP continuously; monitor PAWP and CO hourly. Be alert to the following indicators of decreased cardiac output: decreased BP, increased HR, increased PAP, increased PAWP, decreased measured CO, and decreased RAP.
- Monitor ECG continuously for evidence of dysrhythmias and ST- and T-wave changes. Observe for bradyarrhythmias during sheath removal. Run a 12/18-lead ECG daily.
- Monitor urinary output hourly for the first 4 h, and thereafter according to agency protocol. Consult physician for hourly output <0.5 ml/kg/h for 2 consecutive hours.
- Measure creatinine kinase–myocardial band (CK-MB) immediately after PTCA procedure and then q8h for 24 hours; report elevations. Optimally CK-MB will be 0%-5% of total CK.
- Monitor patient responses to antianginal and coronary vasodilator medications given for hypotension; report BP below desired range. Hypotension also can occur as a result of vessel occlusion. Treat hypotension immediately, as prescribed. Usually, fluids are given and the patient is placed in supine position.
- When patient first sits up, ensure that it is done in stages to minimize the likelihood of postural hypotension. Monitor VS at frequent intervals during this stage.
- Monitor patient continuously for bleeding at sheath insertion site. Monitor Hct level for decrease from baseline values.
- Monitor patient for evidence of cardiac tamponade: hypotension, tachycardia, pulsus paradoxus, jugular venous distention, elevation and plateau pressuring of PAWP and RAP and, possibly, an enlarged heart silhouette on chest x-ray.
- When heparin and antiplatelet drugs are discontinued, monitor patient closely for indicators of coronary occlusion: ST-segment elevation on ECG, angina, hypotension, tachycardia, dysrhythmias, and diaphoresis.
- Monitor peripheral pulses (radial and pedal) and color and temperature of extremities q4h for first 4 h.
- Monitor patient's mental alertness on an ongoing basis.

Altered peripheral tissue perfusion (or risk for same): Involved limb, related to interruption of arterial blood flow secondary to presence of angioplasty sheath or risk of clot formation in vessel after sheath removal

Desired outcome: Upon admission to CCU and continuously there-after, patient has adequate tissue perfusion in the involved limb as evidenced by warm skin, peripheral pulses >2+ on a 0-4+ scale, normal skin color, ability to move the toes, and complete sensation.

- Monitor circulation to affected limb q30min for 2 h and then q2h thereafter. Assess pulses, temperature, color, sensation, and mobility of toes. Be alert to weak or thready pulses, coolness and pallor of the extremity, and patient complaints of numbness and tingling. Consult physician immediately if any of these signs or symptoms is present.
- Inspect sheath site for signs of external or subcutaneous bleeding.
- Keep sandbag at insertion site until discontinued by physician.
- Maintain immobilization of limb at least 6 h or until discontinued by physician.
- Keep HOB no higher than 15 degrees to prevent kinking of sheath.
- Monitor sheath patency by evaluating for continuous IV infusion into the involved vessel.
- Instruct patient to notify staff immediately if numbness, tingling, or pain occurs at the affected extremity.

ADDITIONAL NURSING DIAGNOSES

See discussion of intraaortic balloon pump in "Cardiogenic Shock" under **Altered protection**, p. 372. As appropriate, see nursing diagnoses and interventions in "Hemodynamic Monitoring," p. 37; "Psychosocial Support," p. 88; and "Psychosocial Support for the Patient's Family and Significant Others," p. 100.

Acute myocardial infarction

PATHOPHYSIOLOGY

Acute myocardial infarction (AMI) is necrosis of myocardial tissue due to relative or absolute lack of blood supply to the myocardium. Most AMIs are caused by atherosclerosis (e.g., fat deposits, fibrosis, calcification, and platelet aggregation), which results in a progressive narrowing of the coronary artery, thrombus formation, and ultimately, occlusion of blood flow. Occlusion also can be caused by coronary artery spasm. The site of infarction is determined by the location of the arterial occlusion.

ASSESSMENT

HISTORY AND RISK FACTORS Familial history of CAD, age >65 yr, male sex (risk for females increases after menopause), cigarette smoking, hypercholesterolemia, hypertension, diabetes, obesity, increased stress, and sedentary life-style. The patient may report a history of crescendo or unstable angina.

CLINICAL PRESENTATION Substernal, pressurelike chest pain that can radiate anywhere within the 6-dermatome pathway, from the jaw to the epigastrium. Classically, the pain radiates to the left arm, down the inner aspect along the ulnar nerve. The chest pain differs from angina in that it is constant and unrelieved by rest, position, or nitrates; duration is ≥30 min. Other associated signs and symptoms include nausea, vomiting, dyspnea, orthopnea, anxiety, apprehension, diaphoresis, cyanosis, unexplained weakness and fatigue, and denial. However, sometimes the presentation can be less "typical." Patients may present with only vague symptoms of GI upset or epigastric distress. A patient may have no chest discomfort and only arm or shoulder blade pain. Approximately 25% of AMIs are "silent," with vague symptoms that are not at all suggestive of typical AMI signs.

PHYSICAL ASSESSMENT HR may be increased because of enhanced sympathetic tone, or the patient may have dysrhythmias such as bradycardia, AV block, or ventricular ectopy. BP may be decreased because of a decrease in cardiac output; an increase in temperature may occur because of the inflammatory process. Auscultation may reveal presystolic gallop (S_4); pericardial friction rub; murmurs; crackles; and split S_1, S_2, and S_3 heart sounds if failure has occurred.

DIAGNOSTIC TESTS

ECGs: The first ECG is done immediately and is used to determine suitability for thrombolytic therapy. ECGs are then done in a series (24 h apart). Characteristic changes in certain "lead groups" identify the area and evolution of infarct. Changes include:

Q waves: Are indicative of MI and meet one of two criteria: either they are wide (>.04 sec) or deep (>25% of the total voltage of the QRS).

ST-segment changes: Will be elevated in the lead over or facing the infarcted area. Reciprocal changes (ST-segment depressions) will be found in leads 180 degrees from the area of infarction.

T-wave changes: May occur hours to weeks after infarction. Within the early hours of infarction, "giant" upright T waves may be seen in leads over the infarct. Within several hours to days, the T wave becomes inverted. Gradually over time, the ST segment becomes isoelectric and the T wave may remain inverted. T-wave changes may last for weeks and return to normal or remain inverted for the rest of the patient's life.

Serum enzyme levels: Elevation of CK will peak within 24 h after MI. CK elevation alone, however, is not indicative of an MI because it can be elevated for a variety of reasons, such as trauma or surgery. Isoenzyme levels are more diagnostic of cardiac muscle damage. Generally a CK-MB level that is >10% of the total CK is indicative of myocardial muscle damage. This criterion, however, may vary from one institution to another. If the patient's history is strongly suggestive of MI and CK total and MB are within normal limits, then testing for lactic dehydrogenase (LD) isoenzyme may be helpful. LD_1 is more specific for MI than LD_{2-5}. If the total LD is elevated and LD_1 is the predominant isoenzyme, this is diagnostic of MI.

Serum lipid tests
Cholesterol analysis: A total cholesterol test measures the circulating levels of free cholesterol and cholesterol esters, reflecting the level of the forms of cholesterol that appear in the body. Total cholesterol is the only cholesterol routinely measured. Concentrations vary with age. Most cardiologists prefer patients to have a cholesterol level of <200 mg/dl.

Lipoprotein-cholesterol fractionation: Measures the major lipids in the serum. These include very low-density lipoproteins (VLDL), low-density lipoproteins (LDL), and high-density lipoproteins (HDL). Cholesterol in HDL is inversely related to the incidence of CAD: the higher the HDL, the lower the incidence of CAD. Normal HDL levels range from 29 to 77 mg/100 dl; normal LDL levels range from 62 to 185 mg/100 ml. High LDL levels increase the risk of CAD.

Triglyceride analysis: This test analyzes the storage form of lipids, which constitute 95% of fatty tissue. Although not in itself diagnostic of CAD, serum triglyceride analysis enables early identification of those individuals who may have increased risk of CAD. Triglyceride values are age related, but a generally accepted range is 10-190 mg/dl in individuals age 50-59 yr.

Serum magnesium level: Often drops in AMI associated with increased dysrhythmias.

Leukocyte count and erythrocyte sedimentation rate (ESR):   Although these levels are not diagnostic of MI, they are increased in patients with MI because of the inflammatory process.

Chest x-ray: Usually reveals cardiomegaly and signs of left ventricular failure (interstitial pulmonary edema), but findings also may be normal.

Technetium pyrophosphate: May help to localize area of infarction and demonstrate necrotic tissue. IV pyrophosphate will bind with calcium, which is found in high concentrations within the cells of necrotic tissue, and appears as a darkened area or "hot spot" on the scan up to 10 days after MI.

Multiple-gated acquisition (MUGA) scanning: IV injection of the isotope technetium pertechnetate to evaluate left ventricular function and detect aneurysms, wall-motion abnormalities, and intracardiac shunting. In the stress MUGA test the same test is performed at rest and after exercise.

Echocardiography: To detect abnormalities of left ventricular wall motion, measure ejection fraction, evaluate valve function, and estimate LVEDP. Normal ejection fraction is >60% (approximate).

Positron emission tomography (PET):   Use of isotopes to assess metabolic activity of areas of infarction to determine if viable, but jeopardized, tissue is present. Viable tissue has metabolic activity as seen by increased uptake of the glucose tracer and decreased uptake of the blood flow tracer, which is ammonia.

Hemodynamic monitoring: Used in a patient with a complicated MI that results in failure with possible progression to cardiogenic shock. Pulmonary artery and capillary pressures are measured, along with cardiac output determinations and SVR calculations. With AMI, the following are likely to be found: increased PAP, increased PAWP, decreased CO, and increased SVR.

Coronary angiography: To identify extent of CAD, "culprit" lesions, and suitability for CABG or angioplasty.

Indium-111 antimyosin imaging: Technique in which antibodies (antimyosin) are labeled with radioactive Indium-111 and injected to permit visualization of damaged areas.

COLLABORATIVE MANAGEMENT

Relief of acute pain: IV NTG is titrated until relief of chest pain occurs while ensuring that systolic pressure remains >90 mm Hg. IV morphine sulfate may be used in conjunction with nitrates to relieve chest pain and reduce anxiety, preload, and sympathetic tone. Usual dosage is 2-4 mg initially, in 2 mg increments.

Oxygen: Usually 2-4 L/min *via* nasal cannula or mask, titrated to maintain Sao$_2$ at ≥96%-98%.

Thrombolytic therapy: With streptokinase, anistreplase (APSAC, Eminase), or alteplase (Activase) to lyse the clot in selected patients (see "Caring for Patients Undergoing Coronary Artery Thrombolysis," p. 374).

Reduction of cardiac workload: Achieved with bed rest, beta-blockers, and calcium channel blockers.

Prevention, recognition, and treatment of dysrhythmias: Advanced cardiac life support (ACLS) algorithms (see Appendix 1) or agency protocol used.

Antiplatelet/anticoagulant therapy: For prevention of thrombus, which is an important part of management. ASA decreases platelet aggregation, and heparin prevents clot formation.

Management of fluid imbalance: To optimize preload. Oral and IV fluids are given for dehydration; diuretics and vasodilators are given for volume overload. Hemodynamic monitoring often is used to guide intervention.

Percutaneous transluminal coronary angioplasty: May be performed in individuals with residual stenosis after thrombolytic therapy (see p. 271).

Coronary artery bypass graft (CABG): May be indicated when medical treatment (e.g., nitrates, calcium channel blockers, thrombolysis, and angioplasty) is unsuccessful or disease progression is evident. The patient is evaluated by angiography before surgery, and the decision for surgery is based on the patient's symptoms and angiography results. Surgical indications include (1) stable angina with 50% stenosis of the left main coronary artery, (2) stable angina with three-vessel coronary artery disease, (3) unstable angina with three-vessel disease or severe two-vessel disease, (4) recent myocardial infarction, (5) ischemic heart failure with cardiogenic shock, and (6) signs of ischemia or impending MI after angiography procedure.

The surgical technique for CABG involves use of a conduit, such as a saphenous vein graft (SVG), internal mammary artery (IMA), cadaveric saphenous vein graft (CSVG), brachial vein, or Gore-Tex graft to bypass the obstructed portion of the coronary artery. The saphenous vein is by far the most common of these, with a patency rate far superior to the brachial vein or Gore-Tex graft. The operative procedure involves use of general anesthesia, cardiopulmonary bypass, a medial sternotomy incision, one or more incisions (e.g., on the leg for saphenous vein) for the graft, and placement of pulmonary artery, systemic arterial, and left atrial catheters for postoperative monitoring. Postoperatively the patient is monitored for the following complications: low cardiac output syndrome, hemorrhage, cardiac tamponade, dysrhythmias, atelectasis, hypertension/hypotension, neurologic dysfunction, paralytic ileus, GI bleeding, infection or sepsis, renal failure, or postpericardiotomy syndrome. The mortality rate for CABG is 2%.

NURSING DIAGNOSES AND INTERVENTIONS

Note: The following nursing diagnoses address care for the individual with uncomplicated MI. For patients with complicated AMI, see additional sections in "Acute Cardiac Tamponade," p. 154; "Congestive Heart Failure," p. 293; "Dysrhythmias and Conduction Disturbances," p. 307; "Acute Pericarditis," p. 345; and "Cardiogenic Shock," p. 367.

Pain (chest) related to biophysical injury secondary to decreased oxygen supply to the myocardium
Desired outcomes: Within 2 h of intervention, patient's subjective evaluation of chest pain improves as documented by a pain scale. Nonverbal indicators, such as grimacing, are absent.
- Assess characteristics of chest pain, including location, duration, quality, intensity, presence of radiation, precipitating and alleviating factors, and associated symptoms. Devise a pain scale with patient, rating discomfort from 0 (no pain) to 10. Also be alert to nonverbal indicators, such as grimacing and diaphoresis.
- Assess BP and HR with each episode of chest pain. Although BP may increase initially related to increased sympathetic tone, myocardial damage can decrease heart function, resulting in decreased cardiac output and low BP. HR also may increase because of sympathetic tone, or patient may have dysrhythmias such as bradycardia, heart block, or tachycardia.
- Obtain a 12/18-lead ECG daily for 3 days to document the evolutionary changes seen with MI. In addition, if chest pain recurs, obtain a 12/18-lead ECG during the chest pain to aid in evaluating whether the pain is caused by further ischemia or infarction.
- Titrate NTG drip until complete relief of chest pain occurs, while also maintaining systolic BP at >90 mm Hg. Usually, a 50 μg IV bolus is followed by IV drip. See this nursing diagnosis, p. 273, in "Chest Pain" for dosing and titration guidelines. Administer morphine sulfate as prescribed to reduce chest pain, preload, sympathetic tone, and patient's anxiety.
- To determine and document the CK rise associated with MI, CK total and MB are assessed q8h for 24 h, or per hospital protocol. The CK rises within 8 h, peaks within 24 h, and returns to normal in 2 days.
- Administer oxygen by nasal cannula at 2-4 L/min as prescribed, or based on ABG results.
- Give thrombolytic agent as prescribed. See section "Caring for Patients Undergoing Coronary Artery Thrombolysis," p. 374, for additional information.
- Instruct patient to report decreases or increases in chest pain.

- Provide care in a calm, efficient manner that will reassure patient and minimize anxiety and thus chest pain.
- Regulate visitation in accordance with patient's comfort level.
- Enforce activity restrictions; maintain patient on bed rest to decrease oxygen demand.

Decreased cardiac output related to electrical factors (altered rate, rhythm, or conduction) secondary to cardiac injury and infarcted tissue
Desired outcome: Within 24 h of treatment, patient is in sinus rhythm and the incidence of dysrhythmias is reduced.

- Orient patient to the monitor, its purpose, the alarms, and the need for continuous monitoring.
- Monitor patient continuously in modified chest lead (MCL) V_1 to detect ventricular ectopy versus aberrancy. Monitor on V_2 if supraventricular dysrhythmias are present or if it is imperative to identify axis deviations. Keep alarms on at all times (e.g., 50-100).
- Assess apical HR hourly. Monitor for irregularities in rhythm.
- Document rhythm strip every shift and prn if dysrhythmias occur. Measure PR segment, QRS complex, and QT interval with each strip. Note and report any deviations from the patient's baseline. Normal intervals are PR 0.10-0.20 sec and QRS 0.10 sec. The QT interval is rate related, and the upper limits of normal usually correspond to approximately one half the R-R interval.
- Administer antidysrhythmic agents as prescribed. Prophylactic lidocaine is used in some agencies for the first 24 h after MI. If it is used, the usual protocol is a bolus of 1-1.5 mg/kg initially, followed by a drip of 1-4 mg/min, and another bolus 10 min after the initial bolus, using half the initial dose.
- Monitor serum potassium for levels >5 mEq/L or <3.5 mEq/L. Hypokalemia or hyperkalemia can cause dysrhythmias. Replace potassium as prescribed.
- Deliver oxygen *via* nasal cannula at 2-4 L/min or as prescribed. Oxygen may be beneficial for treating dysrhythmias caused by ischemia.
- See "Dysrhythmias and Conduction Disturbances," p. 300, for more information.

Decreased cardiac output related to negative inotropic changes in the heart secondary to myocardial injury
Desired outcomes: Within 24 h of treatment, patient has adequate cardiac output, as evidenced by systolic BP $\geq$90 mm Hg; CO $\geq$4 L/min; CI $\geq$2.5 L/min/m^2; HR $\leq$100 bpm; RR 12-20 breaths/min with normal pattern and depth (eupnea); orientation to time, place, and person; warm and dry skin; and urinary output $\geq$0.5 ml/kg/h. PAWP remains $\leq$18 mm Hg.

- Assess for and document the following as evidence of myocardial dysfunction with decreasing cardiac output: presence of jugular venous distention, dependent edema (i.e., sacral), hepatomegaly, fatigue, weakness, decreased activity level, and SOB with activity. In addition, assess and document the following:
  - *Mental status:* Be alert to restlessness and decreased responsiveness.
  - *Lung sounds:* Monitor for crackles, rhonchi.
  - *Heart sounds:* Note presence of gallop, murmur, and increased HR.

- □ *Urinary output:* Be alert to output <0.5 ml/kg/h.
- □ *Skin:* Monitor for pallor, mottling, cyanosis, coolness, diaphoresis.
- □ *Vital signs:* Note BP <90 mm Hg systolic, HR >100 bpm, RR >20 breaths/min, and temperature >38.5° C (101.4° F). The temperature of patients with MI may spike as a result of the body's reaction to necrotic tissue.
- If a pulmonary artery catheter is present, record hemodynamic readings q1-2h and prn. Be alert to PAWP >18 mm Hg, CO <4 L/min, and CI <2.5 L/min/m^2.
- Keep accurate I&O records and weigh patient daily. Be alert to fluid volume excess. A 1 kg acute weight gain can signal retention of 1 L of fluid.
- Help minimize cardiac workload by administering prescribed beta-blockers, positioning patient in Fowler's or semi-Fowler's position, and encouraging bed rest.
- Have patient perform active ROM exercises, along with level I activities (see Table 4-1) to help prevent deleterious effects of bed rest on oxygen supplies.
- Administer and titrate prescribed medications: nitrates and afterload reducing agents, such as nitroprusside, and preload reducing agents, such as nitroglycerin, to maintain SVR within 900-1,200 dynes/sec/cm^{-5} and PAWP ≤18 mm Hg; diuretics, such as furosemide and metolazone, to keep PAWP ≤18 mm Hg and urine output ≥0.5 ml/kg/h; and inotropic agents, such as dopamine and dobutamine, to keep systolic BP >90 mm Hg.

Knowledge deficit: Myocardial infarction and its implications for life-style changes

Desired outcome: Within the 24-h period before discharge from CCU, patient and significant others verbalize an understanding of heart attack and the necessary life-style changes that must be made.

- Discuss the following with patient and significant others, providing both oral instructions and written materials:
  - □ Anatomy and functions of the heart muscle.
  - □ Coronary arteries and the atherosclerotic process.
  - □ Definition of "heart attack."
  - □ Healing process of the heart and the role of collateral circulation.
- Assist patient with identifying his or her own risk factors.
- Assist patient with devising a plan for risk-factor modification (e.g., diet, smoking cessation, and stress reduction techniques).
- Provide guidelines for a diet low in cholesterol and saturated fat (see Tables 4-3 and 4-4); refer patient to nutritionist.
- Discuss post-MI activity progression (e.g., a progressive walking program). See Tables 4-1 and 4-2.
- Discuss guidelines for resuming post-MI sexual activity. Explain that sexual activity requires the same amount of oxygen as that needed to walk briskly up two flights of stairs; consequently, patients usually are instructed to wait 2 wk after hospital discharge before resuming sexual activity.
- **Teach patient about medications that will be taken after hospital discharge, including name, purpose, dosage, schedule, precautions, and potential side effects.**

TABLE 4-3 Low-cholesterol dietary guidelines

Foods to avoid	Foods allowed
Egg yolks (no more than 3/wk)	Egg whites; cholesterol-free egg substitutes
Foods made with many egg yolks (e.g., sponge cakes)	Lean, well-trimmed meats; minimize servings of beef, lamb, and pork
Fatty cuts of meat, fat on meats	Fish (except shellfish), chicken and turkey (without the skin)
Skin on chicken and turkey	
Luncheon meats or cold cuts	
Sausage, frankfurters	Dried peas and beans as meat substitutes
Shellfish (e.g., lobster, shrimp, crab)	
Whole milk, cream, whole milk cheese	Nonfat (skim) or lowfat (2%) milk
Ice cream	Low-fat cheeses
Commercially prepared foods with *hydrogenated* shortening, which is saturated fat	Ice milk and sherbet
	Polyunsaturated oils for cooking and food preparation: canola, corn, safflower, cottonseed, sesame, and sunflower
Coconut and palm oils and products made with them (e.g., cream substitutes)	
Butter, lard, hydrogenated shortening	Margarines that list one of the above oils as their first ingredient
Meats and vegetables prepared by frying	Foods prepared "from scratch" with the above suggested oils
Seasonings containing large amounts of sugar and saturated fats	Meats (in acceptable quantity) and vegetables prepared by broiling, steaming, or baking (never frying)
Sauces and gravies	
Salad dressings containing cream, cheeses, or mayonnaise	Spices, herbs, lemon juice, wine, flavored wine vinegars

TABLE 4-4 Guidelines for a diet low in saturated fat

Foods to avoid	Foods to choose
Red meat, especially when highly "marbled"; salami, sausages, bacon	Lean cuts of meat, fresh fish, poultry from which skin was removed before cooking; meats that have been grilled
Whole milk, whipping cream	Lowfat or skim milk
Tropical oils (coconut, palm oils; cocoa butter)	Monosaturated cooking oils, such as olive or canola oil
Candy	Fresh fruit, vegetables
Sweet rolls, donuts	Whole grain breads, cereals
Ice cream	Nonfat yogurt, sherbet
Salad dressings	Vinegar, lemon juice
Peanut butter, peanuts, hot dogs, potato chips	Unbuttered popcorn
Butter	Margarine (safflower oil listed as the first ingredient)

For patients undergoing coronary artery bypass graft

Risk for decreased cardiac output related to negative inotropic changes secondary to intraoperative subendocardial ischemia and administration of myocardial depressant drugs

Desired outcomes: Within 2 h after return to ICU, patient exhibits adequate cardiac output as evidenced by normal sinus rhythm on ECG, measured CO 4-7 L/min, CI 2.5-4 L/min/m^2, peripheral pulses >2+ on a 0-4+ scale, warm and dry skin, and urine output ≥0.5 ml/kg/h. Patient is awake, alert, and oriented.

- Monitor ECG continuously for presence of dysrhythmias, which can alter cardiac output.
- Assess I&O, CO, and CI hourly for evidence of decreasing output.
- For other interventions, see this nursing diagnosis under "Intraaortic Balloon Pump," p. 369, in "Cardiogenic Shock."

Risk for fluid volume deficit related to loss of fluid through normal and abnormal routes secondary to postoperative diuresis and excessive bleeding

---

Note: Diuresis is common in the early postoperative period because of the hormonal changes that accompany surgery.

Desired outcome: Patient is normovolemic as evidenced by intake equal to output plus insensible losses, RAP ≥4 mm Hg, PAWP ≥6 mm Hg, and urinary output between 30 and 120 ml/h.

- Measure I&O hourly. Consult physician for imbalance in I&O ratio (i.e., urinary output ≥120 ml/h and chest tube drainage ≥100 ml/h). Replace excessive chest tube drainage with packed RBCs as prescribed.
- Monitor RAP and PAWP hourly. Report PAWP <6 mm Hg and RAP <4 mm Hg.
- As prescribed, administer IV fluids in the early postoperative period to equal the amount of diuresis.
- Monitor clotting studies (i.e., PT, PTT, activated clotting time [ACT], and platelet count) immediately postoperatively and then q12h for 24 h. Be alert to prolongation of PT, PTT, ACT; decreased platelet count; and low fibrinogen value. Optimal values are: PT 11-15 sec, PTT 30-40 sec (activated), ACT ≤120 sec, platelet count 150,000-400,000 μl, and fibrinogen 200-400 mg/dl.
- Replace clotting factors as prescribed with platelets, fresh frozen plasma, cryoprecipitate, protamine, or aminocaproic acid.
- Assess chest x-ray immediately after surgery and daily for signs of bleeding into the pericardial sac and mediastinum, as evidenced by an increase in the cardiac silhouette.

Hypothermia related to prolonged cooling of body during surgery

Desired outcomes: Patient's body temperature is returned to normal at a rate not greater than 1° C/h as evidenced by warm extremities and absence of shivering. Within 8 h of treatment, oxygen saturation is ≥95%, CO is 4-7 L/min, SVR is ≥900 dynes/sec/cm^{-5}, HR is 60-100 bpm, and BP is within patient's normal range.

Note: The danger of postoperative hypothermia in heart surgery is that the patient will warm too quickly and shiver, causing hypertension or hypotension, increased or decreased SVR, metabolic acidosis, and hypoxia. Each of these problems can increase cardiac workload and may potentiate ischemia, dysrhythmias, or hemorrhage in the early postoperative period.

- On a continuous basis, measure core temperature *via* rectal, tympanic, or thermodilution catheter. If temperature is <36° C (96.8° F), initiate warming measures such as warm blankets, thermal garment, heating lamps, heating blankets, or warm inspired gases.
- Continue to monitor patient during rewarming phase, maintaining rewarming rate at 1° C/h.
- Monitor skin temperature, particularly that of the extremities, q30min-1h during rewarming. Once extremities are warm, patient should be close to normothermia and warming measures should be discontinued.
- Monitor BP, pulse, CO, and SVR continuously during rewarming for sudden changes related to rewarming. SVR may fall along with BP as the peripheral vascular bed dilates. This can precipitate sudden hypotension.
- If shivering due to hypothermia develops, treat immediately with warming measures and drug therapy as prescribed. Drugs used to treat shivering may include morphine sulfate, diazepam or other benzodiazepines, or, in extreme instances, a neuromuscular blocking agent (e.g., vecuronium). During shivering episodes, monitor VS for changes and assess oxygen saturation continuously with oximeter.

Impaired gas exchange (or risk for same) related to altered oxygen supply, alveolar-capillary membrane changes, and altered oxygen-carrying capacity of the blood secondary to CNS depression from anesthesia, atelectasis, and decreased hemoglobin

Desired outcomes: Within 12-24 h of treatment, patient has adequate gas exchange as evidenced by Pao_2 ≥80 mm Hg, $Paco_2$ 35-45 mm Hg, pH 7.35-7.45, presence of normal breath sounds, and absence of adventitious breath sounds. RR is 12-20 breaths/min with normal pattern and depth (eupnea).

- During intubation period, provide supportive measures to ensure optimal aeration: perform suctioning when its need is determined by auscultatory findings, provide chest physiotherapy to posterior and lateral lobes as prescribed, turn patient q2h, and maintain HOB at an elevation of 45 degrees, if tolerated.
- Assess breath sounds, RR, and amount and character of mucus production hourly during the first 12 hours after surgery. Be alert to crackles and rhonchi, labored breathing, and subjective complaints of breathing difficulties. Copious, tenacious secretions place the patient at risk for airway obstruction caused by mucus plugging.
- Monitor Spo_2. Be alert to sustained levels <90%.
- Assess ABG values upon admission and prn during periods of respiratory distress. Consult physician for significant findings, including a decreasing Pao_2, increased $Paco_2$, and the presence of acidosis or alkalosis.

- Consult physician regarding need for ventilation changes if the afore-mentioned assessments suggest their need.
- As prescribed, perform weaning and extubation as early as possible. Use nonopiate analgesics (e.g., ketorolac [Toradol]) and closely monitor the effects of incremental doses of opiate analgesics and sedatives in order to avoid excessive sedation during the weaning process.
  □ Explain weaning procedure to patient. Stay with patient during first 15 min after each ventilatory change and reassure patient about his or her ability to breathe independently. Instruct patient to take slow, deep breaths.
  □ Monitor patient's RR, tidal volume, expiratory pressure, BP, HR, and ECG during weaning. Consult physician for changes, inasmuch as they may be indicative of weaning intolerance.
  □ Assess for indicators that suggest hypoxemia during weaning: agitation, irritability, tachycardia, and diaphoresis.
- After extubation, turn patient q2h. Have patient deep breathe and cough q2h and use incentive spirometry hourly. As prescribed, perform chest physiotherapy qid.
- As soon as tolerated, have patient dangle lower extremities over the side of bed and sit in chair.
- Instruct patient to sit upright as much as possible and to perform deep-breathing exercises. In addition, teach patient the following procedure for basal expansion exercises, which are indicated for patients recovering from chest surgery for whom pain on the surgical side inhibits bilateral chest expansion:
  1. With patient sitting upright, position your palms on the midaxillary lines in the area of the eighth ribs. Instruct patient to inhale as you apply moderate pressure.
  2. Instruct patient to attempt to move your hands outward while expanding the lower ribs.
  3. Instruct patient to maintain maximum inspiration for 1-2 sec to achieve optimal aeration of the alveoli.
  4. Have patient exhale in a relaxed, passive manner.
  5. Teach patients to perform this exercise independently by positioning their own palms against the eighth ribs.
- Explain that performing this technique correctly and at frequent intervals will promote mobility of the lower portion of the chest wall.

ADDITIONAL NURSING DIAGNOSES

As appropriate, see nursing diagnoses and interventions in "Nutritional Support," p. 12; "Mechanical Ventilation," p. 24; "Hemodynamic Monitoring," p. 37; "Prolonged Immobility," p. 78; "Psychosocial Support," p. 88; "Psychosocial Support for the Patient's Family and Significant Others," p. 100.

Congestive heart failure/pulmonary edema

PATHOPHYSIOLOGY

Left heart failure (commonly called congestive heart failure [CHF]) occurs when the left ventricle is unable to maintain a cardiac output sufficient to meet the needs of the body. It often begins when the diseased left ventricular myocardium cannot pump the blood returning from the lungs into systemic circulation. It also can occur because of systemic hypertension. Pressure increases in the lungs due to accumulation of blood. If the pressure exceeds pulmonary capillary oncotic pressure (>30 mm Hg), fluid will flood the pulmonary interstitial spaces. This results in pulmonary edema, which causes impairment of oxygen and carbon dioxide exchange. As pressure continues to increase in the lungs, pressure in the right side of the heart increases because of backflow of pressure in the pulmonary vasculature (see Figure 4-1 for a depiction of the pathophysiology of left heart failure). This can precipitate right heart failure. Right heart failure results most commonly from increased pulmonary vascular resistance as stated, but it also can occur with primary right ventricular AMI. See Figure 4-2 for the pathophysiology of right heart failure.

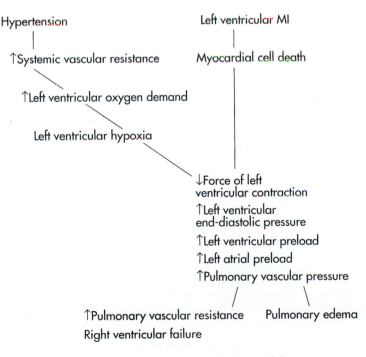

Figure 4-1: Pathophysiology of left heart failure.

↑Pulmonary vascular resistance

↑Force of right ventricular contraction

↑Oxygen demand

Right ventricular hypoxia

↓Force of contraction

↑Right ventricular end-diastolic pressure

↑Right ventricular preload

↑Right atrial pressure

Venous congestion, ↑venous pressure

Peripheral edema

Figure 4-2:   Pathophysiology of right heart failure.

ASSESSMENT

HISTORY AND RISK FACTORS Familial history of coronary artery disease, age >65 yr, male sex (risk for females increases after menopause), cigarette smoking, hypercholesterolemia, hypertension, diabetes, obesity, increased stress, and sedentary life-style. Other important data include noncompliance with low-sodium diet or medications and orthopnea, nocturia, decreased exercise tolerance, and increasing SOB.

Left-sided heart failure (pulmonary edema)
CLINICAL PRESENTATION Anxiety, air hunger, nocturnal dyspnea, dyspnea on exertion, orthopnea, moist cough with frothy sputum, tachycardia, diaphoresis, cyanosis or pallor, insomnia, palpitations, weakness, fatigue, anorexia, and changes in mentation.

PHYSICAL ASSESSMENT Decreased BP, tachycardia, dysrhythmias, crackles, bronchial wheezes, S_3 or summation gallop, and pulsus alternans (alternating strength of the peripheral pulse caused by the failing heart muscle).

MONITORING PARAMETERS Decreased CO/CI; elevated PAP, PAWP, and SVR.

Right-sided heart failure (cor pulmonale)

CLINICAL PRESENTATION Fluid retention, peripheral edema, decreased urinary output, abdominal tenderness, nausea, vomiting, and anorexia.

PHYSICAL ASSESSMENT Hepatosplenomegaly, dependent pitting edema, jugular venous distention, positive hepatojugular reflex, ascites.

MONITORING PARAMETERS Elevated RAP and CVP.

DIAGNOSTIC TESTS

Chest x-ray: Will reveal pulmonary clouding, increased interstitial density, engorged pulmonary vasculature, and cardiomegaly.

Serum electrolyte levels: May reveal hyponatremia (dilutional); hyperkalemia if glomerular filtration is decreased; or hypokalemia, which can result from use of diuretics.

Serum enzyme levels: Liver function test results may be abnormal because of hepatic venous congestion.

Serum bilirubin levels: May reveal hyperbilirubinemia in the presence of liver dysfunction.

Circulation time: Although this test is not usually performed on patients with heart failure, circulation time often is increased at rest in the presence of heart failure. In mild cases of heart failure, circulation time may be normal at rest but increased with exercise. Sodium dehydrocholate is given IV, and the time is measured until the patient begins to experience a bitter taste in his or her mouth.

CBC count: May reveal decreased Hgb and Hct levels in the presence of anemia or dilution.

ABG values: May reveal hypoxemia due to the decreased oxygen available from fluid-filled alveoli and respiratory alkalosis because of the increase in respiratory rate, causing patient to blow off more CO_2.

Digitalis levels: The patient with CHF may have been treated with digitalis in the past. With CHF the patient is predisposed to digitalis toxicity due to the low cardiac output state, which also causes decreased renal excretion of the drug.

COLLABORATIVE MANAGEMENT

Treatment of underlying cause and precipitating factors

Left-sided heart failure: Atherosclerotic heart disease, AMI, dysrhythmias, cardiomyopathy, increased circulating volume, systemic hypertension, aortic stenosis, aortic regurgitation, mitral regurgitation, coarctation of the aorta, atrial septal defect, ventricular septal defect, cardiac tamponade, and constrictive pericarditis.

Right-sided heart failure: Left-sided heart failure, pulmonary hypertension, atherosclerotic heart disease, AMI, dysrhythmias, pulmonary embolism, fluid overload or excess sodium intake, COPD, mitral stenosis, and pulmonary stenosis.

Bed rest and stress reduction.

Low-calorie diet (if weight control is necessary) and low-sodium diet: Extra salt and water are held in the circulatory system, causing increased strain on the heart. Limiting sodium (Table 4-5) will reduce the amount of fluid retained by the body. In addition, fluids may be limited to 1,500 ml/day.

T A B L E   4 - 5   Low-sodium dietary guidelines

Foods high in sodium*	Foods low in sodium
Beans and frankfurters	Bread
Bouillon cubes	Cereal (dry or hot); read labels
Canned or packaged soups	Fresh fish, chicken, turkey, veal, beef,
Canned, smoked, or salted meats;	and lamb (if limiting fats, avoid the
salted fish	latter two)
Dill pickles	Fresh fruits and vegetables
Fried chicken dinners and other	Fresh or dried herbs
fast foods	Gelatin desserts
Monosodium glutamate (e.g., Ac-	Oil, salt-free margarine
cent)	Peanut butter
Olives	Tabasco sauce
Packaged snack foods	Low-salt tuna packed in water
Pancake or waffle mix	
Processed cheese	
Seasoned salts (e.g., celery, onion,	
garlic)	
Sauerkraut	
Soy sauce	
Vegetables in brine or cans	

Additional suggestions
  Do not add table salt to foods.
  Season with fresh or dried herbs.
  Avoid salts or powders that contain salt.
  Do not buy convenience foods; remember that fresh is best.
  Read all labels for salt, sodium, or sodium chloride content.

*Many of these foods now are available in low-salt or salt-free versions.

Pharmacotherapy

Morphine: To induce vasodilatation and decrease venous return, preload, sympathetic tone, anxiety, myocardial oxygen consumption, and pain.

Diuretics: To reduce blood volume and decrease preload.

Inotropic agents: Digitalis to strengthen contractions; dopamine, dobutamine, or amrinone to support BP and enhance contractility (see Appendix 7).

Vasodilators: Nitrates (oral, topical, or IV) to dilate venous or capacitant vessels, thereby reducing preload and cardiac and pulmonary congestion. Nitroprusside, hydralazine, captopril, or prazosin hydrochloride will dilate the arterial or resistant vessels and reduce afterload, thus increasing forward flow (see Appendix 7).

Treatment of acute pulmonary edema: Immediate interventions include oxygen and possible ET intubation; diuretic therapy; and pharmacologic therapy, including inotropic agents, vasodilators, and morphine.

NURSING DIAGNOSES AND INTERVENTIONS

Fluid volume excess related to compromised regulatory mechanism secondary to decreased cardiac output

Desired outcome: Within 24 h of treatment, patient becomes normovolemic as evidenced by absence of adventitious lung sounds, decreased peripheral edema, increased urine output, weight loss, PAWP ≤ 18 mm Hg (reasonable outcome for these patients), SVR $\leq 1,200$ dynes/sec/cm^{-5}, and CO ≥ 4 L/min.

- Auscultate lung fields for presence of crackles and rhonchi or other adventitious sounds.
- Monitor I&O closely. Report positive fluid state or decrease in urine output to <0.5 mg/kg/h.
- Weigh patient daily; report increases in weight. An acute gain in weight of 1 kg can signal a 1 L gain in fluid.
- Note changes from baseline assessment to detect worsening of heart failure, such as increased pedal edema, increased jugular venous distention, development of S_3 heart sound or new murmur, and dysrhythmias.
- Monitor hemodynamic status q1-2h and prn. Note response to drug therapy as well as indicators of the need for more aggressive therapy, including increasing PAWP and SVR and decreasing CO.
- Administer diuretics (furosemide), positive inotropes (dopamine), and vasodilators (nitroprusside) as prescribed. (See Appendix 7 for more information about inotropic and vasoactive drugs.)
- Limit oral fluids as prescribed, and offer patient ice chips or frozen juice pops to decrease thirst and discomfort of dry mouth.
- Maintain bed rest restrictions to facilitate fluid movement from interstitial spaces in dependent extremities to the intravascular spaces.

Impaired gas exchange related to alveolar-capillary membrane changes secondary to fluid collection in the alveoli and interstitial spaces

Desired outcome: Within 24 h of initiation of treatment, patient has improved gas exchange as evidenced by Pao$_2$ ≥ 80 mm Hg, RR 12-20 breaths/min with normal pattern and depth (eupnea), and absence of adventitious breath sounds.

- Monitor respiratory rate, rhythm, and character q1-2h. Be alert to RR >20 breaths/min, irregular rhythm, use of accessory muscles of respiration, or cough.
- Auscultate breath sounds, noting presence of crackles, wheezes, and other adventitious sounds.
- Provide supplemental oxygen as prescribed.
- Monitor Spo$_2$ for decreases to $<90\%$-92%.
- Assess ABG findings; note changes in response to oxygen supplementation or treatment of altered hemodynamics.
- Suction patient's secretions as needed.
- Establish a protocol for deep breathing, coughing, and turning q2h.
- Place patient in semi-Fowler's or high Fowler's position to maximize chest excursion.
- If mechanical ventilation is necessary, monitor ventilator settings, ET tube function, and respiratory status.

Activity intolerance related to imbalance between oxygen supply and demand secondary to decreased functioning of the myocardium

Desired outcome: Within the 12- to 24-h period before discharge from CCU, patient exhibits cardiac tolerance to increasing levels of activity as evidenced by RR <24 breaths/min, normal sinus rhythm on ECG, HR ≤120 bpm (or within 20 bpm of resting HR), BP within 20 mm Hg of patient's normal range, and absence of chest pain.

- Maintain prescribed activity level, and teach patient the rationale for activity limitation.
- Organize nursing care so that periods of activity are interspersed with extended periods of uninterrupted rest.
- To help prevent complications of immobility, assist patient with active/passive ROM exercises, as appropriate. Encourage patient to do as much as possible within prescribed activity allowances. For interventions related to a progressive exercise program, see Table 4-1 and "Prolonged Immobility," p. 78.
- Note patient's physiologic response to activity, including BP, HR, RR, and heart rhythm. Signs of activity intolerance include chest pain, increasing SOB, excessive fatigue, increased dysrhythmias, palpitations, HR response >120 bpm, systolic BP >20 mm Hg from baseline or >160 mm Hg, and ST-segment changes.
- If activity intolerance is noted, instruct patient to stop the activity and rest.
- Administer medications as prescribed, and note their effect on patient's activity tolerance. Examples of medications include prophylactic NTG tablets, paste, or patch to reduce preload.
- As needed to help prevent muscle loss and wasting, refer patient to physical therapy department.

Knowledge deficit: Disease process with CHF and the prescribed diet and medications

Desired outcome: Within the 24-h period before discharge from CCU, patient and significant others verbalize understanding of patient's disease, as well as the prescribed diet and medication regimens.

- Teach patient the physiologic process of CHF, discussing in terms appropriate to the patient how fluid volume increases because of poor heart functioning.
- Teach patient about the importance of a low-sodium diet and medications to help reduce volume overload. Provide patient with a list of foods that are high and low in sodium (see Table 4-5). Teach patient how to read and evaluate food labels.
- Teach patient the signs and symptoms of fluid volume excess that necessitate medical attention: irregular or slow pulse, increased SOB, orthopnea, decreased exercise tolerance, and steady weight gain (≥1 kg/day for 2 successive days).
- Advise patient about the need to keep a journal of daily weight. Explain that an increase of ≥1 kg/day on 2 successive days of normal eating necessitates notification of physician.
- If patient is taking digitalis, teach the technique for measuring pulse rate. Provide parameters for withholding digitalis (usually for pulse rate <60/min) and notifying the physician.
- Instruct patient regarding the prescribed activity progression after hospital discharge and signs of activity intolerance that signal the need for rest and use of prophylactic NTG to reduce congestion of the heart and lungs. General activity guidelines are as follows:

T A B L E   4 - 6   Activity progression after hospital discharge

Week	Distance	Time
1-2	¼ mi	Leisurely; twice daily
2-3	½ mi	15 min
3-4	1 mi	30 min
4-5	1½ mi	30 min
5-6	2 mi	40 min

- Get up and get dressed every morning.
- Space your meals and activities to allow time for rest and relaxation.
- Perform activities at a comfortable, moderate pace. If you get tired during any activity, stop to rest for 15 min before resuming.
- Avoid activities that require straining (e.g., lifting >30 lbs, push-ups, pull-ups, straining during bowel movement). Use laxatives as needed.
- Plan at least two periods a day of walking outside when the weather is nice, following the guidelines in Table 4-6.
- Start out slowly (e.g., 200-400 ft), and work up to ¼ mi in the first week. Progress according to your own ability. Let the way you feel be your guide. Walk a minimum of 3 times a week on nonsuccessive days. Exercise should be fun. Enjoy!
- Warning signals to stop your activity and rest: chest pain, shortness of breath, dizziness or faintness, unusual weakness.

ADDITIONAL NURSING DIAGNOSES

Also see nursing diagnoses and interventions in "Hemodynamic Monitoring," p. 37; "Prolonged Immobility," p. 78; "Psychosocial Support," p. 88; and "Psychosocial Support for the Patient's Family and Significant Others," p. 100.

Cardiomyopathy

PATHOPHYSIOLOGY

Cardiomyopathy is a subacute or chronic disorder usually of unknown or obscure etiology. It can occur secondary to infection, virus, toxins, or nutritional deficiencies. Cardiomyopathy affects the myocardium and is classified according to its effects.

Functional classification

Dilated (previously referred to as "congestive"):   The significant feature of this disease process is dilatation rather than congestion; therefore the term "congestive" has been replaced with "dilated" cardiomyopathy. The majority of cases are termed idiopathic because of the unknown origin of the disease process. Heart failure occurs secondary to decreased systolic ejection fraction. There is little or no hypertrophy of the ventricles.

T A B L E 4 - 7   Hemodynamic presentation with cardiomyopathy

Pressure	Effect	Normal values
Right atrial pressure	Increased	4-6 mm Hg
Pulmonary artery pressure	Increased	20-30/8-15 mm Hg
Pulmonary wedge pressure	Increased	6-12 mm Hg
Cardiac output	Decreased	4-7 L/min
Cardiac index	Decreased	2.5-4 L/min/m^2
Pulmonary vascular resistance	Unchanged or increased	60-100 dynes/sec/cm^{-5}
Systemic vascular resistance	Increased	900-1,200 dynes/sec/cm^{-5}

Hypertrophic or obstructive: Characterized by an abnormally stiff left ventricle during diastole, which restricts ventricular filling. There may be hypertrophy of the ventricular septum, which leads to obstruction of the ventricular outflow tract. This is called idiopathic hypertrophic subaortic stenosis (IHSS). Although cardiac function may remain normal for varying periods of time, deterioration and poor ventricular compliance usually occur.

Restrictive or constrictive: The ventricular walls are rigid from fibrosis, and there is inadequate diastolic filling, resulting in abnormal diastolic function.

Ischemic: Results from coronary artery disease. There is >70% luminal narrowing of at least one coronary artery, as well as multiple ventricular wall motion abnormalities. Cardiomegaly is present, and left ventricular ejection fraction (LVEF) is decreased.

ASSESSMENT

CLINICAL PRESENTATION Decreased contractility and low cardiac output lead to fatigue, weakness, hypotension, ischemic chest pain, low urine output, altered mental status, palpitations, and syncope. Pulmonary congestion associated with decreased contractility can lead to SOB, dyspnea on exertion, orthopnea, peripheral edema, anorexia, and nausea.

PHYSICAL ASSESSMENT Presence of S_3 or S_4 heart sounds or a summation gallop, valvular murmurs of mitral and tricuspid regurgitation, murmur of IHSS, increased venous pressure pulsations, crackles, decreased BP, increased HR, and presence of dysrhythmias. Peripheral hypoperfusion may be present and will manifest as diminished pulses, cool skin, and mottling or cyanosis. In addition, hepatomegaly and mild to severe cardiomegaly may be present, causing a displaced and diffuse PMI.

MONITORING PARAMETERS See Table 4-7.

DIAGNOSTIC TESTS

Cardiac catheterization: Does not confirm cardiomyopathy but can be used to rule out other disorders, such as ischemic heart disease. Findings may include decreased cardiac output, ventricular wall mo-

tion, and ejection fraction; increased filling pressure; and valvular regurgitation.

Endocardial biopsy: May be necessary to identify the type of pathologic agent causing the cardiomyopathy. It can be done during cardiac
catheterization.

Chest x-ray: May detect cardiomegaly with enlarged left ventricle,
pulmonary venous congestion, and characteristic lines of interstitial
edema.

ECG: May reveal dysrhythmias, such as sinus tachycardia, atrial fibrillation, and ventricular ectopy. Other changes may include left ventricular hypertrophy, left bundle-branch block, left anterior hemiblock,
left axis deviation, nonspecific ST-segment changes, and Q waves that
resemble those that occur with myocardial infarction.

Echocardiography: To assess degree of left ventricular impairment
and dilatation of the cardiac chambers. Ventricular wall and septal contractility can be evaluated, as well as valvular motion. Two-
dimensional echo can detect thrombus formation and estimate ejection fraction.

Radionuclide studies: May show diffuse left ventricular hypokine-
sis, left ventricular ejection fraction <40%, and elevated end-diastolic
and systolic volumes.

COLLABORATIVE MANAGEMENT

Pharmacotherapy: To maintain or reestablish hemodynamic stability.

Vasodilators: To decrease preload and afterload, thus improving cardiac output.

Diuretics: To reduce preload and pulmonary congestion.

Inotropic therapy: To enhance contractility (see Appendix 7).

Antidysrhythmic agents: To control dysrhythmias (see Table 4-8).

Calcium channel blockers: To produce vasodilatation and decrease
cardiac workload.

Beta-blockers: For hypertrophic cardiomyopathy, to decrease outflow obstruction during exercise and reduce inappropriate sympathetic
cardiac stimulation.

Anticoagulants: To prevent thrombus formation, inasmuch as these
patients often are at risk because of their predisposition for atrial fibrillation.

Potassium supplements: To replace potassium lost in the urine as a
result of diuresis.

Hemodynamic monitoring: To guide and evaluate therapeutic interventions.

Activity level: Initially reduced to decrease oxygen demand, but then
increased gradually to prevent complications of immobility.

Intraaortic balloon pump: In the presence of a failing myocardium,
may be used to decrease afterload and increase coronary artery perfusion (see discussion, p. 365).

Heart transplantation: For conditions refractory to medical therapy
such as vasodilators and inotropic agents. Each institution has criteria
that must be met before transplantation is considered as alternative
treatment.

T A B L E 4 - 8   Antidysrhythmic drugs

Class I: Local anesthetics and other drugs that decrease automaticity of ventricular conduction, delay ventricular repolarization, decrease conduction velocity, increase conduction *via* AV node, and suppress ventricular automaticity. Class IA decreases depolarization moderately and prolongs repolarization. Class IB decreases depolarization and shortens repolarization. Class IC significantly decreases depolarization with minimal effect on repolarization.

A	B	C
disopyramide (PO)	lidocaine (IV, IM)	encainide (PO)
procainamide (PO, IV, IM)	mexiletine (PO)	propafenone (PO)
quinidine (PO, IV)	phenytoin (PO)	
	tocainide (PO)	

Class II: Beta-blockers that slow sinus automaticity, slow conduction *via* AV node, control ventricular response to supraventricular tachycardias, and shorten the action potential of Purkinje fibers.

> acebutolol (PO)
> atenolol (PO)
> esmolol (IV)
> metoprolol (PO, IV)
> propranolol (PO, IV)
> timolol (PO)

Class III: Increase the action potential and refractory period of Purkinje fibers, increase ventricular fibrillation threshold, restore injured myocardial cell electrophysiology toward normal, and suppress reentrant dysrhythmias.

> amiodarone (PO, IV)
> bretylium (IV, IM)
> sotalol HCl (PO, IV)

Class IV: Calcium channel blockers that depress automaticity in the SA and AV nodes, block the slow calcium current in the AV junctional tissue, reduce conduction *via* the AV node, and are useful in treating tachydysrhythmias due to AV junction reentry.

> diltiazem (PO)
> verapamil (IV)

Unclassified: Depresses activity of the AV node

> adenosine (IV)

NURSING DIAGNOSES AND INTERVENTIONS

Decreased cardiac output related to negative inotropic changes in the heart secondary to myocardial cellular destruction and dilatation

Desired outcomes: Within the 24-h period before discharge from CCU, patient has adequate cardiac output as evidenced by systolic BP $\geq$90 mm Hg; CO 4-7 L/min; CI 2.5-4 L/min/m^2; RR 12-20 breaths/min; HR $\leq$100 bpm; urinary output $\geq$0.5 ml/kg/h; intake equal to output plus insensible losses; warm and dry skin; and orientation to time, place, and person. PAWP is $\leq$18 mm Hg and RAP is 4-6 mm Hg.

- Assess for and document the following factors as evidence of decreasing cardiac output: presence of jugular venous distention, dependent edema, hepatomegaly, fatigue, weakness, decreased activity level, and SOB with activity. In addition, assess and document the following:

- □ *Mental status:* Be alert to restlessness and decreased responsiveness.
- □ *Lung sounds:* Monitor for crackles, rhonchi, wheezes.
- □ *Heart sounds:* Note presence of gallop, murmur, and increased HR.
- □ *Urinary output:* Be alert to output <0.5 ml/kg/h.
- □ *Skin:* Monitor for pallor, mottling, cyanosis, coolness, diaphoresis.
- □ *Vital signs:* Note BP <90 mm Hg systolic, HR >100 bpm, RR >20 breaths/min, and elevated temperature.

- If a pulmonary artery catheter is present, record hemodynamic readings q1-2h and prn. Be alert to PAWP >18 mm Hg and RAP >6 mm Hg. Although normal PAWP is 6-12 mm Hg, these patients may need increased filling pressures for adequate preload, with wedge pressure at 15-18 mm Hg.
- Measure CO/CI q2-4h and prn. Optimally, CO should be within 4-7 L/min and CI should be 2.5-4 L/min/m^2.
- Keep accurate I&O records and weigh patient daily, noting trends. Individuals with cardiomyopathy often are on strict fluid restriction (e.g., 1,000 ml/day).
- Help minimize patient's cardiac workload by assisting patient with ADL when necessary.
- Monitor for compensatory mechanisms, including increased HR and BP due to sodium and water retention.
- Administer medications as prescribed, including nitrates and other vasodilators, diuretics, inotropic agents, and anticoagulants. Observe for the following desired effects:
  - □ *Vasodilators:* Decreased BP, decreased SVR, increased CO/CI.
  - □ *Diuretics:* Decreased PAWP.
  - □ *Inotropes:* Increased CO/CI, increased BP.
- Be alert to the following undesirable effects:
  - □ *Vasodilators:* Headache, nausea, vomiting, dizziness.
  - □ *Diuretics:* Weakness, hypokalemia (see p. 681).
  - □ *Inotropes:* Dysrhythmias, headache, angina.
- Position patient according to his or her comfort level.

Activity intolerance related to imbalance between oxygen supply and demand secondary to decreased myocardial contractility

Desired outcome: Within the 12- to 24-h period before discharge from CCU, patient exhibits cardiac tolerance to increasing levels of activity as evidenced by RR <24 breaths/min, normal sinus rhythm on ECG, BP within 20 mm Hg of patient's normal range, HR within 20 bpm of patient's resting HR, peripheral pulses >2+ on a 0-4+ scale, and absence of chest pain.

- Monitor BP and VS; report changes such as dysrhythmias or decreasing BP.
- Observe for and report any signs of decreased cardiac output, such as oliguria, changes in mentation, or decreased BP.
- Assess peripheral pulses and rate on a scale of 0-4+.
- Plan nursing care so that patient is assured of extended periods of rest (at least 90 min).
- Monitor patient's physiologic response to activity, reporting any symptoms of chest pain, new or increasing SOB, increases in HR

>20 bpm above resting HR, and increase or decrease in systolic BP >20 mm Hg.

• To prevent complications of immobility, perform or teach patient and significant others active, passive, and assistive ROM exercises. For a discussion of in-bed exercise program, see Table 4-1 and interventions in "Prolonged Immobility," p. 78. Consult physician to ensure that exercises are within patient's prescribed limitations.

ADDITIONAL NURSING DIAGNOSES

Also see nursing diagnoses and interventions in "Hemodynamic Monitoring," p. 37; "Prolonged Immobility," p. 78; "Psychosocial Support," p. 88; and "Psychosocial Support for the Patient's Family and Significant Others," p. 100.

Dysrhythmias and conduction disturbances

PATHOPHYSIOLOGY

Dysrhythmias are abnormal rhythms of the heart's electrical system. They can originate in any part of the conduction system, such as the sinus node, atrium, AV node, His-Purkinje system, bundle branches, and ventricular tissue. Although a variety of diseases may cause dysrhythmias, the most common are CAD and AMI. Other causes include electrolyte imbalance, changes in oxygenation, and drug toxicity. Cardiac dysrhythmias may result from the following mechanisms.

Disturbances in automaticity: May involve an increase or decrease in automaticity in the sinus node (i.e., sinus tachycardia or sinus bradycardia). Premature beats may arise *via* this mechanism from the atria, junction, or ventricles. Abnormal rhythms, such as atrial or ventricular tachycardia, also may occur.

Disturbances in conductivity: Conduction may be too rapid, as in conditions caused by an accessory pathway (e.g., Wolff-Parkinson-White syndrome) or too slow (e.g., AV block). Reentry is a situation in which a stimulus reexcites a conduction pathway through which it already has passed. Once started, this impulse may circulate repeatedly. For reentry to occur there must be two different pathways for conduction: one with slowed conduction and one with unidirectional block.

Combinations of altered automaticity and conductivity: Observed when several dysrhythmias are noted (e.g., first-degree AV block [disturbance in conductivity] and premature atrial complexes [PACs], a disturbance in automaticity.

ASSESSMENT

HISTORY AND RISK FACTORS CAD, recent MI, electrolyte disturbances (especially potassium and magnesium), drug toxicity.

CLINICAL PRESENTATION Can vary on a continuum from absence of symptoms to complete cardiopulmonary collapse. General indicators include alterations in LOC, vertigo, syncope, seizures, weakness, fatigue, activity intolerance, SOB, dyspnea on exertion, chest pain, palpitations, sensation of "skipped beats," anxiety, and restlessness.

PHYSICAL ASSESSMENT Increase, decrease, or irregularity in HR, BP, and RR; dusky color or pallor; crackles; cool skin; decreased urine output;

paradoxic pulse and abnormal heart sounds (e.g., paradoxic splitting of S_1 and S_2), and apical-radial pulse deficit.

ECG AND HEMODYNAMIC MEASUREMENTS Decreased cardiac output, elevated PAP. Some ECG findings seen with various dysrhythmias include abnormalities in rate such as sinus bradycardia or sinus tachycardia, irregular rhythm such as atrial fibrillation, extra beats such as PACs and premature junctional complexes (PJCs), wide and bizarre-looking beats such as premature ventricular complexes (PVCs) and ventricular tachycardia (VT), a fibrillating baseline such as ventricular

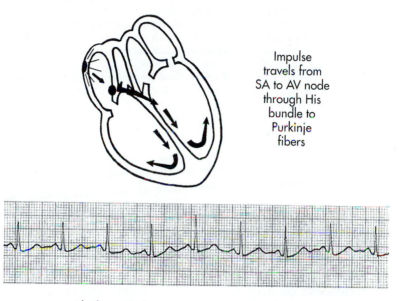

Impulse travels from SA to AV node through His bundle to Purkinje fibers

- Rhythm: regular

- Atrial rate: 60-100 bpm

- Ventricular rate: 60-100 bpm

- P waves: before each QRS

- QRS: normal and of normal width

- PR interval: normal

- P: QRS: 1:1

Significance: Usual, normal rhythm and conduction.

Intervention: None.

Figure 4-3: Normal sinus rhythm. (Illustration from Sheehy SB: *Emergency nursing: principles and practice,* ed 3, St Louis, 1992, Mosby.)

fibrillation (VF), and a straight line as with asystole. Figures 4-3 through 4-23 give an overview of common rhythms, dysrhythmias, and conduction disturbances and their treatment.

DIAGNOSTIC TESTS

12/18-lead ECG: To detect dysrhythmias and identify possible etiology.

Serum electrolyte levels: To identify electrolyte abnormality, which can precipitate dysrhythmias. The most common are hyperkalemia and hypokalemia.

Drug levels: To identify toxicities (e.g., of digoxin, quinidine, procainamide, aminophylline) that can precipitate dysrhythmias.

Ambulatory monitoring (e.g., 24-h Holter monitor or cardiac event recorder):   To identify subtle dysrhythmias and associate abnormal rhythms by means of the patient's symptoms.

Electrophysiologic study (EPS):   Invasive test in which two to three catheters are placed into the heart, giving the heart a pacing stimulus at varying sites and of varying voltages. The test determines origin of dysrhythmia, inducibility, and effectiveness of drug therapy in dysrhythmia suppression.

Exercise stress testing: Used in conjunction with 24-h Holter monitoring to detect advanced grades of PVCs (those caused by ischemia) and to guide therapy. During the test, ECG and BP readings are taken while the patient walks on a treadmill or pedals a stationary bicycle; response to a constant or increasing workload is observed. The test continues until the patient reaches target heart rate or symptoms such as chest pain, severe fatigue, dysrhythmias, or abnormal BP occur.

ABG values: To document trend of hypoxemia.

COLLABORATIVE MANAGEMENT

Antidysrhythmic drugs: See Table 4-8.

Implantable cardioverter-defibrillator (ICD):   To treat lethal cardiac dysrhythmias. It is recommended for patients who are at risk for sudden cardiac death because of VT or VF that cannot be suppressed with pharmacologic therapy. In addition, patients who have survived sudden cardiac death but who do not have an inducible dysrhythmia are candidates. The pulse generator, which is powered by lithium batteries, is surgically inserted into a "pocket" formed in the umbilical region. The ICD is programmed to deliver the electrical stimulus at a predetermined rate and/or after assessing the morphology of the ECG.

The surgical procedure for ICD insertion usually is accomplished *via* one of two approaches. A median sternotomy incision may be used, allowing other forms of cardiac procedures (e.g., valvular surgery, endocardial mapping, aneurysmectomy, CABG) to be performed concurrently. The lateral thoracotomy incision is reserved for patients who have undergone CABG and, subsequently, are prone to adhesions. With the transvenous approach, an incision is made into the subclavian vein, through which the leads are placed. Postoperative complications include atelectasis, pneumonia, seroma at the generator "pocket," pneumothorax, thrombosis, and infection. Lead migration and lead fracture are the two most common structural problems.

Ablation: A procedure in which a catheter is placed in the heart *via* cardiac catheterization and an electrical heat stimulus is applied to the

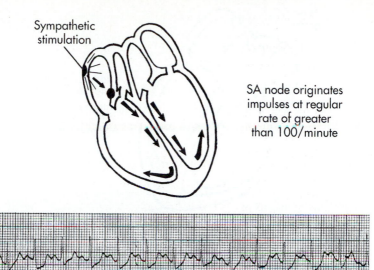

Sympathetic stimulation

SA node originates impulses at regular rate of greater than 100/minute

- Rhythm: regular

- Atrial rate: >100 bpm; usually <160 bpm

- Ventricular rate: >100 bpm; usually <160 bpm

- P waves: before each QRS

- QRS: normal duration

- PR interval: normal

- P: QRS: 1:1

Significance: Increased rate usually caused by sympathetic stimulation. Causes may include pain, fever, anxiety, hypovolemia, heart failure, caffeine intake, use of theophylline or sympathomimetic agents.

Intervention: Treat cause.

Figure 4-4: Sinus tachycardia. (Illustration from Sheehy SB: *Emergency nursing: principles and practice,* ed 3, St Louis, 1992, Mosby.)

area in which the dysrhythmia originates. The heat stimulus causes controlled, localized necrosis of the area.

Dietary guidelines: Patients with recurrent dysrhythmias are usually placed on a diet that restricts or reduces caffeine and is low in fat and cholesterol (see Tables 4-3 and 4-4).

Text continued on p. 307.

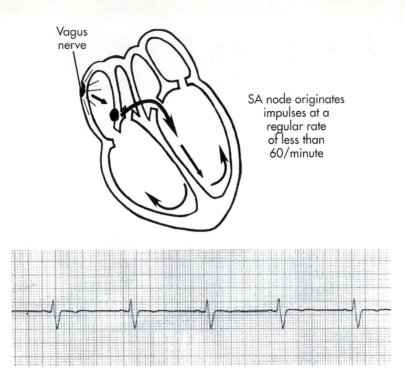

Vagus nerve

SA node originates impulses at a regular rate of less than 60/minute

- Rhythm: regular

- Atrial rate: <60 bpm

- Ventricular rate: <60 bpm

- P waves: before each QRS

- QRS: normal duration

- PR interval: normal

- P: QRS: 1:1

Significance: Slow rate usually caused by increased parasympathetic stimulation. Causes may include vagal stimulation, beta-adrenergic blocking agents and other drugs, AMI, IICP. This rhythm may be "normal" in some people.

Intervention: No treatment necessary unless patient's BP drops and/or LOC is altered or PVCs occur. Initial treatment is atropine and oxygen. See "Bradycardia Algorithm" in Appendix 1.

Figure 4-5: Sinus bradycardia. (Illustration from Sheehy SB: *Emergency nursing: principles and practice,* ed 3, St Louis, 1992, Mosby.)

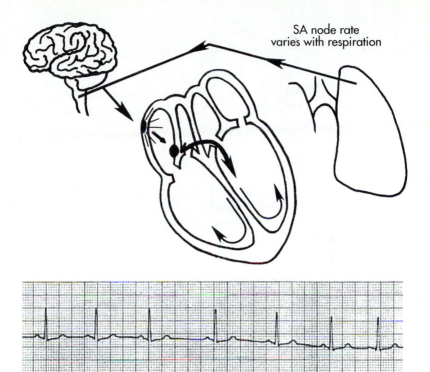

SA node rate
varies with respiration

- Rhythm: irregular

- Atrial rate: 60-100 bpm

- Ventricular rate: 60-100 bpm

- P waves: before each QRS

- QRS: normal duration

- PR interval: normal

- P: QRS: 1:1

Significance: This rhythm usually increases in rate with inspiration and decreases with expiration. It can be a normal finding in children. As an abnormal finding it may be caused by drugs, IICP, or heart disease.

Intervention: Observation; usually no treatment necessary.

Figure 4-6: Sinus dysrhythmia. (Illustration from Sheehy SB: *Emergency nursing: principles and practice*, ed 3, St Louis, 1992, Mosby.)

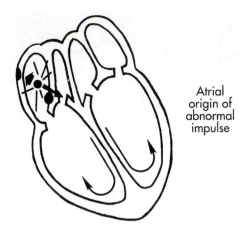

Atrial
origin of
abnormal
impulse

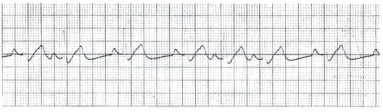

- Rhythm: irregular

- Atrial rate: depends on underlying rhythm

- Ventricular rate: depends on underlying rhythm

- P waves: early beat P looks different from sinus P

- QRS: normal duration

- PR interval: variable in premature complexes

- P: QRS: 1:1

Significance: PACs come from an ectopic atrial focus. Causes often are the same as sinus tachycardia. May progress to atrial fibrillation or atrial tachycardia.

Intervention: Observation. Limit caffeine, alcohol, and smoking. If symptoms occur (decreased BP, dizziness), treatment may include beta-blockers, verapamil, or diltiazem.

Figure 4-7: Premature atrial complexes (PACs). (Illustration from Sheehy SB: *Emergency nursing: principles and practice,* ed 3, St Louis, 1992, Mosby.)

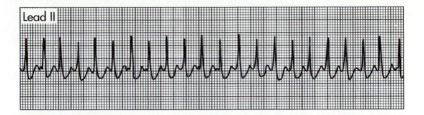

- Rhythm: regular

- Atrial rate: 160-240 bpm

- Ventricular rate: depends on AV conduction ratio

- P waves: may be difficult to identify because of fast rate

- QRS: normal; may be wide if aberrant conduction is present

Significance: Can precipitate chest pain and ischemia. Patients often experience dizziness, diaphoresis, and nausea.

Intervention: Vagal maneuvers, verapamil, adenosine. Less commonly used agents include digoxin and beta blockers. See "Tachycardia Algorithm" in Appendix 1.

Figure 4-8:   Atrial tachycardia. For illustration of electrical activity, see Figure 4-4. (From Grauer K, Cavallaro D: *ACLS vol 1: certification preparation,* ed 3, St Louis, 1993, Mosby.)

Surgical procedures
Left ventricular aneurysmectomy and infarctectomy: Excision of possible focal spots of ventricular dysrhythmias.
Myocardial revascularization: Performed alone or in conjunction with electrophysiologic mapping, with excision or cryoablation of the dysrhythmia focus.
Encircling ventriculotomy: Excises the diseased portion of the ventricle without compromising myocardial blood supply.
Stellate ganglionectomy and block: Alters the electrical stability of the myocardium and predisposition to ventricular dysrhythmias.

NURSING DIAGNOSES AND INTERVENTIONS
Decreased cardiac output related to altered rate, rhythm, or conduction or negative inotropic changes secondary to cardiac disease
Desired outcomes: Within 15 min of development of serious dysrhythmias, patient has adequate cardiac output as evidenced by BP ≥90/60 mm Hg, HR 60-100 bpm, and normal sinus rhythm on ECG. PAP is 20-30/8-15 mm Hg; PAWP is ≤18 mm Hg (a reasonable outcome for these patients); RAP is ≤7 mm Hg; and CO is 4-7 L/min.

Text continued on p. 311.

Pacemaker site varies in the atria

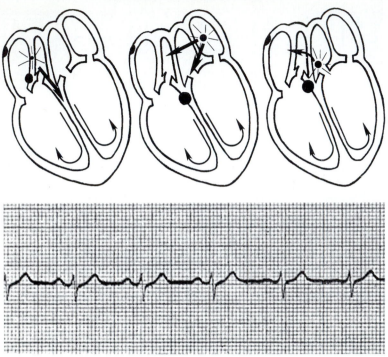

- Rhythm: irregular

- Atrial rate: usually 60-100 bpm

- Ventricular rate: usually 60-100 bpm

- P waves: before each QRS

- QRS: normal duration

- PR interval: usually normal; some variation

- P: QRS: 1:1

Significance: An ectopic atrial focus. Causes may include drugs, COPD, inflammatory disorders.

Intervention: Observation. If cause can be determined, treat cause. If patient is receiving digoxin, check serum level.

Figure 4-9:   Wandering atrial pacemaker. (Illustration from Sheehy SB: *Emergency nursing: principles and practice*, ed 3, St Louis, 1992, Mosby.)

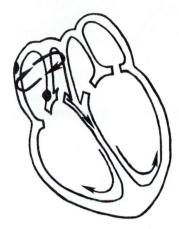

Circus movement
in atria;
variable
degree of block

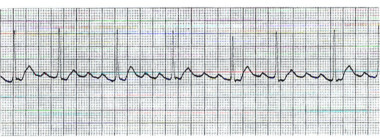

- Rhythm: regular if block is regular; may be irregular

- Atrial rate: 240-350 bpm

- Ventricular rate: depends on AV conduction

- P waves: saw-toothed; F waves

- QRS: normal

- PR interval: not measurable

- P: QRS: P>QRS

Significance: An atrial ectopic focus. AV conduction ratios can be variable, usually at least 2:1. The ineffective atrial contraction can cause pulmonary or cerebral emboli.

Intervention: Digitalis, verapamil, or beta-blockers.

Figure 4-10: Atrial flutter. (Illustration from Sheehy SB: *Emergency nursing: principles and practice,* ed 3, St Louis, 1992, Mosby.)

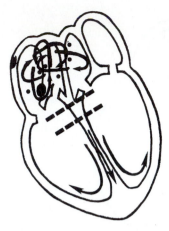

Chaotic impulses
from atria;
variable
degree of block

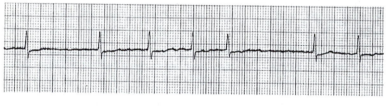

- Rhythm: irregularly irregular

- Atrial rate: >350 bpm

- Ventricular rate: variable

- P waves: coarse or fine fibrillatory waves

- QRS: normal

- PR interval: not measurable

- P: QRS: P>QRS

Significance: Chaotic atrial firing and ineffective atrial contraction. Cardiac output usually drops because of loss of atrial "kick." Ineffective atrial contraction makes clot formation a danger.

Intervention: Patients in chronic AF with a controlled ventricular response usually do not require intervention. For new-onset AF with a rapid ventricular response, digitalis or verapamil may be used.

Figure 4-11: Atrial fibrillation (AF). (Illustration from Sheehy SB: *Emergency nursing: principles and practice,* ed 3, St Louis, 1992, Mosby.)

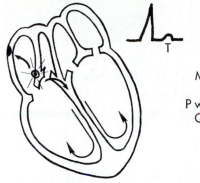

Middle nodal
impulse:
P wave hidden in
QRS complex

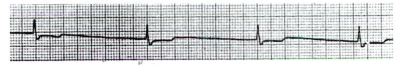

- Rhythm: regular

- Atrial rate: cannot be determined

- Ventricular rate: 40-60 bpm

- P waves: inverted before or after QRS or not present

- QRS: normal

- PR interval: <0.12 sec if P precedes QRS

- P: QRS: P≤QRS

Significance: AV node assumes primary pacing function from atria.

Intervention: Usually no specific therapy indicated. If patient becomes symptomatic because of a slow rate, see "Bradycardia Algorithm" in Appendix 1.

Figure 4-12: Junctional rhythm (JR). (Illustration from Sheehy SB: *Emergency nursing: principles and practice,* ed 3, St Louis, 1992, Mosby.)

- Monitor patient's heart rhythm continuously; note BP and symptoms if dysrhythmias occur or increase in occurrence.
- If a pulmonary artery catheter is present, note PAP, PAWP, and RAP; and monitor for a reduced cardiac output in response to dysrhythmias.
- Document dysrhythmias with rhythm strip. Use a 12/18-lead ECG as necessary to identify the dysrhythmia.

Text continued on p. 315.

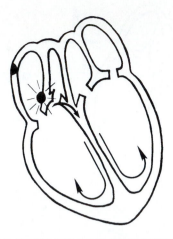

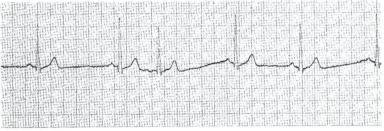

- Rhythm: irregular

- Atrial rate: unable to determine

- Ventricular rate: depends on underlying rhythm

- P waves: before, during, and after QRS

- QRS: normal

- PR interval: <0.12 sec if present

- P: QRS: P≤QRS

Significance: Less common than PACs; may precede blocks.

Intervention: Observation. Usually no treatment is necessary. If indicated, therapy is similar to that for PACs.

Figure 4-13:   Premature junctional complexes (PJCs). (Illustration from Sheehy SB: *Emergency nursing: principles and practice,* ed 3, St Louis, 1992, Mosby.)

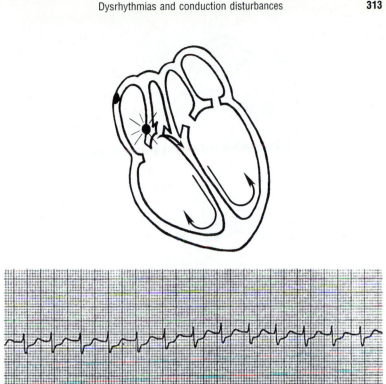

- Rhythm: regular

- Atrial rate: cannot determine

- Ventricular rate: 100-250 bpm

- P waves: inverted before or after QRS

- QRS: normal

- PR interval: unable to determine

- P: QRS: P<QRS

Significance: This rhythm is essentially the same as JR, except that an increase in sympathetic stimulation results in increased HR. Causes may include heart disease, electrolyte disturbances, COPD, or hypoxia.

Intervention: See "Tachycardia Algorithm" in Appendix 1.

Figure 4-14: Junctional tachycardia (JT). (Illustration from Sheehy SB: *Emergency nursing: principles and practice,* ed 3, St Louis, 1992, Mosby.)

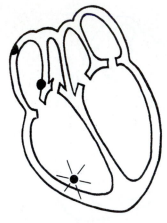

One ventricular
pacemaker fires
rapidly

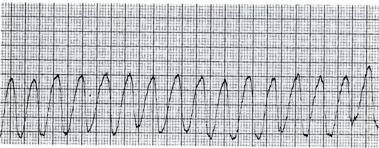

- Rhythm: slightly irregular

- Atrial rate: unable to determine

- Ventricular rate: 150-250 bpm

- P waves: none visible

- QRS: wide (>0.12 sec)

- PR interval: unable to determine

- P: QRS: absent

Significance: Cardiac output falls significantly, cannot be tolerated
for long, and will deteriorate into VF and asystole.

Intervention: See "Tachycardia Algorithm" and "Ventricular Fibrillation/
Pulseless Ventricular Tachycardia (VF/VT) Algorithm" in
Appendix 1.

Figure 4-15:   Ventricular tachycardia (VT). (Illustration from Sheehy SB:
Emergency nursing: principles and practice, ed 3, St Louis, 1992, Mosby.)

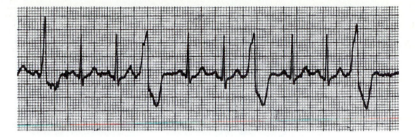

- Rhythm: irregular

- Atrial rate: not determined with PVCs

- Ventricular rate: depends on underlying rhythm

- P waves: not seen

- QRS: wide (>0.12 sec); bizarre

- PR interval: not determined

- P: QRS: P<QRS

Significance: PVCs signal an irritable focus in the ventricle. Causes may include AMI, hypoxia, hypovolemia, electrolyte imbalance. PVCs may be monomorphic (same form repeated) or polymorphic (more than one type present) and may occur in patterns. They may precipitate lethal dysrhythmias.

Intervention: PVCs are common in AMI, and there is controversy regarding treatment. Antidysrhythmic agents (lidocaine) are most beneficial in young patients with normal left ventricular function. Treatment should include correction of electrolyte abnormality, specifically hypokalemia and hypomagnesemia.

Figure 4-16: Premature ventricular complexes (PVCs). For illustration of electrical activity, see Figure 4-15. (Illustration from Sheehy SB: *Emergency nursing: principles and practice,* ed 3, St Louis, 1992, Mosby.)

- Monitor patient's laboratory data, particularly electrolyte and digoxin levels. Serum potassium levels <3.5 mEq/L or >5 mEq/L can cause dysrhythmias.
- Administer antidysrhythmic agents as prescribed; note patient's response to therapy.
- Provide oxygen as prescribed. Oxygen may be beneficial if dysrhythmias are related to ischemia.
- Maintain a quiet environment, and administer pain medications

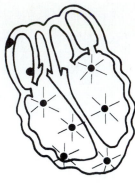

Ventricular
ectopic
sites firing
so fast that
quivering
results

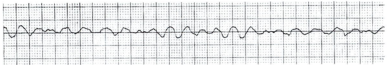

- Rhythm: irregular

- Atrial rate: unable to determine

- Ventricular rate: rapid

- P waves: not seen

- QRS: absent; fibrillatory waves

- PR interval: none

- P: QRS: none

Significance: Most common cause of sudden cardiac death. VF produces
no cardiac output.

Intervention: See "Ventricular Fibrillation/Pulseless Ventricular Tachycardia (VF/VT) Algorithm" in Appendix 1.

Figure 4-17:   Ventricular fibrillation (VF). (Illustration from Sheehy SB:
Emergency nursing: principles and practice, ed 3, St Louis, 1992, Mosby.)

promptly. Both stress and pain can increase sympathetic tone and
cause dysrhythmias.
- If life-threatening dysrhythmias occur, initiate immediate unit protocols or standing orders for treatment, as well as CPR and ACLS
algorithms (see Appendix 1) as necessary.

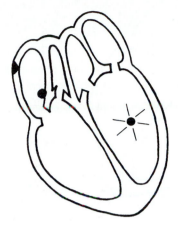

Slow impulses
from ectopic
site in
ventricle

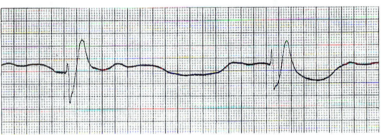

- Rhythm: regular or irregular

- Atrial rate: none

- Ventricular rate: <40 bpm

- P waves: none

- QRS: wide (>0.12 sec); bizarre

- PR interval: none

- P: QRS: none

Significance: Usually lethal. Pulse may be present but usually is not.

Intervention: See "Pulseless Electrical Activity (PEA) Algorithm" in Appendix 1.

Figure 4-18: Idioventricular rhythm. (Illustration from Sheehy SB: *Emergency nursing: principles and practice,* ed 3, St Louis, 1992, Mosby.)

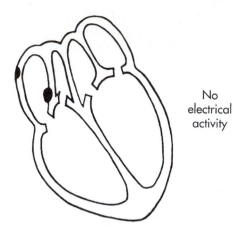

No
electrical
activity

- No electrical activity

- May see a rare, wide, bizarre QRS

Significance: Mortality rate >95%. Always confirm asystole in 2 leads.

Intervention: See "Asystole Algorithm" in Appendix 1.

Figure 4-19:   Asystole. (Illustration from Sheehy SB: *Emergency nursing: principles and practice,* ed 3, St Louis, 1992, Mosby.)

- When dysrhythmias occur, stay with patient; provide support and re-assurance while performing assessments and administering treatment.
- Administer inotropic agents (see Appendix 7) as prescribed to support patient's BP and cardiac output.

Knowledge deficit: Mechanism by which dysrhythmias occur and life-style implications

Desired outcome: Within the 24-h period before discharge from CCU, patient and significant others verbalize knowledge about causes of dysrhythmias and the implications for modification of patient's lifestyle.

- Discuss causal mechanisms for dysrhythmias, including resulting symptoms. Use a heart model or diagrams, as necessary.
- Teach the signs and symptoms of dysrhythmias that necessitate medical attention: unrelieved and prolonged palpitations, chest pain, SOB,

Text continued on p. 323.

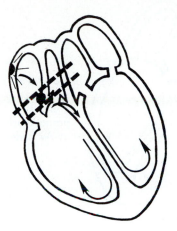

SA node
originates
impulse;
partial block
at AV node

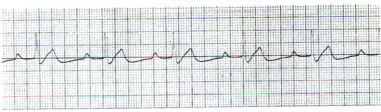

- Rhythm: regular

- Atrial rate: 60-100 bpm

- Ventricular rate: 60-100 bpm

- P waves: present; precede each QRS

- QRS: normal

- PR interval: prolonged (>0.2 sec)

- P: QRS: 1:1

Significance: Impulse conduction is delayed through the AV node. Causes are varied and may include heart disease, ischemia, digitalis toxicity, drug effect, and myocarditis.

Intervention: Observation; usually no treatment needed.

Figure 4-20:   First-degree AV block. (Illustration from Sheehy SB: *Emergency nursing: principles and practice*, ed 3, St Louis, 1992, Mosby.)

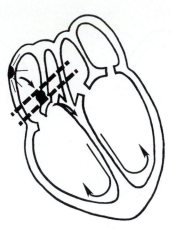

SA node
originates
impulse;
partial block
at AV node

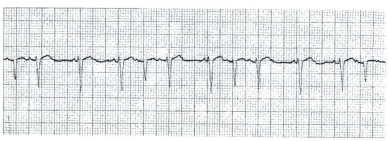

- Rhythm: irregular

- Atrial rate: exceeds ventricular rate

- Ventricular rate: less than sinus rate

- P waves: one P wave precedes each QRS except during nonconducted
  P waves, which occur regularly

- QRS: normal

- PR interval: lengthens progressively with each cycle until one is
  nonconducted

Significance: Usually a transient block that does not progress to complete
heart block.

Intervention: Observation; treatment usually not necessary.

Figure 4-21:   Second-degree AV block (Mobitz I, Wenckebach). (Illustration from Sheehy SB: *Emergency nursing: principles and practice,* ed
3, St Louis, 1992, Mosby.)

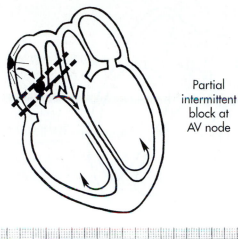

Partial
intermittent
block at
AV node

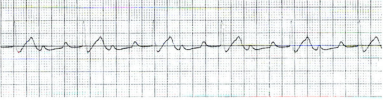

- Rhythm: irregular

- Atrial rate: exceeds ventricular rate

- Ventricular rate: depends on degree of block

- P waves: 2 or more for each QRS

- QRS: normal duration

- PR interval: normal or prolonged on the conducted complex

- P: QRS: P>QRS

Significance: This block may occur with anterior wall AMI and may progress rapidly to complete heart block.

Intervention: Observation if patient is asymptomatic. If symptoms occur, see "Bradycardia Algorithm" in Appendix 1.

Figure 4-22: Second-degree AV block (Mobitz II). (Illustration from Sheehy SB: *Emergency nursing: principles and practice,* ed 3, St Louis, 1992, Mosby.)

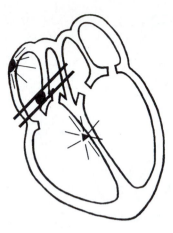

Complete
block at
AV node;
may have
ventricular
independent
pacemaker

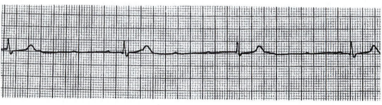

- Rhythm: usually regular

- Atrial rate: exceeds ventricular rate

- Ventricular rate: <60 bpm

- P waves: occur at regular intervals

- QRS: <0.12 sec if pacemaker is in the AV node; >0.12 sec if ventricular

- PR interval: no relationship between P and QRS

- P: QRS: no relationship

Significance: No conduction of SA node impulses. The atria ventricles beat independently of each other. The slow rate can cause myocardial ischemia.

Intervention: Pacemaker insertion necessary. See "Bradycardia Algorithm" in Appendix 1.

Figure 4-23:   Third-degree AV block. (Illustration from Sheehy SB: *Emergency nursing: principles and practice,* ed 3, St Louis, 1992, Mosby.)

rapid pulse (>150 bpm), dizziness, and syncope. Teach patient and significant others how to check pulse rate for a full minute.

- Teach patient and significant others about medications that will be taken after hospital discharge, including drug name, purpose, dosage, schedule, precautions, and potential side effects. Stress that patient will be maintained on long-term antidysrhythmic therapy and that it could be life threatening to stop or skip these medications without physician approval, because doing so may decrease blood levels effective for dysrhythmia suppression.

- Advise patient and significant others about the availability of support groups and counseling; provide appropriate community referrals. Patients who survive sudden cardiac arrest may experience nightmares or other sleep disturbances at home. Explain that anxiety and fear, along with periodic feelings of denial, depression, anger, and confusion, are normal following this experience.

- Stress the importance of leading a normal and productive life, even though patient may fear breakthrough of life-threatening dysrhythmias. If patient is going on vacation, advise him or her to take along sufficient medication and to investigate health care facilities in the vacation area.

- Advise patient and significant others to take CPR classes; provide addresses of community programs.

- Teach the importance of follow-up care; confirm date and time of next appointment, if known. Explain that outpatient Holter monitoring is performed periodically.

- Explain that individuals with recurrent dysrhythmias should follow a general low-fat and low-cholesterol diet (see Tables 4-3 and 4-4) and reduce intake of products containing caffeine, including coffee, tea, chocolate, and colas.

- As indicated, teach patient relaxation techniques, which will reduce stress and enable patient to decrease sympathetic tone (see next nursing diagnosis).

Health-seeking behavior: Relaxation technique effective for stress reduction and facilitation of decreased sympathetic tone

Desired outcome: Within the 24-h period following instruction, patient verbalizes and demonstrates the following relaxation technique.

- Explain that to decrease sympathetic tone, some patients with dysrhythmias may benefit from practicing a relaxation response. Many different techniques can be used, including use of breathing alone or in conjunction with muscle group contraction and relaxation. Other techniques incorporate use of imagery. The following is a relaxation response that can facilitate a hypometabolic state of decreased sympathetic nervous system outflow. Give patient the following instructions:
  1. Sit quietly in a comfortable position. Close your eyes.
  2. Relax all your muscles, starting at your feet and progressing to your facial muscles.
  3. Breathe through your nose. As you breathe out, say the word "one" silently to yourself. Become aware of your breathing and continue this process for approximately 20 min.
  4. Do not worry whether you are achieving a deep level of relaxation. Maintain a passive attitude and permit relaxation to occur

at its own pace. Expect distractions to occur, but just ignore them. Continue breathing and repeating the word "one."
- Encourage patient to practice this technique once or twice a day. Reassure him or her that relaxation is a learned skill that takes practice and becomes easier over time.

For patients with an implantable cardioverter-defibrillator

Knowledge deficit: ICD procedure and follow-up care
Desired outcomes: Within the 24-h period before the procedure, patient and significant others describe rationale for the procedure and method of insertion. Within the 24-h period before discharge from CCU, patient and significant others describe postinsertion care and need for continued physician and nurse follow-up.
- Assess patient's understanding of his or her medical condition (dysrhythmias) and the amount of detailed information desired.
- Discuss the following with the patient and significant others:
  - Type of dysrhythmia patient has, using rhythm strip and heart model to promote understanding.
  - Need for temporary transvenous pacemaker insertion before ICD procedure (i.e., to induce ventricular tachycardia or ventricular fibrillation or for emergency use should the patient require pacing before insertion of ICD).
  - Use of general anesthesia throughout procedure.
  - Testing of the ability of the ICD to terminate lethal dysrhythmias, which will occur in the operating room after implantation, before the incision is closed. Explain that the patient will be given extra systoles *via* the temporary pacemaker to induce clinical rhythm.
  - Reassurance that should the mechanism fail to terminate the dysrhythmia, the patient can be paced in an overdrive mode to abort the dysrhythmia.
  - Continuous observation of patient in a cardiac care unit for 48-72 h, with ongoing monitoring of BP, HR, and RR.
  - Importance of deep breathing, coughing (as necessary), and incentive spirometry exercises, which will be implemented immediately after surgery. Explain that patient is at increased risk for respiratory tract infection because of the thoracic surgery, which tends to cause patient to avoid deep breathing and coughing to guard against pain. Have patient return demonstrations of breathing exercises that will be implemented immediately after surgery. Reassure patient that analgesics can be administered before pulmonary toilet exercises.
  - Discharge instructions: Follow-up visit within 10-14 days, need for obtaining "home defibrillator," and importance of CPR/defibrillator classes for significant others.
- Describe the procedure should ICD device deliver a "shock": the patient should be taken to the emergency department *via* ambulance, and the physician should be notified at once. Teach patient to record the number of "shocks" experienced.
- Explain use of the home defibrillator, which is available commercially from several companies. It is designed to allow the nonmedical person to effect defibrillation, and its purpose is to convert lethal dysrhythmias should the ICD fail.

- Explain that "shocks" during sinus rhythm may indicate a lead fracture in the ICD system. Usually this is detected while the patient is being monitored (e.g., by ECG in physician's office, hospital monitor, or Holter monitor).

Risk for infection related to invasive procedure into thorax

Desired outcome: Patient is free of infection as evidenced by normothermia, WBC count ≤11,000 μl, negative culture results, and absence of the clinical indicators of infection at the incision site and of the respiratory tract.

- Because of the thoracic incision site, the patient is at risk for atelectasis and pneumonia after the ICD insertion procedure. Encourage and assist with deep breathing, coughing (if needed), and incentive spirometry exercises q2h, and encourage early ambulation to the chair. As indicated, assist patient with splinting the incision site with hands or pillow to promote optimal excursion. Provide prescribed analgesics 20 min before scheduled breathing exercises to facilitate compliance. For more information, see this nursing diagnosis in "Acute Pneumonia," p. 242.
- Assess incision site q2h for warmth, erythema, swelling, and drainage. The presence of a seroma, which has the same symptoms as incision site infection, is confirmed by decubitus chest x-rays or CT scan.
- Monitor patient's temperature q2-4h, being alert to elevation >38.6° C (101.5° F).
- Monitor CBC count for elevation of WBCs.
- Consult physician for significant findings.
- Teach patient and significant others the signs and symptoms of infection, both of the incision site (see above) and respiratory tract: cough, sputum production, fever, dyspnea, chills, headache, myalgia. Explain that the older adult may be confused and disoriented and may run low-grade fevers, but few other indicators are present.

Altered sexuality pattern (or risk for same) related to fear of inducing dysrhythmias during sexual activity

Desired outcome: Within the 24-h period before discharge from CCU, patient and significant other verbalize understanding of interventions during and alternatives for sexual intercourse.

- Assess patient for symptoms (dysrhythmias) during presurgical sexual experiences.
- Explain the following interventions or alternatives that can be made if patient continues to experience dysrhythmias during sexual intercourse:
  - □ Patient may need to take a less dominant role.
  - □ Patient may find that taking a prescribed vasodilator before engaging in sexual intercourse will prevent dysrhythmias.
  - □ Suggest that during periods of time when dysrhythmias are a problem, less stressful forms of sexual activity, such as caressing and hugging, are positive alternatives.
- As appropriate, advise patient that stressful situations, such as extramarital relations or unfamiliar environment, may contribute to symptoms during sexual activity.
- Explain that the device may "shock" at any time. If the patient's significant other is in contact with the patient's body at that time,

the shock may be experienced as a tingling sensation by the significant other.

ADDITIONAL NURSING DIAGNOSES

The patient with ICD is at risk for pneumothorax. As indicated, see "Pneumothorax," p. 261, for information related to this disorder. Also see nursing diagnoses and interventions in "Hemodynamic Monitoring," p. 37; "Psychosocial Support," p. 88; and "Psychosocial Support for the Patient's Family and Significant Others," p. 100.

Valvular heart disease

PATHOPHYSIOLOGY

Valvular heart disease involves obstruction to forward flow (stenosis) or insufficiency of the valve, allowing backward flow (regurgitation). One or more valves may be affected by one or both processes. When the effectiveness of a valve is compromised, symptoms of valvular incompetence may develop or the heart may begin to show signs of failure.

Usually, stenosis of a valve is caused by sclerosing, thickening, and calcification of the valve leaflets. A stenotic valve obstructs blood flow from the affected atria or ventricle, which leads to heart chamber hypertrophy. With a stenotic aortic or pulmonic valve, intramyocardial wall tension increases; this increase enables the heart to pump more blood through the highly resistant valve opening. If the stenosis is unrelieved, the ventricle eventually fails. When the left ventricle fails, blood backs up into the left atrium and pulmonary capillary bed, leading to pulmonary congestion and edema. In addition, with ventricular hypertrophy and high intramyocardial wall tension, blood flow to the endocardium may be diminished. These patients therefore may have angina and ventricular dysrhythmias. Both mitral and tricuspid stenosis can be severely debilitating, causing easy fatigability and limited activity.

Regurgitation of a valve may be caused by rheumatic heart disease, dilatation of the valve ring, or damage to the nearby valve structures. Regurgitation results in increased volume into the affected chamber (see Figure 4-24).

ASSESSMENT

See Table 4-10.

DIAGNOSTIC TESTS

Cardiac catheterization: A ventriculogram may assist in visualization of blood flow. Measurement of chamber pressures assists in determining type of disorder present and the degree of severity.

Echocardiography: To determine ventricular function, chamber size, and valve function.

- *Doppler flow studies:* Continuous wave or pulsed wave frequencies used to determine blood flow.

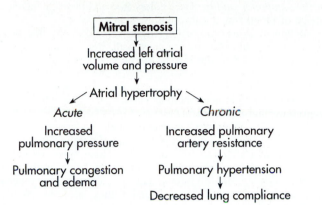

Mitral stenosis
↓
Increased left atrial
volume and pressure
↓
Atrial hypertrophy

Acute

Increased
pulmonary pressure
↓
Pulmonary congestion
and edema

Chronic

Increased pulmonary
artery resistance
↓
Pulmonary hypertension
↓
Decreased lung compliance

Tricuspid stenosis
↓
Decreased systemic venous return
to the right ventricle
↓
Increased right atrial
volume and pressure
↓
Systemic venous congestion
↓   ↓
Liver enlargement   Peripheral
↓   edema
Ascites

Aortic regurgitation
↓
Blood leaks into left
ventricle during diastole
↓
Increased volume in left ventricle
↓
Left ventricular dilatation
↓
Left ventricular failure

Mitral regurgitation
↓
Decreased CO ← Blood backs into left atrium
during left ventricular systole
↓
Increased left atrial pressure
↓
Increased pulmonary vascular pressure
↓
Potential pulmonary edema

Figure 4-24:   Disease progression with valvular disorders.

Color flow mapping studies: Uses colors (red and blue) to enhance the image of blood flowing through the heart.

Transesophageal echocardiography: Uses an endoscope that produces an image unimpeded by the chest wall. Because the esophagus is close to the heart, the images are clear and undistorted.

SURGICAL INTERVENTIONS

Methods of surgical treatment include valve repair (valvuloplasty), commissurotomy, and replacement.

Valve replacement: Performed in patients with moderate to severe calcification, mixed stenosis and insufficiency, and pure insufficiency; procedure has a mortality rate of about 6%. Three types of valve replacement are used for replacement: homografts, heterografts, and artificial grafts. Homografts are human cadaver valves that have been specially treated for surgical use. Because they are not readily available, they seldom are used. A heterograft is a valve from an animal, usually a pig or cow, that has been prepared for surgical use. These valves are readily available and in common use. Artificial valves are made from stainless steel, carbon, and other durable materials, such as plastic. Tissue grafts are advantageous because they are natural and thus blood elements do not tend to form on them. Their disadvantage is their short duration of use, which is about 5-8 yr. There is a tendency for clots to form on artificial valves, and therefore the patient must receive lifetime anticoagulant therapy; however, the valve can be used for 10-15 yr. Postoperative care of the patient who has had valve surgery is similar to that of the patient who has undergone CABG (see p. 281). It is important to note, however, that patients undergoing valve surgery are at increased risk for thrombosis and embolism (particularly with mechanical mitral valves and in patients with atrial fibrillation) and for valvular endocarditis.

Postoperative considerations specific to these patients are discussed under the nursing diagnoses and interventions.

Percutaneous balloon valvuloplasty: For dilatation of stenotic heart valves. Candidates for this procedure (1) are at high risk for surgery, (2) refuse surgery, (3) are older adults (often >80 yr of age), or (4) are informed of treatment choices and choose this procedure over others. The procedure parallels the technique for PTCA (see p. 271). The femoral artery and vein are cannulated, and the patient receives anticoagulation therapy with heparin. For aortic valve dilatation a catheter is passed into the femoral artery to measure supravalvular and left ventricular pressures before valvuloplasty. A balloon valvuloplasty catheter is then passed over a guidewire into the left ventricle. It is inflated three times for 12-30 sec at a pressure of 12 atm. Additional heparin is administered, and the valve gradient is remeasured. To reach the mitral valve the balloon valvuloplasty catheter is passed *via* the femoral vein and through the atrial septum to the mitral valve opening. The inflation procedure is the same.

With both aortic and mitral dilatation, significant improvement has been demonstrated in the valve gradient and in blood flow across the valve. Complications that have been observed include embolization to the brain, disruption of the valve ring, acute valve regurgitation, valvular restenosis, hemorrhage at the catheter insertion site, guidewire perforation of the left ventricle, and dysrhythmias.

Commissurotomy: A procedure in which the stenotic valve is opened by a dilating instrument. When performed early in the course of the disease, chances of success are good, although the procedure may result in valve regurgitation and recurrent stenosis.

NURSING DIAGNOSES AND INTERVENTIONS

Altered protection related to risk of bleeding/hemorrhage secondary to anticoagulation

---

Note: Patients undergoing aortic valve replacement are at a higher risk for postoperative hemorrhage than those undergoing CABG.

Desired outcome: Throughout hospitalization, patient is free of symptoms of bleeding or hemorrhage as evidenced by RAP ≥4 mm Hg, PAWP ≥6 mm Hg, BP within patient's normal range, CO ≥4 L/min, CI ≥2.5 L/min/m^2, urine output ≥0.5 ml/kg/h, urine specific gravity 1.010-1.030, and chest tube drainage ≤100 ml/h.

- Measure chest tube drainage hourly. Report chest tube drainage >100 ml/h. Maintain patency of chest tubes at all times.
- Monitor clotting studies. Be alert to and report prolonged PT, PTT, and ACT and decreased platelet count. Optimal values are as follows: PT 11-15 sec, PTT 30-40 sec (activated), and ACT ≤120 sec. For patient with prolonged PT, PTT, or ACT, administer IV protamine sulfate as prescribed.
- Assess VS hourly, and monitor patient for physical indicators of hemorrhage or hypovolemia: RAP <4 mm Hg, PAWP <6 mm Hg, decreased BP, decreased measured CO/CI, urine output <0.5 ml/kg/h, increased urine specific gravity, and excessive chest tube drainage (>100 ml/h). Be alert to a decreased Hct. Optimal values are: Hct ≥37% (female) and ≥40% (male).
- Assess postoperative chest x-ray for a widened mediastinum, which may indicate hemorrhage and possible cardiac tamponade.
- As prescribed, administer platelets, fresh-frozen plasma, or cryoprecipitate to replace clotting factors and blood volume.
- Administer packed RBCs as prescribed to replace blood volume.
- To correct hyperfibrinolytic state (increased fibrin degradation products), administer aminocaproic acid slowly per IV bolus as prescribed (see Table 6-4).

Decreased cardiac output (or risk for same) related to negative inotropic changes secondary to intraoperative subendocardial ischemia and administration of myocardial depressant drugs

---

Note: After cardiac surgery some myocardial depression is always present, usually lasting 48-72 h. Patients with long-standing aortic stenosis or ventricular failure due to mitral valve disease are at an even greater risk for postoperative low cardiac output.

Desired outcomes: Within 48-72 h of this diagnosis, patient has adequate cardiac output as evidenced by normal sinus rhythm on ECG, measured CO of 4-7 L/min, CI ≥2.5 L/min/m^2, BP within patient's normal range, PAP 20-30/8-15 mm Hg, PAWP 6-12 mm Hg (or range specified by physician), Svo_2 60%-80%, SVR 900-1,200 dynes/sec/ cm^{-5}, peripheral pulses >2+ on a 0-4+ scale, warm and dry skin, and hourly urine output ≥0.5 ml/kg/h. Patient is awake, alert, and oriented.

- Monitor BP, PAP, RAP, Svo_2, HR, and heart rhythm continuously. Monitor PAWP, SVR, and CO hourly. Be alert to and report the following: elevation in PAWP, decreased CO, decreased Svo_2, or elevated SVR.
- Monitor urinary output, noting output that is <0.5 ml/kg/h for 2 consecutive hours.
- Monitor peripheral pulses and color and temperature of extremities q2h.
- Provide oxygen therapy as prescribed.
- Maintain an adequate preload (i.e., PAWP >6 mm Hg, RAP >4-6 mm Hg) *via* administration of IV fluids.

Note: With aortic stenosis and severe left ventricular hypertrophy, a high filling pressure (i.e., PAWP >18 mm Hg) may be necessary to ensure an adequate cardiac output.

- Maintain a normal or reduced afterload (SVR <1,200 dynes/sec/ cm^{-5}) by administering prescribed IV vasodilating drugs, such as nitroprusside and NTG.
- Maintain normal sinus rhythm by administering antidysrhythmic agents as prescribed. Atrial fibrillation is common in aortic and mitral valve disease and may result in a 20% decrease in CO. If a junctional rhythm or bradycardia occurs, a pacemaker usually becomes necessary.
- Administer inotropic agents as prescribed to maintain CI ≥2.5 $L/min/m^2$ and systolic BP >90 mm Hg. Commonly used agents include dobutamine, dopamine, and amrinone. Monitor for side effects, including tachydysrhythmias, ventricular ectopy, headache, and angina.

Altered cerebral tissue perfusion (or risk for same) related to impaired blood flow to the brain secondary to embolization resulting from cardiac surgery

---

Note: Air embolism, particulate embolism from calcified valves, and thrombotic emboli from prosthetic valves may lodge in the brain, leading to varying degrees of stroke.

Desired outcome: Throughout hospitalization, patient has adequate or baseline brain perfusion as evidenced by orientation to time, place, and person; equal and normoreactive pupils; and ability to move all extremities, communicate, and respond to requests (or comparable to patient's preoperative baseline).

- Monitor patient immediately after surgery and hourly for signs of neurologic impairment: diminished LOC, pupillary response, ability to move all extremities, and response to verbal stimuli.
- Assess patient's orientation and ability to communicate, answer yes-no questions, point to objects, write a response on a piece of paper, write sentences and appropriate requests, identify

family members, and identify where he or she is. Inform other health-care personnel about patient's LOC and communication deficits.
- If CNS impairment is suspected, administer urea solutions, mannitol, and corticosteroids as prescribed.
- In the presence of CNS impairment, implement the following measures:
  □ Assist patient with turning and moving as needed. Teach patient to use unaffected extremities to assist with moving.
  □ Perform ROM to all extremities qid. Have patient assist as much as possible.
  □ Progress patient's activity level, as tolerated, with the assistance of a physical therapist.
- When patient is able to take oral foods and fluids, assess patient's ability to swallow. If patient's voice is hoarse or patient coughs when swallowing, consult physician. Patient may require NPO status and an enteric tube until the swallowing reflex has improved.

Knowledge deficit: Risk of infective endocarditis after valve surgery and precautions that must be taken to prevent it

---

Note: All patients with valve surgery are at risk for infective endocarditis (IE) as a result of bacteria entering the bloodstream and traveling to the heart, leading to destruction of a new tissue valve or obstruction of a new artificial valve.

Desired outcome: Within the 24-h period before discharge from CCU, patient verbalizes knowledge about the risk of IE after valve surgery and the precautions that must be taken to prevent it.
- Teach patient about IE (see "Acute Infective Endocarditis," p. 333), describing what it is, how it develops, and how it may affect the repaired valve.
- Teach patient that antibiotics are prescribed as a prophylaxis against endocarditis after valve surgery. Explain that they must be taken before any dental work or examination by instrument is undertaken, including teeth cleaning, fillings, extractions, cystoscopy, endoscopy, or sigmoidoscopy. Caution patient to notify dentists and other physicians about the valve surgery so that antibiotics can be prescribed before any invasive procedure.
- Instruct patient to cleanse all wounds and apply antibiotic ointments to help prevent infection.

For patients undergoing percutaneous balloon valvuloplasty

Knowledge deficit: Procedure for percutaneous balloon valvuloplasty (PBV) and postprocedural assessment

Desired outcome: Within the 24-h period before PBV, patient verbalizes rationale for the procedure, the technique, and postprocedural care.
- Assess patient's understanding of aortic stenosis and the purpose of valvuloplasty. Evaluate patient's style of coping and the degree of information desired.
- As appropriate for patient's coping style, discuss with patient and significant others the valvuloplasty procedure, including:
  □ Location of diseased valve, using heart drawing.

- Use of local anesthesia and sedation during procedure.
- Insertion site of catheter: femoral artery and vein.
- Use of fluoroscopy during procedure. Evaluate patient for a history of sensitivity to contrast material.
- Postprocedural observations made by nurse: BP, HR, ECG, pulses, and catheter insertion site.
- Importance of lying flat 6-12 h postprocedure to minimize the risk of bleeding.

Decreased cardiac output (or risk for same) related to altered preload and negative inotropic changes associated with valve regurgitation or hemorrhage secondary to PBV; or related to altered rate, rhythm, or conduction associated with dysrhythmias secondary to PBV

Desired outcome: Throughout the postoperative course, patient has adequate cardiac output as evidenced by normal sinus rhythm; CO 4-7 L/min; CI ≥2.5 L/min/m^2; HR 60-100 bpm; RAP 4-6 mm Hg; PAWP 6-12 mm Hg; PAP 20-30/8-15 mm Hg; BP within patient's normal range; urinary output ≥0.5 ml/kg/h; peripheral pulses >2+ on a 0-4+ scale; orientation to time, place, and person; and absence of new murmurs, pulsus paradoxus, or jugular vein distention.

- Monitor ECG continuously after procedure. Document any changes. Consult physician for dysrhythmias, and treat according to type of dysrhythmia and hospital protocol.
- Monitor CO/CI, HR, RAP, PAWP, and PAP hourly or as prescribed. Report a fall in CO/CI, change in HR, and increase or decrease in RAP, PAWP, or PAP.
- Monitor Hct and electrolyte values. Observe for a decrease in Hct or any change in electrolyte levels (particularly potassium) that could precipitate dysrhythmias. Optimal values are: Hct >37% (female) or >40% (male) and serum potassium 3.5-5 mEq/L.
- Assess heart sounds immediately after procedure and q4h. Report the development of a new murmur.
- Monitor patient for evidence of cardiac tamponade: hypotension, tachycardia, pulsus paradoxus, jugular vein distention, elevation and plateau pressuring of PAWP and RAP and, possibly, an enlarged heart silhouette on chest x-ray. For more information, see "Acute Cardiac Tamponade," p. 152.

Altered protection related to risk of hemorrhage or hematoma formation secondary to heparinization with PBV

Desired outcomes: Throughout the postoperative course, patient has minimal or absent bleeding or hematoma formation at the catheter insertion site. PTT is within therapeutic anticoagulation range (per physician or agency protocol).

- Monitor catheter insertion site for evidence of bleeding. Report hematoma formation, and outline the bleeding on the dressing for subsequent comparison.
- Keep patient's catheterized leg straight for the prescribed amount of time.
- Monitor heparin drip as prescribed. Usually heparin drip is maintained until 1-2 h before the sheaths are removed.
- Monitor PTT for therapeutic range, which is usually 1½ times that of normal.

- When IV or invasive lines (arterial or venous sheaths) are removed, apply firm pressure either manually or with a mechanical clamp for 30 min.

ADDITIONAL NURSING DIAGNOSES

See "Pulmonary Emboli" for **Knowledge deficit,** p. 258. Also see "Percutaneous Transluminal Coronary Angioplasty" in "Acute Chest Pain" for **Altered peripheral tissue perfusion (or risk for same),** p. 277. See all nursing diagnoses in the discussion of "Coronary Artery Bypass Graft" in "Acute Myocardial Infarction," p. 286. Also see nursing diagnoses and interventions in "Hemodynamic Monitoring," p. 37; "Prolonged Immobility," p. 78; "Psychosocial Support," p. 88; and "Psychosocial Support for the Patient's Family and Significant Others," p. 100.

Acute infective endocarditis

PATHOPHYSIOLOGY

Infective endocarditis (IE) is infection of the endocardium (the innermost layer of the heart), which often involves the natural or prosthetic valve. It is caused by bacteria, viruses, fungi, or rickettsiae. Four mechanisms are known to contribute to the development of IE. One is a congenital or acquired defect of the heart valve or the septum. Frequently it is accompanied by a jet-Venturi stream of blood flowing from a high- to low-pressure area through a narrow opening. This occurs when there is a septal defect or a stenotic or insufficient valve. The low-pressure sink beyond the narrowed jet-flow site provides an area that is ideal for colonization by any infecting organism. The second mechanism is the formation of a sterile platelet fibrin thrombus at the low-pressure site, which gives rise to vegetation. Third, a bacteremia occurs as a result of colonization in the vegetation. Finally, a high level of agglutinating antibodies promotes the growth of the vegetation. Fungal infections result in the largest vegetations.

Portals of entry for the infecting organism include the mouth and GI tract, upper airway, skin, and external genitourinary (GU) tract. Any heart valve can become infected, but the aortic and mitral valves are more common sites than the right-sided pulmonic and tricuspid valves. Tricuspid valve involvement, however, is almost exclusively found in cases of IV drug abuse. Once the infection process begins, valvular dysfunction, manifested by insufficiency with regurgitant blood flow, can occur, ultimately resulting in a decrease in cardiac output. The vegetation may become so large that it obstructs the valve orifice, mimicking valvular stenosis and further reducing cardiac output. At times, pieces of the vegetation may break off and embolize to vital organs. In severe cases the affected valve may necrose, develop an aneurysm, and rupture, or the infection may extend through the myocardium and epicardium to cause a pericarditis (see "Acute Pericarditis," p. 342). If the conduction system is affected by the spreading infection, bundle-branch block may occur. Most complications of IE occur suddenly, with a dramatic change in the clinical picture. Mortality rates between

---

T A B L E   4 - 9   Antibiotic prophylaxis with infective endocarditis

---

Regimen for dental, oral, or upper respiratory tract procedures
Standard regimen for those at risk who can take oral medications
    amoxicillin   3 g PO 1 h before procedure*
If allergic to amoxicillin/penicillin
    erythromycin ethylsuccinate   800 mg PO 2 h before procedure* *or*
    erythromycin stearate   1 g PO 2 h before procedure* *or*
    clindamycin   300 mg PO 1 h before procedure*
Alternate regimen for those unable to take oral medications
    ampicillin   2 g IV or IM 30 min before procedure
If allergic to amoxicillin/penicillin
    clindamycin   300 mg IV 30 min before procedure* *or*
    vancomycin   1 g IV 1 h before procedure (no repeat dose needed)
Regimen for those considered at high risk but not candidates for standard regimen
    ampicillin   2 g IV or IM† *and*
    gentamicin   1.5 mg/kg (not >80 mg) IV 30 min before procedure† *and*
    amoxicillin   1.5 mg orally q6h after initial dose of other medications

Regimen for genitourinary/gastrointestinal procedures
Standard regimen
    ampicillin   2 g IM or IV† *and*
    gentamicin   1.5 mg/kg (not >80 mg) IV 30 min before procedure† *and*
    amoxicillin   1.5 g orally q6h after initial dose of other medications
If allergic to ampicillin/amoxicillin/penicillin
    vancomycin   1 g IV over 1 h before procedure† *and*
    gentamicin   1.5 mg/kg (not >80 mg) 1 h before procedure‡
Alternative low-risk patient regimen
    amoxicillin   3 g PO 1 h before procedure*

Adapted from Dajani AS et al: Prevention of bacterial endocarditis: recommendations by the American Heart Association, *JAMA* 264:2919-2922, 1990.
*Give half of original dose q6h after initial dose.
†Optional to give same dose IV or IM q8h after initial dose.
‡May repeat once, 8 h after initial dose.

20% and 50% have been reported with IE. Recurrence of the infection occurs at a rate of 10%-20%.

ASSESSMENT

HISTORY AND RISK FACTORS Invasive procedures, such as temporary pacemaker insertion, PA catheter insertion, transurethral resection, endoscopy, surgery, or dental work, place the patient with a pre-existing valvular disorder at greater risk of bacteremia development that can lead to IE. Recent increases in IV drug abuse have led to increased incidences in IE, especially IE involving the tricuspid valve. An immunosuppressed patient (i.e., one with a transplant, carcinoma, burns, or diabetes mellitus) also is at risk for IE.

To prevent recurrence of IE or reduce the risk of initial occurrence in the individual with an abnormal heart valve, the American Heart Association recommends prophylactic antibiotics before and after invasive procedures or dental work. See Table 4-9.

CLINICAL PRESENTATION (ACUTE INFECTIVE STAGE) Fever, diaphoresis, fatigue, anorexia, joint pain, weight loss, and abdominal pain. The severity of symptoms varies, depending on the infective organism. For example, *Staphylococcus aureus* will produce more severe symptoms than will *Streptococcus viridans*.

PHYSICAL ASSESSMENT A new or changed murmur may be heard as a result of the valvular dysfunction. (See Table 4-10 for a description of the types of murmurs that can be heard, depending on the valve affected and the type of dysfunction present.) If heart failure has resulted from the valvular disorder, fine crackles may be auscultated at the bases of the lungs and an S_3 or S_4 heart sound may be heard. The skin is often pale, but if right-sided heart failure is present because of valvular insufficiency, jaundice of the skin and sclera may occur, as well as edema, neck vein distention, a positive hepatojugular reflex, and ascites. Late assessment findings include anemia, petechiae, and clubbing of the fingers.

Classic findings

Splinter hemorrhages: Small red streaks on the distal third of the fingernails or toenails.

Janeway lesions: Painless, small, hemorrhagic lesions found on the fingers, toes, nose, or earlobes, probably occurring as the result of immune complex deposition with inflammation.

Osler's nodes: Painful, red, subcutaneous nodules found on the pads of the fingers or on the feet, probably occurring as a result of emboli producing small areas of gangrene or vasculitis.

Roth's spots: Retinal hemorrhages with pale centers seen on fundoscopic examination.

Note: If emboli of the vegetations occur in other areas, signs and symptoms of CVA, peripheral obstruction, or myocardial, renal, or mesenteric infarct will be seen.

HEMODYNAMIC MEASUREMENTS Invasive monitoring devices are used cautiously with these patients to prevent further valvular dysfunction, embolization, and infection. However, when warranted, a PA catheter may be used to assess hemodynamic function. Elevations of PAP or RAP can be expected in most patients with IE. In addition, reduced CO usually is present.

DIAGNOSTIC TESTS

Blood cultures: Provide the definitive diagnosis of the infecting organism. If the results are negative, the patient may be past the acute infective phase and cultures may be repeated later. Organism sensitivity to various antibiotics is essential in guiding therapy.

Echocardiography: Reveals valvular involvement and vegetation size and defines the severity of the valvular dysfunction. M-mode, two-

T A B L E   4 - 1 0   Assessment findings with valvular heart disease

Valve dysfunction	Murmur	Pathology	Hemodynamic changes
Aortic stenosis	Systolic, blowing murmur at second ICS, RSB; may radiate to the neck	Reduced flow across aortic valve with ↑ LV volume and pressure, with diminished CO; LV hypertrophy eventually occurs	↑ LV pressure; ↑ PAEDP; ↓ CO and aortic pressure with a narrow pulse pressure reflecting the decreased stroke volume
Aortic insufficiency	Diastolic blowing murmur at second ICS, RSB, beginning immediately with S_2	Regurgitant blood flow from aorta to LV during diastole	↑ LV pressure and PAEDP; ↓ CO; ↑ systolic BP and widened pulse pressure
Mitral stenosis	Loud, long, diastolic rumbling murmur at fifth ICS, MCL; may radiate to axilla; S_1 is loud and there is an opening snap with S_2	Reduced flow across mitral valve with left atrial and pulmonary congestion	↑ mean PAP; ↓ CO
Mitral insufficiency	Systolic murmur at fifth ICS, MCL	Regurgitant blood flow from LV to left atrium, resulting in pulmonary congestion	Giant V waves in the PA occlusive tracing; ↑ systolic PAP; ↓ CO; mean PAP may be normal

Pulmonic stenosis	Systolic blowing murmur at second ICS, LSB; may radiate to neck	Reduced flow across pulmonic valve with ↑ RV volume and pressure, with diminished LV return, resulting in ↓ CO	↑ RV systolic pressure, mean RAP, PAEDP, and mean PAP
Pulmonic insufficiency	Diastolic murmur at second ICS, LSB that starts later and is lower pitched than aortic murmur	Regurgitant blood flow from pulmonary artery to RV during diastole, resulting in RV overload	↑ systolic RV pressure with wide pulse pressure; LVEDP and CO often normal but may ↓ if disorder is severe
Tricuspid stenosis	Diastolic murmur at fourth ICS	Reduced flow across tricuspid valve with ↑ right atrial and venous congestion	CVP ↑ with accentuated A wave on the RA waveform
Tricuspid insufficiency	Pansystolic murmur at fourth ICS, LSB that increases in intensity with inspiration	Regurgitant blood flow from RV to RA; right atrial and venous congestion occurs	↑ CVP with prominent V wave on the RA tracing; normal or low PAP, LVEDP, and CO

CVP, Central venous pressure; *ICS*, intercostal space; *LSB*, left sternal border; *LV*, left ventricle/ventricular; *LVEDP*, left ventricular end-diastolic pressure; *MCL*, midclavicular line; *PA*, pulmonary artery; *PAP*, pulmonary artery pressure; *PAEDP*, pulmonary artery end-diastolic pressure; *RA*, right atrium; *RAP*, right atrial pressure; *RSB*, right sternal border; *RV*, right ventricle/ventricular.

TABLE 4-11   ECG changes frequently found with ventricular and atrial hypertrophy

Chamber	ECG change
Left ventricular enlargement	"R" voltage increases in V_{4-6}; "S" voltage increases (deeper inflection) in V_{1-2}; the sum of "S" in V_1 or V_2 and "R" in V_5 or V_6 will be >35 mm, or "R" in any V lead will be >25 mm
Left atrial enlargement	"P mitrale" in leads II, III, aV_F, and V_1; P wave is m-shaped with a duration >0.1 sec
Right ventricular enlargement	"R" voltage increased in V_1, V_2; "S" voltage increased in V_5, V_6; sum of "R" in V_1 or V_2 and "S" in V_5 or V_6 will be ≥35 mm
Right atrial enlargement	"P pulmonale" in leads II, III, aV_F, and V_1; P wave is >2.5 mm voltage and <0.1 sec duration

dimensional, or Doppler echocardiograms may be used. Transesophageal echocardiograms may be more useful in detecting vegetation, especially with prosthetic valves.

ECG: Although ECG is not useful in diagnosing IE, it frequently is performed to determine if conduction system defects are present. AV node or bundle of His may be affected as the area of infection spreads. Right or left atrial or ventricular enlargement may be seen as a result of prolonged hemodynamic effects on chamber size or muscle wall thickness (Table 4-11). Atrial dysrhythmias frequently are seen as that chamber enlarges from volume overload. Premature atrial complexes (PACs), paroxysmal atrial tachycardia (PAT), supraventricular tachycardia (SVT), atrial flutter, or atrial fibrillation may be seen on the ECG or monitor strip. Also see Figures 4-4 through 4-23.

Hematology studies: Will show an increase in the WBC count and eosinophil rate. Frequently, anemia is present.

Cardiac enzyme levels: Will be elevated if a myocardial infarction occurs due to emboli of vegetations that migrate to the coronary arteries.

ABG values: Evaluated to determine the degree of pulmonary dysfunction as a result of the cardiac disorder.

Additional studies: May be performed to assess for embolization to other organs. Studies such as renal, mesenteric, or peripheral arteriograms or CT scan may be done.

COLLABORATIVE MANAGEMENT

Antibiotic treatment: Patients usually require 4-6 wk of IV antibiotics. Antibiotic selection is based on the results of the blood culture and sensitivity studies.

Fluid and sodium limitations: Often required to promote optimal hemodynamics. Specific restrictions must be individualized and based on severity of symptoms and impairment of hemodynamic function.

Bed rest: Recommended initially, with activity limitations throughout the remainder of the treatment.

Diet: High in protein and calories to prevent cardiac cachexia.

Pharmacotherapy

Diuretics and vasodilators: May be required to decrease the symptoms of congestive heart failure by decreasing preload.

Positive inotropic agents (e.g., digoxin, dobutamine, amrinone): May be needed to increase contractility and cardiac output. For more information, see Appendix 7.

Nitroprusside, nitroglycerin: To reduce afterload.

Sedation: May be necessary to allay patient's anxiety during this long period of hospitalization.

Oxygen therapy: Administered as needed at an Fio_2 rate that maintains Pao_2 >60 mm Hg and oxygen saturation at >95%. Pulse oximetry is used continuously or intermittently to verify satisfactory oxygen saturation.

Treatment of other signs and symptoms: If heart failure has resulted from the valvular disorder, see "Congestive Heart Failure," p. 291, for treatment of those signs and symptoms. See "Cardiogenic Shock," p. 362, for the medical treatment that may be necessary if the valvular dysfunction deteriorates to the point that it is life threatening.

Prophylaxis regimen: Provides prophylactic antibiotics for those individuals at risk who undergo dental, oral, upper respiratory tract, genitourinary, or gastrointestinal procedures. See Table 4-9.

Surgical valve replacement: Required when hemodynamic function deteriorates or if the infection does not respond to antibiotic therapy. See "Valvular Heart Disease," p. 327. An abscess or infected tissue may be surgically removed if there is no response to long-term antibiotics.

NURSING DIAGNOSES AND INTERVENTIONS

Decreased cardiac output related to altered preload, afterload, or contractility secondary to valvular dysfunction

Desired outcomes: Within 72 h after initiation of therapy, patient has adequate hemodynamic function with controlled atrial fibrillation as evidenced by normal sinus rhythm, HR ≤100 bpm, BP ≥90/60 mm Hg, stable weight, intake equal to output plus insensible losses, RR ≤20 breaths/min with normal depth and pattern (eupnea), and absence of S_3 or S_4 heart sounds, crackles, distended neck veins, and other clinical signs of heart failure. Optimally, the following normal parameters will be achieved: CO 4-7 L/min, CVP 2-6 mm Hg, PAP 20-30/8-15 mm Hg, RAP 4-6 mm Hg, and MAP 60-105 mm Hg.

• Assess heart sounds q2-4h. A change in the characteristics of a heart murmur may signal progression of valvular dysfunction, which can occur with insufficiency, stenosis, or dislodgment of vegetation.

• Assess for the presence of an extra heart sound. A new S_3 or S_4 sound may signal heart failure.

• Monitor heart rhythm continuously. Report dysrhythmias or conduction defects, which may indicate the spread of infection to the conduction system or atrial volume overload.

• Monitor for signs of left-sided heart failure secondary to valvular dysfunction: crackles, S_3 or S_4 sounds, dyspnea, tachypnea, digital

clubbing, decreased BP, increased pulse pressure, increased left ventricular end-diastolic pressure (LVEDP), and decreased CO.

- Monitor for signs of right-sided heart failure secondary to valvular
  dysfunction: increased CVP, distended neck veins, positive hepatojugular reflex, edema, jaundice, ascites.
- Monitor I&O hourly, and measure weight daily. To help prevent
  miscalculations of patient's weight, use the same scale and amount
  of clothing and weigh patient at the same time of day. Notify
  physician if patient's weight increases by more than 1 kg (2 lbs)
  per day.
- If patient's PAP or RAP is high, decrease preload by limiting fluid
  and sodium intake and administering diuretics and venous dilators
  as prescribed.
- If patient's MAP is high, decrease afterload with prescribed arterial
  dilators.
- If afterload is low, increase afterload with vasopressors, as prescribed.

Note: See "Cardiogenic Shock," p. 365, for a discussion of preload and
afterload medications.

- If afterload is low, prevent further reductions caused by vasodilatation (e.g., by avoiding administration of morphine sulfate or rapid
  warming of the patient with hypothermia).
- Increase contractility with positive inotropes, as prescribed.
- Limit patient's activities to reduce myocardial oxygen needs; schedule patient care activities to patient's tolerance.
- Help patient reduce stress by teaching stress-reduction techniques,
  such as imagery, meditation, or progressive muscle relaxation. For
  description of a relaxation technique, see **Health-seeking behavior,**
  p. 323.
- Provide sedation as needed.
- Prevent orthostatic hypotension by changing patient's position
  slowly.

Impaired gas exchange related to alveolar-capillary membrane
changes with decreased diffusion of oxygen secondary to pulmonary
congestion

Desired outcome: Within 24 h of initiation of oxygen therapy and
during the weaning process, patient has adequate gas exchange as evidenced by RR ≤20 breaths/min with normal pattern and depth (eupnea), mixed venous oxygen saturation (Svo_2) 60%-80%, Pao_2 ≥80
mm Hg, arterial oxygen saturation ≥95%, and natural skin color.

- Assess rate, effort, and depth of patient's respirations. Tachypnea
  may indicate pulmonary congestion, inasmuch as the RR increases
  to compensate for the decreased depth caused by pulmonary congestion or airway obstruction.
- Assess color of skin and mucous membranes, being alert to pallor
  as a signal of impaired oxygenation.
- Auscultate lungs q2h. Report presence of crackles (which are most
  often found at the lung bases), rhonchi, and wheezing.
- If hemodynamic monitoring with oximetry is used, assess Svo_2.
  Svo_2 will fall below normal levels when oxygen uptake is in-

creased as a result of increased metabolic demands or if extraction is increased as a result of reduced oxygen delivery. This change occurs before there is a change in symptoms, and it correlates with cardiac output.

- Monitor ABG values for evidence of hypoxemia (Pao_2 <80 mm Hg), respiratory acidosis ($Paco_2$ >45 mm Hg, pH <7.35), or respiratory alkalosis ($Paco_2$ <35 mm Hg, pH >7.45), which may be present with pulmonary congestion.
- Deliver humidified oxygen, as prescribed.
- Assess arterial oxygen saturation with a transcutaneous pulse oximeter. Normal oxygen saturation is 95%-99%. Levels of 90%-95% necessitate frequent assessment. Levels <90% require aggressive interventions to increase oxygen saturation. This is accomplished by increasing Fio_2, decreasing preload, and increasing the number of coughing and deep-breathing exercises.
- Unless contraindicated, place patient in high Fowler's position to facilitate gas exchange.
- Schedule coughing, deep breathing, and incentive spirometry q2-4h to prevent atelectasis.

Risk for infection related to presence of invasive catheters and lines and inadequate secondary defenses secondary to prolonged antibiotic use

Desired outcomes: Patient is free of secondary infection as evidenced by urine that is clear with characteristic odor, by wound healing within acceptable time frame, and by absence of erythema, warmth, and purulent drainage at insertion sites for IV lines. On resolution of acute stage of IE, patient remains normothermic with WBC count ≤11,000 μl, negative culture results, and HR ≤100 bpm. SVR is ≥900 dynes/sec/cm^{-5}, CO is ≤7 L/min, and Svo_2 is 60%-80%. Patient and significant others verbalize rationale for antibiotic therapy and identify where and how to obtain guidelines.

- Ensure strict aseptic technique for insertion site care for all invasive monitoring devices and IV lines.
- Change tubing, collection containers, and peripheral needles and catheters q48-72h, per agency protocol.
- Provide mouth care q4h to minimize the potential for fungal infections.
- For patients with indwelling urinary catheters, cleanse urinary meatus with soap and water during the daily bath. Inspect urine for evidence of infection, such as casts, cloudiness, or foul odor. Be alert to patient complaints of burning with urination.
- Monitor temperature, WBC count, and HR. Increases may be signs of infection.
- Calculate SVR whenever CO measurements are obtained. Septic shock is demonstrated by an increase in CO, a drop in SVR, and increased Svo_2 during the early stages.
- Teach patient and significant others the importance of reporting signs and symptoms of recurring infections (e.g., fever, malaise, flushing, anorexia) or heart failure (e.g., dyspnea, tachypnea, tachycardia, digital clubbing, edema, ascites, weight gain, jaundice).
- Stress the importance of prophylactic antibiotics before invasive procedures such as dental examinations or surgery. The American Heart

Association publishes general guidelines for prophylactic antibiotic treatment for preventing IE (see Table 4-9).

Altered renal, gastrointestinal, peripheral, cardiopulmonary, and cerebral tissue perfusion (or risk for same) related to interrupted arterial blood flow secondary to emboli caused by vegetations

Desired outcome: Patient has adequate perfusion as evidenced by urine output ≥0.5 ml/kg/h; 5-34 bowel sounds/min; peripheral pulses >2+ on a 0-4+ scale; warm and dry skin; BP ≥90/60 mm Hg; RR 12-20 breaths/min with normal pattern and depth (eupnea); normal sinus rhythm on ECG; and orientation to time, place, and person.

Note: Unlike peripheral venous emboli, these emboli are caused by the vegetations; therefore there is nothing that can be done by physicians or nurses to prevent their occurrence.

- Monitor I&O at frequent intervals. Be alert to urinary output <0.5 ml/kg/h for 2 consecutive hours. Report oliguria, because it may be a sign of renal infarct.
- Monitor bowel sounds q2h. Report hypoactive or absent bowel sounds, because they may be the result of mesenteric infarct.
- Assess peripheral pulses, color, and temperature of extremities. Be alert to pulses ≤2+ (on a 0-4+ scale) and extremities that are pale and cool, inasmuch as these findings may denote embolization to the extremities.
- Monitor patient for confusion, changes in sensorimotor capabilities, or changes in cognition. Alterations can occur with cerebral emboli.
- Assess for chest pain, decreased BP, SOB, ischemic or injury pattern on 12-lead ECG, or elevated cardiac enzyme levels. These may be signs of myocardial infarction due to emboli of vegetations that have migrated to the coronary arteries (see "Acute Myocardial Infarction," p. 278).
- Assess for and report appearance of splinter hemorrhages, Osler's nodes, Janeway lesions, and Roth's spots (see "Assessment," p. 335).

ADDITIONAL NURSING DIAGNOSES

As appropriate, see nursing diagnoses and interventions in "Nutritional Support," p. 12; "Hemodynamic Monitoring," p. 37; "Prolonged Immobility," p. 78; "Psychosocial Support," p. 88; "Psychosocial Support for the Patient's Family and Significant Others," p. 100; "Congestive Heart Failure," p. 293; and "Cardiogenic Shock," p. 367.

Acute pericarditis

PATHOPHYSIOLOGY

Pericarditis is the general term for an inflammatory process involving the epicardial surface of the heart and the protective covering, the pericardium. The inflammatory process can occur as the result of a myocardial infarction, an infection, or an immunologic, chemical, or mechanical event. Often early pericarditis manifests as a dry irritation, whereas late pericarditis (after 6 wk) involves pericardial effusions that

T A B L E   4 - 1 2   **Conditions associated with the development of pericarditis**

Autoimmune cardiac injury	Neoplasms
· Dressler's syndrome (post-MI)	Radiation injury
· Postpericardiotomy syndrome	Rheumatologic disease
Drug induced	· Rheumatic fever
· procainamide, hydralazine	· Rheumatoid arthritis
Idiopathic	· Systemic lupus erythematosus
Infection	Trauma
Myocardial infarction	Uremia

can lead to cardiac tamponade if severe. Most often pericarditis is seen in the ICU as a secondary finding in the critically ill patient. Because symptoms can be masked by the primary condition, astute assessment and recognition are essential for appropriate treatment. Occasionally patients are admitted to the ICU with cardiac decompensation caused by the effusions.

The initial pathophysiologic findings of pericarditis include infiltration of polymorphonuclear leukocytes, increased vascularity, and fibrin deposit. The inflammation may spread from the pericardium to the epicardium or pleura. Eventually, the visceral layer develops exudates, and in some cases adhesions may develop. (See Table 4-12 for conditions that are associated with the development of pericarditis.) Large effusions can lead to cardiac tamponade (see p. 152). The excess fluid compresses the heart and impairs filling of the chambers. In addition, ejection of the left ventricle is impaired.

ASSESSMENT

CLINICAL PRESENTATION The chief complaint is chest pain, but location and quality can vary. Usually the pain is aggravated by a supine position, coughing, deep inspiration, and swallowing. Dyspnea develops because of shallow breathing to prevent pain.

Early indicators: Fatigue, pallor, fever, and anorexia.

Late indicators (evident after development of effusions):   Increased dyspnea, crackles, and neck vein distention. Heart sounds will be distant, and the pulmonic component of the second heart sound will be accentuated. Joint pain may be present when inflammation is generalized.

PHYSICAL ASSESSMENT Auscultation of heart sounds often will reveal an intermittent friction rub composed of one, two, or three components: atrial systole, ventricular systole, and rapid ventricular filling. The rub is heard best with the patient sitting and leaning forward and the diaphragm of the stethoscope positioned at the left lower sternal border.

Note: A friction rub may not be heard, even in the presence of pericarditis.

Pulsus paradoxus: BP should be checked for a paradox >10 mm Hg pressure. Normally the systolic pressure is slightly higher during

T A B L E 4 - 1 3   ECG changes with pericarditis

Stage	Time of change	Pattern
1	Onset of pain	ST segments have a concave elevation in all leads except aV_L and V_1; T waves are upright
2	1-7 days	Return of ST segments to baseline with T-wave flattening
3	1-2 wk	Inversion of T waves without R or Q changes
4	Weeks to months	Normalization of T waves

the inspiratory portion of the respiratory cycle. When effusions are present, arterial systolic BP will be decreased during inspiration and the difference will be >10 mm Hg. For procedure, see "Acute Cardiac Tamponade," p. 155.

ECG FINDINGS During acute episodes, atrial dysrhythmias such as PAT, PACs, atrial flutter, or atrial fibrillation may occur. Late dysrhythmias include ventricular ectopy or bundle-branch blocks if the inflammatory process involves the ventricles. Diffuse ST-segment elevation can be documented as described in Table 4-13.

HEMODYNAMIC MEASUREMENTS If a pulmonary artery catheter is in place, it will reveal elevated CVP, PAP, and PAWP. As effusions increase, cardiac output will decrease. If adhesions are present, the filling of the chambers may be restricted, resulting in low volumes and pressures.

DIAGNOSTIC TESTS

ECG: Will show ST- or T-wave changes, which often are confused with ischemic changes. In pericarditis they are more diffuse and follow a four-stage pattern (see Table 4-13).

Echocardiography: Will show absence of echoes in the areas of effusion. This test, which is essential for quantifying and evaluating the trend of effusions, will appear normal if the pericarditis is present without effusions. Transesophageal echocardiography may be helpful in identifying some areas of effusion.

CT scan: Will differentiate restrictive pericarditis from constrictive myopathy *via* the appearance of thickened pericardium on the cross-sectional views of the thorax, which occurs with pericarditis.

Cardiac enzyme levels: May reveal elevation of the CK and MB bands if the epicardium is inflamed.

Cardiac technetium pyrophosphate scan: May show a diffuse regional uptake ("hot spot") in an area of epicardial inflammation.

Hematologic studies: ASO titer is elevated when the cause of the pericarditis is an immunologic disorder. If the pericarditis is the result of an infection, blood cultures will identify the infecting organism.

COLLABORATIVE MANAGEMENT

Bed rest: Enforced until pain and fever have disappeared. Activity limitations continue if effusions are present.

Pharmacotherapy
Nonsteroidal antiinflammatory drugs (NSAIDs): Preferred for reducing inflammation, particularly if the patient has had MI or cardiac surgery, inasmuch as these medications do not delay healing as do corticosteroids. In addition, these medications have fewer side effects than do steroids. Examples include aspirin 650 mg q3-4h, indomethacin 25-75 mg q6h, or ibuprofen.
Prednisone: Given if there is no response to NSAIDs. It is begun at 60-80 mg qd for 5-7 days and then tapered gradually.

Note: In the presence of effusions, anticoagulants are contraindicated because of the high risk of cardiac tamponade, which can result from bleeding into the pericardium.

Subxiphoid pericardiocentesis: Performed if effusions persist and cardiac status begins to decompensate. It removes fluid that is compressing the heart. Echocardiography is used to guide the catheter tip and assess the amount of effusion remaining. The pericardial catheter may be removed after the fluid has been withdrawn or may be left in place for several days to allow for gradual removal of fluid. Usually ≥100 ml is withdrawn q4-6h. The catheter is flushed with saline q4-6h after withdrawal of the effusion to prevent clotting. Strict aseptic technique is essential for preventing infection.
Pericardiectomy: To prevent cardiac compression or relieve the restriction. It may be necessary in chronic pericarditis for patients with recurrent effusions or adhesions.

NURSING DIAGNOSES AND INTERVENTIONS

Ineffective breathing pattern related to guarding due to chest pain
Desired outcome: Within 48 h of this diagnosis, patient demonstrates RR 12-20 breaths/min with normal depth and pattern (eupnea) and verbalizes that chest pain is controlled.
- Assess the character and intensity of the chest pain. Provide prescribed pain medication as needed.
- Teach patient to avoid aggravating factors such as a supine position. Encourage patient to alter his or her position to minimize the chest pain. The following positions may be helpful: side-lying, high-Fowler's, or sitting and leaning forward.
- Assess lung sounds q4h. If breath sounds are decreased, encourage patient to perform incentive spirometry exercises q2-4h along with coughing and deep-breathing exercises.
- To facilitate coughing and deep breathing, support patient's chest by splinting with pillows, or teach patient to press his or her arms against the chest for added support.

Activity intolerance related to bed rest, weakness, and fatigue secondary to impaired cardiac function, ineffective breathing pattern, or deconditioning
Desired outcome: Within 72 h of this diagnosis, patient exhibits cardiac tolerance to increasing levels of exercise as evidenced by peak HR ≤20 bpm over patient's resting HR, peak systolic BP ≤20 mm Hg over patient's resting systolic BP, systolic BP during peak exercise

≤20 mm Hg under patient's resting systolic BP, Svo_2 ≥60%, RR <24 breaths/min, normal sinus rhythm, warm and dry skin, and absence of crackles, murmurs, and chest pain during or immediately after activity.

Note: Steroid myopathy may develop in patients who receive high doses or long-term treatment with steroids. Muscle weakness occurs predominantly in the large proximal muscles. Patients experience difficulty in lifting objects and moving from a sitting position to a standing position.

- Assess the patient for evidence of muscle weakness; assist with activities as needed.
- Modify the activity plan for the patient with post-MI pericarditis who is receiving steroids. A lower activity level may help prevent thinning of the ventricular wall and reduce the risk of an aneurysm or rupture of the ventricle.
- Teach patient to resume activities gradually, as prescribed, allowing for adequate periods of rest between activities.
- For other interventions, see this nursing diagnosis in "Prolonged Immobility," p. 78.

ADDITIONAL NURSING DIAGNOSES

See "Acute Cardiac Tamponade" for **Decreased cardiac output,** p. 154. See "Renal Transplantation" for **Knowledge deficit:** Immunosuppressive medications and their side effects, p. 407; **Impaired skin integrity,** p. 409; and **Risk for infection,** p. 409. For other nursing diagnoses and interventions, see "Prolonged Immobility," p. 78.

Hypertensive crisis

PATHOPHYSIOLOGY

Hypertension is sustained elevation of the resting arterial pressure. In 1993 the American Heart Association (AHA) defined hypertension as elevation of BP above 140/90 mm Hg. More than 63 million Americans have hypertension. Because fatal stroke or other cardiac event can occur as a result of hypertension, the impact of this disease on mortality is greater than that of any other health problem. Table 4-14 describes the blood pressure classifications and the recommendations for follow-up.

Most often hypertension occurs as a primary disorder of unknown etiology. Secondary hypertension is the result of other disorders that alter the mechanisms that control BP. Many factors contribute to the development of secondary hypertension: (1) increase in secretion of catecholamines, (2) increase in secretion of renin by the kidneys, (3) increase in serum sodium and blood volume, (4) increase in plasma and extracellular fluid volume, (5) reduction in kidney perfusion pressure, (6) impairment of control mechanisms in the kidney, and (7) alteration in adrenal cortical hormone secretion. Table 4-15 lists the causes of secondary hypertension.

Hypertensive crisis is seen in about 1% of the population with hypertension. When it occurs, there is a threat of immediate vascular

T A B L E   4 - 1 4   Classification of blood pressure for adults and recommendations for follow-up

Category	Systolic pressure (mm Hg)	Diastolic pressure (mm Hg)	Follow-up
Normal	<130	<85	Recheck in 2 yr
High normal	130-139	85-89	Recheck in 1 yr*
Hypertension			
Stage I (mild)	140-159	90-99	Confirm within 2 mo
Stage II (moderate)	160-179	100-109	Evaluate or refer to source of care within 1 mo
Stage III (severe)	180-209	110-119	Evaluate or refer to source of care within 1 wk
Stage IV (very severe)	≥210	≥120	Evaluate or refer to source of treatment immediately

From the Joint National Committee: The Fifth Report of the Joint National Committee on Detection, Evaluation, and Treatment of High Blood Pressure (JNCV), *Arch Intern Med* 153:154-183, 1993.
*Begin instructions on life-style modification, including:
1. Lose weight if overweight.
2. Limit alcohol intake <1 oz ethanol/day (24 oz beer, 8 oz wine, or 2 oz whiskey).
3. Reduce sodium intake to <100 mmol/day (2.3 g sodium or 6 g sodium chloride).
4. Maintain adequate dietary potassium, calcium, and magnesium intake.
5. Stop smoking.
6. Reduce dietary saturated fat and cholesterol intake for general cardiovascular health.

necrosis, which can occur if the diastolic pressure exceeds 120 mm Hg, although necrosis also has been seen with mean arterial pressures (MAP) ≥150 mm Hg.

The rapidity of the rise in pressure may be more destructive than the actual BP level recorded. If left untreated, hypertensive crisis is fatal in 75% of affected persons within 1 yr. With current treatment techniques, there is a 30% 1-yr mortality rate and a 50% 5-yr mortality rate. Hypertensive crisis can lead to hypertensive encephalopathy as cerebral blood vessels dilate because of their inability to effect autoregulation. Blood flow is increased, and the excessive pressure drives fluid into the perivascular tissue, resulting in cerebral edema. The extreme pressure can cause arteriolar damage, as demonstrated by fibrinoid necrosis of the intima and media of the vessel wall. Although any organ is vulnerable, the eyes and kidneys are most likely to suffer damage, leading to blindness and renal failure.

Patients with hypertension who are admitted to the ICU may have a rebound elevation of the BP if their usual antihypertensive regimen is interrupted. In addition, a loss of BP control can occur because of the nature of the primary disorder, trauma, or the stress of the ICU. Complications of hypertension include nephrosclerosis, aortic dissec-

T A B L E 4 - 1 5   Causes of secondary hypertension

Renal disease	Endocrine disorders	Congenital disorders	Pregnancy-induced disorders	Drug-induced disorders
Acute glomerulonephritis	Cushing's syndrome	Adrenal hyperplasia	Pregnancy-induced hypertension (PIH)	Cyclosporine
Chronic pyelonephritis	Hyperparathyroidism	Coarctation of the aorta	Preeclampsia	Oral contraceptives
Hydronephrosis	Pheochromocytoma		Eclampsia	Steroids
Renal tumors	Primary aldosteronism			
Renovascular hypertension				

tion, coronary artery disease, congestive heart failure, strokes, and peripheral vascular disease.

Pheochromocytoma is a chromaffin-cell tumor of the adrenal medulla that causes secretion of high levels of catecholamines (epinephrine and norepinephrine). The surge of catecholamines causes episodic elevations of blood pressure, increased metabolism, and hyperglycemia. These surges can occur as often as 25 times a day or as infrequently as every 2 mo. While pheochromocytoma accounts for only 0.5% of all new cases of hypertension, it is found in a much larger proportion of individuals who experience hypertensive crisis. The tumor is most often benign (90% of cases).

ASSESSMENT

HISTORY AND RISK FACTORS Psychologic stress, diet high in sodium, and cigarette smoking increase the risk of developing high BP. Hypertension is a familial disease; genetic and environmental factors contribute to its etiology. Hypertension is a risk factor for angina and MI. See "Acute Chest Pain," p. 269, and "Acute Myocardial Infarction," p. 278.

CLINICAL PRESENTATION

Early Indicators: Although most patients are free of symptoms, vague discomfort, fatigue, dizziness, and headache can occur.

Late indicators (nearly always present during a hypertensive crisis): Throbbing suboccipital headache, irritability, confusion, somnolence, stupor, visual loss, focal deficits, and coma. The patient also may have signs of heart failure, including dyspnea on exertion, orthopnea, and paroxysmal nocturnal dyspnea. If coronary artery disease is present, angina may occur as a result of increased myocardial oxygen consumption caused by the high vascular resistance, which is evidenced by high BP. Renal symptoms include hematuria, nocturia, and azotemia. Nausea and vomiting also may occur.

PHYSICAL ASSESSMENT An accurate cuff pressure must be obtained, with three resting measurements taken at least 3-5 min apart. A well-calibrated manometer with a properly fitting cuff or an automatic blood pressure recorder should be selected for use. The bladder of the cuff must encircle the arm and cover two thirds of the length of the upper portion of the arm. Note when the patient last smoked or used any nicotine product, how much caffeine was consumed during the previous 4 h, and whether adrenergic stimulants (e.g., OTC decongestants or bronchodilators) have been used within the past 24 h, because these substances elevate BP.

Cardiac assessment: Evaluates for left ventricular hypertrophy, which results from the need of the heart to pump against the high SVR or afterload. A left ventricular heave may be palpated with the palm of the hand at the mitral area (fifth ICS at the MCL). A fourth heart sound or S_4 gallop may be auscultated in the same site with the stethoscope bell. If cardiac failure is present or the left ventricle is enlarged, the apical impulse will be felt nearer to the anterior axillary line (AAL) instead of the MCL. In addition, crackles may be auscultated in the presence of cardiac failure. Pulsus alternans, an alteration in pulse pressure with a regular rhythm, may be palpated at any of the major pulse points. All peripheral pulses should be palpated bilaterally. With coarctation of the aorta, the femoral pulses will be bilaterally weak with a slow up-stroke, whereas the radial and brachial pulses will be normal or bounding.

Eye assessment: A fundoscope is used to determine whether hemorrhage, fluffy cotton exudates, or arterial-venous nicking of the vessels has occurred. When these changes occur, visual perception is decreased. Nurses should assess the patient's ability to read and recognize objects and people.

Neurologic assessment: May reveal evidence of a residual neurologic deficit from a cerebral infarct or ischemic event, as manifested by a positive Babinski's reflex (up-going toe), hemiparesis, hemiplegia, ataxia, confusion, or cognitive alterations.

Pheochromocytoma assessment: Paroxysmal elevations of BP associated with palpitations, tachycardia, headache, diaphoresis, pallor, warmth or flushing, tremor, excitation, fright, nervousness, feelings of impending doom, tachypnea, abdominal pain, nausea, and vomiting. Episodes also are associated with hyperglycemia and hypermetabolism. Postural hypotension and paradoxic response to antihypertensive medications may occur.

DIAGNOSTIC TESTS

The definitive test for hypertension is BP measurement. Once hypertension has been documented, many tests may be performed to determine the amount of end-organ damage or to diagnose the condition responsible for the development of secondary hypertension.

ECG: Left ventricular hypertrophy (LVH) is demonstrated by an increase in voltage in the LV precordial lead (V_{5-6}). In addition, a strain pattern of ST-segment depression and T-wave inversion reflects repolarization abnormalities due to the endocardial fibrosis that accompanies hypertrophy. General voltage criteria for LVH are (1) "R" in V_5 or V_6 plus "S" in V_1 >35 mm or (2) voltage of "R" in any precordial lead >25 mm.

Echocardiography: LVH with or without dilatation will be demonstrated on echo by an increase in the wall thickness with or without increased chamber size.

Chest x-ray: If dilatation of the left ventricle is present, the cardiac silhouette will be enlarged. If failure is present, there will be evidence of pulmonary congestion and pleural effusions. Notching of the aorta and a distended aortic root are indicative of coarctation of the aorta. If widening of the aorta is seen, dissection is suspected (see p. 358).

Urinalysis/urine culture: Urinalysis results will be normal until hypertension causes renal impairment. Specific gravity may be low (<1.010), and proteinuria may be present. Glomerulonephritis is suspected if the urine contains granular or red cell casts or if the patient has hematuria. Pyelonephritis is suspected if there is bacterial growth in the urine. Elevations of the 24-h urine vanillylmandelic acid (VMA) and urinary catecholamines (10-50 times normal) are indicative of pheochromocytoma, a rare catecholamine-producing tumor found in or near the adrenal glands. The VMA level is elevated only during episodes of hypertension. If the patient has Cushing's disease, the urine cortisol or ACTH level will be elevated.

Blood chemistry determinations: If renal parenchymal disease is present, the patient may have serum creatinine >1.3 mg/dl and BUN >20 mg/dl. The RBC count may fall because of hematuria.

Radiographic studies to detect pheochromocytoma: Angiography may identify an adrenal medulary tumor. An intravenous pyelogram with nephrotomography or CT scan may identify the adrenal tumor.

COLLABORATIVE MANAGEMENT

Treatment of hypertensive crisis: Necessitates immediate and rapid reduction in pressure.

Nitroprusside: Drug of choice because of its almost immediate vasodilatation effects. It is supplied in 50 mg vials, which must be reconstituted with 2-3 ml of sterile water, mixed in a 250 ml bag of D_5W, and infused *via* mechanical controller device. Usual initial dose is 10-25 μg/min, with increases of 5-10 μg q5min. Until oral treatment is effective, the maintenance dose for nitroprusside ranges from 0.25-10 μg/kg/min. This drug has a short action time, and BP will rise almost immediately if the drip is stopped. Direct arterial pressure monitoring is essential for the titration of this drug, with constant vigilance to prevent hypotension. When oral antihypertensives begin to affect the BP, nitroprusside weaning requires care to prevent hypotensive episodes. Because nitroprusside is unstable in light, the bag should be wrapped with the aluminum foil provided by the manufacturer. Nitroprusside is metabolized to thiocyanate, which can cause fatigue, nausea, tinnitus, blurred vision, and delirium. Serum thiocyanate levels should be drawn after 48 h of use and regularly thereafter. Levels <10 mg/dl are considered safe.

Diazoxide: A vasodilator. It is administered in a bolus of 50-150 mg, which may be repeated, or given 15-30 mg/min per IV infusion. Within minutes the SVR drops by about 25%, but the HR can increase by 30 bpm, which can lead to angina in the individual with coronary artery disease. The effects can last for hours.

Labetalol hydrochloride: A fast-acting alpha- and beta-blocker, which also can be used to treat the patient in hypertensive crisis. It is less likely to cause hypotension than is diazoxide. It is administered by IV push slowly, beginning with a 20-80 mg dose. This can be repeated q10min, or a continuous infusion of 2 mg/min can be administered. The usual cumulative dose is 50-200 mg. Keep the patient supine during the injection and for up to 1 h afterward. Maintain BP checks q5min × 6 and then q30min × 4. Monitor for bronchospasm, heart block, or orthostatic hypotension.

Nitroglycerin: A coronary and peripheral vasodilator. It is supplied in a 50-mg vial, which is added to a 250-ml glass bottle of D_5W. The solution may be concentrated to prevent fluid overload if higher doses are needed to control the BP. Nitroglycerin is administered *via* an infusion controller starting at 5 μg/min. Onset of action is rapid, so BP must be monitored closely during titration of the drug. Increase by 5-10 μg q3-5 min. Headache is the most common side effect and requires analgesic administration.

Hydralazine: A potent vasodilator. It is administered as a 10- to 20-mg IV bolus or a 10- to 40-mg IM injection. The onset of action is 10-30 min, with a duration of 2-6 h. Adverse effects include tachycardia, headache, vomiting, and aggravation of angina.

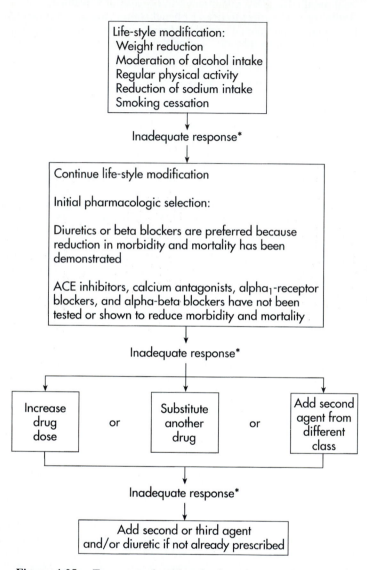

Figure 4-25: Treatment algorithm for hypertension. Asterisk indicates that the patient achieved goal blood pressure or is making considerable progress toward that goal. ACE indicates angiotensin-converting enzyme (From the Joint National Committee: The Fifth Report of the Joint National Committee on Detection, Evaluation, and Treatment of High Blood Pressure [JNC V], *Arch Intern Med* 153:154-183, 1993.)

Enalapril: An angiotensin-converting enzyme (ACE) inhibitor. Usual dose is 0.625-1.25 mg IV bolus, administered over a 5-min period. If an inadequate response is seen, 0.625 mg may be repeated in 1 h. Thereafter, the initial dose may be repeated q6h. Patients on diuretics should receive the lower standard dose. Peak effect from the first IV dose will be observed at 4 h, but for subsequent doses, the peak effect occurs 1 h after administration. Enalapril should be used with caution in individuals with renal failure or bilateral renal artery stenosis.

Methyldopate: An adrenergic blocking agent. Onset of action is 30-60 min. Usual dose is a 250- to 500-mg infusion over 1 h. Mix the drug in 100 ml D_5W or prepare a solution of 10 mg/1 ml. Use with caution in individuals with renal or liver disease.

Phentolamine: An alpha-adrenergic blocking agent. While this drug reduces afterload, it has minimal effect in reducing BP except for secondary hypertension caused by pheochromocytoma. A dose of 5-15 mg is administered *via* IV push. Onset of action is 1-2 min. Use this drug with caution in individuals with coronary artery disease.

Nifedipine: A calcium channel blocking agent, which may be given sublingually by piercing the capsule to provide rapid treatment of hypertension. Initial dosage is 10 mg given sublingually, and it may be repeated after 30 min.

Oral antihypertensive medications: These drugs are added as soon as the patient is able to take oral medications. Examples include captopril, clonidine, and labetalol.

Life-style alterations: Behavioral changes are the cornerstones of medical treatment for early and established hypertension. Normal body weight should be maintained. Alcohol consumption should be <1 oz ethanol a day. Daily intake of sodium for the average adult should be modified to 2 or 3 g for the person with hypertension. Smoking cessation is imperative to halt the injury to the intima of the coronary and peripheral vessels, which leads to the development of atherosclerosis, and to reduce the workload of the heart. A regular aerobic program has been proved beneficial in maintaining better control of blood pressure. This should consist of 30 min of exercise 3-5 times per week at a target heart rate of 60%-80% maximum.

Pharmacotherapy: Maintenance pharmacotherapy for hypertension traditionally has been approached in a stepwise fashion. This approach has been accepted and promoted by the American Heart Association. After an adequate trial of step 1, the patient is advanced to step 2 if the BP remains refractory to treatment. An adequate trial of various medications for each step is attempted. Figure 4-25 identifies the algorithm, and Table 4-16 lists the medications, usual dosage, schedule, and potential side effects of the antihypertensive agents commonly used.

Surgical treatment: Although there is no surgical intervention for primary hypertension, several forms of secondary hypertension respond well to the surgical correction of the primary problem. A coarctation of the aorta can be repaired *via* removal of the narrowed area of the vessel with insertion of a Teflon aortic graft. Renal artery stenosis may be corrected by grafting or by renal artery angioplasty. Pheochromocytoma is a rare epinephrine- and norepinephrine-producing tumor

T A B L E 4 - 1 6 Medications used in the treatment of hypertension

Drug type	Medication	Dosage/schedule	Side effects
Diuretics			
Thiazides/related compounds	bendroflumethiazide	2.5-5 mg; qd	Hypokalemia and hyperuricemia in the first two categories; hypercholesterolemia, hypoglycemia, impotence, and indigestion in all categories of diuretics
	benzthiazide	12.5-50 mg; qd	
	chlorothiazide	125-500 mg; q6-12h	
	chlorthalidone	12.5-50 mg; q24-72h	
	cyclothiazide	1-2 mg; qd	
	hydrochlorothiazide	12.5-50 mg; q12-24h	
	hydroflumethiazide	12.5-50 mg; qd	
	indapamide	2.5-5 mg; qd	
	methyclothiazide	2.5-5 mg; qd	
	metolazone	0.5-5 mg; qd	
	polythiazide	1-4 mg; qd	
	trichlormethiazide	1-4 mg; qd	
Loop diuretics	bumetanide	0.25-2.5 mg; q12h	
	ethacrynic acid	25-200 mg; q12h	
	furosemide	20-320 mg; q6-24h	
Potassium-sparing agents	amiloride	5-10 mg; q12-24	Gynecomastia; menstrual abnormalities
	spironolactone	25-200 mg; q8-12h	
	triamterene	100-300 mg; q12h	
Adrenergic-inhibiting agents			
Beta-blockers	atenolol*	25-200 mg; qd	Fatigue, drowsiness, depression, fluid retention, heart failure, impotence, hypoglycemia, flushing, bronchospasm (for all beta-blockers); bronchospasm is diminished with cardioselective (beta$_1$-blockers)
	betaxolol*	5-40 mg; qd	
	bisoprolol*	5-20 mg; qd	
	metaprolol*	50-200 mg; qd-bid	

Category	Drug	Dose	Notes
Beta-blockers with ISA	nadolol	20-240 mg; qd	May cause severe postural hypotension; dose adjustments should be made based on standing BP
	propranolol	40-120 mg; q6-24h	
	timolol	20-40 mg; bid	
	acebutolol*	100-600 mg; bid	
	carteolol	2.5-10 mg; qd	
	penbutolol	20-80 mg; qd	
	pindolol	5-30 mg; bid	
Alpha- and beta-blocker	labetalol	100-600 mg; bid	
Alpha-receptor blockers	doxazosin	1-16 mg; qd	Hypoglycemia, diarrhea, hypotension, flushing First-dose syncope, blurred vision
	phentolamine	50 mg; qid	
	prazosin HCl	1-7 mg; tid	
	terazosin	1-20 mg; qd	
ACE inhibitors	benazepril	10-40 mg; qd-bid	To prevent severe hypotension, reduce dose of patient's diuretic; may cause hyperkalemia in persons with renal failure; may cause acute renal failure in bilateral renal artery stenosis; also may cause profound postural hypotension; dose adjustments should be made based on standing BP
	captopril	6.25-75 mg; bid-tid	
	cilazpril	2.5-5 mg; qd-bid	
	enalapril	2.5-40 mg; qd-bid	
	fosinopril	10-40 mg; qd-bid	
	lininopril	5-40 mg; qd-bid	
	perindopril	1-16 mg; qd-bid	
	quinapril	5-80 mg; qd-bid	
	ramipril	1.25-20 mg; qd-bid	
	spirapril	12.5-50 mg; qd-bid	
Calcium channel blockers	diltiazem	20-90 mg; tid-qid	Constipation; peripheral edema
	verapamil	30-90 mg; tid-qid	

Continued.

T A B L E 4 - 1 6   Medications used in the treatment of hypertension—cont'd

Drug type	Medication	Dosage/schedule	Side effects
Dihydropyridines	amlodipine	2.5-10 mg; qd	Dihydropyridines are more potent peripheral vasodilators than diltiazem and verapamil and may cause more flushing, peripheral edema, tachycardia, dizziness, and headache
	felodipine	5-20 mg; qd	
	isradipine	1.25-5 mg; bid	
	nicardipine	20-40 mg; bid	
	nifedipine	10-40 mg; tid	
Supplemental antihypertensive agents			
Central alpha-receptor blockers	clonidine HCl	0.1-6 mg; bid *or* 0.1-0.3 mg patch/week	Hypotension
	guanabenz	2-32 mg; bid	
	guanfacine	1-3 mg; qd	
	methyldopa	250 mg-1 g; bid-qid	Hemolytic anemia, depression, dry mouth, nasal stuffiness, impotence
Peripheral neuronal inhibitors	guanethidine	10-50 mg; qd	Hypotension, impotence, weight gain
	reserpine	0.1-0.5 mg; qd	Hypotension, hyperacidity, depression
Vasodilators	diazoxide	50-300 mg IV push	Hypotension; fluid retention
	hydralazine	20-40 mg IV push; 10-50 mg PO q6-12h	Lupus syndrome, angina, sodium retention
	minoxidil	2.5-80 mg PO; q12-24h	Edema, pericardial effusions, increased hair growth
	nitroprusside	0.5 μg/kg/min IV (immediate effects last only 1-5 min)	Hypotension; thiocyanate toxicity (if >20 mg/dl) as evidenced by fatigue, anorexia, weakness, delirium

ACE, Angiotensin-converting enzyme; *ISA,* intrinsic sympathomimetic activity.
*Cardioselective.

found near the adrenal medulla, which results in hypertensive crisis precipitated by stress, postural change, or abdominal pressure. Surgical removal of the tumor(s) returns the patient to a normotensive state.

NURSING DIAGNOSES

Altered cardiopulmonary, cerebral, and renal tissue perfusion related to interruption of arterial flow secondary to vasoconstriction that occurs with interruption of the normal BP control mechanism; or interruption of venous flow secondary to vasodilatation or tissue edema that occurs with loss of autoregulation

Desired outcome: Tissue perfusion is established within 24 h as evidenced by systemic arterial BP 110-160/70-110 mm Hg (or within patient's normal range); MAP 70-105 mm Hg; equal and normoreactive pupils; strength and tone of the extremities bilaterally equal and normal for patient; orientation to time, place, and person; urinary output ≥0.5 ml/kg/h; and stable weight. Within 48 h systolic BP is <140 mm Hg and diastolic BP is <90 mm Hg, with MAP 70-105 mm Hg.

- Monitor BP and MAP q1-5min during titration of the medications. As patient's condition stabilizes, perform these assessments q15min-1h. Be alert to sudden drops or elevations in the BP. As the oral medications begin to affect the BP, wean nitroprusside and other potent vasodilators gradually to prevent hypotensive episodes. Continuous monitoring by arterial cannulation or automatic BP apparatus is recommended.
  - □ Correlate cuff pressure with pressure from arterial cannulation.
  - □ Determine ideal range for BP control and maximal nitroprusside dose with physician. Usually the following guidelines are used: systolic BP <140-160 mm Hg, MAP <110 mm Hg, or diastolic BP <90 mm Hg.
  - □ If hypotension develops, decrease or stop nitroprusside infusion until the pressure rises.
- Assess patient for neurologic deficit by performing hourly neurostatus checks. Be alert to sensorimotor deficit if MAP is >140 mm Hg. As patient's condition stabilizes and BP becomes controlled, perform neurostatus checks at least q4h.
- Monitor patient for changes in fundoscopic examination. Consult physician if hemorrhages or fluffy cotton exudates are present.
- Assess patient for evidence of decreasing renal perfusion by monitoring I&O and weighing patient daily. Consult physician if urinary output is <0.5 ml/kg/h for 2 consecutive hours or of weight gain ≥1 kg (2 lbs). Also be alert to azotemia (increasing BUN), decreasing creatinine clearance, and increasing serum creatinine. Optimal laboratory values are: BUN ≥20 mg/dl, creatinine clearance ≥9.5 ml/min, and serum creatinine ≤1.5 mg/dl.

Pain related to headache secondary to cerebral edema occurring with high perfusion pressures

Desired outcomes: Patient's subjective evaluation of pain improves within 12-24 h, as documented by a pain scale. Nonverbal indicators, such as grimacing, are absent or diminished.

- Monitor patient for headache pain at frequent intervals. Devise a pain scale with patient, rating discomfort from 0 (no pain) to 10 (severe pain).

- Provide pain medications as prescribed. A variety of analgesics may be used, ranging from acetaminophen with codeine to morphine, depending on the severity of the symptoms. Assess effectiveness of the pain medication, using the pain scale to determine degree of relief obtained.
- Teach patient relaxation techniques to use in conjunction with the medications. Guided imagery, meditation, progressive muscle relaxation, and music therapy often are effective. See **Health-seeking behavior,** p. 323.
- Maintain a quiet, low-lit environment that is free of extensive distraction and stimulation. Limit visitations, as indicated.

Sensory/perceptual alterations related to decreased visual acuity secondary to retinal damage occurring with high perfusion pressures; related to pain secondary to cerebral edema

Desired outcome: Within 24-48 h of this diagnosis, patient reads print, recognizes objects or people, and demonstrates coordination of movement.

- Assess patient for signs of decreased visual acuity by monitoring patient's ability to read and recognize objects or people. Evaluate patient's coordination of movement to determine depth perception. Perform a fundoscopic examination q8h for evidence of findings discussed on p. 350. Consult physician for significant findings.
- If patient has decreased visual acuity, assist with feeding and other ADL and keep patient's personal effects within his or her visual field.
- Reassure patient and significant others that visual problems usually resolve when the BP is lowered sufficiently.

ADDITIONAL NURSING DIAGNOSES

For other nursing diagnoses and interventions, see the following as appropriate: "Hemodynamic Monitoring," p. 37; "Psychosocial Support," p. 88; and "Psychosocial Support for the Patient's Family and Significant Others," p. 100.

Aortic aneurysm/dissection

PATHOPHYSIOLOGY

An aneurysm is any abnormal dilatation of an artery. When the aorta is involved, the complications can be life threatening owing to the potential for disruption of blood flow to a large portion of the body, including vital organs such as the brain, heart, kidneys, and gastrointestinal tract. A true aneurysm involves all three layers of the arterial wall (intima, media, and adventitia). There are two forms of true aneurysm: fusiform (a concentric, spindle-shaped deformity) or saccular (an eccentric, balloon-shaped deformity). A false aneurysm is a pulsatile hematoma caused by disruption of the intimal layer or the intimal and medial layers only.

   Most often, aneurysms develop at the site of an atherosclerotic lesion, which initially involves only the intimal layer of the aorta. As the lesion becomes more complicated, there is hemorrhage into the media, which weakens and dilates the arterial wall. With advancing age, the elastin in the aorta is decreased, which further weakens the vessel wall. Acute hypertension may decrease flow into the media, leading to ischemia, which further weakens this layer. The abdominal, thoracic, or ascending arch of the aorta may be affected. A familial tendency toward development of aortic aneurysm has been identified.

After the area of the aorta has been weakened, the law of Laplace promotes further weakening of the wall: as the aortic diameter expands, the tension increases, producing even more dilatation. The rate at which the aneurysm increases is not predictable; however, the likelihood of rupture or dissection increases dramatically when the size exceeds 6 cm.

Rupture of an abdominal aneurysm may lead to extravasation of blood either anteriorly into the peritoneal cavity or posteriorly into the retroperitoneal space. Anterior bleeds often occur rapidly and are associated with a high mortality rate due to rapid circulatory collapse. Posterior bleeds may lead to tamponade on the spinal cord, with neurologic deficits. Either form of rupture can lead to mesenteric ischemia. Surgical repair is the only treatment for rupture.

An *aortic dissection* is a longitudinal tear in the medial layer of the aortic wall caused by the driving pressure of a column of blood. The column of blood drives the dissection distally with the force of systole, and the diastolic recoil within the aorta forces the dissection in the proximal direction. Precipitating factors include medial necrosis from other disorders, trauma (e.g., blunt injury due to vehicular accident), or hypertension (see p. 346). The three types of aortic dissections first described by DeBakey are differentiated by the site of the intimal tear and the direction of dissection. In type I, which accounts for 60%-80% of all cases, the tear begins in the ascending aorta and the dissection extends beyond the aortic arch. Type II is the rarest form, with the intimal tear and entire dissection confined to the ascending aorta. Type III occurs in 20%-30% of all cases and involves a tear in the descending aorta, with distal dissection only.

Aortic dissection is a sudden and very serious threat to life because the disruption of the vessel may continue along any arterial branch of the aorta, compromising organs such as the heart, brain, and kidneys if the coronary, subclavian, innominate, and renal arteries are involved. Approximately 2,000 episodes occur annually, with a mortality rate approaching 100% if the dissection is left untreated.

ASSESSMENT

HISTORY AND RISK FACTORS Hypertension, connective tissue disorders (e.g., Marfan's or Ehlers-Danlos syndrome), coarctation of the aorta, blunt chest trauma, medial necrosis of the aorta, pregnancy, family history of aortic aneurysm.

CLINICAL PRESENTATION The major symptom is a sudden onset of severe, tearing chest or abdominal pain that is unrelieved by position or respiratory change. The pain may radiate to the back if the dissection is moving distally or to the neck if the dissection is moving proximally. With rupture of an abdominal aneurysm, pain will occur along the flank or lumbar back. Vasovagal responses such as diaphoresis, apprehension, nausea, vomiting, and faintness may occur. Signs of congestive heart failure may be seen if the dissection involves the coronary arteries or the aortic valve. Neurologic deficits such as confusion, sensorimotor changes, and lethargy may be the result of a dissection along the branches of the ascending aorta. Urine output will fall if the dissection extends to the renal arteries.

PHYSICAL ASSESSMENT Pulse deficits or BP differences between extremities are classic findings. A drop in BP or pulse at a site helps identify the location of the dissection, inasmuch as both will be decreased beyond the area of dissection. Usually the skin is pale and cool and there is sluggish capillary refill due to poor tissue perfusion. If bleeding extends to the pericardium, cardiac tamponade can occur (see p. 152).

DIAGNOSTIC TESTS

Chest/abdominal x-ray: Will demonstrate widening of the aortic arch or descending aorta. Film taken with patient in upright position is necessary to demonstrate widening of the mediastinum.

Echocardiography of the aortic arch or descending aorta or transesophageal echocardiography: Will locate the site of dissection, inasmuch as the hemorrhage within the vessel will be an area of absent echoes and the total diameter of the vessel will be enlarged.

Aortography or digital subtraction angiography: Will locate actual site of the tear and dissection *via* use of contrast material.

CT scan: Often as useful as an aortogram in locating the dissection; its advantage over an aortogram is that it is noninvasive.

COLLABORATIVE MANAGEMENT

Antihypertensive therapy: Initiated as soon as possible to prevent further aortic dissection. Usually nitroprusside is started, as described in "Hypertensive Crisis," p. 351. An MAP of 70-80 mm Hg is desired. After control of the pressure is achieved, oral antihypertensive therapy is begun, along with gradual weaning from the IV infusion.

Propranolol therapy: To reduce velocity of the left ventricular ejection, HR, and BP. Usually it is administered intravenously in increments of 1 mg at 5-min intervals until the HR is reduced to 60-80 bpm. The maximal initial dosage should not exceed 0.15 mg/kg body weight. Additional dosages of 2-6 mg q4-6h then are administered until the condition can be managed with oral medications.

Absolute bed rest: To prevent further dissection. This may continue for weeks until the dissection has stabilized.

Pain relief: Usually achieved with IV morphine sulfate, 2-10 mg.

Sedation: To prevent sympathetic stimulation, which can increase BP. Diazepam 2-10 mg may be given q4-6h.

Long-term medical management: Aimed at maintaining systolic BP under 130 mm Hg to prevent redissection.

Surgical treatment: Recommended for proximal dissection, distal dissection when vital organ compromise occurs, impending rupture, or when pain and BP are refractory to medications. The surgery involves removal of the dissected vessel sections and replacement of the vessel sections with Teflon grafts.

NURSING DIAGNOSES AND INTERVENTIONS

Altered peripheral, cardiopulmonary, renal, and cerebral tissue perfusion related to interruption of arterial blood flow secondary to narrowed aortic lumen

Desired outcome: Within 48 h of this diagnosis, patient has adequate tissue perfusion as evidenced by distal pulses bilaterally equal and >2+ on a 0-4+ scale; brisk capillary refill (<2 sec); warm skin; bilaterally equal sensations in the extremities; bilaterally equal systolic BP; BP within patient's normal range; HR ≤100 bpm; normal sinus rhythm on ECG; urine output ≥0.5 ml/kg/h; equal and normoreactive pupils; and orientation to time, place, and person.

- Perform bilateral assessment of BP and distal pulses (particularly radial, femoral, and dorsalis pedis) hourly during initial phase of dissection, and then q4h as the patient's condition stabilizes. Note changes in strength or symmetry of distal pulses. Correlate cuff pressures with arterial monitor recordings. Be alert to any change in color, capillary refill, and temperature of each extremity. Report significant findings.
- If the difference in systolic BP between the extremities exceeds 10 mm Hg, consult physician immediately.
- Monitor for paresthesias of the extremities, a sign of decreased peripheral perfusion.
- Assess for signs of pericardial tamponade: distended neck veins, muffled heart sounds, decreased systolic BP (<90 mm Hg or >20 mm Hg drop in systolic trend), and paradoxic pulse.
- Assess cardiovascular status by monitoring heart rate and rhythm, ECG, and cardiac enzyme levels. A dissection along the coronary arteries will result in a myocardial infarction.
- Monitor urine output hourly. Consult physician if urine output is <0.5 ml/kg/h for 2 consecutive hours.
- Assess neurologic status hourly. Report restlessness and changes in LOC, pupil size, or reaction to light.
- Use relaxation techniques such as guided imagery or meditation to reduce BP. Avoid techniques that involve exercise, such as progressive muscle relaxation.

Pain related to biophysical injury secondary to necrosis at the aortic media and distal tissue hypoperfusion

Desired outcomes: Within 24-48 h of this diagnosis, patient's subjective evaluation of pain improves, as documented by a pain scale. Nonverbal indicators, such as grimacing, are decreased or absent.

- Monitor patient at frequent intervals for the presence of discomfort. Devise a pain scale with patient, rating discomfort from 0 (no pain) to 10 (severe pain). Medicate with analgesics as prescribed and rate relief obtained, using the pain scale.
- Teach patient relaxation techniques to use in conjunction with analgesics. Examples include guided imagery and meditation. Avoid progressive muscle relaxation, which may increase cardiac and aortic workload. For guidelines, see **Health-seeking behavior,** p. 323.
- During episodes of pain, assess for a change in peripheral pulses or altered hemodynamics (i.e., BP, PAP, PAWP, CO, SVR), because such changes often are associated with an increase in aortic dissection.

- Control BP during episodes of pain by titrating nitroprusside to maintain specified parameters.
- Immediately consult physician for any increase in the severity of pain, because it may indicate the need for emergency surgery.

ADDITIONAL NURSING DIAGNOSES

For other nursing diagnoses and interventions, see the following as appropriate: "Hemodynamic Monitoring," p. 37; "Prolonged Immobility," p. 78; "Psychosocial Support," p. 88; "Psychosocial Support for the Patient's Family and Significant Others," p. 100; and "Chest Trauma," p. 142.

Cardiogenic shock

PATHOPHYSIOLOGY

Cardiogenic shock is a state in which impaired cardiac function results in a profound reduction in peripheral blood flow that is incompatible with life. Usually, cardiogenic shock is caused by a massive MI that renders 40% or more of the myocardium dysfunctional because of necrosis or ischemia. As a result cardiac output is reduced and all tissues suffer from inadequate perfusion. With decreased perfusion to the heart, coronary flow is reduced, which further impairs cardiac function, decreasing cardiac output even more. Cardiogenic shock occurs with 15%-20% of all MIs and carries a mortality rate of 80% or more. Other causes of cardiogenic shock include depressed cardiac function, postcardiac surgery, massive pulmonary embolus, severe valvular dysfunction, end-stage cardiomyopathy, congestive heart failure, and cardiac tamponade.

The first stage of shock is characterized by increased sympathetic discharge as the baroreceptors at the carotid sinus and aortic arch become stimulated by the drop in BP. The release of epinephrine and norepinephrine is a compensatory mechanism that increases cardiac output by increasing the heart rate and contractility of the uninjured myocardium. Vasoconstriction, a mechanism that increases BP, occurs. The second or middle stage of shock is characterized by decreased perfusion to the brain, kidney, and heart. Lactate and pyruvic acid accumulate in the tissues, and metabolic acidosis occurs due to anaerobic metabolism. Blood is diverted from the skin, gut, and skeletal muscles to the vital organs: brain, heart, and kidneys. In the late stage of shock, which usually is irreversible, compensatory mechanisms become ineffective and multiple organ failure occurs.

At the cellular level, injury begins with hypoxia and loss of adenosine triphosphate (ATP), the energy source for all cellular functions. This leads to condensations in the mitochondria and swelling of the endoplasmic reticulum. The final phase of cellular damage is marked by swelling, rupture of the membrane, and complete cellular degradation. Cellular changes are similar in all body organs and types of tissue.

ASSESSMENT

CLINICAL PRESENTATION The assessment section under "Acute Myocardial Infarction" (see p. 278) describes the early stage of cardiogenic shock. As cardiogenic shock progresses, mentation is decreased due to poor cerebral perfusion. This is evidenced by agitation, restlessness, lethargy, confusion, or unresponsiveness. Urine output drops to <0.5 ml/kg/h as renal perfusion pressure drops and the kidneys attempt to compensate by triggering the renin-angiotensin system to retain more fluid.

PHYSICAL ASSESSMENT HR is elevated and the pulses are equal bilaterally, but they are weak and often irregular. Pulsus alternans may be palpated. Systolic BP is <90 mm Hg or at least 30 mm Hg below the patient's normal resting level. The skin is cold, clammy, and mottled due to compromised peripheral perfusion. Cardiac auscultation usually reveals S_3 or S_4 sounds because of the overdistended and noncompliant ventricle. Crackles are auscultated over the lung fields due to pulmonary congestion; hyperventilation is common.

HEMODYNAMIC MEASUREMENTS Cuff pressures are highly inaccurate during shock, mandating the use of arterial pressure monitoring. PAP monitoring is essential for guiding therapy during the early stage of shock. Arterial systolic and mean arterial pressures are decreased, with a decreased or narrow pulse pressure. Because contractility is greatly reduced, the stroke volume, ejection fraction, and cardiac output are decreased. RAP, PAP, PAEDP, and PAWP all are elevated as evidence of increased preload secondary to pulmonary congestion. SVR is increased because of vasoconstriction, which occurs as a compensatory mechanism when flow to an organ is reduced.

An oximetric catheter may be used to provide continuous measurement of the oxygen saturation of the mixed venous blood (Svo_2) in the pulmonary artery. The Svo_2 reflects the adequacy of oxygen supply in meeting tissue demands. When tissue demand is increased (as in exercise) or supply is decreased (as in cardiogenic shock), the Svo_2 will fall below the normal range of 60%-80%. The Svo_2 has a positive correlation with the cardiac output; thus continuous monitoring of Svo_2 provides an indirect but continuous assessment of CO. For detailed parameters for assessment, see Table 4-17.

DIAGNOSTIC TESTS

The diagnosis of cardiogenic shock is made by physical assessment and analysis of the hemodynamic profile. The primary problem, myocardial infarction, is diagnosed by enzyme changes and ECG (see discussion, p. 279). Other diagnostic tests are useful in assessing the effect of hypoperfusion on other organs.

ABG values: Hypoxemia (Pao_2 <80 mm Hg) and metabolic acidosis (pH <7.35, $Paco_2$ usually <35 mm Hg) are seen due to impaired oxygen diffusion in the alveoli and tissue lactic acidosis from anaerobic metabolism.

Serum chemistry values: Moderate hyperglycemia may be found as a result of epinephrine-induced glycogenolysis. Because the pancreas is hypoperfused, inadequate insulin is released to meet this need. Serum lactate levels may be elevated due to anaerobic metabolism. Elec-

T A B L E   4 - 1 7   Hemodynamic profile of shock

Values	RAP (mm Hg)	RVP (mm Hg)	PAP (mm Hg)	PAWP (mm Hg)	SVR (dynes/sec/cm^{-5})	Svo$_2$ (%)	CO (L/min)	CI (L/min/m^2)
Normal shock	4-6	25/0-5	20-30/8-15	6-12	900-1,200	60-80	4-7	2.5-4
Cardiogenic	6-10	40-50/6-15	50/25-30	25-40	>1,200	≤50	<4	≤1.5
Hypovolemic	0-2	15-20/0-2	15-20/2-8	2-6	>1,200	65	<4	2.5
Neurogenic	0-2	20-25/0-2	20-25/0-8	0-6	≤1,000	60-80	≥4-7	≥2.5
Septic								
Early	0-2	20-25/0-2	20-25/0-8	0-6	≤900	≥60	>7	≥4
Late	0-4	25/0-4	25/4-10	>12	>1,200	≤60	<4	<2.5

trolyte studies may reveal hypernatremia, which is reflective of a water deficit; hypokalemia, which may be associated with the cause of shock; or hyperkalemia, which may be seen with renal failure secondary to the shock state.

Urinalysis: Urine sodium, osmolality, and creatinine levels are reflective of the patient's renal status.

Coagulation profile: Although coagulation studies often are abnormal, there is no established pattern with cardiogenic shock.

ECG: While not specific for cardiogenic shock, dysrhythmias may occur due to infarction or injury to areas of the conduction system and/or myocardium or due to electrolyte imbalance.

COLLABORATIVE MANAGEMENT

Oxygen therapy: For oxygenation of the tissues. If dyspnea, hypoxemia, acidosis, or pulmonary congestion worsens, intubation and mechanical ventilation will be necessary. Morphine sulfate 2 mg IV push may assist in reducing pulmonary congestion, thereby relieving dyspnea and increasing Pao_2.

Correction of acidosis: Sodium bicarbonate delivered by IV push and guided by serial ABG checks to assess effectiveness of treatment.

Correction of electrolyte imbalance: Replacement of potassium, sodium, chloride, or calcium as indicated by serum chemistry findings.

Hemodynamic monitoring: Arterial and pulmonary artery catheters are inserted to guide pharmacologic therapy.

Diuretics: To decrease preload and improve stroke volume and cardiac output. Diuretics such as furosemide 40-200 mg IV push or ethacrynic acid 25-100 ml IV push may be given. Morphine sulfate also reduces preload. Nitrates such as oral, topical, or IV nitroglycerin and IV nitroprusside (Nipride) may be used to decrease filling pressures *via* venous dilatation.

Note: It may be necessary to increase preload if the patient is hypovolemic. In this situation, fluids are increased cautiously, the patient is monitored carefully, and diuretics are discontinued or avoided.

Positive inotropic agents: To improve contractility of the uninjured myocardium and to increase cardiac output. Dopamine infusions at 2-20 μg/kg/min are titrated to accomplish the desired effect. Higher doses increase HR and SVR, which increase the myocardial workload. Dobutamine infusions of 2-20 μg/kg/min increase contractility and decrease preload with less of an increase in HR, but they may decrease renal perfusion. Amrinone infusions of 1-10 μg/kg/min provide the same inotropic effect.

Vasopressors: To increase BP to an adequate mean level (usually $\geq$70 mm Hg) that will perfuse the tissues. This is accomplished by stimulating the alpha-adrenergic receptors in the blood vessels, which causes vasoconstriction. Vasopressors that may be used include dopamine, norepinephrine, epinephrine, phenylephrine, and methoxamine (see Appendix 7).

Intraaortic balloon pump (IABP):   A counterpulsation device that assists the failing heart by decreasing afterload and increasing coronary artery perfusion. It may be used in cardiogenic shock, heart failure, unstable angina, precardiac and postcardiac surgery, refractory ventricular dysrhythmias, cardiomyopathy, and post-PTCA complications, as well as in patients awaiting heart transplantation. IABP is a temporary measure that supports the heart and circulation for up to 30 days. It is used as an adjunct to medical therapy.

Balloon insertion can be performed emergently at the bedside or under controlled conditions during fluoroscopic examination. A local anesthetic agent is injected over the femoral artery, the introducer sheath is inserted, and the balloon is passed through the sheath into the thoracic aorta. The catheter is placed so that the balloon is below the left subclavian artery and above the renal artery. If the balloon migrates in either direction, arterial flow can be obstructed. The balloon is then unwrapped and connected to the pump console. Pumping is timed according to the ECG or arterial pressure waveform. Balloon inflation occurs with diastole, and deflation occurs with systole.

The patient derives benefits from both phases of balloon pumping. Balloon inflation, the first phase, is termed "diastolic augmentation." During this phase there is an increase in blood flow antegrade and retrograde within the aorta. Coronary artery blood flow is increased, resulting in increased oxygen supply to the myocardium. There also is increased blood flow to the kidneys, improving urinary output. Systolic unloading or balloon deflation is the second phase. Aortic pressure decreases rapidly, reducing afterload and resistance to blood flow out of the left ventricle and decreasing ventricular wall tension. With reduced afterload the ventricle empties more completely, stroke volume rises, and myocardial oxygen use diminishes. Clinical signs of the balloon's benefits include increased BP, increased measured cardiac output, increased urinary flow, improved mental alertness, warm extremities, palpable peripheral pulses, decreased chest pain, and improvement of the ECG changes that denote ischemia.

Complications of IABP therapy include aortic dissection, thrombus formation, impaired circulation to the involved leg, sepsis, obstruction to the left subclavian artery blood flow, obstruction to the renal and mesenteric arteries, and paraplegia (due to spinal artery thrombosis). In addition, problems such as pneumonia and dermal ulcers can occur as a result of prolonged immobility.

Note: Pulmonary artery balloon counterpulsation (intrapulmonary artery balloon pump) is available for support of the right ventricle after cardiac surgery. The catheter usually is inserted during surgery and involves creation of an artificial diverticulum on the pulmonary artery. During systole the balloon is deflated and right ventricle stroke volume is directed into the diverticulum, which reduces afterload. During diastole the balloon inflates and the cardiac output is propelled into the pulmonary vessels.

Heart-assist device: A mechanical ventricular assist device (VAD) is used to support the patient with massive left ventricular and/or right ventricular dysfunction. The ˙VAD provides a conduit that diverts blood from the ventricle to an artificial pump. The VAD can maintain circulation and decreased myocardial workload to promote ventricular recovery. Candidates for this device include individuals with acute ventricular dysfunction; shock after cardiotomy, angio-plasty, or myocardial infarction; cardiac arrest; or massive pulmonary embolism.

In general, the right ventricle recovers within 5 days and the left ventricle recovers within 10 days. This device is used as a temporary measure to promote rest and healing of the damaged myocardium. Left ventricular assistance is provided through either percutaneous cannu-lation of the femoral artery or direct cannulation of the atrium and as-cending aorta, whereas a right VAD is used in the right atrium and the main pulmonary artery. In individuals with right and left ventricular failure, biventricular assistance is available. As the patient's overall condition improves, the goal is gradual weaning of the patient from the device by decreasing the flow rate.

Complications of the assist device include coagulopathy, bleeding, embolization, infection, sepsis, right ventricular failure (with left-sided heart assist only), and renal failure. Because of the critical nature of these patients' condition and their need for constant monitoring by means of multiple assessment modalities, highly specialized nursing care is imperative.

Emergency cardiac catheterization: To determine patient's suit-ability for emergency PTCA, CABG, or arthrectomy.

Emergency coronary artery bypass graft: To reperfuse areas with reversible injury patterns. This procedure will not be as beneficial if the tissue already is necrotic as evidenced by Q waves on the ECG (see discussion, p. 281). At the time of surgery a left ventricular an-eurysmectomy may be performed to remove the thin-walled, dysfunc-tional sac.

Emergency percutaneous transluminal coronary angioplasty: To reperfuse areas of the myocardium with reversible injury pattern (see discussion, p. 271).

Thrombolytic therapy: For reperfusion of the injured and unin-farcted myocardium (see discussion, p. 374).

Heart transplantation: To replace the failing heart with a suitably matched donor organ. The recipient is screened carefully to ensure that all other organs are still functional.

NURSING DIAGNOSES AND INTERVENTIONS

Decreased cardiac output related to increased afterload, increased preload, or decreased contractility secondary to loss of $\geq 40\%$ of myo-cardial functional mass

Desired outcome: Before weaning from assist device or pharmaco-logic agents is attempted, the patient's hemodynamic function is as near the acceptable limits as possible as evidenced by CO ≥ 4 L/min, BP $\geq 90/60$ mm Hg, SVR $\leq 1,200$ dynes/sec/cm^{-5}, and PAWP ≤ 12 mm Hg.

- On a continuous basis, monitor arterial BP, PAP, Svo$_2$, and heart rate and rhythm. Titrate vasoactive drugs to achieve a CO between 4-7 L/min, arterial BP $\geq 90/60$, and PAWP ≤ 12 mm Hg.
- Assess cardiac output and SVR q1-4h and after every change in phar-macologic therapy. Consult physician if SVR increases ($> 1,200$ dynes/sec/cm^{-5}), inasmuch as nitroprusside or similar medication may be needed to decrease excessive afterload.

T A B L E   4 - 1 8 Fluid challenge guidelines in cardiogenic shock

Assessment	PAWP (mm Hg)	Fluids
CO low and PAWP low or normal	<6	200 ml infused over 10 min
	6-12	100 ml infused over 10 min
	≥12	50 ml infused over 10 min
PAWP increases during infusion	>6	Return to KVO rate
	≤3	Continue infusion
Assess PAWP after 10 min	If >3 or <6	Repeat challenge

KVO, Keep vein open.

- Auscultate lung sounds q1-2h and monitor urinary output. Report changes, including an increase in crackles and decreased urine output, because additional diuretics may be necessary.
- To prevent further decreases in BP, do not increase the angle of the HOB more than 30 degrees.
- Treat ventricular dysrhythmias with prescribed lidocaine, procainamide hydrochloride, or bretylium infusions.
- Be prepared to employ pacing if bradycardia or a second- or third-degree heart block is found. Either temporary transcutaneous or transvenous pacing may be used.
- If preload is low, administer prescribed crystalloid IV fluids according to fluid challenge protocol (see Table 4-18 for sample protocol). Document patient's hemodynamic response.
- If medical management is ineffective, prepare patient for insertion of IABP (see p. 365) or left VAD (see "Heart-Assist Device," p. 366).

Altered cerebral, renal, peripheral, and cardiopulmonary tissue perfusion related to interrupted arterial blood flow to vital organs secondary to inadequate arterial pressure

Desired outcome: Within 96 h of this diagnosis, patient has adequate tissue perfusion as evidenced by orientation to time, place, and person; equal and normoreactive pupils; normal reflexes; urine output ≥0.5 ml/kg/h; warm and dry skin; peripheral pulses >2+ on a 0-4+ scale; brisk capillary refill (<2 sec); and BP >90/60 mm Hg or within patient's normal range.

- Check neurologic status q1-2h to assess cerebral perfusion. Be alert to changes in LOC, orientation, perception, motor activity, reflexes, and pupillary response to light. Consult physician for any changes.
- Monitor I&O hourly to assess renal perfusion; report urine output <0.5 ml/kg/h for 2 consecutive hours. Assess extremities q1-2h, noting changes in skin color, temperature, capillary refill, BP, and distal pulses.
- Titrate vasoactive drugs to maintain systolic BP >90 mm Hg.

Impaired gas exchange related to alveolar-capillary membrane changes secondary to pulmonary congestion; and related to altered oxygen-carrying capacity of the blood secondary to acidosis occurring with anaerobic metabolism

Desired outcome: Before weaning from supplemental oxygen or ventilatory assistance is attempted, the patient has adequate gas exchange as evidenced by Pao_2 ≥80 mm Hg, RR 12-20 breaths/min with normal depth and pattern (eupnea), oxygen saturation ≥95%, and Svo_2 60%-80%.

- At least hourly, assess rate, depth, and effort of patient's respirations for tachypnea or labored breaths. Also inspect skin and mucous membranes for pallor or cyanosis (a late sign of hypoxia). Consult physician promptly for significant findings.
- Auscultate lung fields q1-2h. Be alert to crackles, rhonchi, or wheezes.
- Monitor ABG values for hypoxemia (Pao_2 <80 mm Hg) or metabolic acidosis (pH <7.35 and HCO_3^- <24 mEq/L).
- Deliver humidified oxygen as prescribed.
- Monitor transcutaneous oxygen saturation with a pulse oximeter. Consult physician if oxygen saturation falls below 90%.
- Monitor Svo_2. When cardiac output drops, Svo_2 will decrease, indicating increased oxygen extraction, which occurs when perfusion is decreased. Alert physician to Svo_2 <60%.
- If patient's condition continues to deteriorate, prepare patient for intubation and mechanical ventilation.

For patients undergoing intraaortic balloon pump procedure

Decreased cardiac output (or risk for same) related to negative inotropic changes and rate, rhythm, and conduction alterations secondary to ischemia or injury

Desired outcomes: Within 24 h of this diagnosis, patient has adequate cardiac output as evidenced by BP within patient's normal range; normal sinus rhythm on ECG; HR 60-100 bpm; peripheral pulses >2+ on a 0-4+ scale; warm and dry skin; hourly urinary output ≥0.5 ml/kg/h; measured CO 4-7 L/min; CI ≥2.5 $L/min/m^2$; PAWP ≤12 mm Hg; SVR ≤1,200 $dynes/sec/cm^{-5}$; Svo_2 60%-80%; and patient awake, alert, oriented, and free from anginal pain.

- Monitor BP, PAP, RAP, Svo_2, and heart rate and rhythm on a continuous basis. Monitor PAWP, SVR, and CO/CI hourly. Be alert to and report to physician the following: elevation in PAWP, decreased CO, ST-segment changes, ectopic heartbeats, decreased Svo_2, or elevated SVR.
- Monitor hourly urinary output, noting output that is <0.5 ml/kg/h for 2 consecutive hours. Monitor BUN and creatinine values daily. Be alert to increased BUN (>20 mg/dl) and serum creatinine (>1.5 mg/dl), which can occur with low urinary output and acute tubular necrosis.
- Monitor bilateral peripheral pulses and color and temperature of extremities q2h.
- Provide oxygen therapy or maintain ventilator settings as prescribed.
- Regulate IV inotropic agents, such as dobutamine, dopamine, and amrinone, to maintain CI ≥2.5-4 $L/min/m^2$. Monitor for side effects, including tachydysrhythmias, ventricular ectopy, headache, and angina. (See Appendix 7 for more information.)
- Regulate afterload-reducing agents such as nitroprusside and nitroglycerin to maintain SVR <1,200 $dynes/sec/cm^{-5}$. Monitor for drug

side effects, including hypotension, headache, dizziness, nausea, vomiting, and cutaneous flushing.

- Administer diuretic agents as prescribed for elevated PAWP (>12 mm Hg). Monitor for signs and symptoms of hypokalemia (e.g., weakness, dysrhythmias), a potential side effect of diuretics.
- Provide a quiet environment conducive to stress reduction.
- Administer prescribed pain medications as needed to reduce sympathetic response, which increases afterload.
- Monitor Hgb and Hct values daily for decrease, which may signal bleeding and reduced blood volume, along with reduced oxygen-carrying capacity of the blood.

Altered peripheral tissue perfusion (or risk for same):   Involved leg, related to interrupted arterial blood flow secondary to arterial wall dissection by sheath or thrombus formation

Desired outcome: Throughout duration of hospitalization, patient has adequate perfusion in the involved leg as evidenced by peripheral pulses >2+ on a 0-4+ scale, normal color and sensation, warmth, full motor function, and absence of bleeding, abdominal pain, and tingling in the involved leg.

- Monitor circulation in affected leg q30min × 4 and q2h thereafter if assessment is within normal limits. Assess pulses, temperature, color, sensation, and mobility of the toes in the involved leg. Consult physician immediately for significant changes.
- Instruct patient to notify staff member if pain, numbness, or tingling occurs in the involved leg.
- Provide protection to heel of involved foot, using sheepskin, occlusive opaque dressing, or heel protector. Place lamb's wool between the toes to minimize the pressure of the toes against each other.
- To enhance perfusion in the involved leg, have patient perform passive foot exercises without bending leg at the hip. The following should be performed qid: foot flexion/extension, foot circles, quadriceps setting. A pneumatic compression device may be beneficial.
- Administer IV dextran or heparin as prescribed to prevent clots from forming on the balloon. Monitor patient for signs of bleeding, including decreased Hct (optimal values are ≥37% [female] or ≥40% [male]), abdominal pain, hematuria, oral bleeding, or blood-tinged mucus.
- Monitor PTT if heparin is used (optimal value is 30-40 sec [activated]). Therapeutic anticoagulation is usually 1½ times that of normal. Maintain adequate hydration (2-3 L/day) to minimize risk of clot formation.
- Keep HOB at 30 degrees or less to prevent upward migration of catheter, which would occlude subclavian artery.
- Assess for the following signs of balloon migration: decreased left radial pulse, sudden decrease in urine output (<0.5 ml/kg/h), flank pain, and dizziness.
- When the balloon is no longer needed, maintain regular balloon inflation to prevent clot formation until balloon can be removed.

Impaired tissue integrity (or risk for same) related to external factors (pressure and immobilization) and internal factors (altered circulation and decreased protein intake due to NPO status)

Desired outcome: Throughout hospitalization, patient's tissue remains intact.

- Position patient on protective bed (e.g., Flexicare, Medicus, or Kin-Air). These beds reduce the capillary pressure to less than closing pressure, thereby enhancing blood flow to dependent areas. In addition, they also circulate air around the patient to promote evaporation of moisture.
- Reposition patient q2h, particularly at night when spontaneous movement is diminished. When turning patient, keep involved leg extended and log roll patient onto side.
- Ensure meticulous skin care to keep skin clean and dry. Inspect vulnerable areas (e.g., coccyx, ischial tuberosity, calcaneus, and malleoli) at least tid.
- Ensure that patient's diet is high in protein and calories to promote nitrogen balance. If patient's oral intake is inadequate or in the event of intubation, confer with physician regarding need for nutritional support such as enteral feedings or parenteral nutrition.
- As patient's condition improves, teach patient how to move in bed while minimizing flexion of involved hip.
- See "Wound and Skin Care," p. 57, for more information.

Ineffective breathing pattern related to fatigue and decreased energy secondary to heart failure and related to decreased lung expansion secondary to medically imposed position (HOB no higher than 30 degrees)

Desired outcomes: Within 4 h of this diagnosis, patient has an effective breathing pattern as evidenced by Pao_2 ≥80 mm Hg, Spo_2 >90%, absence of adventitious breath sounds, and RR 12-20 breaths/min with normal pattern and depth (eupnea).

- Monitor breath sounds q2h. Assess anterior and posterior lung fields for adventitious (e.g., crackles, rhonchi) or absent sounds.
- Monitor oxygen saturation by pulse oximetry. Be alert to levels <90%.
- Monitor respiratory rate, rhythm, and breathing pattern hourly.
- Be alert to indicators of atelectasis (e.g., dyspnea, elevated temperature, weakness, absent or decreased breath sounds) and respiratory infection (elevated temperature, SOB, increased sputum production or coughing, altered color of sputum).
- Monitor temperature q4h and WBC count daily for signs of infection. Be alert to low-grade fever of ≤37.8° C (≤100° F) and increased WBC count.
- Provide supplemental oxygen and chest physiotherapy as prescribed.
- Encourage patient to perform deep-breathing exercises or incentive spirometry q1-2h while awake to promote gas exchange, followed by coughing to raise secretions, if indicated.
- If coughing is ineffective in raising secretions, employ suction as indicated, using aseptic technique.
- Reposition patient at least q2h to minimize stasis of lung secretions.
- Monitor patient's fluid volume status to ensure that hydration is adequate to keep secretions thin and mobile. Unless contraindicated, maintain patient's fluid intake at 2-3 L/day.
- As often as it is allowed, elevate HOB 30 degrees to promote effective breathing pattern.

- If patient continues to exhibit ineffective breathing pattern in spite of these measures, prepare for ET intubation and mechanical ventilation.

Altered protection related to risk of bleeding/hemorrhage secondary to mechanical coagulopathy and IV anticoagulants

Desired outcome: Throughout hospitalization, patient has no symptoms of bleeding as evidenced by secretions and excretions negative for blood and absence of abdominal pain or ecchymoses. Hct is ≥37% (female) or ≥40% (male), PTT is in the range of therapeutic anticoagulation established by physician or protocol, ACT is ≤120 sec, and platelet count is 150,000-400,000 μl.

- Monitor PTT, ACT, and platelet level daily. Be alert to levels not within therapeutic range. Note that anticoagulation and decreased platelet level increase the risk of bleeding and hemorrhage.
- Monitor Hct and Hgb daily. Decreased levels may signal the presence of bleeding.
- Test GI drainage and stool daily for blood.
- Protect patient from injury. Pad side rails, if necessary, and turn patient carefully. Use sponge-tipped applicators for oral care.
- Test gastric pH q4h. Administer gastric acid–neutralizing drugs, such as antacids or histamine H_2-receptor antagonists (see Table 8-13, p. 555) as prescribed to maintain gastric pH >5.

Note: Also see **Risk for infection,** which appears in the next section, "For Patients with a Heart-Assist Device," p. 373.

For patients with a heart-assist device

Altered protection related to risk of bleeding secondary to therapeutic anticoagulation and effects of cardiopulmonary bypass or VAD on blood components

Desired outcome: Throughout duration of hospitalization, patient has no symptoms of internal or external bleeding as evidenced by secretions and excretions negative for blood; chest tube drainage within acceptable amounts (<100 ml/h); and absence of ecchymoses and abdominal or back pain.

- Monitor Hct daily for a decrease in value. Optimal values are as follows: Hct ≥37% (female) or ≥40% (male).
- Test gastric drainage and stool daily for blood; report positive results.
- Monitor daily clotting studies (PT, PTT), platelets, and ACT. Report elevations of PT (>11-15 sec), PTT (>30-40 sec), or ACT above desired range, which will depend on whether patient has received anticoagulants. Anticoagulation of patients with a heart-assist device in place is desirable but may not be feasible if the patient is bleeding actively from the surgical site. Monitor platelets and be alert to a decrease to <100,000 μl, which represents a significant drop and the increased risk of bleeding.
- Inspect all drainage for evidence of bleeding.
- Administer coagulation factors as prescribed (e.g., platelets, fresh-frozen plasma, cryoprecipitate, vitamin K, protamine sulfate, and aminocaproic acid).
- Test gastric pH q4h, and administer prescribed antacids to maintain pH >5.

- Administer prophylactic acid-neutralizing drugs (i.e., antacids) as prescribed, as well as H_2-receptor antagonists, which block the release of histamine (see Table 8-13, p. 555).

Risk for disuse syndrome related to imposed restrictions against movement secondary to presence of assist device or debilitated state

Desired outcome: Patient maintains baseline ROM without evidence of muscle atrophy or contracture formation.

- Be aware that patient can be turned gently from side to side when the heart-assist device is in place. Do this q2h, observing assist device cannulas closely to ensure that tension is not placed on them during patient repositioning.
- Provide passive ROM to extremities qid.
- See "Prolonged Immobility," p. 78, for more information.

Decreased cardiac output (or risk for same) related to altered preload and negative inotropic changes secondary to reduced right ventricular contraction occurring with left heart–assist device

---

Note: This is a complication of the left heart–assist device, particularly when the outflow cannula is located in the left ventricle. When the left ventricle is decompressed, septal wall motion is diminished, thereby reducing right ventricular contraction. Patients who have pulmonary hypertension or impaired right ventricular function due to AMI or cardiopulmonary bypass are especially prone to this problem.

Desired outcome: Within 24 h of this diagnosis, patient's cardiac output is adequate as evidenced by measured CO 4-7 L/min, RAP 4-6 mm Hg, PVR 60-100 dynes/sec/cm^{-5}, and LAP $\geq$10 mm Hg.

- Monitor patient for a decrease in CO with associated increases in RAP and PVR, which are diagnostic of the complication just described.
- Ensure that patient attains prescribed IV fluid intake to maintain a minimal LAP of 10 mm Hg. An adequate preload is necessary to prevent a vacuum effect from the device, which would aggravate this problem.

Risk for infection related to inadequate primary defenses secondary to presence of multiple invasive lines, movement restrictions, and stasis of body fluids

Desired outcome: Patient is free of infection as evidenced by normothermia, WBC count $\leq$11,000 μl, negative culture results, and absence of erythema, swelling, warmth, tenderness, and purulent drainage at incision or cannulation sites.

- On a daily basis, monitor temperature, WBC count, and all incisions and cannulation sites for evidence of infection. Be alert to low-grade fever of approximately 37.8° C (100° F); WBC count >11,000 μl; and incision that is erythematous, warm, swollen, and tender to the touch or that has purulent discharge.
- Culture any suspicious drainage or secretions; report positive findings.
- Change IV tubing q72h (or per agency protocol), using aseptic technique.
- Change all dressings over catheter insertion sites per agency proto-

col, using aseptic technique. Apply antimicrobial ointment (e.g., povidone-iodine).
- Administer prophylactic IV antibiotics as prescribed.
- Provide nutritional support to ensure that nitrogen balance is attained.
- Monitor breath sounds q2h. Assess for the presence of crackles, rhonchi, or signs of consolidation. If extubation has occurred, establish hourly deep-breathing and coughing exercises.
- If patient is incapable of raising secretions independently, perform suctioning as often as need is determined by auscultation. Inspect the mucus, noting color and consistency. Be alert to secretions that are yellow, green, or thickened.
- Provide gentle chest physiotherapy as prescribed. Percussion and vibration can be performed over the posterior and lateral lung lobes during every positioning change, or at least qid.

Altered nutrition: Less than body requirements related to decreased intake secondary to oral intubation; or increased need secondary to debilitated state and impaired tissue perfusion with concomitant nitrogen malabsorption

Desired outcome: Within the 24- to 48-h period before discharge from ICU, patient has adequate nutrition as evidenced by a balanced nitrogen state, stable weight, urine nitrogen 10-20 g/24 h, thyroxine-binding prealbumin 20-30 mg/dl, and retinol-binding protein 4-5 mg/dl.
- Provide nutrition *via* tube feedings or total parenteral nutrition to ensure minimum of 1-5 g protein/kg/day and a calorie intake of 100 kcal/kg/day, along with other essential elements. Have dietitian monitor daily calorie and protein intake.
- Weigh patient daily for trend. Report continuing decreases in weight.
- Monitor 24-h urinary nitrogen q3days for increase in excretion.
- Monitor I&O hourly. Report positive or negative fluid state of 300 ml/h.
- Assess patient for signs of cardiac cachexia: muscle atrophy, weakness, anorexia, and weight loss.
- For more information, see section "Nutritional Support," p. 1.

ADDITIONAL NURSING DIAGNOSES

Also see the following, as appropriate: "Mechanical Ventilation," p. 24; "Hemodynamic Monitoring," p. 37; "Prolonged Immobility," p. 78; "Psychosocial Support," p. 88; and "Psychosocial Support for the Patient's Family and Significant Others," p. 100.

Caring for patients undergoing coronary artery thrombolysis

PATHOPHYSIOLOGY

Acute thrombus formation with coronary artery occlusion is the most common cause of AMI. During the initial phase of injury, the development of necrosis typically starts with the subendocardial layer and spreads to the epicardial layer of heart muscle. Early reperfusion of an ischemic myocardium can prevent or reduce myocardial injury.

Therefore, the ability to dissolve (lyse) fresh coronary thromboses early in the course of infarction is essential in order to salvage myocardial tissue and preserve ventricular function. The goal of thrombolysis is to reduce infarct size, improve left ventricular function, and minimize morbidity and mortality. Thrombolytic therapy is a safe and effective way to establish reperfusion for patients with AMI secondary to complete or partial coronary arterial thrombotic occlusion.

Thrombolytic agents act to dissolve or lyse existing clots. A clot, or thrombus, is formed when deposits of fibrin collect within the artery and form an insoluble matrix. The fibrin clot eventually is broken down by the naturally occuring enzyme, plasmin. Thrombolytic agents work to accelerate this natural process by converting plasminogen to plasmin, which rapidly dissolves the fibrin clot. However, plasmin also breaks down circulating clotting proteins, thus producing excessive fibrin/fibrinogen degradation products (FDPs). The presence of large amounts of FDPs results in significant systemic anticoagulation and can trigger bleeding complications. First-generation thrombolytics (streptokinase, anistreplase, urokinase) are nonfibrin selective and activate both fibrin-bound and nonfibrin-bound plasminogen. Alteplase, a second-generation thrombolytic, is fibrin selective and preferentially activates fibrin-bound plasminogen.

Indications that lysis has taken place include decreased chest pain, rapid resolution of ST-segment depression, and a new onset of dysrhythmias. Up to 80% of patients are reported to have had reperfusion dysrhythmias, primarily accelerated idioventricular rhythm and PVCs. Bradycardia and heart block also are seen.

After clot lysis occurs, thrombin is released into the circulation. The thrombin induces platelet clumping and increases the potential for reocclusion. Use of thrombolytic agents results in excessive circulating thrombin and increases the risk of coronary artery reocclusion. Heparin and antiplatelet agents are used as adjuncts to thrombolytic therapy to inhibit the action of free thrombin and prevent reocclusion.

ASSESSMENT

HISTORY AND RISK FACTORS Presence of cardiac risk factors (see "Acute Myocardial Infarction," p. 278). Assess patient for absolute and relative contraindications for thrombolytic therapy (Table 4-19). Assess for recent (within 6 mo) streptococcal infection when use of streptokinase or anistreplase is anticipated. Assess for aspirin allergy, since antiplatelet therapy with aspirin usually is initiated.

SUBJECTIVE FINDINGS Candidates for thrombolytic therapy include patients with clear symptoms of AMI: usually, sudden onset of chest pain/pressure that is unrelieved by sublingual nitrates and lasts >30 min but <6-12 h. The pain may radiate to the neck, jaw, and arms. Intermittent, severe chest pain over hours or days can indicate subtotal occlusion secondary to coronary thrombosis, and these patients also may be considered for thrombolytic therapy. Diaphoresis, nausea, vomiting, anxiety, and other symptoms consistent with the diagnosis of AMI may be present.

Selection of candidates for thrombolytic therapy relies heavily on clinical history and physical examination. The presentation of aortic

T A B L E 4 - 1 9 Contraindications for thrombolytic therapy

Minor relative contraindications
- Recent (within 10 days) minor trauma, including CPR
- History of cerebrovascular disease
- Pregnancy
- Likelihood of left-sided heart thrombus (e.g., atrial fibrillation, severe left ventricular dyskinesia)
- Acute pericarditis
- Hemostatic defect, including those associated with liver/renal dysfunction, anticoagulant therapy
- Diabetic hemorrhagic retinopathy, other hemorrhagic ophthalmic conditions
- Advanced age (>75 yr); controversial: patient's physiologic status rather than absolute chronologic age should be used to guide patient selection

Major relative contraindications
- Recent (within 10 days) major surgery, serious trauma, obstetric delivery, organ biopsy, puncture of noncompressible vessels
- GI/GU bleeding within 10 days
- Uncontrolled hypertension: SBP >180 or DBP >110 mm Hg

Absolute contraindications
- Known hypersensitivity to thrombolytic agents
- Active internal bleeding
- Recent (within 2 mo) CVA
- Recent (within 2 mo) intracranial neoplasm, arteriovenous malformation/aneurysm
- Recent (within 2 mo) intracranial/intraspinal surgery or trauma
- Bleeding diathesis
- Severe uncontrolled hypertension: DBP >120 mm Hg

dissection and acute pericarditis is similar to that of AMI, and these diagnoses must be excluded before proceeding with thrombolytic therapy.

OBJECTIVE FINDINGS The patient may experience tachycardia, bradycardia, irregular pulse, hypotension, and other findings consistent with AMI (see p. 278). Assess patient for absolute and relative contraindications for thrombolytic therapy (Table 4-19). Assess for and note all venipuncture attempts and superficial injuries that could become active bleeding sites after thrombolysis. Perform a careful baseline neurologic assessment for comparison of subsequent examinations, which are indicated to detect neurologic changes associated with acute CVA.

DIAGNOSTIC TESTS

ECG: 12- or 18-lead ECG is performed to determine presence, location, and extent of myocardial injury. Localized ST-segment elevation of 1 mm in 2 contiguous leads, significant Q waves, and T-wave inversion are findings associated with AMI. ST-segment elevation that decreases after administration of sublingual NTG suggests coronary artery spasm (Prinzmetal's angina) and thrombolytic therapy is not indicated.

Laboratory studies: Serum enzymes, electrolytes, CBC, and clotting studies are evaluated before initiating thrombolytic therapy. A heparin-lock device is used for specimen collection. Do not delay therapy for confirmation of laboratory values.

COLLABORATIVE MANAGEMENT

Thrombolytics: Prompt identification of candidates for thrombolytic therapy and rapid initiation of therapy increase the effectiveness of all thrombolytic agents. Because time is crucial, initiation of thrombolytic therapy may occur in the prehospital setting or in the emergency department of a smaller hospital before transfer to a definitive care center. In these settings the thrombolytic agents are administered peripherally. In other cases thrombolytic agents are started in the catheterization laboratory where they are administered *via* the intracoronary route while the patient is undergoing fluoroscopic examination. Ideally, thrombolytic therapy is initiated within 30 min of the patient's arrival to the hospital's emergency department. Patients with AMI must be identified expediently and treated rapidly. Currently four thrombolytic agents are in general use: streptokinase, anistreplase (Eminase), urokinase, and alteplase (tissue-type plasminogen activator). Table 4-20 compares these agents.

First-generation thrombolytics
- *Streptokinase:* An enzyme derived from group C beta-hemolytic streptococcus, it acts as a catalyst for the conversion of plasminogen to plasmin, which lyses the clot. Streptokinase can be administered intravenously or *via* the intracoronary route. Because it is an antigen, patients who have had previous exposure to streptococcal organisms may have built up antibodies against streptokinase. Therefore, steroids or antihistamines are administered before streptokinase therapy to prevent a hypersensitivity reaction. Usual dosage is 1.5 million IU, given IV as a continuous infusion over 60 min.
- *Anistreplase:* A plasminogen activator that induces clot lysis with fewer systemic lytic effects than does streptokinase. Allergic and anaphylactic reactions are possible. Usual dose is 30 IU by IV injection over 2-5 min.
- *Urokinase:* An enzyme derived from human renal cells. It activates plasminogen directly to form plasmin. At the present time urokinase is not FDA-approved for peripheral thrombolytic therapy in acute coronary arterial occlusion. However, it is used for intracoronary infusion and administered in cardiac catheterization laboratories. Urokinase is more expensive than streptokinase but is less likely to result in hypersensitivity reactions. Both urokinase and streptokinase have some systemic lytic effects and may result in bleeding complications in other areas of the body.

Second-generation thrombolytic
- *Alteplase:* Produced by the body and converts plasminogen to plasmin after binding to the fibrin clot. This mechanism of action is advantageous because there are no systemic lytic effects. In addition, it is nonantigenic. It has a shorter half-life than do

T A B L E   4 - 2 0   Comparison of agents used for coronary thrombolysis

	First-generation agents		Second-generation agent
	Streptokinase (Kabikinase, Streptase)	Anistreplase, APSAC (Eminase)	Alteplase t-PA, (Activase)
Effectiveness			
Recanalization rate	31%-62%	51%-53%	71%
Patency rate	55%-57%	50%-68%	67%-92%
Diminished with increasing clot age	Yes	Yes	No
Safety			
Clot-specific activity	No	No	Yes
Systemic anticoagulation	Yes	Yes	Limited
Duration of hemostatic compromise	24-36h	24-48h	12-24h
Reocclusion rate	15%	14%	16.3%
Dosage/effects			
Dosage	1.5 million IU, IV infusion over 30-60 min*	30 U, IV direct injection over 2-5 min	100 mg, IV infusion over 3h*

Drug source	Bacterial protein	Bacterial protein and human plaminogen	Recombinant DNA
Antigenic properties		Yes	No
Incidence of drug-induced hypotension	4%-25%	4%-25%	Not observed
Incidence of intracranial bleeding	0.3%-0.5%	0.6%	0.4%-0.5%
Mortality			
Early (5-6 wk)	8%	6.4%	4.6%
Late (1 yr)	10.5%	11.1%	7.4%
Cost			
To hospital (per dose)	$600	$2,100	$2,600
Estimated nursing time to prepare/administer	45 min	15 min	60 min

Modified from Majoros K: Comparisons and controversies in clot buster drugs, *Crit Care Nurs Quart* 16(2):58, 1993; and Keen J, Baird M, Allen J: *Mosby's critical care and emergency drug reference*, St Louis, 1994, Mosby.
*Other dosing regimens are used.

the other enzymes and has been shown in initial studies to be more effective than streptokinase and urokinase in lysing coronary thromboses. The usual dose is 100 mg given intravenously as a 10-mg bolus followed by a continuous infusion of 50 mg/h for 1 h and then 20 mg/h for 2 h.

Adjunctive therapy: Standard therapy for AMI is initiated, including oxygen administration, continuous ECG monitoring, nitrates, IV analgesia, beta-blockade, and other therapies as indicated. Heparin and antiplatelet agents are given concurrently with thrombolytic therapy to prevent reocclusion.

Coronary angiography: May be performed to assess for patency or reocclusion. Because of the systemic lytic effects of all thrombolytics, it is best to wait 24-48 h after initial thrombolytic therapy. See discussion in "Acute Myocardial Infarction," p. 281.

NURSING DIAGNOSES AND INTERVENTIONS

Knowledge deficit: The atherosclerotic process and the rationale, procedure, and expected outcomes of thrombolytic therapy

Desired outcome: Before initiation of the thrombolytic therapy, patient verbalizes basic knowledge about the atherosclerotic process and thrombolytic therapy.

- Assess patient's knowledge about the atherosclerotic process and the rationale, procedure, and expected outcome of thrombolytic therapy. Explain the goal of therapy: to reduce injury to the heart muscle.
- Explain the need for monitoring and close postprocedural observation.
- Provide emotional support during the procedure, keeping the patient informed about the events that are taking place.
- After the procedure, discuss potential long-term outcomes and the possibility of reocclusion, including interventions the patient can take to prevent it: take prescribed antiplatelet medications, exercise, comply with dietary modifications, and manage or eliminate risk factors such as smoking, hyperlipidemia, hypertension, stress, and obesity.
- Before discharge, instruct patient to report any signs and symptoms of MI that occur after hospitalization: unrelenting chest heaviness or pressure; pain that radiates to the arm, neck, or jaw; accompanying nausea and diaphoresis; and lightheadedness or dizziness.

Altered protection related to risk of bleeding/hemorrhage secondary to nonspecific thrombolytic effects of therapy

Desired outcome: Symptoms of bleeding complications are absent as evidenced by BP within patient's normal range, HR ≤100 bpm, blood-free secretions and excretions, natural skin color, baseline or normal LOC, and absence of back and abdominal pain, hematoma, headache, dizziness, and vomiting.

- When patient is admitted, obtain a thorough history, assessing for the following:
  - Risk factors for intracranial hemorrhage: uncontrolled hypertension, cerebrovascular pathology, CNS surgery within previous 6 mo.

- □ Bleeding risks: recent or active GI bleeding, recent trauma, recent surgery, bleeding diathesis, advanced liver or kidney disease
- □ Risk of systemic embolization: suspected left-sided heart thrombus
- □ History of streptococcal infection or previous streptokinase therapy
- Monitor clotting studies per agency protocol. Regulate heparin drip to maintain PTT at 1½-2 times control levels or according to protocol. *Never* discontinue heparin without physician's directive.
- Apply pressure dressing over puncture site if cardiac catheterization was performed. Inspect site at frequent intervals for evidence of hematoma formation. Immobilize extremity for 6-8 h after catheterization procedure.
- Avoid unnecessary venipunctures, IM injections, or arterial puncture. Obtain laboratory specimens from heparin-lock device.
- Monitor patient for indicators of internal bleeding: back pain, abdominal pain, decreased BP, pallor, and bloody stool or urine. Report significant findings to physician.
- Monitor patient for signs of intracranial bleeding q2h: change in LOC, headache, dizziness, vomiting, and confusion.
- Test all stools, urine, and emesis for occult blood.
- Use care with oral hygiene and when shaving patient. For more information about safety precautions, see **Altered protection** in "Pulmonary Emboli," p. 257.

Risk for injury related to potential for allergic or anaphylactic reaction to streptokinase or anistreplase secondary to antigen/antibody response

Desired outcome: Patient has no symptoms of allergic response as evidenced by normothermia, RR 12-20 breaths/min with normal pattern and depth (eupnea), HR ≤100 bpm, BP at baseline or within normal limits, natural skin color, and absence of itching, urticaria, headache, muscular and abdominal pain, and nausea.

- Before treatment, question patient about history of previous streptokinase therapy or streptococcal infection. Consult physician for positive findings.
- Administer prophylactic hydrocortisone as prescribed.
- Monitor patient during and for 48-72 h after infusion for indicators of allergy: hypotension (brief or sustained), urticaria, fever, itching, flushing, nausea, headache, muscular pain, bronchospasm, abdominal pain, dyspnea, or tachycardia. These indicators can appear immediately after or as long as several days after streptokinase therapy.
- If hypotension develops, increase rate of IV infusion/administer volume replacement as prescribed. Prepare for vasopressor administration if there is no response to volume replacement.
- Treat allergic response with diphenhydramine or other antihistamine, as prescribed.

Decreased cardiac output (or risk for same) related to alterations in rate, rhythm, and conduction secondary to increased irritability of ischemic tissue during reperfusion (usually occurs within 1-2 h after initiation of therapy)

Desired outcomes: Within 12 h of initiation of thrombolytic therapy, patient has adequate cardiac output as evidenced by normal sinus rhythm on ECG, peripheral pulses >2+ on a 0-4+ scale, warm and dry skin, and hourly urine output ≥0.5 ml/kg/h. Patient is awake, alert, and oriented without palpitations, chest pain, or dizziness.

- Monitor ECG continuously during thrombolytic therapy for evidence of dysrhythmias. Consult physician for significant dysrhythmias.
- With any dysrhythmia, check VS and note accompanying signs and symptoms such as dizziness, lightheadedness, syncope, and palpitations.
- Ensure availability of emergency drugs and equipment: lidocaine, atropine, isoproterenol, epinephrine, defibrillator-cardioverter, external and transvenous pacemaker.
- Administer lidocaine infusion as prescribed.
- Evaluate patient's response to medications and emergency treatment.

Decreased cardiac output (or risk for same) related to inotropic changes in the heart secondary to reocclusion and myocardial ischemia

---

Note: Reocclusion occurs in up to 16% of patients within 24-48 h after thrombolysis.

Desired outcomes: Within 48 h of initiation of thrombolytic therapy, patient has adequate cardiac output as evidenced by normal sinus rhythm on ECG, peripheral pulses >2+ on a 0-4+ scale, warm and dry skin, and hourly urine output ≥0.5 ml/kg/h. Patient is awake, alert, and oriented without palpitations, chest pain, or dizziness.

- Monitor patient for signs of reocclusion: chest pain, nausea, diaphoresis, and dysrhythmias. Consult physician for any signs of reocclusion.
- Obtain 12/18-lead ECG if reocclusion is suspected.
- Anticipate and prepare patient for cardiac catheterization, PTCA, or repeated thrombolytic therapy.
- For other interventions, see this nursing diagnosis under "Acute Myocardial Infarction," p. 283.

Selected Bibliography

American Heart Association: *Textbook of advanced cardiac life support,* Dallas, 1994, The Association.

American Heart Association: *1993 Heart and stroke facts statistics,* Pub no 55-0502, Dallas, 1993, The Association.

Baas LS: Pericarditis. In *Teaching patients with acute conditions,* Springhouse, PA, 1992, Springhouse.

Baas LS, editor: *Essentials of cardiovascular nursing,* Rockville, MD, 1991, Aspen.

Baas LS, Meissner JE: Cardiovascular care. In *Illustrated manual of nursing practice,* ed 2, Springhouse, PA, 1994, Springhouse.

Cheitlin MD, Sokolow M, McIlroy MB: *Clinical cardiology,* ed 6, Norwalk, CT, 1993, Appleton-Lange.

Chernow B: The pharmacologic approach to the critically ill patient, ed 3, Baltimore, 1994, Williams & Wilkins.

Cimini DM: Indium-III antimyosin antibody imaging: a promising new technique in the diagnosis of MI, *Crit Care Nurse* 12(6):44-51, 1992.

Cole P: Thrombolytic therapy: then and now, *Heart Lung* 20(5 part 2):542-551, 1991.

Collins MA: When your patient has an implantable cardioverter defibrillator, *Am J Nurs* 94(3):34-39, 1994.

Cone M: Cardiopulmonary support in the intensive care unit, *Am J Crit Care* 1(1):98-108, 1992.

Cronin LA: Beating the clock: saving the heart with thrombolytic drugs, *Nursing 93* 23(8):34-42, 1993.

Daily E: Clinical management of patients receiving thrombolytic therapy, *Heart Lung* 20(5 part 2):552-565, 1991.

Dajani AS et al: Prevention of bacterial endocarditis: recommendations by the American Heart Association, *JAMA* 264:2919-2922, 1990.

Dunnington CS: Sotalol hydrochloride (Betapace): a new antiarrhythmic drug, *Am J Crit Care* 2(5):397-406, 1993.

Futterman LG, Lemberg L: Radiofrequency catheter ablation for supraventricular tachycardias, *Am J Crit Care* 2(6):500-505, 1993.

Grauer K, Cavallaro D: *ACLS vol 2: a comprehensive review,* ed 3, St Louis, 1993, Mosby Lifeline.

Gunnar R et al: Guidelines for the early management of patients with acute myocardial infarction, *J Am Coll Cardiol* 16(2):249-292, 1990.

Interqual: The ISD-A review system with adult ISD criteria, August 1992, North Hampton, NH and Marlboro, MA, Interqual.

Joint National Committee: The Fifth Report of the Joint National Committee on Detection, Evaluation, and Treatment of High Blood Pressure (JNC V), *Arch Intern Med* 153:154-183, 1993.

Keen J, Baird M, Allen J: *Mosby's critical care and emergency drug reference,* St Louis, 1994, Mosby.

Kim MJ, McFarland GK, McLane AM: *Pocket guide to nursing diagnoses,* ed 6, St Louis, 1995, Mosby.

Kinney MR, Packa DR, Dunbar SB: *AACN's clinical reference for critical care nursing,* ed 3, St Louis, 1993, Mosby.

Majoros K: Comparisons and controversies in clot buster drugs, *Crit Care Nurs Quart* 16(2):58, 1993.

Mastrisciano L: Unstable angina: an overview, *Crit Care Nurse* 12(2):30-39, 1992.

McCance KL, Huether SE: *Pathophysiology: the biologic basis for disease in adults and children,* St Louis, 1990, Mosby.

Porterfield LM: The cutting edge in arrhythmias, *Crit Care Nurse* (suppl) June 1993.

Rapaport E: Overview: rationale of thrombolysis in treating acute myocardial infarction, *Heart Lung* 29(5 part 2):538-541, 1991.

Saver CL: Decoding the ACLS algorithms, *Am J Nurse* 94(1):27-36, 1994.

Sheehy SB: *Emergency nursing: principles and practice,* ed 3, St Louis, 1992, Mosby.

Sifri-Steele C, Meyer LT: Implementing changes in standards of care for patients with unstable angina: Wellen's syndrome, *Crit Care Nurse* 13(2):23-28, 1993.

Steuble BT: Cardiovascular disorders. In Swearingen PL: *Manual of medical-surgical nursing care,* ed 3, St Louis, 1994, Mosby.

Thelan L et al: *Textbook of critical care nursing: diagnosis and management,* ed 2, St Louis, 1994, Mosby.

Thompson EJ: Transesophageal echocardiography: a new window on the heart and great vessels, *Crit Care Nurse* 13(5):55-66, 1993.

RENAL-URINARY DYSFUNCTIONS

Acute renal failure

PATHOPHYSIOLOGY

Acute renal failure (ARF) is a syndrome characterized by an abrupt deterioration of renal function, resulting in the accumulation of metabolic wastes, fluids, and electrolytes, usually accompanied by a marked decline in urinary output. If it is undetected or treated inadequately, ARF can lead to parenchymal damage and progress to chronic renal failure. ARF is caused by decreased renal perfusion, parenchymal damage, or obstruction. It is categorized as prerenal, intrarenal, and postrenal (Table 5-1).

Prerenal failure is the result of decreased blood flow to the kidneys. The events leading to prerenal insults cause decreased renal vascular perfusion and usually are associated with systemic hypoperfusion. If renal hypoperfusion exceeds the adaptive mechanisms of autoregulation and renin release, ischemic damage occurs, leading to parenchymal (intrarenal) involvement. Intrarenal involvement usually results from a prolonged mean arterial pressure of <75 mm Hg. Failure of autoregulation enhances the sympathetic response and, coupled with the renin-angiotensin system, causes severe afferent arteriole constriction. This results in a further decrease in glomerular blood flow and glomerular hydrostatic pressure and decreases the glomerular filtration rate. The amount of cellular damage depends on the duration of ischemic episode. Mild reversible injury occurs with ≤25 min of ischemia; more severe damage results after 40-60 min of ischemia; and irreversible damage may occur with 60-90 min of ischemia.

The most common cause of ARF is acute tubular necrosis (ATN). ATN is the result of nephrotoxic injury or a prolonged compromise in renal perfusion (ischemic injury). In the acutely ill adult both factors may be operative because renal ischemia tends to potentiate the injury produced by nephrotoxins. Toxic ATN, caused by nephrotoxic agents, is an insult or injury to the tubular cell. Toxic ATN results in tubular

---

T A B L E 5 - 1 Causes of acute renal failure

Prerenal (decreased renal perfusion)	Intrarenal (parenchymal damage; acute tubular necrosis)	Postrenal (obstruction)
Hypovolemia	**Nephrotoxic agents**	**Calculi**
· GI losses	· Antibiotics (ami-	**Tumor**
· Hemorrhage	noglycosides, sulfon-	**Benign prostatic hy-**
· Third space (intersti-	amides, methicillin)	**pertrophy**
tial) losses (burns,	· Diuretics (e.g., furo-	**Necrotizing papillitis**
peritonitis)	semide)	**Urethral strictures**
· Dehydration from	· Nonsteroidal antiin-	**Blood clots**
diuretic use	flammatory drugs	**Retroperitoneal fibro-**
Hepatorenal syndrome	(e.g., ibuprofen)	**sis**
Edema-forming condi-	· Contrast media	
tions	· Heavy metals (lead,	
· Congestive heart fail-	gold, mercury)	
ure	· Organic solvents (car-	
· Cirrhosis	bon tetrachloride, eth-	
· Nephrotic syndrome	ylene glycol)	
Renal vascular disor-	**Infection (gram-**	
ders	**negative sepsis), pan-**	
· Renal artery stenosis	**creatitis, peritonitis**	
· Renal artery thrombo-	**Transfusion reaction**	
sis	**(hemolysis)**	
· Renal vein thrombosis	**Rhabdomyolysis with**	
	myoglobinuria (se-	
	vere muscle injury)	
	· Trauma	
	· Exertion	
	· Seizures	
	· Drug related: heroin,	
	barbiturates, IV am-	
	phetamines, succinyl-	
	choline	
	Glomerular diseases	
	· Poststreptococcal glo-	
	merulonephritis	
	· IgA nephropathy (e.g.,	
	Berger's disease)	
	· Lupus glomerulone-	
	phritis	
	· Serum sickness	
	Ischemic injury	

T A B L E 5 - 2   Common nephrotoxic agents

Drugs	*X-ray contrast media*
Antineoplastics	*Biologic substances*
methotrexate	myoglobin
cisplatin	tumor products
Antibiotics	*Chemicals*
cephalosporines	ethylene glycol
aminoglycosides	pesticides
tetracycline	organic solvents
Nonsteroidal antiinflammatory drugs	*Heavy metals*
ibuprofen	lead
ketorolac	mercury
	gold

cell necrosis, cast formation, and tubular obstruction. The basement membrane usually is not injured, and it often is nonoliguric in nature. Oliguria may occur with both toxic ATN and ischemic ATN. Common nephrotoxic agents are found in Table 5-2.

Fluid, electrolyte, and acid-base disorders that occur with ARF include hypervolemia, hyperkalemia, hyperphosphatemia, hypocalcemia, and metabolic acidosis (Table 5-3). Phosphate levels rise because of impaired excretion of phosphorus by the renal tubules with continued GI absorption. Hypocalcemia results from the lack of active vitamin D, which would otherwise stimulate absorption of calcium from the GI tract. High phosphorus levels also inhibit the absorption of calcium. In turn, hypocalcemia triggers the parathyroid glands to secrete parathyroid hormone (PTH), which mobilizes calcium from the bone.

Generally, there are three identifiable phases or stages of ARF. The first phase usually is characterized by oliguria, a drop in the 24-h urinary output to ≤400 ml. This phase lasts approximately 7-14 days, depending on the underlying pathologic condition. Approximately 30% of patients, however, have a syndrome of nonoliguric renal failure. The diuretic phase is evidenced initially by a doubling of the urinary output from the previous 24-h total. During this phase the patient may produce as much as 3-5 L of urine in 24 h. The recovery phase is marked by a return to a normal 24-h volume (1,500-1,800 ml). Usually, renal function continues to improve and may take 6 mo to 1 yr from the initial insult to return to baseline functional status.

ASSESSMENT

ARF can dramatically affect fluid, electrolyte, and acid-base balances. HISTORY AND RISK FACTORS Chronic illness (e.g., hypertension, diabetes), recent infections (e.g., streptococcal), recent episodes of hypotension (major bleeding, major surgery), exposure to nephrotoxic drugs or other agents (e.g., **carbon tetrachloride**, diuretics, aminoglycoside antibiotics, dyes), recent blood transfusion, urinary tract disorder, toxemia of pregnancy or abortion, **recent** severe muscle damage (rhabdomyolysis with myoglobinuria), burn trauma.

T A B L E 5 - 3 Altered electrolyte balance in ARF

Condition/cause	Nursing implications

Hyperkalemia
Decreased ability to excrete K^+; K^+ release with catabolism
	• Monitor ECG for tall and peaked T waves, loss of P waves, prolonged PR interval, widened QRS, and cardiac arrest (more likely seen with K^+ >6.5 mEq/L).
	• Monitor serum K^+ levels for values ≥5 mEq/L.
	• Monitor patient for such indicators as paresthesias, muscle weakness or flaccidity, and HR <60 bpm.
	• Teach patient and significant others the indicators of hyperkalemia and the importance of notifying nurse promptly if they occur.
	• Provide a list of foods high in potassium (see Table 10-12) and stress the importance of avoiding these foods.
	• Implement the following to help minimize the cellular release of potassium:
	  ▫ Ensure that patient consumes only the amount of protein prescribed by physician; enforce sound infection control techniques to minimize risk of infection; and treat fevers promptly. Catabolism of protein, which occurs in these situations, causes potassium to be released from the tissues.
	  ▫ Ensure that patient consumes the allotted amounts of carbohydrates, and limit strenuous patient activity as prescribed, both of which will spare protein.
	• Be aware that hyperkalemia can be a fatal complication, especially during the oliguric phase of ARF, because of its adverse effect on cardiac status. Keep emergency supplies (i.e., manual resuscitator, crash cart, and emergency drug tray) readily available.
	• For more information, see "Hyperkalemia," p. 389.

Hypokalemia Prolonged, inadequate oral intake; use of potassium-losing diuretics without proper replacement; excessive loss from vomiting, diarrhea, or gastric or intestinal suctioning	• Monitor ECG for prolonged PR interval, flattened or inverted T wave, depressed ST segment, presence of U wave, and ventricular dysrhythmias; ECG changes are more likely to occur at serum levels <3 mEq/L. • Be alert to serum K^+ <3.5 mEq/L. • Monitor patient for muscle weakness, soft and flabby muscles, paresthesias, decreased bowel sounds, ileus, weak and irregular

T A B L E 5 - 3   Altered electrolyte balance in ARF—cont'd

Condition/cause	Nursing implications
	pulse, and pulse and distant heart sounds. Neuromuscular symptoms are seen at serum levels of approximately 2.5 mEq/L.
	· Teach patient and significant others the indicators of hypokalemia and the importance of notifying nurse promptly if they occur.
	· Provide a list of foods high in potassium (see Table 10-12), and assist with planning menus that incorporate them.
	· Administer potassium-sparing diuretics (e.g., spironolactone, triamterene) as prescribed.
	· Administer oral or IV potassium supplements as prescribed; for oral route, administer with at least 4 oz water or juice to minimize gastric irritation.
	· For more information, see "Hypokalemia," p. 681.
Hypernatremia Kidneys' inability to excrete excess sodium; decreased water intake; increased water losses *via* osmotic diuresis; excessive parenteral administration of sodium-containing solutions (e.g., sodium bicarbonate, 3% sodium chloride)	· Monitor serum sodium levels for serum Na$^+$ >147 mEq/L.
	· Monitor VS and I&O hourly; weigh patient daily.
	· Be alert to dry mucous membranes, flushed skin, firm and rubbery tissue turgor, hyperthermia, oliguria, or anuria.
	· Assess sensorium for restlessness and agitation; institute seizure precautions as indicated.
	· Administer prescribed IV replacement fluids.
	· Administer diuretics, as prescribed.
	· For more information, see "Hypernatremia," p. 679.
Hyponatremia Loss through vomiting, diarrhea, profuse diaphoresis; use of potent diuretics; salt-losing nephropathies; administration of large amount of sodium-free IV fluids (may be associated with fluid volume excess or postobstructive diuresis)	· Monitor for serum Na$^+$ <137 mEq/L.
	· Monitor I&O hourly; record weight daily for trend.
	· Assess patient for abdominal cramps, diarrhea, nausea, dizziness when changing position, postural hypotension, cold and clammy skin, and apprehension.
	· Provide parenteral replacement therapy as prescribed.
	· Institute a safe environment for individuals with altered LOC.
	· For more information, see "Hyponatremia," p. 677.

Continued.

T A B L E   5 - 3   Altered electrolyte balance in ARF—cont'd

Condition/cause	Nursing implications
Hypocalcemia Poor absorption of dietary calcium; precipitation of calcium out of the tissues in the presence of elevated phosphorus level; inadequate absorption and utilization of calcium occurring with lack of conversion of vitamin D to its usable form	• Monitor for serum Ca^{2+} <8.5 mg/dl. • Monitor for numbness and tingling around the mouth, muscle twitching, facial twitching, and tonic muscle spasms. Assess for Trousseau's sign (carpopedal spasm) and Chvostek's sign (spasm of lip and cheek). • Administer calcium and vitamin D supplements as prescribed. Reinforce the necessity of taking these medications as prescribed. • Teach patient and significant others the indicators of hypocalcemia. • Teach the importance of continued medical follow-up to check serum calcium levels. • For more information, see "Hypocalcemia," p. 688.
Hyperphosphatemia Abnormal retention of phosphates due to the kidneys' inability to excrete excess phosphorus	• Monitor for serum phosphorus >4.5 mg/dl. • Although most foods contain generous amounts of phosphate, those especially high in phosphate include beef, pork, dried beans, dried mature peas, and dairy products (see Table 10-13). Monitor patient's diet accordingly. • Administer phosphate binders as prescribed. Assess for constipation, which may result from use of phosphate binders. • Teach patient and significant others the relationship between calcium and phosphate levels in the body. • Emphasize that maintaining good phosphate control and calcium balance may help control itching and prevent future problems with bone disease. • Reinforce the need for follow-up visits to check serum phosphate levels. • For more information, see "Hyperphosphatemia," p. 697.
Hypermagnesemia Administration of magnesium-containing medications to patients with impaired renal function	• Monitor serum Mg^{2+} for levels >2.5 mEq/L. • Assess for diaphoresis, flushing, hypotension, drowsiness, weak-to-absent DTRs, bradycardia, lethargy, and respiratory impairment. • Teach the above indicators to patient and significant others.

T A B L E 5 - 3   Altered electrolyte balance in ARF—cont'd

Condition/cause	Nursing implications
	• Avoid giving medications that contain magnesium (see Table 10-15). Emphasize to patient that such medications should not be taken without physician's approval.
	• For more information, see "Hypermagnesemia," p. 704.
Metabolic acidosis	
Kidneys' inability to excrete excess acid produced by normal metabolic processes. Marked tissue trauma, infection, and diarrhea may contribute to a more rapid development of acidosis (often associated with K^+ >5 mEq/L)	• Monitor for HCO_3^- <22 mEq/L and pH <7.35.
	• Monitor I&O, LOC, and VS. Be alert to Kussmaul's respirations, SOB, anorexia, headache, nausea, vomiting, weakness, apathy, fatigue, and coma.
	• Institute seizure precautions in the presence of altered LOC.
	• Administer IV fluids and bicarbonate as prescribed.
	• Teach patient the importance of dietary restrictions, particularly of protein, and of maintaining adequate carbohydrate intake to prevent worsening acidosis.
	• Stress that patient should report to physician increased temperature and other signs of infection.
	• Teach patient the importance of taking sodium bicarbonate as prescribed and of maintaining dialysis schedule (both hemodialysis and peritoneal dialysis help correct acidosis).
	• For more information, see "Metabolic Acidosis," p. 720.
Uremia	
Failure of the kidneys to excrete urea, creatinine, uric acid, and other metabolic waste products	• Monitor patient for chronic fatigue, insomnia, anorexia, vomiting, metallic taste in the mouth, pruritus, increased bleeding tendency, muscular twitching, involuntary leg movements, decreasing attention span, anemia, muscle wasting, and weakness.
	• Teach patient and significant others that the indicators of uremia develop gradually and are very subtle. Explain the importance of notifying nurse of sudden worsening of the symptoms that may be present.
	• Monitor and record dietary intake of protein, potassium, and sodium.
	• Use lotions and oils to lubricate patient's skin and relieve drying and cracking.

Continued.

T A B L E 5 - 3   Altered electrolyte balance in ARF—cont'd

Condition/cause	Nursing implications
	• Provide oral hygiene at frequent intervals, using a soft-bristled toothbrush and mouthwash, to help combat patient's thirst and the metallic taste caused by uremia. Chewing gum and hard candy also may help alleviate thirst and the unpleasant taste.
	• Encourage isometric exercises and short walks, if patient is able, to help maintain patient's muscle strength and tone, especially in the legs.
	• Teach significant others that because of patient's decreasing concentration level, they should communicate with patient by using simple and direct statements.
	• Teach patient to maintain good nutrition by ingesting the allotted amounts of carbohydrates and high–biologic value protein to support cell rebuilding and decrease waste products from protein breakdown.
	• Explain that profuse bleeding can occur with uremia and that knives, scissors, and other sharp instruments should be used with caution.
	• Stress that OTC medications, such as aspirin and ibuprofen, may enhance bleeding tendency.
	• Emphasize the importance of follow-up visits to evaluate the progression of uremia.
	• Stress that dialysis schedule should be maintained to decrease the symptoms of uremia and correct many of the metabolic abnormalities that occur.

CLINICAL PRESENTATION

Prerenal: Oliguria, urinary Na <20 mEq/L, elevated specific gravity, increased urine osmolality, normal sediment or presence of hyaline and granular casts, elevated plasma BUN/creatinine ratio (20:1).
Intrarenal: May have oliguria or be nonoliguric, urinary Na >20 mEq/L, low specific gravity, decreased urinary osmolality, presence of RBC casts and cellular debris in urine, decreased plasma BUN/creatinine ratio (10:1).

FLUID VOLUME ALTERATIONS

Excess: Peripheral edema, jugular vein distention, S_3 and S_4 gallops, crackles, increased BP, oliguria.
Deficit: Decreased BP, poor skin turgor, flushed skin, dry mucous membranes, oliguria.

ELECTROLYTE IMBALANCES Dysrhythmias, altered mental status, GI disturbances, neuromuscular dysfunction.

METABOLIC ACIDOSIS Weakness, disorientation, SOB, Kussmaul's respirations, CNS depression.

UREMIC MANIFESTATIONS Accumulation of urea, creatinine, uric acid; anemia and bleeding tendencies; fatigue and pallor; increased BP, congestive heart failure, pericarditis with tamponade, pulmonary edema; anorexia, nausea, vomiting, diarrhea; behavioral changes; decreased wound healing ability; increased susceptibility to infection.

PHYSICAL ASSESSMENT

Cardiovascular: S_3 and S_4 gallops, pericardial friction rub, jugular vein distention, tachycardia, dysrhythmias, increased BP, pulsus paradoxus in the presence of fluid volume excess, edema (peripheral, periorbital, sacral), capillary fragility, purpura.

Respiratory: Crackles, hyperventilation.

Neuromuscular: Weakness, lethargy, muscle irritability, muscle tenderness, asterixis.

Cutaneous: Pallor; presence of uremic frost in persons with severe uremia.

DIAGNOSTIC TESTS

Serum BUN, creatinine, uric acid, and electrolyte levels: Creatinine is the most reliable indicator of renal function. BUN is influenced by hydration, catabolism, presence of bleeding, infection, fever, and antianabolic agents (corticosteroids). BUN, creatinine, and uric acid levels will be elevated in the presence of ARF, as will potassium, phosphorus, and possibly magnesium.

Creatinine clearance test: For clinical purposes this is the most reliable estimation of glomerular filtration rate. Accuracy depends on complete collection. Creatinine clearance decreases with age. Normal creatinine clearance is 95-125 ml/min. In the presence of ARF it usually is <50 ml/min.

Urinalysis: The presence of sediment-containing tubular epithelial cells, cellular debris, and tubular casts supports a diagnosis of ARF. Large amounts of protein and many RBC casts are common in ARF when it is secondary to parenchymal (intrarenal) disease. Sediment is normal when the causes are categorized as prerenal.

Urinary sodium: A prerenal cause is signaled by a sodium count <10 mEq/L.

CBC and coagulation studies (PT, PTT): To evaluate for hematologic complications. Baseline Hct may be low as a result of ARF, and Hct and Hgb will fall steadily if the patient has bleeding or hemodilution from fluid overload.

ABG values: Because patients with ARF have metabolic acidosis, $Paco_2$ and plasma pH values will be low.

Ultrasonography: Identifies hydronephrosis, fluid collection, and masses.

Intravenous pyelograms (IVP), both retrograde and antegrade: To diagnose partial or complete obstruction.

Renal scan: Provides information about renal perfusion.

Renal angiography and venography: Assess for the presence or absence of thrombotic or stenotic lesions in the main renal vessels.

COLLABORATIVE MANAGEMENT
Prerenal acute renal failure
Volume replacement: Replacement solutions include free water plus electrolytes lost through the urine, wounds, drainage tubes, diarrhea, and vomiting. Usually losses are replaced on a volume-for-volume basis. Maintenance fluids total approximately 1,500 ml/24 h. With a moderate fluid deficit (5% weight loss), at least 2,400 ml is given over a 24-h period. A severe deficit (>5% weight loss) requires a replacement of at least 3,000 ml/24 h.
Diuretics (furosemide [Lasix] and ethacrynic acid [Edecrin]):   Decrease filtrate reabsorption and enhance water excretion. They may be used, after adequate hydration, to increase urine output or in an attempt to prevent onset of oliguria. If volume overload is present, diuretics are used to prevent pulmonary edema. Osmotic diuretics, such as mannitol, may be used to increase intravascular volume, promote renal blood flow, increase glomerular filtration rate, and stimulate urinary output. See Table 5-4 for additional information on diuretics.
Dopamine: Low doses, usually ≤ 2 μg/kg/min, to stimulate dopaminergic receptors, encourage renal vasodilatation, and promote renal blood flow. Slightly higher doses (e.g., 3-6 μg/kg/min) are used in mildly hypotensive patients to stimulate dopaminergic and beta$_1$-receptors, resulting in improved BP and cardiac output. Doses >7 μg/kg/min lack renal vasodilatory effects and may cause damaging renal vasoconstriction.

Intrarenal acute renal failure
Removal or discontinuation of toxic agent: (e.g., aminoglycosides, dye load, chemicals).
Dialytic therapy: Maintains homeostasis (see discussion, p. 410).
Nutrition therapy: Involves a diet high in carbohydrates to prevent endogenous protein catabolism and muscle breakdown, low in sodium for individuals who retain sodium and water, high in sodium for those who have lost large volumes of sodium and water as a result of diuresis or other bodily drainage, low in potassium if the patient is retaining potassium, and low in protein to maintain daily requirements while minimizing increases in azotemia. Nutrition is delivered *via* oral, enteral, or total parenteral nutrition (TPN). (See Table 10-11, p. 674, for a list of foods high in sodium and Table 10-12, p. 683, for a list of foods high in potassium.)
Blood transfusions: Packed RBCs are given if indicated to maintain a stable Hct. There are two major hematologic complications of renal failure:
Anemia: Caused by decreased erythropoietin, low-grade GI bleeding from mucosal ulceration, blood drawing, and shortened life of the RBCs.
Prolonged bleeding time: Caused by decreased platelet adhesiveness. As renal failure progresses, anemia becomes more profound and platelet adhesiveness decreases further.
Pharmacotherapy
Antihypertensives: See Table 4-16, p. 354).

T A B L E 5 - 4   Diuretic use in acute renal failure

Types	Mechanisms of action	Potential fluid and electrolyte abnormalities
Osmotic diuretics mannitol urea	Increase osmotic pressure of the filtrate, which attracts water and electrolytes and prevents their reabsorption	Hyponatremia Hypokalemia Rebound volume expansion
Loop diuretics furosemide ethacrynic acid bumetanide	Inhibit reabsorption of Na^+ and Cl^- at the ascending loop of Henle in the medulla; they produce a vasodilatory effect on the renal vasculature	Hypokalemia Hyperuricemia Hypocalcemia Hypomagnesemia Hyperglycemia and impairment of glucose tolerance Dilutional hyponatremia Hypochloremic acidosis
Thiazides bendroflumethiazide benzthiazide chlorothiazide sodium hydrochlorothiazide hydroflumethiazide methyclothiazide polythiazide trichlormethiazide	Inhibit reabsorption of Na^+ in the ascending loop of Henle at the beginning of the distal loop	Hypokalemia Dilutional hyponatremia Hypercalcemia Metabolic alkalosis Hypochloremia Hyperuricemia Hyperglycemia and impaired glucose tolerance
Thiazide-like diuretics chlorthalidone indapamide metolazone quinethazone	Action same as thiazides	Same as thiazides
*Potassium-sparing diuretics** amiloride HCl spironolactone triamterene	Inhibit aldosterone effect on the distal tubule, causing Na^+ excretion and potassium reabsorption	Hyperkalemia Hyponatremia Dehydration Acidosis Transient increase in BUN
Carbonic anhydrase inhibitors acetazolamide sodium dichlorphenamide methazolamide	Block the action of the enzyme carbonic anhydrase, producing excretion of sodium, potassium, bicarbonate, and water	Hyperchloremic acidosis Hypokalemia Hyperuricemia

Note: Loop or osmotic diuretics (or a combination of both) are used in patients with ARF to prevent hypervolemia and to stimulate urinary output.
*Used with caution in patients with oliguria.

Phosphate binders (aluminum hydroxide antacids and calcium carbonate antacids): Bind phosphorus and control hyperphosphatemia. They are given with meals.

Sodium bicarbonate: Controls metabolic acidosis and promotes shift of potassium back into the cells.

Sodium polystyrene sulfonate (Kayexalate): Oral or rectal preparation that exchanges sodium for potassium in the GI tract to help control hyperkalemia.

Water-soluble vitamin supplements: For patients receiving dialytic therapy. Water-soluble vitamins are diffused across the membrane and are removed during dialysis.

Recombinant human erythropoietin (rHuEPO): IV preparation given 3×/wk after dialysis in doses of 50-500 U/kg to correct anemia of chronic renal failure. Maintenance doses are given 3×/wk to maintain Hct levels of 33%-38%. Adverse reactions include development or worsening of hypertension; clotting of vascular access; depletion of iron stores; and slight increases in predialysis levels of BUN, creatinine, and potassium in individuals with Hct <30%.

Note: See Table 5-5 for a list of drugs that require dosage modification for patients with ARF. Drugs that require dosage modification in renal failure are those that are excreted primarily by the kidneys. Dosage must be governed by clinical responses, as well as serum levels, if available. Drugs that should be avoided (Table 5-6) are those that are nephrotoxic; those (or their metabolites) that are toxic to other organs if they accumulate; those that aggravate uremic symptoms; and those that accentuate metabolic derangements of renal failure.

Postrenal acute renal failure

Relief of obstruction: Achieved *via* catheterization with indwelling urinary catheter, ureteral stent to relieve obstruction before surgical intervention, lithotripsy to disintegrate stones, or prostatectomy if benign prostatic hypertrophy is the cause of the obstruction.

Monitoring of fluid and electrolyte balance: Postobstructive diure-

---

T A B L E   5 - 5   Drugs that require dosage modification in renal failure

Antimicrobials	Cardiovascular agents	Analgesics	Sedatives	Miscellaneous
amikacin	digitoxin	meperidine	meprobamate	cimetidine
amphotericin B	digoxin	methadone	phenobarbital	clofibrate
ethambutol	guanethidine			insulin
gentamicin	procainamide			neostigmine
kanamycin				
lincomycin				
penicillins				
sulfonamides				
tobramycin				
vancomycin				

T A B L E 5 - 6   Drugs to avoid in renal failure

amiloride
aspirin
cisplatin
lithium carbonate
magnesium-containing medications (see Table 10-15)
nitrofurantoin
nonsteroidal antiinflammatory drugs (e.g., ibuprofen)
phenylbutazone
spironolactone
tetracycline

sis may result in hypovolemia (see p. 669), hyponatremia (see p. 677), hypokalemia (see p. 681), hypocalcemia (see p. 688), and hypomagnesemia (see p. 700). See Table 5-3 for factors leading to altered electrolyte balance in ARF.

Culturing of urine and administration of antibiotics: If indicated.

NURSING DIAGNOSES AND INTERVENTIONS

Fluid volume excess related to compromised regulatory mechanism secondary to acute renal failure

Desired outcome: Within 24-48 h of onset, patient becomes normovolemic as evidenced by balanced I&O, urinary output ≥0.5 ml/kg/h, body weight within patient's normal range, BP within patient's normal range, CVP 2-6 mm Hg, HR 60-100 bpm, and absence of edema, crackles, gallop, and other clinical indicators of fluid overload.

Note: Although patient is retaining sodium, his or her serum sodium level may be within normal limits or decreased from baseline due to the dilutional effect of the fluid overload.

- Document I&O hourly. Consult physician if urinary output falls to <0.5 ml/kg/h.
- Weigh patient daily; consult physician regarding significant weight gain (e.g., 0.5-1.5 kg/24 h).
- Assess for and document the presence of basilar crackles, jugular vein distention, tachycardia, pericardial friction rub, gallop, increased BP, increased CVP, or SOB, any of which are indicative of fluid volume overload.
- Assess for and document the presence of peripheral, sacral, or periorbital edema.
- Restrict patient's total fluid intake to 1,200-1,500 ml/24 h, or as prescribed. Measure all output accurately, and replace milligram for milligram at intervals of 4-8 h, or as prescribed.
- Provide ice chips, chewing gum, or hard candy to help patient quench thirst and moisten mouth.
- Monitor serum osmolality and serum sodium values. These values may be decreased because of the dilutional effect of fluid overload.
- Recognize that if it is delivered, TPN will provide the largest volume of fluid intake for the patient. If total fluid intake is >2,000

ml/day, ultrafiltration with dialysis (see p. 410) or continuous arteriovenous hemofiltration (CAVH) (see p. 414) may be necessary to maintain fluid balance.

- If patient is retaining sodium, restrict sodium-containing foods (see Table 10-11, p. 674) and avoid diluting IV medications with high-sodium diluents. Also avoid sodium-containing medications such as sodium penicillin.

Fluid volume deficit related to active loss secondary to diuresis, vomiting, diarrhea, and hemorrhage; or related to failure of regulatory mechanism with fluid shift to interstitial compartments

Desired outcomes:　Within 24 h of this diagnosis, patient becomes normovolemic as evidenced by balanced I&O; urinary output ≥0.5 ml/kg/h with specific gravity of 1.010-1.020; CVP 2-6 mm Hg; HR 60-100 bpm; BP within patient's normal range; and absence of thirst and other indicators of hypovolemia. Patient's weight stabilizes within 2-3 days.

- Weigh patient daily. Consult physician for weight loss of 1-1.5 kg/24 h.
- Monitor and document I&O hourly. Consult physician if patient's output is <0.5 ml/kg/h. With deficit, intake should exceed output by 0.5-1 L (depending on severity of dehydration) q24h.
- Consult physician for increase in losses from vomiting, diarrhea, or wound drainage or sudden onset of diuresis.
- Observe for and document indicators of dehydration and hypovolemia (e.g., poor skin turgor, dry and sticky mucous membranes, thirst, hypotension, tachycardia, and decreasing CVP).
- Encourage oral fluids if they are allowed. Ensure that IV fluid rates are maintained as prescribed.
- Approximately 20% of patients with ARF have GI bleeding. Monitor Hgb, Hct, and BUN levels. In the presence of bleeding with ARF, Hgb and Hct values will fall steadily (rapidly if there is massive bleeding).

Note:　A patient with ARF has an Hct in the range of 20%-30% because of the anemia that occurs with renal failure. BUN will increase in the presence of GI bleeding without a concomitant rise in serum creatinine level.

- Test all stools, urine, emesis, and peritoneal dialysate drainage for occult blood. Check urine and dialysate drainage at least q8h.
- To minimize the risk of bleeding, keep side rails up and padded, use small-gauge needles for injections, minimize blood drawing, and promote the use of electric razors and soft-bristled toothbrushes. Limit invasive procedures as much as possible. If possible, avoid IM/SC injections for 1 h after hemodialysis. Apply gentle pressure to injection sites for at least 2-3 min.
- Inspect gums, mouth, nose, skin, and perianal and vaginal areas q8h for bleeding. Also inspect hemodialysis insertion and peritoneal access sites for evidence of bleeding q8h. Apply a soft, occlusive sterile dressing to peritoneal, subclavian, or femoral access sites daily to protect skin from irritation and bleeding due to catheter movement.

Altered nutrition: Less than body requirements related to catabolic state and excessive metabolic needs secondary to ARF; and related to anorexia and psychologic aversion to dietary restrictions
Desired outcomes: Within 72 h of this diagnosis, patient has adequate nutrition as evidenced by a caloric intake that ranges from 35-45 calories/kg normal body weight, a daily protein intake that consists of 50%-75% of high–biologic value proteins, and a nitrogen intake of 4-6 g more than nitrogen loss (calculated from 24-h urinary urea excretion and protein intake).

- Infuse enteral feedings and TPN as prescribed.
- Assess and document patient's intake of nutrients every shift.
- Weigh patient daily. Consult physician for significant findings (i.e., loss of >1.5 kg/24 h).
- As prescribed, use cooling blanket or antipyretic agents to control fever. Fever increases tissue catabolism, which in turn increases metabolic needs.
- The end products of protein metabolism that accumulate in renal failure are reflected by an increase in BUN level. Low-protein diets are used to decrease the nitrogenous load and attempt to control uremia to some extent. Ensure intake of high–biologic value protein, which contains the more essential amino acids necessary for cell building (e.g., eggs, meat, fowl, milk, and fish).
- Be sure that caloric intake ranges from 35-45 cal/kg normal body weight. The exact amount will vary with age, sex, activity, and the degree of preexisting malnutrition. Foods that may be used to increase caloric intake include honey, hard candy, gumdrops, and sherbet.
- Restrict high-potassium foods such as bananas, citrus fruits, fruit juices, nuts, tea, coffee, legumes, and salt substitute. In ARF the kidneys are unable to excrete potassium effectively. (See Table 10-12 for foods high in potassium.)
- Sodium requirements will vary greatly. If oliguria is present, sodium intake may be restricted in the diet. If diuresis is present, sodium intake may be increased because of excess sodium loss in the urine. Intervene accordingly. (See Table 10-11 for foods high in sodium.)
- Hypocalcemia may be present early in ARF as a result of decreased absorption of calcium from the gut and the presence of hyperphosphatemia. As prescribed, replace calcium orally (e.g., with dairy products) or intravenously, and administer phosphate binders as prescribed.
- If patient is anorexic or nauseated, provide small, frequent meals. Present appetizing food in a pleasant atmosphere; eliminate any noxious odors. As indicated, administer medication with prescribed antiemetic ½ h before meals.

Risk for infection related to inadequate secondary defenses as a result of immunocompromised state associated with ARF; and related to multiple invasive procedures
Desired outcome: At the time of discharge from ICU, patient is free of infection as evidenced by normothermia, negative culture results of dialysate and body secretions, and WBC count ≤11,000/μl.

Note: After the initial insult, infection is the primary cause of death in ARF.

- Monitor and record patient's temperature q8h. If it is elevated (i.e., >37° C [99° F]), monitor temperature q2-4h, and q2h if it is >38° C (101° F). Because ARF may be accompanied by hypothermia, even a slight rise in temperature of 1°-2° may be significant.
- Inspect and record the color, odor, and appearance of all body secretions. Be alert to cloudy or blood-tinged peritoneal dialysis return, cloudy and foul-smelling urine, foul-smelling wound exudate, purulent drainage from any catheter site, foul-smelling and watery stools, foul-smelling vaginal discharge, or purulent sputum. Be aware that uremia retards wound healing, and therefore it is important that all wounds (including scratches resulting from pruritus) be assessed for indicators of infection. Send sample of any suspicious fluid or drainage for culture and sensitivity tests as indicated.
- Monitor WBC count for elevations.
- Ensure sound infection control when manipulating central lines, peripheral IV lines, and indwelling catheters. Be aware that catabolism of protein, which occurs with infection, causes potassium to be released from the tissues.
- Avoid use of indwelling urinary catheter in patients with oliguria and anuria. The presence of a catheter in these patients further increases the risk of infection.
- To help maintain the integrity of the oral mucous membranes, provide oral hygiene q2h.
- Reposition patient q2-4h to help maintain the barrier of an intact integumentary system. Provide skin care at least q8h.
- Encourage good pulmonary hygiene by having patient practice deep-breathing exercises (and coughing, if its need is indicated) q2-4h.

Knowledge deficit: Biochemical alterations associated with ARF
Desired outcome: Within 72 h of admission, patient and significant others verbalize accurate information regarding patient's disease state and the measures that can be taken to prevent its occurrence or minimize its effects.

- Determine patient's and significant others' knowledge about patient's disease process and the biochemical alterations (hyperkalemia, hypokalemia, hypernatremia, hyponatremia, hypocalcemia, hyperphosphatemia, hypermagnesemia, metabolic acidosis, and uremia) that can occur.
- Teach patient and significant others the signs and symptoms of the biochemical alterations (see Table 5-3 and **Altered protection,** p. 401).
- Provide lists of foods high in potassium (see Table 10-12), sodium (see Table 10-11), phosphorus (see Table 10-13), and magnesium (see Table 10-14), which patient should add or avoid when planning meals. In addition, provide a list of medications that contain magnesium (see Table 10-15), which should not be taken without physician approval.

- Explain the importance of consuming only the amount of protein prescribed by physician and avoiding exposure to persons with infection or a febrile illness in order to minimize catabolism of protein, which causes potassium to be released from the tissues. Reinforce that patient should consume the prescribed amount of carbohydrates and limit strenuous activity as prescribed, both of which will spare protein and thus minimize potassium release.
- Teach patient to report to physician an increase in temperature or other signs of infection.
- Reinforce the importance of taking vitamin D and calcium supplements as prescribed.
- Teach the relationship between calcium and phosphate levels. Emphasize that maintaining good phosphate control and calcium balance may help control itching and prevent future problems with bone disease.
- Stress the importance of taking phosphate binders (e.g., Amphojel, Alternagel) as prescribed.
- Teach patient not to take OTC medications without first consulting physician. Aspirin, for example, exacerbates the bleeding tendency caused by uremia.
- Instruct patient about the importance of maintaining the prescribed dialysis schedule, inasmuch as dialysis will help correct acidosis, uremia, and many of the metabolic abnormalities that occur.
- Teach patient to use lotions and oils to lubricate skin and relieve drying and cracking.
- Stress the importance of follow-up monitoring of serum electrolyte levels.

Altered protection related to neurosensory changes secondary to electrolyte imbalance, metabolic acidosis, and uremia

Desired outcomes: Within 48-72 h of onset, patient verbalizes orientation to time, place, and person and maintains his or her normal mobility.

- Monitor patient for the following mentation and motor dysfunctions associated with ARF:
  - Hyperkalemia (during oliguric phase): Muscle weakness, irritability, paresthesias.
  - Hypokalemia (during diuretic phase): Lethargy; muscle weakness, softness, flabbiness; paresthesias.
  - Hypernatremia: Fatigue, restlessness, agitation.
  - Hyponatremia: Dizziness when changing position, apprehension, personality changes.
  - Hypocalcemia: Neuromuscular irritability, tonic muscle spasms, paresthesias.
  - Hyperphosphatemia: Excessive itching, muscle weakness, hyperreflexia.
  - Hypermagnesemia: Drowsiness, lethargy, sensation of heat.
  - Metabolic acidosis: Confusion, weakness.
  - Uremia: Confusion, lethargy, itching, metallic taste, muscle twitching.
- Explain to significant others that patient's decreasing attention level necessitates simple and direct communication efforts.

Prevent infection (see **Risk for infection,** p. 399), control fevers by using cooling blankets and acetaminophen, and maintain adequate nutritional intake (see **Altered nutrition,** p. 399) to minimize tissue catabolism and thus production of nitrogenous wastes, which in turn will decrease azotemia.

- To alleviate unpleasant metallic taste caused by uremia, provide frequent oral hygiene. Because patient with uremia is at increased risk for bleeding, ensure use of soft-bristled brushes. If appropriate, provide chewing gum or hard candy, which may help alleviate the unpleasant metallic taste.
- Encourage isometric exercises and short walks, if patient is able, to help maintain muscle strength and tone, especially in the legs.
- Decrease environmental stimuli, and use a calm, reassuring manner in caring for patient.
- Encourage establishment of sleep/rest patterns by scheduling daytime activities appropriately and promoting relaxation method (see **Health-seeking behavior,** p. 324).
- Assess for decreased tactile sensations in the feet and legs, which may occur with peripheral neuropathy. Be alert to the potential for pressure sores and friction burns, which may occur with peripheral neuropathy.
- Use splints and braces to aid in mobility for patients with severe neuropathic effects.

Constipation related to immobility, restrictions of fresh fruit and fluids, and use of phosphate binders
Desired outcome: Within 48 h of onset, patient has bowel movements of soft consistency.

- Monitor and record the number and quality of patient's bowel movements.
- Administer prescribed stool softeners and bulking agents, such as psyllium husks.
- If these measures fail, administer standard Fleet, oil retention, or tap water enemas as prescribed. Because excess fluid can be absorbed from the gut, avoid using large-volume water enemas.
- Encourage moderate exercise on a routine basis.
- Establish a regular schedule for fluid intake within patient's prescribed limits.
- Provide 4 oz of hot water ½ h before breakfast to stimulate bowel evacuation.
- Administer metoclopramide as prescribed to increase motility in the presence of autonomic neuropathy.

Impaired skin integrity (or risk for same) related to uremia, with resulting pruritus and edema
Desired outcome: Patient's skin remains intact.

- Monitor patient for presence of pruritus with resulting frequent and intense scratching.
- Pruritus decreases with reduced BUN level and control of hyperphosphatemia. Monitor laboratory values of BUN and phosphorus, and report levels outside the optimal range (BUN >20 mg/dl and phosphorus >4.5 mg/dl or 2.6 mEq/L).
- Administer phosphate binders (e.g., Alternagel) as prescribed, and if possible, reduce patient's dietary intake of phosphorus (see Table 10-13, p. 693).

- Ensure that patient's fingernails are cut short and that the nail tips are smooth.
- Because uremia retards wound healing, monitor scratches for indicators of infection.
- Because of reduced oil gland activity in uremia, the patient's skin may be quite dry. Use skin emollients liberally and avoid harsh soaps and excessive bathing.
- Advise patient of the potential for bruising due to clotting abnormality and capillary fragility.
- Pruritus increases in the presence of secondary hyperparathyroidism. Monitor serum calcium and PTH levels, and report elevations (Ca^{2+} >10.5 mg/dl and PTH >30% above the upper limit of the test used).
- As prescribed, administer oral antihistamine, such as diphenhydramine, to relieve itching.

ADDITIONAL NURSING DIAGNOSES

For patients undergoing dialytic therapy, see nursing diagnoses and interventions in "Renal Replacement Therapies," p. 418. Also see the following, as appropriate: "Nutritional Support," p. 12; "Prolonged Immobility," p. 78; "Psychosocial Support," p. 88; and "Psychosocial Support for the Patient's Family and Significant Others," p. 100.

Renal transplantation

Renal transplantation has become an accepted mode of treatment for end-stage renal disease, to a large extent a result of advances in the development of immunosuppressive medications in the late 1960s and the 1970s. Approximately 30%-40% of individuals who need transplantation have chronic renal failure caused by glomerulonephritis; 20%-30% have pyelonephritis or other interstitial disease; 15%-20% have multisystem disease; and approximately 10% have cystic kidney disease. There are two types of transplant donors, living and cadaveric. The 1-yr success rate with live donor transplantation is 90%-95%. The 1-yr success rate with cadaveric transplantation since the advent of cyclosporine has improved to 75%-85%. The majority of patients do not have a suitable (medically or psychologically) live donor and therefore are placed on a cadaveric waiting list. The demand exceeds the supply, with approximately 6,000-7,000 patients awaiting transplantation in the United States alone.

Rejection and infection remain the major complications after transplantation. Rejection is the phenomenon that represents the recipient's immunologic response to the transplanted kidney. There are two types of lymphocytes involved in the rejection response, and either or both may participate: B lymphocytes, which form antibodies (humoral immunity), and T lymphocytes, which produce cell-mediated immunity. The rejection response can be categorized into four distinct types: hyperacute, accelerated acute, acute, and chronic (Table 5-7).

T A B L E   5 - 7   Types of renal rejection

Type	Mechanism	Clinical presentation	Treatment
Hyperacute	Preformed antibodies against donor antigens	Occurs in the operating room; kidney turns blue and becomes soft and flabby	Removal of kidney
Accelerated acute	May be mediated by humoral antibody or primed lymphocytes (possible presensitization in the recipient)	Occurs 48-72 h after transplantation. Abrupt fall in urine output; leukocytosis or leukopenia; tenderness over kidney; decreased flow on renal scan; profound thrombocytopenia	Bolus IV steroids for 3-4 days; antilymphocyte preparations; poor prognosis for reversal
Acute	Cell-mediated T lymphocytes infiltrate renal tissue; humoral-mediated antigen-antibody complexes, platelets, and fibrin aggregates are present in glomerular and peritubular capillaries; may be a combination of cell-mediated and humoral-mediated	Occurs from 1-2 wk to several months after transplantation: fever, leukocytosis, and enlarged and tender kidney, drop in urine output, weight gain (1-1.5 kg/24 h), hypertension, elevated BUN and creatinine	Bolus steroids, antilymphocyte preparations, and monoclonal antibody treatments most effective in reversing this type of rejection; good prognosis
Chronic	Probably a combined effect of antibody and cell-mediated components	Occurs months to years after transplantation; slow, progressive decrease in renal function; hypertension; proteinuria	None known; poor prognosis for graft survival

ASSESSMENT FOR REJECTION
Sudden drop in urine output: Oliguria or anuria may develop.

Note: A sudden drop in output in the first 24 postoperative hours, when a Foley catheter is in place, may signal the presence of clot obstruction, which should be ruled out as the first cause of oliguria.

Elevated temperature: Low-grade, persistent fevers of 37.2°-37.8° C (99°-100° F) can occur with rejection. In the presence of accelerated or acute rejection, the patient may have fevers ranging from 37.8°-40° C (100°-104° F).
Edema: May increase in grade from 1+ (slight indentation over bony areas such as the tibia) to 3+ and 4+, with the degree of indentation increasing significantly.
Hypertension: BP that increases ≥10 mm Hg over baseline.
Weight gain: Increase of 2-3 lbs over a 24-h period.
BUN and creatinine values: Will increase from previous 24-h levels (e.g., BUN 25-52 mg/dl; creatinine 1.3-1.8 mg/dl).
24-h urine collection: Will exhibit a change in components (e.g., decreases in creatinine clearance, total amount of creatinine excreted, and urinary sodium excretion, and an increase in protein excretion).

Note: In the early postoperative period, the urine may remain bloody for several days, causing urinary protein concentration to be falsely elevated due to Hgb breakdown in the urine.

Renal scan: Will exhibit decreased blood flow.
Kidney assessment: Will reveal a firm, large kidney that may be tender on palpation.

DIAGNOSTIC TESTS
Renal scan: Evaluates blood flow to the kidney and rate of excretion of substances into the bladder.
Renal biopsy: Determines presence, type, and severity of rejection.
Renal ultrasound: To rule out possibility of obstruction.

TREATMENT OPTIONS FOR REJECTION
Megadoses of IV methylprednisolone (Solu-Medrol):   Block the production of interleukin-2 (IL-2), thereby barring essential factors for activated T cells; prevent transcription of IL-1. The release of IL-1 and IL-2 is part of the process of helper T-cell and cytotoxic T-cell differentiation, which occurs during the immune response that is triggered when foreign antigens are present in the body. Methylprednisolone also is used for its antiinflammatory properties (Table 5-8).
Antithymocyte or antilymphocyte preparations: See Table 5-8.
Monoclonal antibody (Orthoclone OKT3):   Reacts with and blocks the function of the T3 complex on the surface of the T lymphocytes, causing their entrapment by cells in the spleen and liver and leading to their destruction. The T3 complex is responsible for the ability of the T lymphocyte to identify a transplanted organ as foreign (see Table 5-8).

T A B L E   5 - 8   **Immunosuppressives (standard agents and prophylaxis)**

Drug name	Action	Dosage
azathioprine (e.g., Imuran)	Blocks proliferation of immunocompetent lymphoid cells; affects the rapidly dividing B and T cells	Ranges from 1.5-2 mg/kg/day; IV or PO
corticosteroids (prednisone)	Suppress the body's inflammatory and allergic processes	Varies; total dose tapered to 20-30 mg/day by first postoperative month
cyclophosphamide (e.g., Cytoxan)	See azathioprine	1 mg/kg/day IV or PO
cyclosporine (e.g., Sandimmune)	Interferes with helper T-lymphocyte function; used in combination with corticosteroids and azathioprine	8-14 mg/kg/day PO; 3-4 mg/kg *via* continuous IV infusion
antilymphocyte sera (e.g., ATGAM)	Immunoglobulin preparation that coats the T cells, making them susceptible to phagocytosis	*Prophylaxis:* 10-15 mg/kg IV over 4-6 h for 5-10 days *Rejection:* 10-15 mg/kg IV over 4-6 h for 10-14 days
monoclonal antibody (Orthoclone OKT3)	Reacts with T3 complex on the surface of the T cells, causing their removal from the circulation	5 mg IV push over 30-60 sec for 10-14 days to treat rejection

Note: Each of these agents, when used individually or in combination, leads to an increased incidence of infection and malignancy secondary to their immunosuppressive properties.

Graft irradiation: Destroys lymphocytes within the graft. Irradiation is performed with 150 rad for approximately 3 days in succession.

NURSING DIAGNOSES AND INTERVENTIONS

Fear and anxiety related to threat to health status secondary to potential loss of the kidney from rejection

Desired outcomes: Within 48 h after the transplant, patient verbalizes accurate information about the signs and symptoms of rejection. Patient's fear and anxiety are controlled as evidenced by HR ≤100 bpm, BP within patient's normal range, and RR ≤20 breaths/min. Patient demonstrates ability to relax, discusses anxiety related to the rejection, and exhibits increased involvement in his or her own care.

• Provide opportunities for patient to express fears, concerns, and anxieties about kidney rejection.

- Assess patient's knowledge of the signs and symptoms of rejection. Ensure that patient and significant others can verbalize knowledge of the following indicators of rejection:
  - Persistent, low-grade fever of 37.2°-37.8° C (99°-100° F).
  - Increased swelling of feet, ankles, hands, or face.
  - Weight gain >1 kg/24 h.
  - Painful and swollen kidney.
  - Elevated BP.
  - Decreased 24-h urine output.
- Reassure patient that several medication regimens (e.g., corticosteroids, antilymphocyte preparations, and monoclonal antibody) are available to treat rejection episodes.
- Reassure patient that rejection does not necessarily mean kidney loss. Under most circumstances, rejection can be reversed.
- Reassure patient that retransplantation is a viable option if kidney loss occurs.

Knowledge deficit: Immunosuppressive medications and their side effects

Desired outcome: Within 72 h after initiation of medications, patient and significant others verbalize accurate information regarding the prescribed immunosuppressive agents, the side effects that can occur, and precautions that should be taken.

- Provide patient with verbal and written information for the type of immunosuppressive agent that has been prescribed. Discuss the generic name, trade name, purpose, usual dosage, route, side effects, and precautions (see Table 5-8 for purpose, usual dosage, and route) for the medications discussed below.

Azathioprine (Imuran)

- Major side effects include leukopenia and thrombocytopenia, nausea and vomiting, and diarrhea. In addition, it increases the risk of cancer and can contribute to an increased susceptibility toward infection and hepatotoxicity.
- Report fever, chills, cough, muscle or joint pain, rapid heartbeat, stomach pain with nausea and vomiting, sores in mouth and on lips.
- Blood should be tested at frequent intervals for evaluation of WBCs and platelets. Report jaundice promptly to health care provider.
- Hair loss can occur early in the treatment course, but it usually lessens in occurrence over time.

Corticosteroids

- Major side effects include cushingoid features, edema, hypertension, bone disease, muscle wasting, cataracts, steroid-induced diabetes, acne, GI irritation, and capillary fragility.
- Immediately report swelling of ankles, hands, or face; BP >20 mm Hg over baseline; swollen or bleeding gums; night sweats; change in eyesight; muscle weakness.

Cyclophosphamide (e.g., Cytoxan)

- Major side effects include hemorrhagic cystitis (manifested by hematuria and dysuria); alopecia; and bone marrow depression, often appearing during days 9-14 of treatment.

- Increasing fluid intake and voiding frequently minimizes the potential for hemorrhagic cystitis. WBC count is monitored regularly to detect bone marrow suppression.
- Report presence of rashes or lesions (warts) on skin or genital area.

Cyclosporine (Sandimmune)
- Major side effects include nephrotoxicity, hepatotoxicity, leukopenia, thrombocytopenia, hirsutism, muscle pain, fluid retention, edema, tremors, hypertension, nausea, vomiting, diarrhea, gum hyperplasia, anorexia, and anaphylaxis (rare but can occur with IV route). Immediately report these symptoms.
- Blood levels of cyclosporine are monitored at frequent intervals to ensure maximal absorption of oral solution. This is particularly important for patients experiencing GI malabsorption.
- To make oral solutions more palatable, mix with orange juice or milk and drink immediately. Stir the mixture well and use a glass container because plastic, foam, or paper will absorb the medication.
- Rinse syringe and container with milk or orange juice and drink the remaining solution to ensure that all medication has been taken.
- Take medication 1 h before or 2 h after meals, and if taking twice a day, space the doses 12 h apart.
- Tolerance to the medication, with a decrease in side effects, occurs over time.
- Because of gum hyperplasia, brush teeth with soft-bristled toothbrush and nonabrasive toothpaste after meals and snacks.
- Report nausea and vomiting that occur after dose of cyclosporine and *do not* repeat dose unless told to do so by physician.
- Report headache, breast enlargement, flushing, and presence of any skin lesions.
- Protect skin from freezing temperatures (e.g., by wearing a mitten when taking foods out of the freezer).
- Consult physician before taking OTC medications.

Antilymphocyte sera
- Major side effects include serum sickness (see next entry), local phlebitis, thrombocytopenia, and pruritus.
- Report rashes on the skin or genital area, joint pain and swelling, fever and chills, and night sweats. These indicators may signal serum sickness.

Monoclonal antibody
- Major side effects include chills and fever, headache, photophobia, nausea, vomiting, diarrhea, dyspnea, and bronchospasm.

Caution: Intensive monitoring is required during the first two doses, owing to the high frequency of side effects (first-dose reaction) discussed above. In addition, there is an increased risk of pulmonary edema in the presence of fluid volume excess.

The patient is premedicated with acetaminophen, diphenhydramine, and hydrocortisone to decrease the above symptoms. A chest x-ray must be clear before the first dose is given.

Risk for infection related to inadequate secondary responses as a result of immunosuppression
Desired outcome: Patient is free of infection as evidenced by normothermia; absence of erythema, swelling, and drainage of catheter and wound sites; absence of adventitious breath sounds or cloudy and foul-smelling urine; negative results of urine, wound drainage, and blood cultures; and WBC count 4,500-11,000 μl.

- Assess and record patient's temperature q4h; consult physician for elevations $\geq 37.8°$ C (100° F).
- Assess and document condition of indwelling IV sites and other catheter sites q8h. Be alert to swelling, erythema, tenderness, and drainage. Consult physician for any of these findings.
- As prescribed, obtain blood, urine, and wound cultures when infection is suspected.
- Be alert to WBC count $>11,000$ μl or $<4,500$ μl. A below-normal WBC count with increased band neutrophils on differential (shift to the left) may signal acute infection.
- Inspect graft wound for erythema, swelling, and drainage. Consult physician for significant findings.
- Record volume, appearance, color, and odor of urine. Be alert to foul-smelling or cloudy urine, frequency and urgency of urination, and patient complaints of flank or labial pain, all of which are signs of renal-urinary infection.
- Auscultate lung fields q8h, noting presence of rhonchi, crackles, and decreased breath sounds.
- Use meticulous aseptic technique when dressing and caring for wounds and catheter sites.
- Obtain specimens for urine cultures once a week during patient's hospitalization and once a month after hospital discharge.

Altered oral mucous membrane related to treatment with immunosuppressive medication
Desired outcomes: Patient's oral mucosa, tongue, and lips are pink, intact, and free of exudate and lesions. Patient states that he or she can swallow without difficulty within 24 h after treatment for altered oral mucous membrane.

- Inspect the mouth daily for signs of exudate and lesions; consult physician if they are present. Teach patient to perform self-inspection of mouth.
- Teach patient to brush with a soft-bristled toothbrush and nonabrasive toothpaste after meals and snacks.
- To help prevent monilial infection, provide patient with mycostatin prophylactic mouthwash for "swish and swallow" after meals and at bedtime.

Impaired skin integrity (or risk for same): Herpetic lesions, skin fungal rashes, pruritus, and capillary fragility related to treatment with immunosuppressive medications
Desired outcome: Patient's skin is intact and free of open lesions or abrasions.

- Assess for and document daily the presence of erythema, excoriation, rashes, or bruises on patient's skin.
- Assess for and document the presence of rashes or lesions in the

perineal area, inasmuch as herpetic lesions are common in the immunosuppressed patient.

- Inspect the trunk area daily for the presence of flat, itchy rashes. Skin fungal rashes are common in the immunosuppressed patient.
- Teach patient the importance of daily skin care with water, nondrying soap, and lubricating lotion.
- Use nonallergenic tape when anchoring IV tubing, catheters, and dressings.
- Assist patient with changing position at least q2h; massage areas that are susceptible to breakdown, particularly areas over bony prominences.

ADDITIONAL NURSING DIAGNOSES

As indicated, see "Acute Renal Failure," p. 397. Also see "Organ Rejection" for **Powerlessness** related to actual and perceived inability to control organ rejection episodes, p. 649. For other nursing diagnoses and interventions, see the following sections, as appropriate: "Nutritional Support," p. 12; "Prolonged Immobility," p. 78; "Psychosocial Support," p. 88; and "Psychosocial Support for the Patient's Family and Significant Others," p. 100.

Renal replacement therapies

The patient with renal dysfunction has an increasingly malfunctioning physiologic system. The goal of renal replacement therapy (RRT) is to restore dynamic equilibrium to that system. Indications for RRT in a critical care setting include fluid removal, solute removal, and correction of electrolyte and acid-base abnormalities. RRT uses four principles for solute and water removal: diffusion, osmosis, ultrafiltration, and convection.

Diffusion: Movement of solutes from an area of greater concentration to an area of lesser concentration. Diffusion requires a concentration gradient. During dialysis, high concentrations of waste products and excess electrolytes diffuse into the dialysate, which contains much lower concentrations of these solutes.

Osmosis: Passive movement of water from an area of low solute concentration to an area of high solute concentration. Thus the use of high concentrations of glucose in the peritoneal dialysate causes movement of water from the patient's plasma into the dialysate.

Ultrafiltration: Movement of water from an area of higher pressure to an area of lower pressure. In hemodialysis, negative pressure in the dialysate facilitates the rapid removal of excess water from the blood compartment in which positive pressure exists.

Convection: Removal of a substance with fluid across a semipermeable membrane over time.

INDICATIONS FOR RRT

- Volume excess
- Hyperkalemia and other electrolyte disturbances
- Metabolic acidosis

T A B L E   5 - 9   Comparison of renal replacement therapies

	Peritoneal dialysis	Hemodialysis	CAVH	CVVH
Access route	Catheter, which may be used immediately	Subclavian or femoral catheter or arteriovenous shunt, which may be used immediately	Arterial and venous catheters or shunt Patient's mean arterial pressure drives flow rate	Double-lumen venous catheter Pump used to achieve flow rate
Semipermeable membrane	Peritoneum; approximately 2.2 m^2 (the total area available for diffusion of solutes)	Cuprophan or cellulose acetate; 1-2 m^2	High-efficiency, high-flux material (polysulfone, polyamide, and poly-acrylonitrile)	Same as CAVH
Molecular movement	Diffusion by a concentration gradient	Diffusion by a concentration gradient	Diffusion and convection	Same as CAVH
Water removal	Osmotic pressure, using high glucose concentration	Hydrostatic pressure (pressure gradient across the membrane)	Ultrafiltration—hydrostatic pressure	Same as CAVH
Duration	10-24 h, 3-4/wk, or continuous cycling	4-5 h, 3/wk; maximum of 3-4 h/day	Continuous	Same as CAVH
Efficiency	Slow diffusion; less efficient than hemodialysis	High efficiency	High for fluid removal, moderate solute removal	Same as CAVH
Risk of infection	High	Lower than peritoneal method	High for access infection	Same as CAVH
Major problem	Development of peritonitis	May not be tolerated by the patient with hemodynamic instability	Dehydration and hypotension	Same as CAVH

T A B L E 5 - 10   **Advantages and disadvantages of methods of renal replacement therapy**

Advantages	Disadvantages
Hemodialysis	
Very efficient; requires short, frequent treatments	Special equipment and trained staff
	Heparinization usually required
As needed, fluid and chemical balance may be altered rapidly	Possibility of disequilibrium from too-rapid fluid and biochemical shifts
	Possible difficulty in maintaining vascular access
	Blood loss necessitating transfusion
Peritoneal dialysis	
Simple equipment; rapid initiation of treatment	Time consuming
	Risk of peritonitis and pneumonia
No anticoagulation needed	Desired effects slower to occur
Slow dialysis; less risk of hypotension and rapid fluid and electrolyte shifts	Protein loss
	Some patient discomfort
Hemofiltration	
Physiologic process	Low-efficiency solute removal
Ideal for the patient who is hemodynamically unstable	Large volume fluid replacement
	Potential for electrolyte imbalance
Allows administration of large volumes (e.g., TPN)	Increased responsibilities for ICU nurses
Technically simple	
CVVH effective in patients with MAP <70 mm Hg	

- Uremic intoxication
  - □ Central nervous system (encephalopathy)
  - □ Hematologic (bleeding due to platelet dysfunction)
  - □ Gastrointestinal (anorexia, nausea, vomiting)
  - □ Cardiovascular (pericarditis)
- Need for removal of dialyzable substances (metabolites, drugs, toxins)

DETERMINATION FOR TYPE OF RRT USED

- Availability of hemodialysis, peritoneal dialysis, continuous arteriovenous hemofiltration (CAVH), or continuous venovenous hemofiltration (CVVH) in the institution.
- Type best suited for patient's clinical status. Catabolism, for example, causes rapid rises in BUN, creatinine, and potassium values. The patient needs rapid removal of metabolic wastes (i.e., hemodialysis) (Table 5-9). Advantages and disadvantages of RRT methods are found in Table 5-10. Complications of RRT are found in Table 5-11.
- Blood or peritoneal access route availability.
- Ability to effect safe anticoagulation.

T A B L E 5 - 11 **Complications of renal replacement therapies**

Hemodialysis	Peritoneal dialysis	Hemofiltration
Hypotension	Bowel or bladder perforation	Bleeding
Air embolus		Infection
Angina and dysrhythmias	Hyperglycemic hyperosmolar coma	Volume depletion
		Blood leakage
Blood loss (dialyzer rupture)	Hypernatremia	Decreased ultrafiltration
	Hypovolemia	Filter clotting
Disequilibrium syndrome	Metabolic alkalosis	Electrolyte disturbances
	Peritonitis	Air embolus with CVVH
Hemolysis	**Procedural complications**	
Hemorrhage		
Septicemia	Abdominal distention: failure to drain dialysate	
Bleeding		
Clotting		
High-output heart failure	• Catheter obstruction from clots or fibrin	
Infection	• Catheter becoming wrapped in omentum	
Phlebitis	Cuff erosion	
Venous spasm	Catheter malposition	
	Tunnel infection	

PERITONEAL DIALYSIS

The semipermeable membrane used during peritoneal dialysis is the patient's peritoneum. A special catheter is placed in the peritoneal cavity, and dialysate solution is instilled. Water, electrolytes, and waste products cross between the capillary bed of the peritoneum and the dialysate *via* osmosis and diffusion.

System components

Catheter: Two types are commonly used:
- *Trocar:* A stiff Silastic catheter inserted at the bedside that provides temporary access.
- *Soft Silastic indwelling catheter* (e.g., Tenckhoff): Inserted in the operating room to provide permanent access.

Dialysate: A premixed sterile electrolyte solution with a composition similar to that of normal plasma. The concentration of ionized calcium is high to maintain a positive calcium balance. Hypocalcemia tends to occur in patients with renal failure, and the goal is to maintain serum calcium levels at 8.5-10 mg/dl. Glucose concentrations are variable inasmuch as hypertonic solutions are used to increase osmotic load for greater filtration. Potassium is added according to patient need.

Methods of peritoneal dialysis

Intermittent peritoneal dialysis (IPD): Usually involves 3-4 treatments a week, lasting 8-10 h each session. Hospitalized patients with acute renal failure may undergo dialysis for 24 h every other day.

Continuous ambulatory peritoneal dialysis (CAPD): Involves extension of the time the fluid remains in the abdomen (dwell time) to

4 h during the day and 8 h during the night, with 4-5 exchanges during a day. Dialysis occurs 7 days a week, 24 h a day. This method is the most physiologic form of dialysis.

HEMODIALYSIS

With hemodialysis an artificial semipermeable membrane is used to diffuse water, electrolytes, and waste products from the blood. The patient's blood is heparinized, passed through the dialyzer, and then returned to the circulation. For acutely ill patients, dialysis may be needed from 3 times a week to daily.

System components

Dialyzer (artificial kidney):   Consists of the blood compartment, dialysate compartment, and the semipermeable membrane. Small molecules, such as electrolytes, water, and waste products, pass through this membrane; RBCs, protein, and bacteria, however, are too large to cross.

Dialysate: Electrolyte solution similar to normal plasma. The potassium concentration varies according to patient need. Glucose may be necessary to prevent changes in the patient's serum glucose and osmolality values. Although glucose is a large molecule, it can cross the semipermeable membrane, resulting in hypoglycemia. Use of a glucose bath reduces the risk of hypoglycemia.

Vascular access: Method used to deliver blood to the dialyzer at a rate of at least 200-300 ml/min.

- *Arteriovenous (AV) shunt:* Insertion of a Silastic tube into an artery and a vein, allowing blood to flow from the artery to the vein externally.
- *Subclavian or femoral catheter:* Temporary access catheter (usually double lumen) that is placed in a large vein to enhance blood flow.
- *Arteriovenous (AV) fistula:* Anastomosis of an artery and vein, resulting in dilated vessels for easy cannulation and increased blood flow.
- *Graft:* Bovine, Gore-Tex, or saphenous vein. The graft connects the artery and vein internally in the arm or thigh.
- *Hemasite:* A T-shaped device inserted into an arterialized vein with a Gore-Tex graft. The "T" projects out of the skin, resulting in an external entry point.

CONTINUOUS ARTERIOVENOUS HEMOFILTRATION OR CONTINUOUS VENOVENOUS HEMOFILTRATION

Continuous arteriovenous hemofiltration (CAVH) and continuous venovenous hemofiltration (CVVH) are two types of renal therapy performed to manage fluid overload in critically ill patients. Their advantage over conventional dialytic therapies is that ultrafiltration occurs gradually, thus avoiding drastic volume changes and rapid fluid shifts. Treatment duration may be 24 h or several days, depending on the total amount of fluid to be removed.

Principles

- Use of a highly permeable, hollow fiber filter (e.g., Amicon Diafilter 20).
- Removal of plasma water and unbound substances, such as urea, cal-

cium, sodium, potassium, chloride, vitamins, and unbound drugs, with a molecular weight between 500 and 10,000 daltons.

- Filtration: Movement of fluid across a semipermeable membrane from an area of greater pressure to one of lesser pressure (pressure gradient).
- Convection: Some elements in plasma water (e.g., urea) conveyed across the membrane as a result of the differences in hydrostatic pressure. The removal of large amounts of plasma water results in the removal of large amounts of filterable solutes.

For ultrafiltration to occur, there must be a pressure gradient across the membrane that favors filtration. In CAVH or CVVH this is called transmembrane pressure (TMP), and its major determinants are hydrostatic pressure and oncotic pressure. The higher pressure in the blood compartment is a function of the individual's blood pressure. There is adequate pressure in the blood compartment when the systolic pressure is 50-70 mm Hg. Higher pressures enhance ultrafiltration. Negative pressure for ultrafiltration can be achieved by lowering the collection container 20-40 cm below the hemofilter. The differences in hydrostatic pressure also cause the crossing of some elements, such as glucose and some vitamins. The longer it takes for blood to clear the filter, the more likely that intermediate molecules (vitamins and glucose) will be filtered out of the patient's system. Opposing the hydrostatic pressure is oncotic pressure, which is maintained by plasma proteins that do not pass through the membrane. When hydrostatic pressure exceeds oncotic pressure, filtration of water and solutes occurs.

Indications for continuous arteriovenous hemofiltration or continuous venovenous hemofiltration

- Massive fluid overload: congestive heart failure, acute renal failure, overaggressive fluid resuscitation in multiple trauma.
- Fluid overload in the presence of hemodynamic instability.
- Cardiogenic shock with pulmonary edema.
- Oliguric patient unresponsive to diuretics.
- Patient with anuria who requires large volumes of parenteral fluid: acts as a supplement to hemodialysis to maintain fluid balance.

Method: The hemofilter and lines are primed with normal saline before the treatment is initiated. Blood flows from the arterial (usually femoral or radial) limb of the vascular access through the filter and returns through the venous (usually femoral or cephalic) limb of the access. A continuous infusion of heparin prevents clotting in the lines and filter. Blood is driven through the system by the patient's blood pressure with CAVH, so no pump is used. With CVVH a pump is used to drive the blood flow. As the blood flows through the filter, water, electrolytes, and most drugs not bound to plasma protein diffuse across the membrane and thus become part of the filtrate. If the objective is the removal of large amounts of fluid and solute (urea, potassium, and creatinine), it is necessary to infuse large volumes of filtration replacement fluid (FRF) to maintain electrolyte balance. Nursing responsibilities include initiation of treatment, monitoring of the patient and system, and discontinuing treatment. Tables 5-10 and 5-11 discuss the advantages, disadvantages, and complications of RRTs, including hemofiltration. Table 5-12 discusses troubleshooting major problems with hemofiltration.

T A B L E 5 - 12   **Troubleshooting major problems in hemofiltration**

Problem	Cause	Intervention

Hypotension	Cardiac dysfunction
	Excessive intravascular
	   volume removal
		Cardiotonic and pressor
		   support
		Fluid replacement
		Recalculate UF rate

Poor ultrafiltration	High hematocrit
	Decreased MAP
	Clotted filter
		Predilution fluid replace-
		   ment
		Pressor support to increase
		   MAP
		Flush filter; replace if nec-
		   essary

Clotted hemofilter	Inadequate anticoagulation
	Poor blood flow rates
	Kinks in blood tubing
		Check ACT hourly and
		   adjust heparin infusion
		Pressors or fluid replace-
		   ment to increase MAP
		Check tubing hourly to
		   guard against kinks
		Change filter and restart
		   therapy

COLLABORATIVE MANAGEMENT
For patients undergoing dialysis
Dietary restrictions
Hemodialysis: Between dialysis treatments the main products of protein metabolism and potassium and sodium will accumulate because of the kidneys' inability to excrete excesses of these products. Therefore it is necessary to restrict the intake of protein to decrease the amount of urea generated, to restrict potassium to prevent hyperkalemia, and to restrict sodium to prevent hypernatremia and curb thirst. Recommended guidelines include protein 1-1.2 g/kg/day; sodium 80-100 mEq/day (individualized); and potassium 40-80 mEq/day (individualized).
Peritoneal dialysis: Patients undergoing peritoneal dialysis tend to lose more protein through the peritoneal membrane. Therefore protein restriction is liberalized to 1.2-1.5 g/kg/day to compensate for the extra loss. If peritonitis develops, protein loss can increase from around 10 g/day to 50 g/day. Patients undergoing CAPD may need calorie restrictions due to the added calories they absorb from the glucose contained in the dialysate. If hypertonic solutions are used several times a day, these patients can absorb as much as 600 calories or more from the dialysate. Potassium may be less restricted in these patients because the dialysate is potassium free and allows better diffusion of potassium with less accumulation that would lead to hyperkalemia. Sodium restriction in peritoneal dialysis is approximately 80-100 mEq/day to prevent hypernatremia and control thirst to prevent fluid overload.
Fluid restriction: To prevent fluid overload secondary to the kidneys' inability to excrete excess water. Weight gain between dialysis

T A B L E 5 - 13   Approaches to fluid replacement

Predilution: replacement fluid infused proximal to the filter	Postdilution: replacement fluid infused distal to the filter
Patient population: Those with poor blood flow and elevated BUN and Hct levels	*Patient population:* All types
Replacement fluid infused into arterial line	Replacement fluid infused into venous line
Used to enhance urea clearance to $\geq 18\%$; decreases oncotic pressure, increasing net TMP; moves urea from erythrocytes into plasma	Used to maintain fluid and electrolyte balance
Increases net fluid removal	Less replacement fluid required
Potentially increases filter life	Simplified clearance determination
*Urea clearance 12.5 ml/min	Urea clearance 10.6 ml/min

*If increased urea clearance is desired, predilution mode of fluid replacement is used.

treatments usually is the result of fluid retention. An attempt is made to limit interdialytic weight gain to 1.5-2 kg by limiting fluid intake to 1,500-1,800 ml in 24 h. This restriction also is individualized.

Phosphate binders: To prevent or control hyperphosphatemia, which can occur because of the kidneys' inability to excrete excess dietary phosphates.

Vitamin D analogs (dihydrotachysterol—the active form of vitamin D) and **calcium replacement:** To prevent hypocalcemia and renal osteodystrophy, which may occur due to the body's inability to absorb calcium and maintain serum levels. If hypocalcemia occurs, the parathyroid glands are activated to release parathormone, which releases calcium from the bone to replenish serum levels. Over time this can lead to bone demineralization and osteodystrophy.

Water-soluble vitamins and folic acid: Are dialyzable and necessitate replacement after dialysis.

For patients undergoing continuous arteriovenous or venovenous hemofiltration

The goal is the removal of excess fluid, while maintaining electrolyte balance and adequate fluid intake for homeostasis. In the critically ill adult, catabolic rate is 2-3 times that of normal, and this is balanced with TPN.

TPN: To maintain nutritional requirements.

CAVH: To correct hypervolemic state. Either a shunt or large-bore catheter is used for access.

Predilution fluid replacement: If increased solute removal is required. (See Table 5-13 for differences between predilution and postdilution replacement.)

Filtration replacement fluid (FRF): To maintain fluid and electrolyte balance. (See Table 5-14 for calculation of infusion rate of these

---

T A B L E 5 - 14   Calculation of filtration replacement fluid (FRF) rate

---

Infusion rate

Equals ultrafiltrate plus other losses per hour minus all fluid infused minus net removal rate

Example

Ultrafiltrate = 600 ml/h + Losses (urine, GI) = 100 ml/h − Hyperalimentation 100 ml/h; vasopressors 50 ml/h − Net fluid removal rate 150 ml/h

FRF rate

= (600 + 100) − (100 + 50 + 150)
$$700 \quad - \quad 300$$

FRF rate

= 400 ml/h

---

fluids.) Concentration may vary, depending on the replacement needs of the patient.

Standard fluids infused simultaneously include:
1 L 0.9 NS with 7.5 ml 10% CaCl
1 L 0.9 NS with 1.6 ml 50% $MgSO_4$
1 L 0.9 NS
1 L D_5W with 150 mEq $NaHCO_3$
Final composition of fluid for typical patient:
Sodium: 150 mEq/L
Chloride: 114 mEq/L
Bicarbonate: 37 mEq/L
Magnesium: 1.6 mEq/L
Calcium: 2.5 mEq/L

Heparin infusion solution: To prevent clotting in the circuit.

Vasopressors: To maintain arterial pressure, which is necessary for driving the blood through the hemofilter.

NURSING DIAGNOSES AND INTERVENTIONS

For patients undergoing dialysis

Risk for infection related to invasive procedure used to obtain peritoneal or vascular access for dialysis

Desired outcome: Patient is free of infection as evidenced by normothermia, WBC count ≤11,000 μl, blood and dialysate free of infective organisms, and absence of erythema, purulent drainage, abdominal or access site pain, or cloudy dialysate.

- Assess and document condition of the access site daily. Be alert to the presence of erythema, purulent drainage, or tenderness.
- Peritonitis accounts for a high incidence of failure with peritoneal dialysis. Use strict aseptic technique when cleansing catheter site and connecting and disconnecting dialysate bags. Use an antiseptic solution such as hydrogen peroxide or povidone-iodine to cleanse the access site. Maintain aseptic technique when cleansing and drying the site. Cover the site with a dry, sterile dressing. Because moist

surfaces breed bacteria, change the dressing immediately if it becomes wet.

- Keep all external access devices (shunts, subclavian catheters, femoral catheters, peritoneal catheters) covered with a dry, sterile dressing between treatments.
- Document the appearance of peritoneal dialysis effluent. If peritoneal drainage becomes cloudy or contains flecks of material, send specimen for a culture and obtain a cell count to check for increased white cells in the peritoneal effluent. Consult physician for changes in outflow.
- Report the presence of an elevated temperature, malaise, access site drainage, cloudy dialysate, and abdominal pain.
- Teach patient to notify staff members if symptoms of infection occur.

Altered nutrition: Less than body requirements related to dietary restrictions and protein loss occurring with peritoneal dialysis

Desired outcomes: Patient has adequate nutrition as evidenced by stable weekly body weight. Patient's caloric intake ranges from 35-45 calories/kg body weight/day (may not be appropriate for patient with CAPD, who absorbs calories through the dialysate); high–biologic value protein intake is 50%-75% of patient's daily protein intake. Nitrogen intake is 4-6 g more than nitrogen loss (loss calculated from 24-h urinary urea excretion and intake estimated from protein intake).

- Document food intake; count calories consumed with each meal. Total caloric intake should be 35-45 calories/kg body weight/24 h.
- Consult with physician and dietitian regarding use of nutritional supplements for maintaining caloric intake.
- For patient undergoing peritoneal dialysis, encourage intake of protein (e.g., milk shakes using protein supplements, custards).
- Weigh patient daily. Be alert to losses ≥10% of patient's normal body weight over a 1-wk period. Daily fluctuations reflect body fluid changes.
- For the patient receiving hemodialysis, encourage the intake of foods that are high in calories (e.g., butter, honey, hard candy, tapioca, sherbet, corn syrup, ginger ale, jellies, jams, marshmallows). Patients undergoing peritoneal dialysis absorb extra calories from the glucose in the peritoneal dialysate.
- Concentrate protein intake on high–biologic value protein foods (e.g., meats, milk, fish, fowl, and eggs).
- Minimize the intake of protein from low–biologic value protein foods (e.g., breads, cereals, pastas, grains, fruits, and vegetables).
- For patients receiving hemodialysis in particular, suggest the intake of caloric substances that do not contain protein or electrolytes. Examples of commercial products available include Cal-Powder, Controlyte, Hycal, and Polycose.
- As appropriate, provide a referral to the dietitian, who can teach the patient and significant others meal-planning techniques that will include restrictions while maintaining a high-calorie intake.
- If patient is anorexic or nauseated, provide small, frequent meals. Present appetizing food in a pleasant atmosphere. As indicated, administer prescribed antiemetic ½ h before meals.

Fluid volume excess (or risk for same) related to dietary indiscretions of sodium and fluids and compromised regulatory mechanisms secondary to renal failure

Desired outcome: Within 24-48 h of admission, patient is normovolemic as evidenced by balanced I&O; stable weight; HR ≤100 bpm; BP within patient's normal range; RR 12-20 breaths/min; and absence of edema, crackles, and other physical indicators of hypervolemia.

- Monitor and record I&O q4h and weight daily; report significant findings to physician. Be alert to weight gain of >0.5-1 kg/24 h.
- Assess and record status of VS, lung sounds, and cardiac rate and rhythm. Be alert to crackles, tachycardia, pericardial friction rub, and pulsus paradoxus.
- Assess for presence of peripheral, periorbital, and sacral edema.
- Maintain fluid restrictions, as prescribed.
- Elevate HOB during peritoneal dialysis to relieve pressure of fluid against diaphragm.
- If outflow is poor, change patient's position or irrigate catheter to determine patency.

Risk for fluid volume deficit related to active loss secondary to excess fluid removal during dialysis or bleeding secondary to heparinization

Desired outcomes: Patient is normovolemic as evidenced by balanced I&O, daily weight within 1-2 lbs of calculated dry weight (true body weight without any excess fluid), BP within patient's normal range, CVP ≥2 mm Hg, and HR ≤100 bpm. Hct is 20%-30% (a range expected for the patient receiving dialysis, inasmuch as anemia is associated with renal failure), and there is no evidence of blood loss due to line separation or membrane rupture.

- When using hypertonic dialysate for peritoneal dialysis, assess skin turgor, mucous membranes, CVP, BP, and HR for signs of dehydration, which can occur from excessive fluid loss. Be alert to sudden decrease in BP, tachycardia, poor skin turgor, dry mucous membranes, and change in mental status (e.g., restlessness or unresponsiveness).
- When using hypertonic peritoneal dialysate, check finger-stick glucose q4h. Consult physician for blood glucose levels >200 mg/dl.
- Weigh patient daily for trend. Monitor I&O q8h, and consult physician for output >1,500 ml over intake.
- Monitor Hct results before each hemodialysis. Notify physician if a >2-point drop occurs.
- If hypotension occurs during peritoneal dialysis, stop the dialysis, consult physician, and encourage oral fluids up to 1,000 ml (or per protocol).
- If hypotension occurs during hemodialysis, give normal saline or volume expanders as prescribed, and notify physician.
- During hemodialysis, secure lines and needles with tape to prevent disconnection and dislodgement of needles. Consult physician immediately if blood loss occurs due to line separation or dialyzer rupture. As prescribed, send type and screen to the laboratory.
- Maintain pressure over venipuncture sites for at least 5 min after needles have been removed.

Altered peripheral tissue perfusion (or risk for same):   Access site, related to interruption of vascular flow secondary to clot formation, pressure, obstruction, or disconnection of vascular access device

Desired outcomes: Patient's access site for dialysis has adequate perfusion as evidenced by palpation of thrill, auscultation of bruit, visualization of blood flow, and warmth of shunt tubing or AV fistula. Warmth and brisk capillary refill (<2 sec) are present in the access extremity.

- Confirm patency of access site by palpating for a thrill (vibratory sensation) and auscultating for presence of bruit (buzzing sound) over shunt or AV fistula. Monitor the access extremity for warmth and brisk capillary refill.
- Keep a small section of the shunt tubing exposed for visualization of blood flow. Ensure that the blood appears uniformly red and that the external tubing is warm to the touch. Dark strands or white serum in the tubing can signal clotting.
- Notify physician promptly if patency cannot be confirmed. Streptokinase or embolectomy may be indicated to save the fistula.
- Avoid taking BP, drawing blood, or using restrictive clothing, name bands, or restraints on arm with fistula. Teach patient the importance of these restrictions.
- If using a pressure dressing over the access site, make sure it is snug enough to prevent bleeding but not so tight that it could stop blood flow and promote clot formation. Remove the pressure dressing after it has been on the site for 1-2 h.
- Maintain constant infusion of heparin (e.g., 10 U/ml, or as prescribed, *via* piggyback) through subclavian or femoral line or flush with heparinized saline and cap as prescribed.
- Keep shunt clamps or rubbershod hemostats at bedside to clamp line in the event of accidental disconnection.
- Flush peritoneal catheter before and after dialysis with 30-50 ml normal saline to ensure patency.
- Always check fistula, graft, or shunt for patency after any hypotensive episode.
- If for any reason it is suspected that air has entered the vascular access, clamp the line and place the patient in a left side-lying Trendelenburg position, which will trap air at the apex of the right ventricle of the heart, away from the outflow tract. Call physician *stat,* administer oxygen, and monitor VS carefully.
- For more information, see "Pulmonary Emboli," p. 251.

Altered protection (or risk for same) related to neurosensory alterations secondary to endogenous chemical alteration (dialysis disequilibrium syndrome) occurring with rapid removal of metabolic wastes and changes in serum osmolality

Desired outcome: Patient verbalizes orientation to time, place, and person and does not exhibit signs and symptoms of disequilibrium syndrome: headache, nausea, vomiting, restlessness, asterixis, stupor, coma, or seizures.

- Monitor patient for indicators of disequilibrium syndrome.
- Consult physician for changing LOC and other marked signs of disequilibrium.
- Recognize predisposing factors: BUN >150 mg/dl; hypernatremia (serum sodium >147 mEq/L); severe metabolic acidosis (pH <7.35,

$Paco_2$ <35 mm Hg, HCO_3^- <22 mEq/L); and history of neurologic problems (e.g., seizures). The syndrome often is prevented by short, frequent dialysis exchanges and by increasing the osmolality of dialysate by adding glucose, glycerol, urea, or mannitol or by giving IV mannitol during treatment.

- Monitor BUN levels before and after dialysis to evaluate for changes occurring along with signs and symptoms of disequilibrium.
- Raise and pad side rails, and keep an appropriately sized airway at the bedside as indicated.

Ineffective breathing pattern related to decreased lung expansion secondary to impaired respiratory mechanics occurring with dialysate in the peritoneal cavity

Desired outcome: Patient becomes eupneic within 24 h of this diagnosis.

- Monitor patient's respiratory rate, depth, and pattern, and assess breath sounds when dialysate is dwelling in the peritoneal cavity.
- Elevate the HOB to reduce pressure of fluid against the diaphragm and increase vital capacity.
- Schedule deep-breathing exercises and incentive spirometry q2-4h.
- Get patient up in a chair 3-4 times a day, if possible.

For patients undergoing continuous arteriovenous or venovenous hemofiltration

Decreased cardiac output (or risk for same) related to decreased preload and electrical changes secondary to fluid and electrolyte shifts occurring with hemofiltration

Desired outcomes: Patient's cardiac output is adequate as evidenced by systolic BP ≥100 mm Hg (or within patient's normal range), HR 60-100 bpm, RR 12-20 breaths/min, peripheral pulses >2+ on a 0-4+ scale, brisk capillary refill (<2 sec), and normal sinus rhythm on ECG.

- Assess and document BP, HR, and RR hourly for the first 4 h of hemofiltration, and then q2h. Be alert to indicators of fluid volume deficit, manifested by a drop in systolic BP to <100 mm Hg, tachycardia, and tachypnea.
- Assess and document peripheral pulses and color, temperature, and capillary refill in the extremities q2h. Be alert to decreased amplitude of peripheral pulses and to coolness, pallor, and delayed capillary refill in the extremities as indicators of decreased perfusion.
- Measure and record I&O hourly. Consult physician for a loss of ≥200 ml/h over desired loss.
- Monitor cardiac rhythm continuously; notify physician of decrease in BP of 20 mm Hg from baseline, tachycardia, depressed T waves and ST segments, and dysrhythmias, which can occur with hypovolemia, potassium changes, or calcium changes.
- Ensure prescribed rates of ultrafiltration and replacement fluid infusion (see Table 5-14), and adjust if ultrafiltration rate changes. Use an infusion pump for replacement fluids to ensure precise rate of infusion. Also maintain TPN and IV rates, as well as oral intake, within 50 ml of the values used to calculate the filtration fluid replacement rate. If any parameters change more than 50 ml, recalculate filtration fluid replacement rate and adjust accordingly.
- Monitor serum electrolyte values, being alert to changes in potas-

sium, calcium, phosphorus, and bicarbonate. Compare patient's values with the following normal ranges: potassium 3.5-5 mEq/L, calcium 8.5-10.5 mg/dl, phosphorus 2.5-4.5 mg/dl, and bicarbonate 22-26 mEq/L. (See "Fluid and Electrolyte Disturbances," p. 667, and "Acid-Base Imbalances," p. 706).

Risk for fluid volume deficit related to active loss secondary to excessive ultrafiltration during CAVH or CVVH

Desired outcomes: Patient is normovolemic as evidenced by gradual weight loss (<2.5 kg/day) and urinary output ≥0.5 ml/kg/h in nonoliguric patients. Ultrafiltration rate remains within 50 ml of the desired hourly rate.

- Measure and record I&O q30min for the first 2 h and then hourly. Ensure that it is within desired limits.
- Weigh patient q8h. Be alert to daily loss ≥2.5 kg.
- Record cumulative ultrafiltrate loss hourly. Measure amount in the ultrafiltrate container. The difference between this value and total hourly intake is the cumulative loss per hour.
- Check replacement fluid rate hourly to ensure that it is within prescribed limits, usually 25 ml of the calculated rate.
- Consult physician for unanticipated fluid loss from vomiting, diarrhea, fever, and wound drainage.
- Consult physician for increased filtration rate, which may occur because of increased BP, or increased negative pressure, which may be caused by lowering of the ultrafiltration collection device.
- Monitor VS hourly; consult physician for increased arterial pressure (≥10 mm Hg above baseline), which would increase flow through the hemofilter, thereby increasing the rate of ultrafiltration.
- Adjust the filtration replacement fluid rate as prescribed when ultrafiltration rate increases.
- Maintain intake (oral, IV, TPN) within 25-50 ml of the value used to calculate fluid replacement rate.

Fluid volume excess (or risk for same) related to excessive fluid intake associated with decreased ultrafiltration secondary to hypotension, clogged or clotted filter, or kinked lines

Desired outcome: Patient experiences a gradual fluid loss and becomes normovolemic as evidenced by BP remaining at baseline range; ACT 2-3 times that of the baseline value; CVP 2-6 mm Hg, HR 60-100 bpm, RR 12-20 breaths/min; and absence of edema, crackles, and other physical indicators of hypervolemia.

- Monitor BP q30min for the first 2 h and then hourly. Consult physician for a 10 mm Hg drop in BP, which would decrease the rate of ultrafiltration significantly.
- If ultrafiltration rate is decreased to 50% of the baseline, consult physician and decrease FRF rate as prescribed.
- Check tubes hourly for kinks.
- Maintain constant heparin infusion per infusion pump to maintain ACT at 2-3 times that of the baseline value.
- Monitor clotting time q2h. Use of an activated clotting time device is advisable.
- Inspect vascular access filter and lines for patency hourly. If clotting or clogging with protein is suspected, flush the system with 50 ml normal saline to check patency.

- If clots are present, consult physician. As prescribed, change the filter and recheck ACT to ensure necessary adjustment in heparin infusion rate.
- On an hourly basis, assess for and document the presence of physical indicators of hypervolemia: CVP >6 mm Hg, BP elevated ≥20 mm Hg over baseline, tachycardia, jugular venous distention, basilar crackles, increasing edema (peripheral, sacral, periorbital), and tachypnea.

Knowledge deficit: Hemofiltration procedure

Desired outcome: Patient or significant other verbalizes accurate information about the hemofiltration procedure within 24-48 h of the instruction.

- Assess patient's knowledge of the procedure and intervene accordingly.
- Explain the necessity of vascular access and the sensations that can be anticipated during cannula insertion.
- Explain the importance of and rationale for limited movement of the involved extremity after cannula placement.
- Describe the equipment that will be used for the procedure (e.g., filter, lines, infusion pump).
- Explain that VS will be assessed and blood tests will be performed at frequent intervals to monitor patient's status during the procedure.
- Explain to patient that his or her blood will be visible in the filter and lines.
- Reinforce that a staff member will be close to patient at all times during the procedure and will explain each step as it occurs.
- Explain that the procedure may take 24 h or longer until fluid balance is attained.
- Teach patient that the typical access sites are the femoral artery and femoral vein or the radial artery and cephalic vein.

Impaired physical mobility related to movement restrictions because of access and equipment for hemofiltration

Desired outcomes: Patient exhibits ability to move about in bed with assistance without evidence of disruption of hemofiltration equipment. Patient's skin remains intact, and there is no evidence of muscle atrophy or contracture formation due to imposed immobility.

- Secure access catheters with gauze wraps (elastic wrap may compress access site and cause clotting) and tape to ensure safe movement of the involved limb without disruption of access cannula.
- Explain to patient the need for care and assistance when moving the involved limb.
- Use soft restraints if movement must be restrained markedly.
- Turn and reposition patient at least q2h, maintaining good body alignment.
- Massage bony prominences during every position change to promote comfort and circulation.
- Support involved extremities with pillows.
- Teach patient assisted ROM exercises on uninvolved extremities. Encourage isometric, isotonic, and quadriceps-setting exercises on uninvolved extremities, especially for patients whose CAVH or CVVH lasts >24 h.

Risk for fluid volume deficit related to potential for blood loss secondary to line disconnection or membrane rupture
Desired outcome: Patient's membrane and line connections remain intact, and ultrafiltrate test results are negative for blood.
- Tape and secure all connections within the system.
- Check connections hourly to ensure that they are secure.
- Avoid concealing lines, filter, or connections with linen.
- Position filter and lines close to the access extremity; secure them with gauze wraps and tape to prevent traction on the connections.
- Inspect ultrafiltrate hourly for any signs of blood. If unsure whether ultrafiltrate contains blood, check the solution with an agency-approved test for occult blood.
- If the test is positive for blood, clamp the ultrafiltrate port and consult physician for further interventions.

ADDITIONAL NURSING DIAGNOSES

See "Pulmonary Emboli" for **Altered protection,** p. 257. For more information about fluid and electrolytes, see "Fluid and Electrolyte Disturbances," p. 676. Also see "Prolonged Immobility," p. 78.

Selected Bibliography

Beasioli S, Barbaresi F, Barbiero M: Intermittent venovenous hemofiltration as a chronic treatment for refractory and intractable heart failure, *ASAIO Journal* 38(3):M658-M663, 1992.
Dipiro J et al: *Pharmacotherapy: a pathophysiologic approach,* Norwalk, Conn, 1993, Appleton & Lange.
Horne MM, Jansen PR: Renal-urinary disorders. In Swearingen PL, editor: *Manual of medical-surgical nursing care: nursing interventions and collaborative management,* ed 3, St Louis, 1994, Mosby.
Horne MM, Swearingen PL: *Pocket guide to fluids and electrolytes,* ed 2, St Louis, 1993, Mosby.
Interqual: The ISD-A review system with adult ISD criteria, August 1992, North Hampton, NH, and Marlboro, Mass, Interqual, Inc.
Kim MJ, McFarland GK, McLane AM: *Pocket guide to nursing diagnoses,* ed 6, St Louis, 1995, Mosby.
Lancaster L, editor: *Core curriculum for nephrology nursing,* ed 2, Pitman, NJ, 1991, Anthony J. Janetti.
Leichtman AB, Strom TB: Therapeutic approach to renal transplantation: triple therapy and beyond, *Transplant Proc* 20(suppl 8):1-6, 1988.
Lew SQ, Bosch JP: Continuous renal replacement therapy: an overview, *Nephrol News Issues* 2(9):18-20, 1988.
Moir EJ: Nursing care of patients receiving Orthoclone OKT 3, *Am Nephrol Nurs Assoc J* 16(5):327-328, 366, 1989.
Norris MK, House MA: Organ and tissue transplantation: nursing care from procurement through rehabilitation, Philadelphia, 1991, Davis.
Paradiso C: Hemofiltration: an alternative to dialysis, *Heart Lung* 18(3):282-290, 1989.
Price C: Continuous arteriovenous ultrafiltration: a monitoring guide for ICU nurses, *Crit Care Nurs* 9(1):12-19, 1989.
Schetz M, Lauwers PM, Ferdinande P: Extracorporeal treatment of acute renal failure in the intensive care unit: a critical view, *Intensive Care Med* 15:349-357, 1989.
Sigler MH, Teehan BP: Advantages of continuous renal replacement therapy in acute renal failure, *Nephrol News Issues* 2(9):22-28, 1988.

Wendon J, Smithies M, Sheppard K: Continuous high-volume venous-venous haemofiltration in acute renal failure, *Intensive Care Med* 15:358-363, 1989.

Zorzanello M: Preventing acute renal failure in patients with chronic renal insufficiency: nursing implications, *Am Nephrol Nurs Assoc J* 16(6):433-436, 1989.

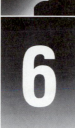

6 NEUROLOGIC DYSFUNCTIONS

Myasthenia gravis

PATHOPHYSIOLOGY

Myasthenia gravis (MG) is a chronic, progressive autoimmune disorder that manifests as weakness and abnormal fatigability of the voluntary striated skeletal muscles. The abnormality occurs at the neuromuscular junction on the postsynaptic membrane, where persons with MG exhibit changes of the structural integrity of the membrane and a marked reduction in the number of acetylcholine receptors (AChR). Acetylcholine (ACh), a neurotransmitter, is synthesized and stored in the terminal expansion of motor nerve axons. Neurotransmission involves the release of ACh into the synaptic cleft and the attachment of ACh to AChR on the postsynaptic membrane. In turn, this interaction activates the muscle action potential, which is responsible for muscle contraction. This process takes only milliseconds and is terminated by the removal of ACh from the neuromuscular junction, in part by the action of acetylcholinesterase, which catalyzes the breakdown of ACh, deactivating it. In approximately 85%-90% of patients with MG, an anti-AChR antibody is present, which is believed to cause structural damage to the postsynaptic AChR, inhibit receptor site synthesis, and cause receptor site blockade. If production of new receptor sites is insufficient, failure of neuromuscular transmission eventually occurs.

MG is associated with an increased rate of occurrence of other autoimmune disorders, including rheumatoid arthritis, thyrotoxicosis, systemic lupus erythematosus, Sjögren syndrome, polymyositis, ulcerative colitis, and pernicious anemia. Studies have shown that the thymus gland, which plays a role in the development of the immune system, undergoes pathologic changes in 80% of persons with MG. MG usually affects women between 15-35 years of age and men after age 40. The peak incidence for women is during the third decade and for men in the fifth decade. The overall ratio of women to men is 3:2. The course of the disease depends on the muscle groups involved and the degree of their involvement. Remissions and exacerbations can occur.

ASSESSMENT

Clinical presentation: Weakness and abnormal fatigability of skeletal muscles that worsen as effort is sustained and the day progresses.
Ocular form: Limited to the eyes and can be mild in nature. This form usually responds poorly to drug therapy but may remit spontaneously. Eye signs include ptosis, diplopia, and inability to maintain upward gaze.
Generalized forms
Mild: Slow onset, usually begins with eye signs and spreads to bulbar (cranial) nerves and skeletal muscles but spares the respiratory muscles. The mild form of MG may remit; however, if it progresses to a moderate or severe form, remission is less likely. If progression occurs, it usually begins within 2 yr of the onset of symptoms. This form responds well to drug therapy.
- *Eye signs:* Ptosis, diplopia, inability to control extraocular muscles.
- *Bulbar signs:* Difficulty chewing, dysphagia, dysarthria, inability to close mouth, nasal regurgitation of fluids, mushy and nasal tone to voice, neck-muscle weakness with head bob, inability to raise chin off chest.
- *Limbs/girdle:* Weakness.

Moderate: Onset slow to moderate with early eye involvement. All muscle groups are involved to varying degrees. This form responds less well to drug therapy. Remission is possible.
- *Eye and bulbar signs:* See "mild" form. This type of MG is associated with severe bulbar signs and symptoms.
- *Skeletal muscle involvement:* Decreased strength in all extremities; inability to maintain position without support.
- *Respiratory muscle involvement:* Diaphragmatic and intercostal weakness, dyspnea, ineffective cough, accumulation of secretions, and potential for respiratory arrest.

Severe or acute fulminating: Rapid onset with severe bulbar and skeletal weakness. Respiratory muscle involvement occurs early. Incidence of myasthenic or cholinergic crisis (see following discussion) is high in this type of MG. Response to treatment is poor, and there is a high mortality rate, usually due to respiratory failure, respiratory infections, or aspiration of food or fluids. See signs and symptoms of "mild" and "moderate" forms.
Myasthenic and cholinergic crises: Patients with any of the generalized forms of MG may experience crisis, either myasthenic or cholinergic. Crisis may occur rapidly or incipiently, ultimately resulting in respiratory failure, which necessitates intubation or tracheostomy with mechanical ventilation. Crisis is a dramatic and frightening occurrence for the patient with MG. This individual is acutely aware of how she or he feels and tends to be knowledgeable about the disease.

It is important for the nurse to listen to and observe the patient closely, because a subjective complaint of increasing anxiety, apprehension, or insomnia may herald the onset of crisis.

Although RR and ABG values can be normal, the patient may be experiencing subtle decreases in chest expansion and air movement due to muscle weakness. These changes may be accompanied by increasing dysphagia, dysarthria, dysphonia, and an accumulation of oropharyngeal secretions, which increases the risk of aspiration.

Myasthenic crisis: Results from the need for more medication because of either tolerance to the medication or an exacerbation of the disease due to infection, trauma, surgery, temperature extremes, stress, endocrine imbalance, or intake of medications with neuromuscular-blocking properties such as sedatives, tranquilizers, narcotics, or antibiotics (e.g., neomycin, kanamycin, gentamicin, streptomycin, tetracycline).

- *Signs and symptoms:* Increasing muscle weakness in spite of normal or increasing drug dosage, increasing anxiety and apprehension, severe ocular and bulbar weakness, and respiratory muscle weakness that occurs rapidly and can lead to respiratory arrest.

Cholinergic crisis: Results from an overdose of anticholinesterase medication, which blocks the AChR sites, causing a neuromuscular depolarizing block.

- *Signs and symptoms:* Increasing muscle weakness, increasing anxiety and apprehension, fasciculations (twitching) around the eyes and mouth, diarrhea and cramping, sweating, pupillary constriction, sialorrhea (excessive salivation), and difficulty breathing and swallowing.

DIAGNOSTIC TESTS

Tensilon test: Edrophonium chloride (Tensilon) is a short-acting anticholinesterase agent that delays hydrolysis of ACh, permitting the ACh released by the nerve to act repeatedly over a longer period of time. In the patient with MG, weakness and muscle fatigue will improve within 30-60 sec of IV Tensilon injection (2-10 mg), and improvement will last up to 5 min.

This test also identifies the type of crisis. In myasthenic crisis the weakness improves with Tensilon, whereas in cholinergic crisis the symptoms worsen.

Caution: Have atropine sulfate at the bedside during Tensilon test to reverse the effects of Tensilon if the patient is in cholinergic crisis.

Serum antibody titer: Elevated serum antibodies against acetylcholine receptors are present in 80%-90% of cases of generalized MG.

Electromyography (EMG): Muscle action potentials are recorded from selected skeletal muscles. The amplitude of the evoked muscle action potentials falls rapidly in persons with MG.

Mediastinoscopy: To evaluate for the presence of thymic abnormalities, which are present in 80% of patients with MG. Of this group 65%-90% have thymic hyperplasia, whereas 10%-15% have gross or microscopic thymomas.

CT scan of the thymus gland: To evaluate for the presence of thymic abnormality (see "Mediastinoscopy," above).

Thyroid studies: To evaluate for hyperthyroidism. Frequently, thyroid abnormalities are present in young women with MG. MG also is associated with a condition known as Hashimoto's thyroiditis, an autoimmune disorder.

Other laboratory studies: Serum creatine phosphokinase (CPK), erythrocyte sedimentation rate (ESR), and antinuclear antibody levels are studied because of the frequent occurrence of other immunologic disorders with MG.

COLLABORATIVE MANAGEMENT

Emergency interventions for myasthenic or cholinergic crisis: Once supportive emergency therapy in an intensive care setting has been instituted, the patient is stabilized, the type of crisis is identified, and specific treatment is begun. Anticholinesterase medications may be withheld or reduced temporarily. A "drug holiday" will improve subsequent patient responsiveness to medication. With the resumption of anticholinesterase medications, dosage, timing, and combinations of medications will need readjustment. In severe MG, plasmapheresis (see below) may hasten improvement in signs and symptoms.

Pharmacotherapy during noncrisis periods: Medications must be given on time to maintain therapeutic effects. Pharmacologic management is patient specific.

Anticholinesterase agents: Such as pyridostigmine bromide (Mestinon), neostigmine bromide (Prostigmin Bromide), and ambenonium chloride (Mytelase). These drugs inhibit the hydrolysis of ACh by acetylcholinesterase at the neuromuscular junction. Generally pyridostigmine is the drug of choice because it is longer acting and has fewer side effects. The patient usually is started on one tablet q3h during the day, and the dose is adjusted as required. Sustained-release preparations usually are given at bedtime to maintain the patient's strength throughout the night and early morning hours.

Corticosteroids (e.g., ACTH and prednisone):   With their use clinical improvement has been shown in 70%-100% of patients with MG. Although the mechanism of action of steroids has not been established, studies have shown that they exert certain direct influences on neuromuscular transmission. In addition, they suppress the action of the immune system at many levels by decreasing the size of the thymus gland and lymphatic tissue, decreasing circulating lymphocyte population, and decreasing antireceptor reactivity of peripheral lymphocytes. Treatment must be continued indefinitely. Indications for their use include weakness that is uncontrolled by anticholinesterase drugs or surgery and patients who refuse surgery. Corticosteroids produce favorable results in patients with all degrees of muscle involvement from ocular to severe respiratory impairment. Corticosteroids are used alone or in conjunction with anticholinesterase drugs.

Immunosuppressive drugs: Cytotoxic drugs such as azathioprine (Imuran) and cyclophosphamide (Cytoxan) may be used alone or in combination with other therapies in situations in which there is a poor response to steroids. Side effects can be serious and include toxic hepatitis, thrombocytopenia, leukopenia, infections, nausea, vomiting, and alopecia. Leukemia and lymphoma also can occur.

Immune globulin: Human immune globulin in high doses is reported to provide rapid but temporary relief of symptoms in some individuals with MG.

Thymectomy: Removal of the thymus gland may lead to clinical improvement, especially in patients with hyperplasia of thymic tissue. Two approaches are used: the transcervical approach or the thoracotomy approach with sternal splitting. Usually, best results are seen with a combination of surgery and medication in patients <50-60 yr with recent onset of moderate, generalized MG. The transcervical approach may be less successful because of the presence of residual thymic tissue, which may lead to reactivation of the MG. Plasmapheresis sometimes is used before surgery to increase strength and allow for a decrease in medication dosage.

Plasmapheresis: Involves a complete exchange of plasma with the removal of abnormal circulating antibodies that interfere with the acetylcholine receptors. Table 6-1 describes potential complications with corresponding nursing assessments and interventions. (For additional information about fluid and electrolyte disturbances, see Chapter 10.)

Radiotherapy: For severe cases of MG when the patient is unresponsive to other therapies. Total body and splenic irradiation have been used.

Respiratory support: ET tube or tracheostomy with mechanical ventilation may be necessary, depending on the degree of involvement of the respiratory muscles. (See "Mechanical Ventilation," p. 19.)

Nutritional support: If patient has dysphagia, enteral or parenteral feedings may be needed. (See "Nutritional Support," p. 1.)

NURSING DIAGNOSES AND INTERVENTIONS

Impaired gas exchange related to altered oxygen supply associated with decreases in chest expansion and air movement secondary to weakness and abnormal fatigability of pharyngeal, diaphragmatic, intercostal, and accessory muscles of respiration

Desired outcomes: Within 12-24 h of initiation of treatment, patient has adequate gas exchange as evidenced by orientation to time, place, and person; RR ≤20 breaths min with normal depth and pattern (eupnea); Pao_2 ≥80 mm Hg; $Paco_2$ ≤45 mm Hg; and oxygen saturation ≥94%.

- Assess patient for indicators of altered respiratory function: diminished or adventitious breath sounds; changes in rate, rhythm, and depth of respirations; changes in skin color; nasal flaring or intercostal or suprasternal retractions; and restlessness, irritability, confusion, or somnolence.
- Monitor ventilatory capability *via* pulmonary function tests. Vital capacity <75% of predicted value, tidal volume <1,000 ml (or <patient's normal/baseline volume), and RR >34 breaths/min are signals of the need for assisted ventilation.
- Monitor ABG and pulse oximetry results. Falling Pao_2 (<60 mm Hg), rising $Paco_2$ (>50 mm Hg), and falling oxygen saturation, coupled with changes in vital capacity, tidal volume, and increasing

T A B L E   6 - 1   Nursing interventions for complications of plasmapheresis

Hypovolemia

Can result from rapid removal of up to 3 L of body fluid during plasmapheresis with volume replacement that is too slow during the procedure

- Perform a baseline assessment of patient's weight, skin turgor, and VS before the procedure is begun. During plasmapheresis, monitor patient for thirst, poor skin turgor, dizziness, confusion, nausea, and flattened neck veins. Assess VS continuously for evidence of hypovolemia, including decreased BP and increased HR. Monitor Hct for elevation, which occurs with hypovolemia. Weigh patient after procedure. Remember that 1 L of fluid equals 1 kg; thus hypovolemia can be reflected readily in weight changes.
- Provide fluids during plasmapheresis as prescribed, *via* oral, enteral, or IV access.
- Monitor and record I&O throughout the procedure. Be alert to oliguria (urinary output <30 ml/h for 2 consecutive hours).
- Protect patients who are dizzy or confused by keeping side rails up and the bed in its lowest position.

Clotting abnormalities

Can result from removal of clotting factors during plasmapheresis

- Assess PT, PTT, and platelet count before and after procedure. Be alert to PT and PTT greater than those of control values and to increased platelet count. Normal ranges are as follows: PT 11-15 sec, PTT 30-40 sec, and platelet count 150,000-400,000 μl.
- Be alert to signs of impaired clotting, such as oozing from arterial puncture, venous access, or IV sites. Monitor patient for epistaxis or other signs of hemorrhage, such as elevated pulse rate, decreasing BP, or changes in patient's mental status.
- Apply firm, continuous (e.g., 10 min) pressure to the arterial puncture site once the catheter or needle is removed. A pressure dressing is recommended.
- Check gastric aspirate and stools for occult blood.
- Instruct patient to alert staff to the presence of bleeding from puncture and other sites.

Hypokalemia

Can result from removal of potassium during the plasma exchange

- Assess serum potassium before, during, and after plasma exchange. Be alert to decreasing levels (<3.5 mEq/L).
- Monitor for physical signs of hypokalemia, including bradycardia, fatigue, leg cramps, nausea, and paresthesias.
- Observe cardiac monitor for signs of cardiac dysrhythmias: ST-segment depression, flattened T wave, presence of U wave, and ventricular dysrhythmias. Report abnormal cardiac rhythms to physician.
- During reinfusion of blood, administer potassium as prescribed to prevent hypokalemia and dangerous dysrhythmias. If prescribed, administer antidysrhythmic agents.

Caution: Patients on prednisone or digitalis therapy are at increased risk for hypokalemia and should be monitored closely for its occurrence.

T A B L E 6 - 1   Nursing interventions for complications of plasmapheresis—cont'd

---

Hypocalcemia

Can result from binding of calcium to acid-citrate-dextrose (ACD), the anticoagulant used during plasmapheresis

- Assess serum calcium levels before, during, and after plasmapheresis. Be alert to decreasing levels (<8.5 mg/dl).
- Monitor patient for signs of hypocalcemia, such as numbness with tingling of fingers and circumoral area, hyperactive reflexes, muscle cramps, tetany, paresthesia, Chvostek's sign (see p. 688), diffuse irritability, emotional instability, impaired memory, and confusion.
- Observe cardiac monitor for evidence of hypocalcemia: prolonged QT interval caused by elongation of ST segment.
- Encourage patient to drink milk before and during the plasma exchange.
- As prescribed, administer calcium gluconate during plasmapheresis if indicators of hypocalcemia occur.

Myasthenic crisis

Can result from removal of circulating anticholinesterase drugs during plasmapheresis

Cholinergic crisis

Can result from removal of antibodies and decreased need for anticholinesterase drugs after plasmapheresis

- In the event of either crisis, have the following available: IV infusion apparatus, medications (edrophonium chloride [Tensilon], neostigmine bromide, atropine, and pralidoxime chloride [Protopam Chloride]), manual resuscitator, oxygen, suction equipment, and intubation tray if intubation is not already in place.
- Monitor patient for evidence of crisis, such as decreased vital capacity (<1 L), inability to swallow, ptosis, diplopia, dysarthria, dysphonia, dyspnea, muscle weakness, and nasal flaring. Stay with patient if these signs appear and notify physician promptly.

RR, indicate the need for ET intubation or tracheostomy and for mechanical ventilation to support respiration. As indicated, prepare patient for this procedure.

Note: If mechanical ventilation already is in place, ventilator settings will vary, depending on patient's size and ABG results. Check ventilator settings at set intervals. Consult with anesthesia and/or respiratory therapy staff members regarding setting changes as patient's needs change.

- Provide pulmonary toilet q2h when patient is awake and prn. In addition, turn patient after each physiotherapy session to facilitate lung expansion, decrease risk of atelectasis, and prevent consolidation of secretions.

Ineffective airway clearance related to ineffective cough; decreased energy; and abnormal fatigability of diaphragmatic, intercostal, pharyngeal, and accessory muscles of respiration

Desired outcome: Within 24-48 h of intervention/treatment, patient's airway is clear as evidenced by absence of adventitious breath sounds.
- Assess breath sounds, effectiveness of patient's cough, and the quality, amount, and color of sputum. Consult physician for significant findings, including patient's inability to raise secretions; for secretions that are tenacious, thick, or voluminous.
- Suction secretions as indicated, using hyperoxygenation before and after procedure.

Note: If patient has a tracheostomy, to prevent aspiration of secretions, always suction the trachea and mouth before deflating tracheostomy cuff. This is especially important in patients with MG because of their increase in saliva (sialorrhea).

- If the patient has a tracheostomy and is receiving oral or enteric feedings, inflate the tracheostomy cuff and elevate HOB before each feeding to prevent aspiration of food. Place patient in semi-Fowler's to high Fowler's position at all times to facilitate chest excursion and decrease risk of aspiration.
- Assess VS for indicators of atelectasis and upper respiratory infection (see **Risk for infection,** which follows). Consult physician for significant findings.
- Increase activity as allowed and tolerated to minimize stasis of secretions and to facilitate expansion of the lung.
- If prescribed, administer or assist with intermittent positive pressure breathing (IPPB) treatments.
- Keep another tracheostomy tube of the same size and an obturator at the bedside in the event of inadvertent extubation.

Risk for infection related to inadequate primary defenses (stasis of secretions), inadequate secondary defenses (suppressed inflammatory response), invasive procedures (e.g., insertion of ET tube), and chronic disease

Desired outcome: Patient is free of infection as evidenced by normothermia; HR 60-100 bpm; pulmonary secretions that are clear, thin in consistency, and odorless; and WBC count ≤11,000 μl.
- Monitor patient for signs of infection, including temperature elevations ≥37.8° C (100° F), tachycardia, and diaphoresis.
- Assess color, consistency, amount, and odor of pulmonary secretions. Consult physician for a change in sputum color (i.e., to green, tan, brown, bloody). Obtain sputum specimens for culture as indicated.
- Monitor CBC results for elevation of WBC count (>11,000 μl).
- Administer antibiotics as prescribed.
- Use meticulous handwashing procedure before caring for patient and sterile technique when performing suctioning and other invasive procedures.
- Protect patient from exposure to persons with infection, particularly upper respiratory infection (URI).
- Turn and reposition patient at least q2h to prevent stasis of secretions.
- See Appendix 8 for more information.

Impaired swallowing related to decreased or absent gag reflex, decreased strength or excursion of muscles involved in mastication, facial paralysis, or mechanical obstruction (tracheostomy tube)

Desired outcome: Patient demonstrates capability for safe and effective swallowing, as evidenced by presence of gag reflex and adequate strength and excursion of muscles involved in mastication, before oral foods and fluids are given or reintroduced.

- Assess patient for the presence of the gag reflex, ability to swallow, and strength and excursion of muscles involved in mastication. As indicated, consult with a speech therapist to determine patient's ability to swallow.
- If patient cannot swallow, confer with physician regarding alternate method of nutritional support, such as enteral or parenteral nutrition (see "Nutritional Support," p. 1).

Note: If the patient has an artificial airway, add a few drops of blue food coloring to tube feedings to facilitate assessment of aspiration.

- After return of patient's gag reflex and ability to swallow, begin oral feedings cautiously.
  - □ When reinstating oral intake, begin with a small quantity of ice chips, which may help stimulate the swallowing reflex, and progress to semisolid foods (e.g., textured food, applesauce) and then to solid foods.
  - □ Elevate HOB ≥70 degrees to facilitate gravity flow through the pylorus and to minimize the potential for regurgitation and aspiration.
  - □ Provide small feedings at frequent intervals (e.g., q4h while patient is awake).
  - □ Avoid cold foods and beverages, which cause bloating and upward pressure on the diaphragm and may impede respiratory excursion.
  - □ Keep suction equipment at the bedside; suction excess secretions as necessary after each feeding. Inspect the buccal surface for residual food particles after each meal. Provide materials for oral hygiene after every meal.
- If patient begins oral feedings with a tracheostomy tube in place, elevate HOB ≥70 degrees to facilitate movement of food through the pylorus and to minimize the potential for regurgitation and aspiration. Inflate tracheostomy tube cuff for 30 min before and after feeding to prevent aspiration in the event that the patient vomits or regurgitates. Progress the diet slowly, as described above.
- If patient is unable to communicate verbally, be alert to signs of respiratory distress that can occur in response to aspiration: dyspnea or change in rate and depth of respirations, restlessness or agitation, pallor, and presence of adventitious breath sounds. If these signs occur, discontinue feeding immediately; ensure that HOB is elevated; and provide oxygen *via* nasal cannula, mask, or ET tube. If a tracheostomy tube is in place, suction through the tube to remove food or secretions that may be obstructing the airway. As prescribed, obtain specimen for ABG analysis or arrange for a chest x-ray.

Sensory/perceptual alterations (visual) related to altered sensory reception associated with diplopia or ptosis
Desired outcomes: Within 48-72 h of this diagnosis, patient relates that vision is adequate to perform ADL.
- Assess for and document signs of weakness of the ocular muscles (i.e., diplopia, ptosis, or incomplete closure of the eye).
- Provide an eye patch or frosted lens for the patient with diplopia; alternate the patch or lens to the opposite eye q2-3h during patient's awake hours.
- Provide eyelid crutches for the patient with ptosis, or loosely tape eyelids open but *only* when providing direct care.
- Administer artificial tears in each eye at least q4-6h to lubricate and protect corneal tissue.
- As indicated, provide assistance with ADL and ambulation to protect patient from injury.
- Keep patient's environment consistent to facilitate location of desired objects.

Knowledge deficit: Thymectomy procedure, including preoperative and postoperative care
Desired outcome: Before surgery, patient verbalizes understanding of the surgical procedure, including preoperative and postoperative care.
- Assess patient's knowledge of thymectomy and its relationship to myasthenia gravis. Provide explanations as indicated.
- Describe the preoperative routine both verbally and with written material. Discuss preoperative medications, application of antiembolic hose, the potential for postoperative discomfort, and the availability of analgesia. Advise patient that the medication regimen may change after surgery, because removal of the thymic tissue may result in improvement in the patient's condition. If the patient will have a thoracotomy approach, explain that chest tubes will be present after surgery; with a transcervical approach, a portable wound drainage system (e.g., Hemovac) will be present to collect wound drainage.
- During the preoperative period, teach coughing and deep-breathing techniques that will be employed after surgery for expanding the lungs and mobilizing secretions into the upper portion of the airway.
- Explain that plasmapheresis may be performed preoperatively to improve the patient's clinical state. (See **Knowledge deficit:** Purpose and procedure for plasmapheresis, which follows.)
- Explain that pulmonary function and ABG studies will be performed preoperatively to provide baseline data that will be used to evaluate respiratory status and again postoperatively to assist in determining the patient's readiness for extubation.
- Prepare patient for the possibility of tracheostomy with assisted ventilation for the preoperative and postoperative periods to prevent respiratory problems that can occur as a result of the stresses of surgery or the risk of myasthenic or cholinergic crisis.
- Before surgery, devise a communication system that uses aids such as a magic slate, hand signals, call bell, or word board, inasmuch as patient is likely to require a ventilator postoperatively. (A communication system already may be in place if a ventilator is in use.)

- Explain that the results of a thymectomy are variable and may not be apparent for several months to years.

Knowledge deficit: Purpose and procedure for plasmapheresis

Desired outcome: Before the first plasma exchange, patient verbalizes knowledge of the purpose and procedure for plasmapheresis.

- Assess patient's previous experience with and knowledge of plasmapheresis.
- As appropriate, teach patient the following about plasmapheresis: Blood is withdrawn *via* an arterial catheter, anticoagulated, and then passed through a cell separator. The plasma portion of the blood that contains the AChR antibodies is removed. RBCs, WBCs, and platelets are mixed with saline, potassium, and plasma protein fraction and then are returned to the body, minus the plasma, *via* a venous access.
- Advise patient that plasmapheresis generally is performed to control severe symptoms until other modalities (medications, thymectomy) take effect, when other treatments have failed, or to increase patient's strength and improve general status before surgery.
- Explain that patient should eat before plasmapheresis and that nutrition will be provided during the procedure.
- Advise patient that the nurse will perform several assessment procedures before, during, and after plasmapheresis (see Table 6-1).
- Advise patient that the procedure may take several hours and that it may be performed as often as 3-4 times a week, depending on patient's condition.
- Explain that the patient's degree of weakness may increase during and after the procedure because of the removal of plasma-bound medications (corticosteroids and anticholinesterase agents). Reassure patient that he or she will be monitored closely during the procedure and will receive appropriate medication after plasmapheresis.

Knowledge deficit: Signs and symptoms of myasthenic and cholinergic crises

Desired outcome: Within 24 h of stabilization of respiratory status, patient and significant others verbalize the signs and symptoms of impending myasthenic and cholinergic crises.

- Assess patient's/family's previous experience with and knowledge of myasthenic and cholinergic crises.
- Explain the differences between *myasthenic crisis:* an exacerbation of the myasthenic symptoms, frequently triggered by an infection; and *cholinergic crisis:* an episode triggered by toxic levels of anticholinesterase medication. The crisis, regardless of type, may manifest similar symptoms, including abdominal cramping, diarrhea, generalized weakness, increased pulmonary secretions, and impaired respiratory function.
- Advise patient/family to report immediately indications of crisis.
- Recommend that emergency respiratory support equipment (resuscitator bag and suction apparatus) should be available in the home if patient has a history of crisis events.
- Advise patient to carry an identification card with diagnosis, medications, medication contraindications, and physician's name and phone number.

- Provide address and phone number of Myasthenia Foundation: 53 West Jackson Blvd., Chicago, IL 60604; 1-800-541-5458.

ADDITIONAL NURSING DIAGNOSES

See "Nutritional Support," p. 12; "Mechanical Ventilation," p. 24; "Psychosocial Support," p. 88; and "Psychosocial Support for the Patient's Family and Significant Others," p. 100. Also see "Renal Transplantation" for **Knowledge deficit:** Immunosuppressive medications and their side effects, p. 407.

Guillain-Barré syndrome

PATHOPHYSIOLOGY

Guillain-Barré syndrome (GBS) is an acute or subacute postinfectious polyneuritis. The frequency of GBS after an infection, along with its occurrence in conjunction with diseases of lymphoid tissue (e.g., Hodgkin's disease), suggests that it is an autoimmune disorder. Statistically, GBS affects 1.5-2 individuals per 100,000 population.

GBS mainly affects the Schwann cell, which synthesizes and maintains the peripheral nerve myelin sheath. The result is the segmental loss of myelin along the peripheral nerve axon. Cellular inflammatory infiltrates that consist of T and B lymphocytes, macrophages, and neutrophils appear in the areas of myelin loss. Studies suggest that the macrophages penetrate the basement membrane and strip apparently normal myelin from intact axons, causing the characteristic signs and symptoms of GBS. The ventral (motor) root axons of the anterior horn cells, which innervate voluntary skeletal muscles, are primarily involved. Dorsal (sensory) root axons of the posterior horn also are affected but to a lesser degree. Recovery of neurologic function depends on proliferation of Schwann's cells and remyelination of axons. Recovery can be expected in 85%-95% of cases, with minor residual deficits occurring in less than half of affected patients.

ASSESSMENT

HISTORY AND RISK FACTORS Respiratory or GI illness 10-14 days before onset of the neurologic symptoms, in which a viral agent such as parainfluenza 2 virus, herpes zoster, measles, mumps, rubella, or varicella is present (50% of cases); recent vaccination (15% of cases), such as for influenza; recent surgical procedure (5% of cases).

CLINICAL PRESENTATION Ascending flaccid motor paralysis is the most common presenting sign and is associated with the early loss of deep tendon reflexes (DTRs). Weakness, which usually precedes the paralysis, is symmetric and generally begins in distal muscle groups and ascends to involve more proximal muscles. Muscles of respiration (intercostals and diaphragm) frequently are involved, and approximately half of all patients will require mechanical ventilation. Complaints of distal paresthesias are common. In more serious or prolonged cases, proprioceptive and vibratory dysfunctions are present. In addition, loss of pain and temperature sensations in a glove-and-stocking distribution has been reported. Sensory complaints usually appear first, with muscle weakness developing rapidly over 24-72 h. Approximately 90% of patients reach the peak of dysfunction within 2 weeks.

Autonomic nervous system involvement (a type of autonomic dysreflexia): Occurs in most patients with GBS: Sinus tachycardia, bradycardia, orthostatic hypotension, hypertension, excessive diaphoresis, bowel and bladder retention, loss of sphincter control, increased pulmonary secretions, syndrome of inappropriate antidiuretic hormone secretion, and cardiac dysrhythmias (a common cause of death).

Cranial nerve involvement with GBS: All cranial nerves except I and II may be involved. See Appendix 4.

PHYSICAL ASSESSMENT Symmetric motor weakness, decreased or absent DTRs, hypotonia or flaccidity of affected muscles, presence of respiratory abnormalities (e.g., nasal flaring, hypoventilation), facial paralysis.

DIAGNOSTIC TESTS

The diagnosis for GBS is based on clinical presentation, history of antecedent illness, and CSF findings.

Lumbar puncture (LP) and CSF analysis: CSF analysis usually shows an elevated protein, without any increase in WBCs. This is referred to as the "albuminocytologic dissociation." This dissociation usually is noted during the course of GBS and is helpful in differentiating GBS from other CNS disorders such as infection. CSF protein, normally between 15-45 mg/100 ml, may peak 4-6 wk after onset of GBS to levels of several hundred mg/ml. This elevation may persist for months. CSF pressure, which is normally between 0-15 mm Hg (90-180 mm H_2O), may be elevated in severe cases.

Electrodiagnostic studies: EMG and nerve conduction velocity (NCV) demonstrate profound slowing of motor conduction velocities and conduction blocks due to the demyelination of peripheral nerves. Although these changes may not appear initially, they will become apparent several weeks into the illness. Evoked potentials (auditory, visual, and brain stem) may be used to distinguish GBS from other neuropathologies.

CBC count: Moderate leukocytosis may occur early in disease, possibly due to the inflammatory process associated with demyelination in GBS, but CBC level will return to normal as the disease runs its course.

Pulmonary function studies: May be performed during initial diagnostic evaluation. Vital capacity (VC) of <1 L indicates a possible need for assisted ventilation.

ABG studies: Performed if VC drops below 1 L or if patient demonstrates dyspnea, confusion, restlessness, nasal flaring, use of accessory muscles of respiration, or breathlessness (noted during a count by the patient from 1-10). A decrease in Pao_2 >10-15 mm Hg or increase in $Paco_2$ of 10-15 mm Hg greater than baseline or normal value signals the need for immediate intubation or tracheostomy.

COLLABORATIVE MANAGEMENT

Respiratory support: ET intubation or tracheostomy with assisted mechanical ventilation, as necessary.

Corticosteroids: May slow or halt demyelinating process and decrease inflammation along the peripheral nerves. Methylprednisolone and oral steroids are used with varied results.

Plasmapheresis: Involves a complete exchange of plasma with the removal of abnormal circulating antibodies that affect the peripheral nerve myelin sheath. Removal of these autoantibodies may lessen the duration and severity of GBS. For nursing interventions for complications of plasmapheresis, see Table 6-1.

Maintenance and monitoring of cardiovascular function: As necessary, cardiac monitoring may be initiated for dysrhythmias, arterial pressure monitoring may be used to evaluate hypertension or hypotension, and antihypertensive agents or vasopressors may be administered to maintain BP within normal levels.

Management of bowel and bladder dysfunction: Nasogastric suction and parenteral infusion may be started for patients with paralytic ileus; an indwelling urinary catheter may be inserted in patients with urinary retention.

Nutritional management: Parenteral feedings are given until return of peristalsis. Tube feedings or gastrostomy feedings are used for patients with severe dysphagia. With recovery of gag reflex and swallowing ability, the diet will progress to semisolid and solid foods, which are more readily swallowed than are liquids.

Management of motor dysfunction: Active and passive ROM exercises are performed at frequent intervals during all phases of GBS. Activity must be balanced with caloric intake to prevent muscle wasting. As the patient's condition stabilizes, physical and occupational therapy personnel should be involved in the planning of the rehabilitation process. The primary goal is maintenance of the patient's mobility and independence.

Caution: ROM must not be done strenuously during the acute phase because this may exacerbate weakness and possibly accelerate the demyelinating process.

NURSING DIAGNOSES AND INTERVENTIONS

Impaired gas exchange related to altered oxygen supply associated with decreased lung expansion secondary to weakness or paralysis of intercostal and diaphragmatic muscles

Desired outcomes: Within 12-24 h of this diagnosis, patient has adequate gas exchange as evidenced by orientation to time, place, and person; RR 12-20 breaths/min with normal pattern and depth (eupnea); HR $\leq$100 bpm; BP within patient's normal range; Pao_2 $\geq$80 mm Hg; $Paco_2$ $\leq$45 mm Hg; and oxygen saturation $\geq$94%.

- Assess neurologic function hourly, or as often as needed. Ascending motor and sensory dysfunctions usually occur rapidly (over 24-72 h) and can lead to life-threatening respiratory arrest.
- Monitor patient's respiratory status and results of diagnostic tests for evidence of distress or other abnormalities. Be alert to and consult physician for the following: adventitious (crackles, rhonchi), decreased, or absent breath sounds; temperature $\geq$37.8° C (100° F); increased HR and BP; tidal volume or vital capacity decreased from

baseline; a decrease in Pao_2 or increase in $Paco_2$ $\geq$10-15 mm Hg from baseline or normal values; abnormal respiratory rate or rhythm; increasing restlessness or anxiety; and confusion.

- In the presence of the aforementioned indicators, be prepared to assist with intubation or tracheotomy.
- Prepare patient for the likelihood of these interventions; explain that they will be temporary measures.
- Maintain mechanical ventilation *via* ET tube or tracheostomy as indicated; check ventilator settings at regular intervals to ensure that they are within prescribed limits. (See "Mechanical Ventilation," p. 19.)
- Continue to monitor ABG results and pulse oximetry. Improvement is indicated by increases in Pao_2 (optimally to $\geq$80 mm Hg) and oxygen saturation and a decrease in $Paco_2$ (optimally to $\leq$45 mm Hg). Consult physician for continued abnormalities.

Ineffective airway clearance related to ineffective cough; decreased energy; increasing paralysis of respiratory, pharyngeal, and facial muscles; and absence of the gag reflex

Desired outcome: Within 12-24 h of this diagnosis, patient's airway is clear as evidenced by absence of adventitious breath sounds, HR 60-100 bpm, BP within patient's baseline range, RR 12-20 breaths/min with normal depth and pattern (eupnea), tidal volume or vital capacity within baseline parameters, Pao_2 $\geq$80 mm Hg, $Paco_2$ $\leq$45 mm Hg, and absence of restlessness.

- Monitor patient for the following: adventitious (crackles, rhonchi), decreased, or absent breath sounds; increased HR and BP; tidal volume or vital capacity decreased from baseline; abnormal respiratory rate or rhythm; decrease in Pao_2 or increase in $Paco_2$; and increasing restlessness or anxiety.
- Suction the airway as determined by auscultation findings. As the paresis or paralysis subsides (usually after 2-4 wk, the usual time of the peak of the dysfunction), cranial nerve function will begin to return (i.e., gag, swallowing, and coughing). Evaluate patient's ability to cough, whether or not he or she has been placed on mechanical ventilation. Assess for the presence of adventitious sounds to determine effectiveness of patient's cough.
- Deliver oxygen and humidification as prescribed.
- Maintain mechanical ventilation as prescribed; confirm that ventilator settings are within prescribed limits. (See "Mechanical Ventilation," p. 19.)
- Unless contraindicated, maintain adequate hydration (up to 2-3 L/day) to minimize thickening of pulmonary secretions.
- Turn and reposition patient at least q2h to prevent stasis of secretions.

Risk for disuse syndrome related to ascending flaccid paralysis and paresthesias

Desired outcomes: Patient maintains baseline/optimal ROM of all joints and baseline muscle size and strength of all muscles.

- Assess neurologic function hourly or as often as indicated. Ascending motor and sensory dysfunction usually occurs rapidly, over 24-72 h. During the stage of GBS crisis when neurologic dysfunction is progressing, assess motor and sensory levels starting with the lower extremities and working upward to determine level of deficit.

▫ Assess muscle symmetry by using a side-to-side comparison.

▫ Assess muscle strength: *For lower extremities,* have patient pull heel of foot toward the buttocks as you provide resistance by holding onto the foot. *For upper extremities,* have patient extend and flex the wrists and arms against your resistance.

▫ Assess DTRs of the Achilles, patellae, biceps, triceps, and brachioradialis. Normal response is +2; report decreased (+1) or absent (0) response.

▫ Assess for the presence of paresthesia, including the location, degree, and whether or not it is ascending.

▫ Assess for the presence or absence of position sense by moving patient's big toe or thumb up and down while patient's eyes are closed. Also note presence or absence of vibratory sense by placing a vibrating tuning fork over bony prominences.

▫ Assess for the presence or absence of response to light touch or pinprick by starting at the feet and working upward to determine the level of dysfunction.

Note: Sensory symptoms usually are milder than are motor complaints, with vibration and position sensations affected most often. However, about a quarter of affected patients will experience pain, requiring analgesia. When light touch, pinprick, and temperature sensations are affected, they most often are found in a glove-and-stocking distribution. Patients frequently experience muscle tenderness and sensitivity to pressure.

▫ Assess for cranial nerve dysfunction (see Appendix 4).

• Record and report sensorimotor deficit, including degree of involvement.

• Turn and reposition patient in correct anatomic alignment q2h or more often if requested by patient. Support patient's position with pillows and other positioning aids.

• To maintain patient's muscle function and prevent contractures, ensure that active or passive ROM exercises are performed q2h during all phases of GBS. Involve significant others in exercises, if appropriate.

• Obtain a physical therapy referral, and begin rehabilitation planning process during the early stages of the disorder.

• As indicated, apply splints to hands-arms and feet-legs to help prevent contracture; alternate splints so that they are on for 2 h and off for 2 h.

• Apply antiembolic stockings as prescribed to help promote tissue perfusion and minimize the risk of thrombophlebitis, deep vein thrombosis, and pulmonary emboli.

• Low air loss or fluidized beds may be used to manage the respiratory, autonomic, and musculoskeletal problems that occur with GBS. Use an air mattress to help maintain skin integrity. For interventions related to maintaining skin integrity, see "Wound and Skin Care," p. 57.

Dysreflexia (or risk for same) related to noxious stimulus

Desired outcome: Patient has no symptoms of autonomic dysreflexia (AD), as evidenced by normal T-wave configuration on ECG, HR 60-

100 bpm, BP within patient's normal range, cool and dry skin, patient's normal strength, and absence of headache and chest and abdominal tightness.

- Assess for signs of AD: cardiac dysrhythmias; HR <60 bpm or >100 bpm; elevated and sustained BP (e.g., ≥250-300/150 mm Hg); facial flushing; increased sweating, possibly due to loss of thermal regulation; extreme generalized warmth; profound weakness; and complaints of severe headache or tightening in the chest and abdomen.
- Place patient on cardiac monitor as prescribed.

Note: Because of the risk of fatal cardiac dysrhythmias in GBS, continuous cardiac monitoring is recommended for the first 10-14 days of hospitalization.

- Monitor patient carefully during activities that are known to precipitate AD: position changes, vigorous coughing, straining with bowel movements, and suctioning.
- Be aware of and implement measures to prevent factors that may precipitate AD:
  - *Bladder stimuli:* Urinary tract infection, cystoscopy, urinary catheter insertion, clogged urinary catheter, urinary calculi.
  - *Bowel stimuli:* Fecal impaction, rectal examination, enemas, suppositories.
  - *Sensory stimuli:* Pressure caused by tight clothing, dressings, bed covers, thigh straps on urinary drainage bags; prolonged pressure on skin surface or over bony prominences; temperature changes, such as exposure to a cool breeze or draft.
- If indicators of AD are present, implement the following:
  - Elevate HOB or place patient in a sitting position to promote decrease in BP.
  - Monitor BP and HR q3-5min until patient stabilizes.
- Determine and remove offending stimulus:
  - For example, if patient's bladder is distended, catheterize cautiously, using sufficient lubricant.
  - If patient has an indwelling urinary catheter, check for obstruction such as granulation in catheter or kinking of tubing. As indicated, irrigate catheter, using no more than 30 ml normal saline.
  - If urinary tract infection is suspected, obtain a urine specimen for culture and sensitivity once crisis stage has passed.
  - Check for fecal impaction. Perform the rectal examination gently, using an ointment that contains a local anesthetic (e.g., Nupercaine).
  - Check for sensory stimuli, and loosen clothing, bed covers, or other constricting fabric as indicated.
- Consult physician if symptoms do not abate within 15-30 min, especially the elevated BP, because the consequences are life threatening: seizures, subarachnoid or intracerebral hemorrhage, fatal cerebrovascular accident.
- As prescribed, administer antihypertensive agents and monitor effectiveness.

Decreased cardiac output (or risk for same) related to decreased afterload secondary to reduced peripheral vascular tone

---

Note: These patients, while normovolemic, may experience a decreased cardiac output due to an enlarged vascular space. This is similar to the vascular response seen in distributive (e.g., anaphylactic or septic) shock.

Desired outcome: Patient has adequate cardiac output as evidenced by BP within patient's normal range; HR 60-100 bpm; urinary output ≥0.5 ml/kg/h; peripheral pulses >2+ on a 0-4+ scale; orientation to time, place, and person; PAWP 6-12 mm Hg; SVR 900-1,200 dynes/sec/cm^{-5}; CO 4-7 L/min; and normal sinus rhythm on ECG.

- Monitor patient for indicators of decreased cardiac output: drop in systolic BP >20 mm Hg from baseline, systolic BP <80 mm Hg, or a continuing drop in systolic BP of 5-10 mm Hg with every assessment; HR >100 beats/min; irregular HR; restlessness, confusion, and dizziness; warm and flushed skin; peripheral edema; and decreasing urinary output <0.5 ml/kg/h for 2 consecutive hours. Monitor hemodynamic pressures, particularly PAWP, CO, and SVR.
- Continuously assess cardiac rate and rhythm per cardiac monitor; report changes in rate and rhythm.
- Implement measures to prevent episodes of decreased cardiac output due to orthostatic hypotension:
  - Change patient's position slowly.
  - Perform ROM exercises q2h to prevent venous pooling.
  - Apply elastic antiembolic hose as prescribed to promote venous return.
  - Avoid placing pillows under patient's knees, "gatching" the bed, or allowing patient to cross the legs or sit with legs in a dependent position.
  - Collaborate with physical therapy personnel in progressing patient from a supine to upright position, with the use of a tilt table.
- As prescribed, administer fluids to treat the hypotension.
- As prescribed, administer vasopressor (e.g., epinephrine) to counteract peripheral vasodilatation.

Sensory/perceptual alterations (or risk for same) related to altered sensory transmission secondary to cranial nerve involvement with GBS
Desired outcome: Patient relates the presence of normal vision, exhibits normal pupillary and gag reflexes, intact corneas, ability to masticate, and full ROM of head and shoulders.

- Assess cranial nerve function (see Appendix 4). Patients with GBS commonly exhibit deficits in cranial nerves III through XII.
- Evaluate cranial nerves III, IV, and V by checking for extraocular eye movements, pupillary light reflex, and degree of ptosis and for the presence of diplopia.
  - If patient experiences a deficit, place objects where patient can see them. Assist patient with ADL as indicated.
  - Cover one eye with a patch or frosted lens if patient is experiencing diplopia; alternate patch or lens q2-3h during patient's waking hours.
  - Use eyelid crutches for patients with ptosis.

- Evaluate cranial nerves V and VII by checking patient's facial sensation and movement, ability to masticate, and the corneal reflex.
  - In the presence of a deficit, assess patient for corneal irritation or abrasion. Apply artificial tear drops or ointments as prescribed. Secure the eyelid in a closed position if corneal reflex is diminished or absent.
- Evaluate cranial nerves IX, X, and XII by checking for pharyngeal sensation and movement (swallowing), the presence or absence of the gag reflex, and control of the tongue.
  - If a deficit is found, provide suctioning during oral hygiene. Do not feed patient an oral diet until the gag reflex returns.
- Assess cranial nerve XI by checking patient's ability to shrug the shoulders and turn the head from side to side.
  - If a deficit is found, position patient's head in a position of comfort and proper anatomic alignment.

Constipation related to hypoperistalsis or paralytic ileus associated with neuromuscular impairment
Desired outcome: Within 3-5 days of this diagnosis, patient has a bowel movement or returns to usual pattern of elimination.

- Assess patient's GI status, noting absence or presence and quality of the following: bowel sounds, abdominal distention, nausea, vomiting, and abdominal discomfort. In the presence of hypoperistalsis or paralytic ileus, patient will exhibit high-pitched, tinkling sounds that will be heard early in obstruction or ileus; or a decrease or absence of sounds occurring with complete obstruction or paralytic ileus.
- If patient is having bowel movements, determine the amount, consistency, and frequency. Question patient about his or her usual pattern of bowel elimination.
- Begin bowel training program based on patient's needs and status of dietary intake. Examples include the following:
  - Provide a high-roughage diet if patient is able to chew and swallow without difficulty; give patient prune juice every evening.
  - Establish a regular time for elimination (e.g., 30 min after meals) and have a bed pan readily available.
  - Facilitate patient's normal bowel habits: ensure privacy; provide warm oral fluids with each attempt at defecation.
  - Administer stool softeners (e.g., docusate sodium) or bulk-building additives such as psyllium.
  - Administer prescribed medicated suppositories.

Caution: Care must be taken to avoid stimulation of autonomic dysreflexia by using generous amounts of anesthetic ointment (e.g., Nupercaine) and ensuring gentle insertion when giving suppository or enema.

  - Provide 2-3 L/day of fluid to prevent dehydration and constipation. This may be contraindicated for patient with impaired renal or cardiac status.

Knowledge deficit: Purpose and procedure for plasmapheresis
Desired outcome: Before the first plasma exchange, patient verbalizes knowledge of the purpose and procedure for plasmapheresis.

- Assess patient's previous experience with and knowledge of plasmapheresis.
- As appropriate, teach patient the following about plasmapheresis: Blood is withdrawn *via* an arterial catheter, anticoagulated, and then passed through a cell separator. The plasma portion of the blood that may contain the autoantibody whose target is the peripheral nerve myelin sheath is removed. RBCs, WBCs, and platelets are mixed with saline, potassium, and plasma protein fraction and then are returned to the body, minus the plasma, *via* a venous access.
- Advise patient that plasmapheresis *may* lessen the duration and severity of the symptoms of GBS.

Note: Benefits of plasmapheresis with GBS have not been determined definitively. Although plasmapheresis is still in the experimental stage with this disorder, some studies have shown a rapid but temporary improvement in symptoms.

- Explain that patient should eat before plasmapheresis and that nutrition will be provided during the procedure.
- Advise patient that the nurse will perform several assessment procedures before, during, and after plasmapheresis. See **Risk for disuse syndrome,** p. 441, for neuroassessment parameters. Also see Table 6-1 for the following complications: hypovolemia, clotting abnormalities, hypokalemia, and hypocalcemia.
- Advise patient that the procedure may take several hours and that it may be performed as often as 3-4 times a week, depending on the patient's condition.

ADDITIONAL NURSING DIAGNOSES

See "Acute Spinal Cord Injury" for **Urinary retention,** p. 189. See "Renal Transplantation" for **Knowledge deficit:** Immunosuppressive medications and their side effects, p. 407. See "Myasthenia Gravis" for **Risk for infection**, p. 434, and **Impaired swallowing,** p. 435. For other nursing diagnoses and interventions, see the following as appropriate: "Nutritional Support," p. 12; "Mechanical Ventilation," p. 24; "Prolonged Immobility," p. 78; "Psychosocial Support," p. 88; and "Psychosocial Support for the Patient's Family and Significant Others," p. 100.

Cerebral aneurysm and subarachnoid hemorrhage

PATHOPHYSIOLOGY

An aneurysm is a localized dilatation of an arterial lumen caused by weakness in the vessel wall; 90% of cerebral aneurysms are saccular or berry (congenital). The other 10% comprise fusiform, septic, miliary, dissecting, and traumatic aneurysms. Saccular aneurysms are believed to result from a congenital hypoplasia of the muscle (medial) layer in the arterial wall, in combination with hypertension and atherosclerosis; 85%-90% occur at the bifurcation of the blood vessels that compose Willis' circle. The remainder occur in the posterior cerebral circulation, often at the bifurcation of the basilar and vertebral arteries.

Most aneurysms are silent until they rupture, although nearly half of the affected population experience some warning sign or symptom as a result of expansion of the lesion and compression of cerebral tissue. When rupture occurs, hemorrhage into the subarachnoid space (SAS) and basal cisterns results. If the patient survives the initial effects of subarachnoid hemorrhage (SAH), which include destruction of brain tissue by the force of arterial blood, intracerebral hemorrhage, and sharply increased ICP, he or she also must survive two of the common causes of morbidity and mortality—rebleeding and cerebral arterial vasospasm. Although bleeding may occur at any time, the risk of rebleeding from an aneurysm is greatest in the first 24-48 h after the initial incident and remains high for the first 2 wk. The patient also is at increased risk for rebleeding between 7-10 days post-SAH, when the normal process of clot dissolution occurs.

Cerebral vasospasm, the constriction of the arterial smooth muscle layer of the major cerebral arteries, causes a dramatic decrease in cerebral blood flow, which in turn leads to cerebral ischemia and progressive neurologic deficit. Vasospasm occurs in as many as 60% of patients with SAH, and its onset is between 4-14 days post-SAH and peaks between 7-10 days. The pathogenesis of cerebral vasospasm is poorly understood but seems to be directly related to the amount of blood in the SAS and basal cisterns. The greater the volume of blood, the more pronounced the vasospasm. It is hypothesized that as the clots in the basal cisterns begin to hemolyze, spasmogenic substances are released that precipitate the onset of vasospasm. In addition to rebleeding and vasospasm, the patient with a ruptured cerebral aneurysm and SAH is at risk for communicating hydrocephalus, hypothalamic dysfunction, and hyponatremia.

Communicating hydrocephalus: Communicating hydrocephalus develops in approximately 20% of patients with SAH. This condition occurs as a result of the presence of blood in the SAS and ventricular system. The hydrocephalus may be *acute* (lasting <24 h), *subacute* (lasting >24 h-1 wk), or *chronic* (lasting >7 days). Blood in the SAS and ventricles obstructs flow of CSF, interfering with its circulation and reabsorption and causing a rise in CSF pressure, with concomitant decrease in neurologic status.

Hypothalamic dysfunction: Hypothalamic dysfunction, seen in approximately one third of patients with hydrocephalus following SAH, may result from mechanical pressure on the hypothalamus from a dilated third ventricle. One manifestation of this dysfunction is an increase in serum catecholamines, which leads to overstimulation of the sympathetic nervous system.

Hyponatremia: Hyponatremia may be caused by cerebral salt-wasting syndrome, syndrome of inappropriate antidiuretic hormone (SIADH), or a combination of factors influencing sodium and water metabolism. Hyponatremia is reported to occur in 10%-50% of patients with SAH. If not identified and corrected early, hyponatremia may lead to intracranial hypertension, cerebral ischemia, seizures, coma, and death. See Table 6-2 for signs and symptoms of cerebral salt wasting and SIADH.

T A B L E 6 - 2   Clinical presentation with cerebral salt-wasting syndrome and syndrome of inappropriate antidiuretic hormone (SIADH)

Cerebral salt-wasting syndrome	*SIADH*
Hypotension	Normotension
Postural hypotension	Normal pulse rate or bradycardia
Tachycardia	Normal or low hematocrit
Elevated hematocrit	Increased glomerular filtration rate
Decreased glomerular filtration rate	Normal or decreased BUN and creatinine
Normal or elevated BUN and creatinine	Normal or low urine output
Normal or low urine output	Normovolemia or hypervolemia
Hypovolemia	Normal hydration
Dehydration	Dilutional hyponatremia
True hyponatremia	Hypoosmolality
Hypoosmolality	Increased body weight
Decreased body weight	

Note: Both hypothalamic dysfunction and hyponatremia are seen more frequently in patients with extensive SAH and are positively correlated with the subsequent development of cerebral vasospasm.

ASSESSMENT

Signs and symptoms before and after rupture depend on the size, site, and amount of bleeding.

Warning signs and symptoms (before bleeding):   Headaches (possibly localized); generalized, transient weakness; fatigue; occasional ptosis and dilated pupil due to palsy of cranial nerve III; diplopia, blurred vision, and pain above and behind the eye.

Clinical presentation after initial bleeding: Meningeal signs (due to presence of blood in the SAS) include headache, nuchal rigidity, fever, photophobia, lethargy, nausea, and vomiting. Patients report that the headache is the worst they have ever experienced, a sensation of a "bullet going off in the head."

Increased intracranial pressure (IICP):   Caused by SAH or intracerebral hemorrhage and the subsequent cerebral edema (Table 6-3; also see "Craniocerebral Trauma," p. 123).

Indicators of hydrocephalus

Acute: Onset within 24 h; loss of pupillary reflexes, sudden onset of coma or persistent coma after initial SAH.

Subacute: Onset within 1-7 days; gradual changes in LOC with confusion, drowsiness, lethargy, and stupor.

Chronic: Onset after 7 days; gradual changes in LOC and orientation with confusion, incontinence, and impaired balance, mobility, and gait; intellectual impairment (slowness, mutism); lack of affect; and presence of frontal lobe reflexes (grasp and sucking), which are abnormal in the adult.

T A B L E 6 - 3   Indicators of increased intracranial pressure

Alterations in consciousness: Increasing restlessness, confusion, irritability, disorientation, increasing drowsiness, lethargy
Bradycardia
Increasing systolic BP with a widening pulse pressure
Irregular respiratory patterns (e.g., Cheyne-Stokes, ataxic, apneustic, central neurogenic, hyperventilation)
Hemisensory changes and hemiparesis or hemiplegia: Due to involvement of hemispheric sensory and motor pathways
Worsening headache
Pupillary changes
Dysconjugate gaze and inability to move one eye beyond midposition: Caused by involvement of cranial nerves III, IV, and VI
Seizures
Involvement of other cranial nerves: Depends on the severity of neurologic insult

Note: If these indicators of IICP are left untreated, the patient will undergo irreversible brain damage or death. If these indicators occur suddenly, there will be displacement of brain substance (herniation), which will progress rapidly to permanent brain damage or death. For additional information about herniation syndromes, see "Craniocerebral Trauma," p. 124.

Hyponatremia: Anxiety, confusion, agitation, disorientation, lethargy, stupor, coma, anorexia, nausea, vomiting, abdominal pain, cold and clammy skin, generalized weakness, and lower extremity muscle cramps. See Table 6-2 for signs and symptoms of cerebral salt wasting and SIADH.
Altered hypothalamic regulatory mechanisms: Vomiting, glycosuria, proteinuria, and hyponatremia. Increased circulating catecholamines can cause flushing, diaphoresis, pupillary dilatation, decreased gastric motility, increased serum glucose, fever, hypertension, tachycardia, cardiac dysrhythmias, ischemia, and infarction.
Physical assessment: Pathologic reflexes due to the presence of blood in the SAS.
Kernig's sign: Resistance to full extension of the leg at the knee when the hip is flexed.
Brudzinski's sign: Flexion of the hip and knee with neck flexion.
Fundoscopic assessment: May reveal retinal hemorrhage(s) at the side of the optic disk. Hemorrhage is caused by blood from the SAS being forced along the optic nerve sheath under high pressure. The patient may complain of blurred vision or blind spots (scotomata).
Hunt-Hess classification system: Permits objective and continuing evaluation of the patient's initial symptoms and their progression. Grading is performed according to symptom presentation and level of consciousness.
Grade 0: Unruptured
Grade I: Asymptomatic or minimal headache, slight nuchal rigidity
Grade Ia: No acute meningeal reactions but with fixed neurologic deficit
Grade II: Moderate to severe headache, nuchal rigidity, possible cranial nerve deficit but no other neurologic deficit

Grade III: Drowsiness, confusion; mild focal deficit
Grade IV: Stuporous, moderate to severe hemiparesis, possible early
 decerebrate rigidity and vegetative disturbances
Grade V: Deep coma, decerebrate rigidity, moribund appearance

DIAGNOSTIC TESTS

CT scan: To identify presence of aneurysm and subarachnoid or intracerebral hemorrhage; and size, site, and amount of bleeding. Scan also may reveal the presence of hydrocephalus due to blocked CSF reabsorption pathways. If the aneurysm is small, it may not appear on the scan.

Cerebral angiography: To confirm diagnosis of ruptured aneurysm and SAH. It is used to show the size, location, and vessels involved, and the presence of other aneurysms, as well as to determine the accessibility of the aneurysm and the presence of hematoma, vasospasm, and hydrocephalus. A four-vessel study involving both carotids and vertebrals is recommended due to the 15%-20% chance of an existing second aneurysm. Very small aneurysms can be missed on angiogram, as are those that do not fill with contrast material due to the presence of vasospasm or a blood clot within the aneurysm.

Lumbar puncture (LP) and cerebrospinal fluid (CSF) analysis: To confirm presence of blood in the CSF, which signals that SAH has occurred. CSF pressure, which normally is 0-15 mm Hg (70-180 mm H_2O), may be as high as 250 mm H_2O, with the pressure proportionate to the degree of bleeding. Protein may be increased as much as 80-130 mg/dl (normal is 15-50 mg/dl). WBC count may be greater than the normal of $\leq$10/mm; and CSF glucose may be low (<40 mg/dl) in the presence of SAH.

Note: Performance of LP in the patient with SAH and IICP carries substantial risk of herniation and rebleeding. It is performed only when results of the CT are nondiagnostic.

Magnetic resonance imaging (MRI): To reveal very small aneurysms that are not visualized with CT or angiography.

Transcranial Doppler (TCD) ultrasonography: To evaluate the flow of blood through cerebral arteries and permit early detection of cerebral vasospasm.

ABG analysis: To detect hypoxemia and hypercapnia and to determine appropriate respiratory therapy.

ECG: To detect cardiac changes and dysrhythmias precipitated by hypothalamic dysfunction.

COLLABORATIVE MANAGEMENT

Respiratory support: To maintain airway and provide intubation and ventilation as necessary. Serial ABG tests are performed to identify hypoxemia (Pao_2 <80 mm Hg) and hypercapnia ($Paco_2$ >45 mm Hg). Hypercapnia is a potent cerebral vasodilator that can increase ICP in patients who are already at risk.

Bed rest, with activity limitation: To help prevent stress and strain. An attempt should be made to keep patient in a quiet, calm, and soothing environment with lowered lights and noise level. Usually, ADL are completed by nursing staff. Active ROM and isometric exercises are restricted during acute and preoperative stages to prevent IICP. Passive ROM is prescribed to prevent formation of thrombi, with subsequent pulmonary emboli.

ICP monitoring: See "Collaborative Management" under "Craniocerebral Trauma," p. 131.

HOB elevation: To help facilitate venous outflow from the intracranial cavity and lower ICP. A 15-45 degree angle usually is prescribed.

Fluid and electrolyte management: Fluids usually are limited to 1,500-1,800 ml/24 h to prevent overhydration, with subsequent cerebral edema and further increases in ICP. Electrolytes are replaced as indicated by patient's clinical data and laboratory values. It is recommended that hyponatremia be treated based on a careful assessment and identification of etiology. If the cause is true hyponatremia (cerebral salt wasting), normal saline, packed RBCs, and colloids are recommended. If the cause is dilutional hyponatremia (SIADH), free water restriction is recommended. Fluid restriction ranges from 500-800 ml/24 h to 1,000-1,500 ml/24 h. If fluid restriction is not an option, sodium replacement is implemented. Also found to be effective is the concurrent administration of a diuretic (furosemide) and replacement of solute with 3% hypertonic saline. Occasionally patients do not tolerate the saline infusion. Medications reported to be useful in the treatment of SIADH under this circumstance include demethylchlortetracycline (demeclocycline-DMC), lithium, glycerol, and phenytoin (Dilantin). All therapies should be administered cautiously with frequent (at least q4h) assessment of fluid and electrolyte status.

Nutrition therapy: Adequate nutritional intake is maintained *via* parenteral nutrition or lipid emulsions, enteral feedings, and oral intake as indicated by patient's neurologic status. See "Nutritional Support," p. 1.

Pharmacotherapy

Sedatives: Phenobarbital is the drug of choice for reducing restlessness and irritability, which can increase BP and ICP.

Antipyretics: Acetaminophen is used to control fever, which increases cerebral metabolic activity. It may be administered along with a hypothermia blanket and chlorpromazine to decrease temperature and control shivering. Usually aspirin is avoided because of its propensity for affecting the clotting cascade.

Analgesics: Acetaminophen for mild pain and codeine sulfate for more severe pain. Although codeine, when given in usual doses, will not depress neurologic indicators, it can cause constipation and thus should be administered with stool softeners to prevent straining.

Stool softeners: Docusate sodium (Colace) is the drug of choice for preventing straining, which can increase ICP.

Corticosteroids: Dexamethasone (Decadron) is the drug most commonly used for its antiinflammatory actions in relieving cerebral edema and decreasing ICP. There is some disagreement as to its effectiveness. It must be administered cautiously, and the patient should be monitored carefully for side effects, including GI tract irritation. Antacids and histamine H_2-receptor antagonists (see Table 8-13, p. 555) may be given to inhibit gastric secretions and reduce the risk of gastric erosion.

Antihypertensives: Hydralazine hydrochloride (Apresoline), reserpine (Serpasil), propranolol (Inderal), nimodipine (Nimotop), labetalol (Normodyne, Trandate), or sodium nitroprusside (Nipride) is administered to reduce BP in patients with persistent hypertension. They may be used in combination with a thiazide diuretic.

Osmotic diuretics: Mannitol (Osmitrol), urea (Ureaphil), and glycerol may be used to reduce ICP and treat cerebral edema *via* diuresis and a slightly hypovolemic state. All must be used with caution due to the risk of electrolyte imbalances and other serious side effects and adverse reactions.

Note: With the rapid movement of extracellular fluid from brain tissue to plasma and the associated decrease in brain volume, there may be an increased potential for rebleeding following the administration of mannitol. In addition, mannitol may cause a rebound increase in ICP approximately 8-12 h after administration due to increased circulating volume. It is suggested that furosemide (Lasix) be used to decrease the rebound effect of mannitol.

Loop diuretics: Furosemide (Lasix) is being used by some physicians because it seems to decrease cerebral edema without causing the rise in intracranial blood volume that occurs with mannitol.

Anticonvulsants: Phenytoin and phenobarbital may be used to control or prevent seizures.

Antifibrinolytics: Epsilon-aminocaproic acid (EACA [Amicar]) or tranexamic acid (TEA [Amikapron]) may be used to prevent lysis of the aneurysmal clot, which occurs normally between 7-14 days postrupture. It delays the spontaneous breakdown of the clot and provides time for further stabilization of the patient in preparation for surgery. EACA usually is administered *via* continuous infusion for the patient with SAH. The length of therapy is determined by the patient's status and readiness for surgery and the physician's preference (Table 6-4).

T A B L E 6 - 4   Nursing implications for administration of epsilon-aminocaproic acid (EACA)

- Be aware that rapid administration may induce hypotension, bradycardia, or cardiac dysrhythmias.
- Monitor for and report the following side effects: nausea, cramps, diarrhea, dizziness, tinnitus, headache, skin rash, malaise, nasal stuffiness, postural hypotension.
- Be alert to clotting or thrombosis, which can be precipitated by this medication. Assess for indicators of thrombophlebitis: calf erythema, warmth, tenderness, or increase in size or positive reaction for Homans' sign. Provide pneumatic compression stockings as prescribed.
- Assess for indicators of pulmonary emboli: chest pain, dyspnea, fever, tachycardia, cyanosis, falling BP, restlessness, agitation.
- Monitor and report blood levels of EACA *via* use of chromatography, which is available in some institutions.
- Consult physician promptly for significant findings.

Note: Use of antifibrinolytic agents remains controversial. The results of research on these agents have been inconclusive.

Investigational therapy to reduce cerebral vasospasm: The following are experimental treatments. To date no completely effective method has been found.

Craniotomy: Performed within 48 h to evacuate the blood clot that is present after SAH in an attempt to prevent vasospasm.

Rauwolfia *alkaloids (reserpine) and kanamycin sulfate (Kantrex):* To decrease circulating serotonin, a vasoactive substance that can promote vasospasm.

Isoproterenol (Isuprel): To block catecholamine release, increase cardiac output, and increase cerebral perfusion.

Theophylline (aminophylline): Used in conjunction with isoproterenol to increase vascular dilatation. When theophylline is used with isoproterenol, lidocaine is added to prevent cardiac dysrhythmias precipitated by the isoproterenol.

Nitroglycerin (Tridil) and phenylephrine (Neo-Synephrine): To dilate cerebral vessels and increase cerebral perfusion.

Sodium nitroprusside (Nipride): To relax smooth muscle and dilate cerebral vessels.

Calcium channel blockers, such as nimodipine and nicardipine: To inhibit calcium influx across the cell membrane of vascular smooth muscles, thereby decreasing peripheral vascular resistance and promoting vasodilatation. Nimodipine and nicardipine selectively affect cerebral vessels.

Methylprednisolone (Solu-Medrol): May reduce severity of ischemic deficit and stabilize cell membranes, thereby decreasing cerebral edema.

Barbiturate coma: To decrease metabolic needs of the brain until the vasospasm subsides and blood flow improves (used rarely). See "Craniocerebral Trauma," p. 133.

Triple H therapy: Each of the following therapies may be used singly or in combination.

Note: Although hypervolemic-hypertensive therapy with hemodilution has been proved to be an effective treatment for vasospasm, it carries great risks, and the patient's BP, ICP, and neurologic status must be monitored closely. If used preoperatively (rare), this therapy may precipitate IICP with rerupture and rebleeding from the aneurysm. When used postoperatively, the patient may experience cerebral edema with cerebral ischemia and subsequent neurologic deficit.

- *Hypervolemia* (saline, whole blood, packed cells, plasma protein fraction [Plasmanate], albumin, and hetastarch [Hespan]): To increase circulating volume to reverse or prevent ischemia due to vasospasm.
- *Hemodilution* (albumin and crystalloid fluids): To decrease blood viscosity.
- *Hypertension* (dobutamine [Dobutrex], phenylephrine [Neo-Synephrine], dopamine [Intropin], isoproterenol [Isuprel], levarter-

enol [Levophed], metaraminol [Aramine]): To increase BP, thereby increasing cerebral perfusion pressure and preventing ischemia and infarction.

Placement of a shunt for treatment of hydrocephalus: Hydrocephalus develops in 20%-25% of patients with subarachnoid hemorrhage from a ruptured cerebral aneurysm. A shunt is placed to drain CSF and thereby prevent enlargement of the ventricles with compression of cerebral tissue and IICP. The method of CSF drainage depends on the type of hydrocephalus. For acute and subacute types a ventricular catheter (ventriculostomy) usually is positioned, whereas for chronic hydrocephalus, one end of a small catheter is positioned into a ventricle, with the other end draining into a body cavity or space (e.g., subarachnoid space, cistern, peritoneum, vena cava, pleura). Major complications include infection and malfunction. If the shunt has a valve for the purpose of controlling drainage or preventing reflux of CSF, the surgeon may request that the valve be pumped periodically to ensure proper functioning. For nursing interventions after shunt placement, see Table 6-5.

Surgical interventions: Surgical treatment is based on the patient's clinical status and the neurosurgeon's preference. Surgical timing is a continuing source of controversy. Some surgeons operate on patients with grade I or II symptoms within a few days of the initial SAH. By doing so, their intent is to avoid rebleeding, an often fatal complication. Others prefer to wait more than 2 wk until the peak time for vasospasm (7-10 days post-SAH) has passed. Use of antifibrinolytic and antihypertensive agents reduces the risk of rebleeding during the presurgical period. Patients with grades III-V symptoms generally are con-

---

T A B L E 6 - 5   Nursing interventions after shunt placement

- After the shunting, assess patient for indicators of IICP (see Table 6-3) caused by either the disease itself or shunt malfunction.
- Position patient on side opposite the insertion site, either flat or with head elevated slightly (as prescribed) to prevent pressure on shunt mechanism.
- Assess VS; LOC (orientation to time, place, person); pupillary light reflex; and motor function.
- Monitor I&O and limit fluids as prescribed.
- Avoid severe head and neck rotation, flexion, or hyperextension to prevent kinking, compression, or twisting of the shunt catheter, which would impede CSF flow.
- If the shunt has a valve for controlling drainage or preventing reflux of CSF, pump the valve to ensure proper functioning, according to surgeon's directive. Usually the valve is located behind or above the ear and is the approximate diameter of a fingertip. Pumping involves gentle, serial compressions of the tissue over the shunt. If the valve is working properly, the emptying and refilling of the valve will be felt with palpation.
- Assess for indicators of meningitis (see p. 486), peritonitis (see p. 562), or septicemia (see p. 623) due to presence of shunt mechanism.

sidered poor surgical risks, especially in the period immediately after SAH. If the condition of these patients is clinically unstable, the trend is to treat them medically until they show improvement and stabilization. Surgery is considered for any patient with a large intracranial clot that causes a life-threatening intracranial shift. It is delayed for patients with cerebral vasospasm until the vasospasm subsides.

Repair of a cerebral aneurysm requires a craniotomy with either clipping or ligation of the neck of the aneurysm, coagulation of the aneurysm, or encasement of the aneurysmal sac in surgical gauze. The method of repair depends on the size, site, and number of perforating arteries, as well as the patient's clinical condition and the surgeon's preference.

While surgical interventions remain the mainstay of treatment of cerebral aneurysms, there are new modalities being used. In selected centers and in selected cases, interventional radiology with use of endovascular balloon therapy is an option. The goal of therapy, achieved either through balloon occlusion of the aneurysm or of the parent vessel, is thrombosis of the aneurysm. Generally, patient selection is limited to poor surgical candidates with surgically difficult or inaccessible aneurysms.

NURSING DIAGNOSES AND INTERVENTIONS

Decreased adaptive capacity: Intracranial, related to compromise of fluid dynamic mechanisms secondary to hemorrhage into the subarachnoid space

Desired outcome: Patient exhibits adequate cerebral perfusion within 24-72 h of treatment, as evidenced by orientation to time, place, and person (or consistent with baseline); equal and normoreactive pupils; BP within patient's normal range; HR 60-100 bpm; RR 12-20 breaths/min with normal depth and pattern (eupnea); bilaterally equal motor function, with extremity strength and tone normal for patient; ICP 0-15 mm Hg; cerebral perfusion pressure 60-80 mm Hg; and absence of headache, vomiting, and other indicators of IICP.

- Assess hourly for indicators of IICP (see Table 6-3) and herniation (see "Craniocerebral Trauma," p. 124).
- Calculate cerebral perfusion pressure (CPP) by means of the formula

$$CPP = MAP - ICP$$

$$\text{where} \quad MAP = \frac{\text{Systolic BP} + 2(\text{Diastolic BP})}{3}$$

CPP <30 mm Hg is incompatible with life. If ICP monitoring is used, assess for IICP (ICP ≥15 mm Hg or elevated above patient's baseline), and consult physician promptly if it occurs (see discussion in "Craniocerebral Trauma," p. 123).

- Assess for and treat conditions that can cause increasing restlessness with concomitant IICP: distended bladder, constipation, hypoxemia, headache, fear, anxiety.
- Implement measures that help prevent IICP and herniation:
  - Maintain complete bed rest.
  - Keep HOB elevated 15-45 degrees or as prescribed to promote cerebral venous outflow.

- Avoid hyperflexion, hyperextension, or hyperrotation of the neck to decrease the risk of jugular vein compression, which can impede venous outflow, thereby increasing ICP.
- Instruct patient to avoid activities that use isometric muscle contractions (pulling or pushing side rails and pushing against the foot board). These activities raise systolic BP, which increases ICP.
- Caution patient about straining with bowel movements because this increases intrathoracic pressure, which in turn increases ICP.
- Instruct patient to exhale through the mouth when moving in bed or having a bowel movement.
- Instruct patient to avoid coughing, because it increases intrathoracic pressure and ICP. Teach patient to open mouth when sneezing to minimize the increase in ICP.
- Maintain a quiet, relaxing environment; decrease external stimuli in the room, such as lights or noise. Limit visitors if appropriate, and encourage them to talk quietly with patient and try to keep conversations as nonstressful for the patient as possible.
- Minimize vigorous activity by assisting with ADL (feeding, bathing, dressing, toileting).
- Maintain a patent airway and adequate ventilation to prevent cerebral hypoxia, which, concomitant with hypoxemia and hypercapnia, can cause dramatic cerebral vasodilatation and an increase in cerebral edema and ICP.
- Monitor ABG values for evidence of hypoxemia (Pao_2 <80 mm Hg) or hypercapnia ($Paco_2$ >45 mm Hg), which can lead to IICP. Administer oxygen *via* nasal cannula, mask, ET tube, or tracheostomy as prescribed.
- Avoid vigorous, prolonged suctioning during period of intubation because this can precipitate hypoxemia, hypercapnia, and anxiety, which in turn can increase ICP.
- Some sources recommend hyperoxygenation of the patient with 100% oxygen during suctioning in order to increase Pao_2 and decrease $Paco_2$, which will help prevent cerebral vasodilatation. Follow this procedure if it is prescribed.
- Limit fluids intake to 1,500-1,800 ml/24 h as prescribed.
- Monitor and record I&O accurately.
- Administer antihypertensive medication as prescribed to keep BP at desired levels.
- Administer stool softeners as prescribed to prevent constipation, which can lead to straining and IICP with herniation.
- As prescribed, administer antitussive agents to prevent coughing and antiemetics to prevent or treat vomiting. Both coughing and vomiting can increase intrathoracic pressure and ICP.
- If IICP occurs suddenly, perform hyperinflation (as prescribed, or per agency protocol) with a manual resuscitator at a rate of ≥50 breaths/min to decrease $Paco_2$.
- If prescribed for acutely increased ICP, administer bolus of mannitol (i.e., 1.5-2 g/kg, as a 15%-25% solution infused over 30-60 min). Because of this relatively high dose and rapid infusion rate, monitor renal status before and during administration, and evaluate fluid and electrolyte status (see Chapter 10), body weight, and total

output before and after the infusion. Consult physician if cerebral spinal fluid pressure is not reduced within 15 min of starting the infusion.

Altered protection related to risk of rebleeding from cerebral aneurysm associated with clotting anomaly secondary to normal fibrinolytic response

Desired outcomes: Patient has no symptoms of rebleeding from ruptured cerebral aneurysm as evidenced by orientation to time, place, and person; equal and normoreactive pupils; BP within patient's normal range; HR 60-100 bpm; RR 12-20 breaths/min with normal depth and pattern (eupnea); bilaterally equal motor function, with extremity strength and tone normal for patient; and absence of headache, papilledema, nystagmus, and nausea. ICP is 0-15 mm Hg; CPP is 60-80 mm Hg.

- Assess for signs and symptoms of IICP with herniation, which can signal that rerupture with rebleeding from cerebral aneurysm has occurred. See preceding diagnosis, **Decreased adaptive capacity.**
- Administer antifibrinolytic agent (i.e., EACA) as prescribed to prevent the normal hemolytic response and stabilize the blood clot around the ruptured aneurysm.
- Monitor administration of EACA. Use an infusion controller or pump to ensure accurate infusion. Initial loading dose of 5 g is followed with 1-1½ g/h, not to exceed 24-36 g in 24 h. Mix with D_5W, normal saline, or lactated Ringer's solution.
- See Table 6-4 for nursing implications for administering EACA.

Decreased adaptive capacity: Intracranial, related to compromise of fluid dynamic mechanisms secondary to cerebral vasospasm associated with ruptured cerebral aneurysm

Desired outcomes: Patient has baseline or normal neurologic status as evidenced by orientation to time, place, and person; equal and normoreactive pupils; BP within patient's normal range; HR 60-100 bpm; RR 12-20 breaths/min with normal depth and pattern (eupnea); bilaterally equal motor function, with extremity strength and tone normal for patient; and absence of headache, papilledema, nystagmus, and nausea. ICP is 0-15 mm Hg or at patient's baseline; CPP is 60-80 mm Hg.

- Assess for indicators of IICP (see Table 6-3) and herniation (see "Craniocerebral Trauma," p. 124), which may occur either abruptly or gradually. Cerebral vasospasm generally affects the major cerebral vessels in the hemisphere or at the site of the ruptured aneurysm and can cause a focal neurologic deficit with or without a major or sudden loss of consciousness. Vasospasm also may be characterized by a gradual onset of confusion and deteriorating LOC associated with focal motor deficits. A headache that worsens over time and increasing BP may precede the onset of more serious neurologic symptoms.
- In the presence of the aforementioned indicators, prepare patient for cerebral angiography or CT scan with contrast medium, the only methods for confirming the presence of vasospasm and ruling out rebleeding.
- Administer the prescribed medications (i.e., mannitol, nitroprusside sodium, nimodipine) and intravenous fluids (e.g., colloids or whole

blood to increase volume, BP, and subsequently cerebral perfusion) for treating cerebral vasospasm.

- If using hypervolemic-hemodilution therapy per protocol or prescription, observe for signs and symptoms of fluid overload: imbalanced I&O, adventitious breath sounds (crackles, rhonchi), respiratory distress, decreased Hct, hyponatremia (serum sodium <137 mEq/L), jugular vein distention, peripheral edema, and increased CVP, RAP, and PAP.

- Continue to treat the IICP (see **Decreased adaptive capacity:** Intracranial, secondary to hemorrhage into the subarachnoid space, p. 455).

Constipation related to prolonged immobility, decreased fluid intake, inadequate intake of fiber, and restriction against Valsalva maneuver for straining

Desired outcome: Patient has bowel movements within his or her normal pattern (or at least q3-5days) without straining.

- Obtain data regarding patient's normal bowel elimination pattern, including date of most recent bowel movement.

- Assess for indicators of constipation, including abdominal distention, cramping, and complaints of fullness or pressure in the abdomen or rectum. Auscultate for bowel sounds.

- Advise patient to defecate whenever the need arises but to refrain from straining because this can increase ICP dramatically, thus increasing the risk of rerupturing and rebleeding from the aneurysm. Instruct patient to exhale slowly when defecating, inasmuch as this will help prevent a sudden increase in ICP.

- Assist patient into semi-Fowler's or high Fowler's position to facilitate bowel elimination, unless this position is contraindicated. Use of a bedside commode is recommended rather than a bed pan, because the physical and emotional stress of getting on a bed pan may increase ICP more than moving with assistance to a commode.

- Teach patient to select foods high in fiber to facilitate bowel elimination.

- Unless contraindicated, offer patient a warm drink to stimulate peristalsis. Record amount on I&O record.

- Administer stool softeners as prescribed.

- Avoid use of rectal thermometers, suppositories, enemas, or digital evacuation of an impaction. This type of stimulus may cause patient to perform a Valsalva-type maneuver, which in turn may increase intrathoracic and intracranial pressures, resulting in the potential for rerupture and rebleeding from the aneurysm.

ADDITIONAL NURSING DIAGNOSES

As appropriate, see nursing diagnoses and interventions in "Nutritional Support," p. 12; "Mechanical Ventilation," p. 24; "Alterations in Consciousness," p. 55; "Prolonged Immobility," p. 78; "Psychosocial Support," p. 88; and "Psychosocial Support for the Patient's Family and Significant Others," p. 100. See "Status Epilepticus" for **Risk for trauma** (oral and musculoskeletal), p. 467. See "Meningitis" for **Pain** related to headache, photophobia, and fever, p. 491. Also see "Diabetes Insipidus" for **Risk for fluid volume deficit,** p. 509. See "Syndrome of Inappropriate Antidiuretic Hormone" for **Risk for injury,** p. 513.

Care of the patient following intracranial surgery

Cranial surgery is performed for the following reasons: removal of a space-occupying lesion such as a tumor, hematoma, or abscess; repair of a vascular abnormality such as an aneurysm or arteriovenous malformation (AVM); drainage of cerebrospinal fluid from the ventricular system; correction of skull fractures; biopsy of tissue to confirm a diagnosis and facilitate treatment; control of seizures; and reduction of pain.

The surgical approach selected by the neurosurgeon depends primarily on the location of the pathologic condition. The *supratentorial* approach is used to remove or correct problems in the frontal, temporal, or occipital lobes, as well as in the diencephalic area (pituitary, hypothalamus). Lesions of the cerebellum and brainstem usually require an *infratentorial* (suboccipital) approach. The *transsphenoidal* approach gains access to the pituitary gland to remove a tumor, control bone pain associated with metastatic cancer, or attempt to arrest the progression of diabetic retinopathy in a patient with diabetes mellitus. After intracranial surgery the major goals of treatment are to maintain cerebral function through control of ICP; recognize, prevent, or treat complications; provide supportive care until the patient can resume ADL; and prepare and plan for rehabilitation.

COMPLICATIONS AFTER INTRACRANIAL SURGERY

Increased intracranial pressure with herniation: Cerebral edema, hemorrhage, infection, and surgical trauma can all lead to IICP with herniation (see Table 6-3). Some cerebral edema is expected after intracranial surgery, and it usually peaks about 72 h after surgery (see "Craniocerebral Trauma," p. 123).

Intracranial bleeding: May be intracerebral, intracerebellar, subarachnoid, subdural, extradural, or intraventricular. Bleeding may be caused by the lengthy and extensive surgical procedure, prolonged anesthesia, preexisting medical problems, or medications.

Stroke: Can occur intraoperatively or postoperatively as the result of fluctuations in BP that lead to cerebral ischemia and infarction. Stroke secondary to cerebral arterial vasospasm may occur after subarachnoid hemorrhage. Air embolism is a possible cause of stroke in the patient undergoing infratentorial surgery in the sitting position. See "Stroke: Cerebral Infarct and Intracerebral Hematoma," p. 470.

Seizures: Generalized or partial seizures can occur as a result of surgical trauma, irritation of cerebral tissue by the presence of blood, cerebral edema, cerebral hypoxia, hypoglycemia, preexisting seizure disorder, or inadequate anticonvulsant levels.

CNS infection: Meningitis, encephalitis, and ventriculitis may occur as a result of bacterial contamination before, during, or after surgery. For example, a gunshot wound to the brain may introduce organisms at the time of injury. After surgery the presence of moist, bloody head dressings (an effective culture medium) or a break in sterile technique during a dressing change may lead to CNS infection. (See "Meningitis," p. 485, and "Infection Prevention and Control," Appendix 8)

Hydrocephalus: May appear preoperatively or occur postoperatively as an acute or chronic complication. Usually it is caused by a slowing or complete stoppage of the flow of CSF through the ventricular system secondary to edema, bleeding, scarring, or obstruction. For a discussion of shunt creation, see "Cerebral Aneurysm and Subarachnoid Hemorrhage," p. 454.

Diabetes insipidus (DI) and syndrome of inappropriate antidiuretic hormone (SIADH):   The result of a disturbance in the hypothalamus or posterior lobe of the pituitary gland. ADH is produced within the supraoptic nuclei of the hypothalamus and stored in the posterior pituitary. This disturbance may result from edema, manipulation, or partial or total removal of the gland. DI is the result of a decrease or loss of production of ADH, which leads to excessive urinary output, with a potential for serious fluid and electrolyte problems (see "Diabetes Insipidus," p. 504). SIADH, a less common problem, is the result of an increase in the release of ADH, which leads to reabsorption of large amounts of water *via* the renal tubules, with concurrent loss of large amounts of sodium. Like DI, SIADH also can cause serious fluid and electrolyte problems (see "Syndrome of Inappropriate Antidiuretic Hormone," p. 511).

Cardiac dysrhythmias: May occur as a result of cerebral hypoxia or ischemia, manipulation of the brainstem, or the irritating effects of blood in the CSF (see "Dysrhythmias and Conduction Disturbances," p. 300).

Hyperthermia: May be caused by injury or irritation of the hypothalamic temperature-regulating centers or the presence of blood in the CSF, or may be an indicator of wound infection, atelectasis, pneumonia, or urinary tract infection. Regardless of the cause, an elevated temperature is detrimental because it increases the metabolic needs of the brain, potentially leading to increased blood flow to the area, with concomitant cerebral edema.

CSF leak: Caused by a channel between the subarachnoid space (SAS) and the outside as a result of a tear or rupture of the dura mater. A CSF leak may be present preoperatively after a skull fracture, or it may occur during surgery. CSF leakage from the ear is called "otorrhea"; from the nose it is called "rhinorrhea." The leakage of CSF indicates an open pathway to the SAS, which carries a serious risk of infection.

Loss of corneal reflex: May be caused by surgical trauma to motor pathways from the frontal lobe or trauma or edema of the brainstem cranial nerve nuclei. It can result in corneal abrasion, ulceration, and blindness if it is not recognized and treated promptly.

Periocular edema: Can occur after supratentorial surgery with manipulation of the scalp or frontal bones of the cranium or retraction of the frontal lobes.

POSTOPERATIVE NEUROLOGIC DEFICITS

Some neurologic deficit(s) may be present preoperatively and should be noted and documented. Deficits that occur after surgery may be due to surgical trauma or the presence of cerebral edema, which will interfere with normal brain function. With time these deficits may improve. The following are some of the neurologic deficits that may be present in the patient after intracranial surgery.

Diminished level of consciousness: The degree of improvement in LOC will depend on the amount of preoperative damage to cerebral tissue. Generally, LOC improves as anesthesia wears off, cerebral edema subsides, and ICP decreases.

Communicative and cognitive deficits: The ability to communicate and understand after surgery depends on the degree of preoperative dysfunction, the site of the lesion, the extensiveness of the surgical procedure, and the degree of postoperative cerebral edema.

Broca's (expressive, motor, nonfluent) dysphasia: A situation or disorder in which an individual can comprehend the situation and follow commands appropriately but cannot articulate wishes and needs.

Wernicke's (receptive, sensory, fluent) dysphasia: A situation or disorder in which an individual does not understand the situation and cannot follow commands appropriately.

Motor and sensory deficits: Motor deficits (weakness or paralysis) are caused by injury or edema to the primary motor cortex and corticospinal (pyramidal) tracts. Generally improvement will be seen as cerebral edema subsides. Early physical therapy is necessary to prevent long-term disabilities such as foot or wrist drop, contractures, and hip rotation. Sensory deficits are caused by injury or edema to the primary sensory cortex or the sensory association areas of the parietal lobe. In addition, damage to the spinothalamic tracts may cause sensory deficits. Examples of sensory deficits include the inability to distinguish objects according to size, shape, weight, texture, and consistency and the inability to distinguish changes in temperature, touch, pressure, and position. As with motor deficits, improvement in sensory perception generally will occur as cerebral edema subsides.

Cranial nerve impairment: The degree and presence of cranial nerve deficit(s) depend on the site of the lesion, preoperative deficit, the degree of postoperative cerebral edema, and the surgical approach. Infratentorial surgery for lesions in the posterior fossa (brainstem and cerebellum) may involve significant cranial nerve manipulation and trauma, with considerable postoperative cranial nerve deficit. Deficit(s) may improve with decreasing cerebral edema or may be permanent. Assessment of cranial nerve dysfunction is an important nursing function. For more information about the function of all the cranial nerves, see Appendix 4.

Respiratory complications: Respiratory complications after intracranial surgery can be particularly serious because any increase in Pa_{CO_2} resulting in hypercapnia will lead to cerebral vasodilatation, with a subsequent increase in intracranial volume, and thus IICP. Respiratory complications include the following:

- Partial or complete airway obstruction due to accumulation of secretions and improper positioning.
- Neurogenic pulmonary edema due to a sudden increase in ICP.
- Cerebral edema that causes compression of brainstem respiratory centers.
- Atelectasis and pneumonia.
- Pulmonary embolus.

Gastrointestinal bleeding (Cushing's ulcer) and paralytic ileus: The development of GI bleeding is associated with cerebral trauma and the postoperative period after neurosurgery. Although the cause is unclear, it is believed that stress from the trauma or surgery can lead to continued vagal stimulation, which in turn leads to a hyperacidic state that causes gastric erosion, ulceration, and ultimately hemorrhage. Gastric erosion, ulceration, and hemorrhage also can be precipitated by medications, especially the corticosteroids (see "Acute Gastrointestinal Bleeding," p. 568). Paralytic ileus is common after abdominal surgery but also may occur after neurologic surgery. Decreased or absent peristalsis may be the result of prolonged anesthesia, immobility, trauma, electrolyte deficiencies, and mechanical obstruction.

Thrombophlebitis, deep vein thrombosis (DVT), and pulmonary embolus: Each of these complications is related to or the result of prolonged bed rest and immobility after intracranial surgery. Other factors, such as a prolonged surgical procedure or preexisting coagulopathies and blood dyscrasias, may influence the postoperative development of these complications.

COLLABORATIVE MANAGEMENT AFTER INTRACRANIAL SURGERY

Respiratory support: Oxygen supplements, intubation, and mechanical ventilation are provided as indicated.

Activity restrictions: Will depend on patient's LOC and general condition.

Positioning: For most patients HOB is elevated 30 degrees to promote venous drainage, thereby reducing ICP.

- In posterior fossa surgery (infratentorial approach), the supporting muscles of the neck are altered. This necessitates turning the patient with the neck in alignment with the head and the support of the head, neck, and shoulders in the process.
- After craniectomy, during which a bone flap is removed, the patient should not be positioned on the side on which bone has been removed. Label patient's head dressing, chart, and bed with this information.
- After procedures in which a large intracranial space has been left due to extensive surgery, patient should not be positioned on operative side immediately after surgery because this may cause a sudden shift in intracranial contents, with subsequent hemorrhage or herniation.

Pharmacotherapy: The following may be prescribed postoperatively:

Corticosteroids (e.g., dexamethasone):   To decrease cerebral edema.

Note: Current research has not resolved the question of whether steroids are effective in the treatment of cerebral edema.

Osmotic diuretics (e.g., mannitol, urea):   To control cerebral edema causing IICP.

Anticonvulsants (e.g., phenytoin, phenobarbital):   To prevent seizures in the immediate postoperative period caused by cerebral edema and irritation due to surgical manipulation of the brain. Anticonvulsants may be continued prophylactically for a period of 1-2 yr after surgery.

Antibiotics: To prevent or treat postoperative infection.

Antipyretics: For prompt treatment of elevated temperature, which, if left untreated, can increase metabolic activity, causing increased use of oxygen and glucose supplies.

Analgesics: To treat or control pain due to headache. Drugs of choice are acetaminophen alone or with codeine sulfate.

Antacids (e.g., Maalox):   To prevent the formation of gastric ulceration occurring from steroid use or as a result of the stress of surgery.

Histamine H_2-receptor antagonists (e.g., ranitidine [Zantac]):   To suppress gastric secretions and thus prevent or facilitate healing of Cushing's ulcer (see Table 8-13, p. 555).

Fluid and electrolyte management: To prevent or treat increasing cerebral edema. Usually fluids are limited to 1,500-1,800 ml/day, depending on patient's body size and overall condition.

Nutritional support: The method and type of nutritional support are determined by the patient's condition and may include any of the following: oral feedings, enteral feedings, supplements, or parenteral nutrition (i.e., TPN, fat emulsion therapy). See "Nutritional Support," p. 1.

Physical medicine consultation: To evaluate patient for physical, occupational, and speech therapy and to begin planning for rehabilitation.

NURSING DIAGNOSES AND INTERVENTIONS

Risk for injury related to potential for development of gastric ulcer (Cushing's) or gastritis secondary to hyperacidic state

Desired outcomes: Result of patient's gastric pH test is >5, and patient has no symptoms of gastric ulcer and gastritis as evidenced by gastric secretions and stool culture that are negative for blood; HR ≤100 bpm; BP within patient's normal range; and absence of midepigastric discomfort.

- Monitor for indicators of GI bleeding or ulceration: midepigastric discomfort, occult or frank blood in stool or gastric secretions, decreasing BP, increasing HR. If these indicators are present, consult physician and prepare for insertion of a gastric tube.
- Monitor Hct or Hgb results daily; report decreasing values. Normal values are as follows: Hct 37%-47% (female) or 40%-54% (male) and Hgb 14-18 g/dl (male) or 12-16 g/dl (female).
- Test gastric drainage pH q4h. Administer H_2-receptor antagonists and/or antacids as prescribed to maintain pH >5.
- Implement measures to prevent ulceration and hemorrhage:
  - As prescribed, administer antacids to prevent gastric ulceration and histamine H_2-receptor antagonists to suppress gastric secretions and promote healing.
  - Administer steroids, aspirin, phenytoin, and other medications that irritate gastric mucosa with a meal or snack.
  - Limit patient's intake of acidic or spicy foods, as well as caffeine-containing substances such as coffee, cola, and chocolate.

ADDITIONAL NURSING DIAGNOSES

See nursing diagnoses and interventions in "Nutritional Support," p. 12; "Prolonged Immobility," p. 78; "Psychosocial Support," p. 88; and

"Psychosocial Support for the Patient's Family and Significant Others," p. 100. See "Craniocerebral Trauma" for **Risk for infection (CNS),** p. 136; **Ineffective thermoregulation,** p. 137; **Risk for disuse syndrome,** p. 138; and **Impaired corneal tissue integrity,** p. 138. Also see "Cerebral Aneurysm and Subarachnoid Hemorrhage" for **Decreased adaptive capacity** secondary to hemorrhage into the subarachnoid space, p. 455; **Decreased adaptive capacity** secondary to cerebral vasospasm, p. 457; and **Constipation,** p. 458. See "Status Epilepticus" for **Risk for trauma** (oral and musculoskeletal), p. 467. See "Meningitis" for **Pain** related to headache, photophobia, and fever, p. 491. See "Diabetes Insipidus" for **Fluid volume deficit,** p. 509. See "Syndrome of Inappropriate Antidiuretic Hormone" for **Risk for injury,** p. 513.

Status epilepticus

PATHOPHYSIOLOGY

Status epilepticus is a state of recurring or continuous seizures of at least 30 minutes' duration in which the patient does not return to full consciousness from the postictal state before another seizure occurs. The two major types of status epilepticus, based on the classification of Gastaut and used by Engel, are generalized status epilepticus and partial status epilepticus. *Generalized status* includes convulsive status (generalized tonic-clonic seizures) and absence status (petit mal seizures). *Partial status* includes simple partial status (focal motor or epilepsia partialis continua) and complex partial status (temporal or nontemporal seizures). The term "nonconvulsive status" also is used to describe absence and complex partial status. Convulsive status (generalized tonic-clonic seizures) is the more common type and is considered a life-threatening medical emergency because of the hypoxia and neuronal metabolic exhaustion that occur. Neuronal death may occur.

A common cause of status epilepticus in persons with epilepsy is noncompliance with medications or a drop in anticonvulsant serum levels caused by alcohol abuse or infection. Other causes for individuals with and without preexisting epilepsy include acute metabolic disturbances (hypoglycemia, hyponatremia, hypocalcemia), cerebrovascular accident, CNS infection (meningitis, encephalitis), CNS trauma or tumors, and alcohol or drug abuse. Prompt treatment is vital in preventing complications such as cardiac dysrhythmias, hyperthermia, aspiration, hypertension, hypotension, anoxia, hyperglycemia, hypoglycemia, dehydration, myoglobinuria, and oral or musculoskeletal injuries. The mortality rate in status epilepticus is 10%-12%.

ASSESSMENT

HISTORY AND RISK FACTORS Epilepsy, drug or alcohol abuse, recent head injury, infection, headaches. If the patient is taking antiepilepsy medications, record the following: drug name, dosage, time last taken, length of time drug has been taken, and any recent medication changes. Determine whether patient is taking any other medications, including name, dose, and time last taken.

Partial status epilepticus

Complex partial status: Manifested as a prolonged confusional state due to continuing or recurring seizures. Automatisms (lip smacking, chewing, swallowing) and speech difficulty may be present. Once this period of status passes, postictal confusion and sleepiness may ensue.

Simple partial status: The second most common form of status epilepticus, it is commonly manifested as focal motor status (epilepsia partialis continua). Usually consciousness remains intact, and motor activity is localized to one area of the body such as the face or hand. It may last for hours or days.

Generalized status epilepticus

Absence status: Characterized by some alteration in consciousness, ranging from a dreamy state to stupor. Automatisms or mild clonic movements, such as fluttering of the eyelids, may be present. Clinically, absence status is difficult to differentiate from complex partial status.

Convulsive status: The most common form of status epilepticus, it is characterized by generalized tonic-clonic seizures without return to full consciousness. This is a life-threatening medical emergency requiring immediate intervention.

DIAGNOSTIC TESTS

Serum drug screen: Rules out drug or alcohol intoxication.

Serum electrolyte, BUN, calcium, magnesium, and glucose values; CBC count: Rule out electrolyte imbalance or metabolic disturbance as the cause of status epilepticus.

Antiepilepsy serum drug level: To determine the amount of drug in patient's system.

ABG analysis: To obtain baseline levels and determine state of oxygenation.

ECG: Evaluates cardiovascular status, especially during administration of drugs such as phenytoin that may lead to hypotension and dysrhythmias.

EEG: Performed during the seizure and can differentiate between absence and complex partial status.

CT scan: To rule out presence of a brain lesion.

COLLABORATIVE MANAGEMENT

Maintenance of alveolar ventilation and other vital functions: Cardiopulmonary function and VS are assessed closely. Oral airway, oxygen, and if necessary, intubation and respiratory support, are initiated.

Prevention of Wernicke-Korsakoff syndrome: 100 mg IV thiamine and 50 ml of 50% glucose are administered if chronic alcohol ingestion or hypoglycemia is suspected.

Pharmacotherapy
Administration of fast-acting anticonvulsant
- IV diazepam (Valium): Given to achieve high serum and brain concentrations. It is not used as a long-acting anticonvulsant.
  —0.2 mg/kg up to 20 mg.
  —Do not infuse faster than 5 mg/min due to respiratory depression that can occur with faster infusion rate.
  —Monitor respiratory and cardiovascular status continuously during administration.
- IV lorazepam (Ativan): Given to achieve high serum and brain concentrations. It is not used as a long-acting anticonvulsant.
  —0.1 mg/kg up to 8 mg.
  —Do not infuse faster than 2 mg/min.
  —Monitor respiratory and cardiovascular status continuously during administration.

Administration of long-acting anticonvulsant
- IV phenytoin (Dilantin): Usual loading dose is 18-20 mg/kg.
  —Do not infuse faster than 50 mg/min, inasmuch as hypotension or dysrhythmias can develop.
  —Flush line with normal saline only. Microcrystallization, which occurs when phenytoin is used with dextrose, also may occur when it is used in saline as a continuous drip.
  —Monitor VS closely.
  —If status persists after 20 mg/kg dose, an additional 5 mg/kg up to a maximum total dose of 30 mg/kg may be given.

Caution: High doses of phenytoin can cause seizure activity; therefore >30 mg/kg is not recommended.

Administration of IV phenobarbital: If patient is allergic to phenytoin.
  —Usual dosage is 20 mg/kg.
  —Do not infuse faster than 50-100 mg/min.

Caution: If given simultaneously with or after lorazepam or diazepam, respiratory depression and hypotension can occur, possibly necessitating ventilatory support.

General anesthesia: Pentobarbital coma
  —Given if administration of fast-acting anticonvulsant, long-acting convulsant, or IV phenobarbital is ineffective in stopping the seizure activity.
  —Loading dose is 5 mg/kg.
  —Maintenance dose is 0.5-3 mg/kg/h to stop seizure activity or maintain burst suppression on EEG.
  —Monitor respiratory and cardiovascular activity continuously.
  —Mechanical ventilation and vasopressors usually are required.
  —Periodic tapering of pentobarbital is done to see if seizures have remitted.
  —Patient may be in a coma for days to weeks.

Paraldehyde, lidocaine, midazolam, or neuromuscular blockade: Alternative therapies to stop the seizure activity. Neuromuscular blockade will stop the movements but not the electrical activity.

Nutritional support: Enteral or parenteral nutrition may be necessary, depending on the duration of the status epilepticus and patient's underlying nutritional state.

NURSING DIAGNOSES AND INTERVENTIONS

Risk for trauma (oral and musculoskeletal) related to seizure activity
Desired outcome: Patient's oral cavity and musculoskeletal system do not exhibit evidence of trauma after the seizure.

- Pad the side rails, keep side rails up at all times, maintain bed in its lowest position, and keep an oral airway at the bedside.
- Perform protective measures during the seizures:
  - □ Put a soft object such as a pillow under patient's head.
  - □ Move sharp or potentially dangerous objects away from patient.
  - □ Loosen any tight clothing.
  - □ Avoid restraining patient, because the force of the tonic-clonic movements could traumatize the patient.
  - □ Avoid forcing airway into patient's mouth when jaws are clenched. Force could break teeth, causing patient to swallow or aspirate them.
  - □ Avoid use of tongue blade, which could splinter.
  - □ Stay with patient; assess and record seizure type and duration. Record any automatic behavior (e.g., lip smacking, chewing movements), motor activity, incontinence, tongue biting, and postictal state.
- After seizure, reorient and reassure patient.

Impaired gas exchange related to altered oxygen supply associated with hypoventilation and bradypnea secondary to depressant effect of seizures on respiratory center
Desired outcome: Within 1 h of treatment/intervention, patient has adequate gas exchange as evidenced by Pao_2 ≥80 mm Hg, $Paco_2$ 35-45 mm Hg, pH 7.35-7.45, and RR 12-20 breaths/min with normal depth and pattern (eupnea).

- Assess patient's respiratory status, including rate, depth, rhythm, and color. Be alert to use of accessory muscles of respiration, rapid or labored respirations, and cyanosis (a late sign of dysfunction).
- Position an oral airway to help maintain open airway. To prevent injury, avoid forcing airway into mouth.
- Keep patient turned to the side to allow secretions to drain; suction as necessary.
- Monitor ABG values to assess oxygenation. Be alert to hypoxemia (Pao_2 <80 mm Hg) and respiratory acidosis ($Paco_2$ >45 mm Hg and pH <7.35).
- Keep intubation equipment readily available for airway and ventilation assistance.
- Administer oxygen as indicated per nasal cannula, mask, or manual resuscitator.
- Administer antiepilepsy medications within prescribed criteria to avoid further depression of respiratory center.

Altered cerebral and cardiopulmonary tissue perfusion related to interrupted blood flow secondary to continuous seizure activity or vasodilatory effects of some antiepilepsy medications

Desired outcome: Within 1 h of treatment/intervention, patient has adequate cerebral and cardiopulmonary perfusion as evidenced by orientation to time, place, and person; normal sinus rhythm on ECG; BP within patient's normal range; RR 12-20 breaths/min with normal depth and pattern (eupnea); and absence of headache, papilledema, and other clinical indicators of IICP.

Note: Metabolic demands of the brain and heart are increased greatly during seizure activity; thus adequate perfusion is essential for organ function.

- Maintain airway and ventilation to ensure maximum delivery of oxygen to the brain cells.
- Monitor VS q2-4min. Respiratory depression, decreased BP, and dysrhythmias can occur with rapid infusion of diazepam and phenytoin. BP must be maintained within normal limits for optimal brain perfusion.
- Monitor cardiac status *via* cardiac monitor. Be alert to dysrhythmias.
- Ensure safe administration of antiepileptic drugs: diazepam at 5 mg/min, lorazepam at 2 mg/min, phenobarbital at 50-100 mg/min, or phenytoin at 50 mg/min. See "Collaborative Management," p. 466, for details.
- Perform baseline and serial neurologic assessments to determine the presence of focal findings that suggest an expanding lesion. (See Table 6-3 for indicators of IICP.)

Noncompliance with prescribed medication regimen related to misunderstanding health care recommendations, not understanding importance of following medication schedule, running out of medication, or stopping medication intentionally because of frustration or denial of the disease

Desired outcome: Within the 24-h period before discharge from the critical care unit, patient verbalizes understanding of the rationale and importance of taking the medication as prescribed, as well as the consequence of noncompliance.

- Once a diagnosis of noncompliance with the medication regimen has been established, determine patient's reason for noncompliance.
- Assess patient's understanding of epilepsy and its treatment.
- Ensure that patient is aware that stopping the antiepilepsy medication can result in serious problems, including status epilepticus. Explain that if patient plans to stop the medication for any reason, he or she should do so with physician's guidance so that it can be done as safely as possible, although the risk of status epilepticus would remain.
- Evaluate the effect epilepsy has on patient's life-style.
- Once the problem has been identified, work with the patient to find a solution. For example, if the patient is experiencing a side effect from the medication, such as gastric upset, suggest that patient try taking the medication after meals. If the gastric upset is a result of increasing the medication, advise patient to increase the dose more slowly.

- Refer patient to regional epilepsy support groups and the Epilepsy Foundation of America (EFA), including regional affiliate and national headquarters.
- As appropriate, refer patient to nurse specialist or social worker at regional center for individual counseling.

Knowledge deficit: Disease process, treatment, and necessary life-style changes for epilepsy

Desired outcome: Within the 24-h period before discharge from the critical care unit, patient verbalizes understanding of epilepsy, including its etiology, pathophysiology, and seizure classification, as well as its treatment and necessary life-style changes.

- Assess patient's understanding of epilepsy.
- As indicated, teach patient about the disease, its cause, pathophysiology, and seizure classification.
- Ask patient to describe the seizure(s) in detail, including warning signals (aura) that occur at the beginning of the seizure. Explain to patient that this aura or warning is the beginning of the seizure and that patient should lie down or get into a safe position to prevent injury.
- Assess patient's knowledge of the antiepilepsy medication, including its name, purpose, schedule, dosage, precautions, and side effects. Teach patient the importance of maintaining a constant blood level of the medication by taking the medication every day as prescribed. Explain that if the medication is missed or taken erratically, he or she cannot attain the blood level that is necessary for preventing seizure breakthrough. If a dose of medication is missed, instruct patient to notify his or her physician.
- Advise patient that a normal life is possible.
- Teach patient that sleep deprivation can precipitate SE and that each individual must know his or her own limits. However, having epilepsy does not mean that it is necessary to get more sleep than do persons who do not have epilepsy.
- Teach patient and significant others the safety interventions that should be made during a seizure (see **Risk for trauma** [oral and musculoskeletal] related to seizure activity, p. 467). In addition, explain the importance of easing patient to the floor and turning patient to a side-lying position.
- Inform patient of the state's driving regulations for persons with epilepsy.
- Teach patient the importance of avoiding dangerous machinery and heights if his or her seizures are not being controlled adequately by medications.

Ineffective individual coping related to frustration secondary to unpredictable nature of the disease

Desired outcome: Within 24-48 h of this diagnosis, patient verbalizes feelings, identifies strengths and ineffective coping behaviors, and demonstrates a responsible role in his or her own care.

- Assess patient's knowledge of the disease and its treatment. See preceding diagnosis, **Knowledge deficit.**
- Encourage patient to express feelings of frustration so that you can evaluate areas of major concern.
- Involve patient in decisions regarding care so that he or she has more

of a sense of control over the disease (e.g., encourage patient to participate in the decision for scheduling the medications).
- Help patient set realistic goals for employment and living arrangements. Refer patient to regional or local Epilepsy Foundation of America as appropriate.
- To involve patient in self-care, encourage him or her to educate others in what to do should a seizure occur.
- Encourage patient's involvement in support groups in which patient can learn coping strategies from other persons with the same disorder.
- For additional interventions, see the same nursing diagnosis in "Psychosocial Support," p. 93.

ADDITIONAL NURSING DIAGNOSES

For other nursing diagnoses and interventions, see the following as appropriate: "Mechanical Ventilation," p. 24; "Psychosocial Support," p. 88; and "Psychosocial Support for the Patient's Family and Significant Others," p. 100.

Stroke: acute cerebral infarct and intracerebral hematoma

PATHOPHYSIOLOGY

Stroke is the leading cause of adult disability and the third leading cause of death. Although strokes can occur at any age, the majority occur in individuals over age 55. The term "stroke" refers to an acute vascular injury to the brain. There are two major categories of stroke—ischemic and hemorrhagic. Subcategories of these major stroke types are shown in Figure 6-1. Each stroke type is defined by the pathophysiologic event. This section deals exclusively with acute cerebral infarct and intracerebral hematoma, the clot that remains following the hemorrhage. Subarachnoid hemorrhage (SAH) and arteriovenous malformations (AVM) are discussed on pp. 446 and 459.

Acute cerebral infarcts (ACIs) comprise 80% of all strokes. Primarily they are caused by thrombi or emboli that interrupt blood flow to the brain and cause an ischemic event that leads to infarction. The ischemic event compromises the Na^+/K^+ pump, leading to neuronal depolarization and neurotransmitter release. These actions cause a massive flux of ions and water, resulting in brain cell edema. Extracellular K^+ and intracellular Ca^{2+} rise, and the pH falls. The resulting high concentration of intracellular Ca^{2+} and lactic acidosis cause cellular metabolic alterations that ultimately lead to cellular death. The lactic acidosis stimulates the vasomotor center, which causes a marked elevation in arterial pressure. This response is known as the CNS ischemic response. Although it can be appreciated during the acute phase of stroke, the ischemic response is most pronounced during a Cushing response just before herniation.

The two most common causes of ACIs are thrombus and embolic clot formation. A thrombus is a clot formed in the artery, usually oc-

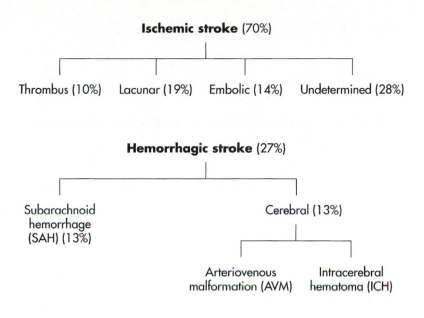

Figure 6-1:   Stroke classification.

curring in branches of low flow with plaque formation. Blood adheres to the rough edges of the plaque and forms a clot that occludes the vessel. Cerebral emboli most commonly are formed in the heart and travel to the brain. Some clots are formed in the carotid or other cerebral arteries and break off and migrate to occlude a smaller artery in the brain. Characteristic deficits are produced, depending on the artery involved (Table 6-6).

Intracerebral hematomas (ICHs) can occur in any location of the brain (Table 6-7). Although various pathophysiologic events can result in ICH, the most common cause is hypertension, usually resulting in the rupture of a small penetrating artery in the basal ganglia. Damage occurs as blood destroys and displaces the brain tissue. Because of the lack of blood flow, ischemia develops in the area that surrounds the already injured brain tissue, resulting in even greater injury. Intracerebral blood sometimes ruptures into the lateral ventricle and puts the patient at risk for communicating hydrocephalus. Lobar hemorrhages are less common and, when found in elders, often are caused by cerebral amyloid angiopathy. Other common causes of hemorrhage include vascular malformations, vasculitis, neoplasms, hematologic disorders, and stimulant abuse (cocaine and amphetamines).

T A B L E 6 - 6   Neuroanatomy related to neurologic deficit

Vessel	Area supplied	Deficit
ICA (internal carotid artery)	Right or left hemisphere	Contralateral motor or sensory deficit, aphasia with dominant hemisphere, neglect with nondominant hemisphere, contralateral visual field deficit (hemianopia), contralateral eye deviation
MCA (middle cerebral artery)	Right or left convex surface of the brain, most of the basal ganglia, internal capsule, putamen, and globus pallidus	Contralateral hemiplegia (arm and face > leg), sensory involvement, aphasia of dominant hemisphere, neglect of nondominant hemisphere (denial of weakness), homonymous hemianopia
ACA (anterior cerebral artery)	Right or left frontal lobe, corpus callosum, caudate nucleus, internal capsule	Weakness or sensory loss of contralateral leg and proximal arm; behavior disturbance: abulia, confusion, memory loss, and urinary incontinence
PCA (posterior cerebral artery)	Midbrain, thalamus, choroid plexus, occipital lobe, and medial temporal lobe	Contralateral visual field deficit, color blindness, impaired depth perception, occasional sparing of central vision, memory loss, sensory loss, nystagmus, pupillary abnormalities, ataxia
Vertebral artery	Medulla and/or cerebellum	Face, nose, or eye ipsilateral numbness with contralateral body numbness, facial weakness, vertigo, ataxia, nystagmus, dysphagia, dysarthria
Basilar artery	Pons, midbrain, and/or cerebellum	Quadriplegia or hemiplegia/paresis, locked-in syndrome (pons), dysarthria, dysphagia, ataxia, nystagmus, vertigo, coma

ASSESSMENT

Each stroke type has a unique presentation based on the pathophysiology and location of the event. A complete and ongoing physical examination is crucial during the initial phase of stroke to detect further deterioration.

T A B L E 6 - 7   Hemorrhagic locations and syndromes

Area	Syndrome
Putamen	Contralateral hemiplegia, hemisensory loss, hemianopia, slurred speech
Thalamic	Contralateral hemiplegia; hemisensory loss; small, poorly reactive pupils; decreased LOC
Pontine	Locked-in syndrome (awake, aware, unable to verbally communicate, quadriplegia), coma
Cerebellar	Occipital headache, ataxia, dizziness, headache, nausea, vomiting
Lobar	Mimics cerebral infarct (e.g., contralateral motor and sensory signs)

HISTORY AND RISK FACTORS Hypertension, smoking, aging, and previous history of transischemic attack (TIA)/stroke are the strongest risk factors. Risk factors for stroke are classified according to those that can be changed and those that cannot be changed. Risk factors that cannot be changed are age ($>$55 yr); race (risk for African Americans is twice that of whites); gender (risk for males is twice that of females); previous history of stroke, TIA, and AMI (increases risk $\times$10); and family history of stroke or AMI. Risk factors that can be changed include hypertension, heart disease, diabetes mellitus, obesity, hypercholesterolemia, sedentary life-style, and smoking.

Cardiac disease is the most common cause of cerebral embolism. Cardiac dysrhythmias predisposing to embolic strokes include atrial fibrillation and sick sinus syndrome. Dilated cardiac myopathy, ventricular thrombus after AMI, and valvular disease are additional causes of cardioembolic stroke. Thrombotic strokes usually are caused by local atherosclerosis of large vessels (e.g., internal cerebral artery [ICA] or middle cerebral artery [MCA]) related to occlusion of small perforating vessels (lacunar infarction).

For acute cerebral infarct/intracerebral hemorrhage

CLINICAL PRESENTATION Individuals with ischemic strokes caused by MCA occlusion in the dominant hemisphere usually are awake with hemiparesis, aphasia, visual field cut, and sensory loss. Individuals with ACI usually do not experience pain other than a headache, nor do they have altered LOC unless the stroke causes mass effects as a result of swelling or involves the brainstem or thalamic regions bilaterally. Individuals with acute hemispheric infarction have elevated arterial BP and often appear drowsy even in the absence of swelling. While both thrombotic and embolic strokes can begin abruptly, the former are more likely to evolve over several hours and may fluctuate over several hours or days. In contrast, the deficit caused by embolic strokes usually is maximal at onset and often occurs during activity.

For intracranial hematoma

CLINICAL PRESENTATION Dependent on the size and location of the hematoma. For example, a relatively small hemorrhage into the brainstem may produce quadriplegia and coma, whereas a hematoma of similar size in the basal ganglia may produce hemiparesis without altered LOC. Generally, the larger the hematoma (as measured by CT scan), the worse the prognosis.

Neurologic findings with ICH are similar to those with ACI. However, individuals with ICH are more likely to have altered LOC, vomiting, headache, very high BP, and IICP. Furthermore, the neurologic deficit may evolve over minutes to a few hours, requiring intubation and ICP monitoring. Neurosurgical consultation is often necessary.

For both stroke types

PHYSICAL ASSESSMENT The Glasgow Coma Scale (Appendix 3) is often used to evaluate patients with stroke in critical care. Since this scale primarily measures LOC, it should not be the only measure of neurologic function. The NIH stroke scale (Table 6-8) provides a better measurement of deficits and is quick and easy to use. It also guides the examiner in evaluating cognitive, language, and motor deficits that are unique to stroke. Comprehensive neurologic assessment assists the critical care nurse in detecting declines in neurologic status and responses to interventions.

COMPLICATIONS The most serious are those that affect the central nervous system (CNS) and cardiopulmonary systems.

CNS: IICP associated with extension of the infarct or hematoma and its associated edema, which may cause midline shift and herniation; IICP associated with hydrocephalus following ICH; and seizures, which occur most commonly within the first 24 h but may present at any time.

Cardiopulmonary: ECG changes, including QT prolongation, ST-segment depression, T-wave inversion, and U waves. Ventricular ectopy is also common. Dysrhythmias are not always associated with underlying heart disease. Cardiac dysrhythmias following stroke may be caused by release of catecholaminergic neurotransmitters into the systemic circulation, causing both hypertension and cardiac muscle damage. Individuals with new ECG changes have a less favorable prognosis. ECG monitoring for the first 24-72 h is recommended, along with evaluation of CPK-MB isoenzymes.

The most common causes of death within the first month after stroke are MI, pneumonia, and sepsis. Other complications include pulmonary embolism, deep vein thrombosis, skin breakdown, and depression. Neurogenic pulmonary edema is rare and more commonly occurs with traumatic head injury.

DIAGNOSTIC TESTS

CT scan: Performed within the first 24 h, primarily as a method of differentiating ischemic from hemorrhagic stroke. It is often normal with ACI during the first 24 h. ICH is always seen on CT scan.

MRI and magnetic resonance arteriogram (MRA): Noninvasive tests that provide detailed information regarding the area of injury or its vascular supply.

T A B L E 6 - 8 **National Institutes of Health stroke scale**

		Baseline	30 min	1 h	2 h	24 h	48 h	7-10 days
1.a. Level of consciousness	Alert 0 Drowsy 1 Stuporous 2 Coma 3							
1.b. LOC questions	Answers both correctly 0 Answers one correctly 1 Incorrect 2							
1.c. LOC commands	Obeys both correctly 0 Obeys one correctly 1 Incorrect 2							
2. Best gaze	Normal 0 Partial gaze palsy 1 Forced deviation 2							
3. Best visual	No visual loss 0 Partial hemianopia 1 Complete hemianopia 2 Bilateral hemianopia 3							
4. Facial palsy	Normal 0 Minor 1 Partial 2 Complete 3							

Continued

T A B L E 6 - 8 National Institutes of Health stroke scale—cont'd

		Baseline	30 min	1 h	2 h	24 h	48 h	7-10 days
5. Best motor arm	No drift — 0 Drift — 1 Can't resist gravity — 2 No effort against gravity — 3 No movement — 4							
6. Other arm	For brainstem stroke — 0-4 (Use same scale as above)							
7. Best motor leg	No drift — 0 Drift — 1 Can't resist gravity — 2 No effort against gravity — 3 No movement — 4							
8. Other leg	For brainstem stroke — 0-4 (Use same scale as above)							
9. Limb ataxia	Absent — 0 Present in upper or lower — 1 Present in both — 2							
10. Sensory	Normal — 0 Partial loss — 1 Dense loss — 2							

11. Neglect	No neglect Partial neglect Complete neglect	0 1 2					
12. Dysarthria	Normal articulation Mild to moderate dysarthria Near unintelligible or worse	0 1 2					
13. Best language	No aphasia Mild to moderate aphasia Severe aphasia Mute	0 1 2 3					
14. Change from previous examination	Same Better Worse	S B W					
15. Change from baseline	Same Better Worse	S B W					

From the National High Blood Pressure Education Program, National Institutes of Health, and National Heart, Lung, and Blood Institute: NIH Pub No 93-1088, January 1993.

Doppler studies: Include transthoracic echocardiogram to evaluate heart structure and function; transesophageal echocardiogram and carotid Doppler or duplex to evaluate blood flow and presence or degree of stenosis in the extracranial carotid arteries; and transcranial Doppler to evaluate the intracranial vessels and give information on the velocity of blood flow in the anterior and posterior cerebral circulation. The latter is also used for evaluating vasospasm, determining brain death *via* detection of cerebral circulatory arrest, intraoperative monitoring, and locating emboli.

Cerebral angiography: Invasive procedure used to visualize the cerebral blood vessels. It provides more specific information on the cause of stroke by identifying the blood vessel involved. In clinical trials, cerebral angiography is being used in conjunction with thrombolytics in patients with ACI to identify the site of acute vessel occlusion, with subsequent injection of a thrombolytic agent to dissolve the clot and restore blood flow to the brain. Cerebral angioplasty is also being investigated.

Laboratory studies: Hematology, chemistry, and coagulation profiles as well as evaluations for syphilis (e.g., *via* VDRL, RPR, FTA), sedimentation rate to assess for infection or vasculitis, and drug screen (e.g., cocaine, amphetamine).

Less common laboratory tests may include determinations of lupus anticoagulant, anticardiolipin antibody, and hemoglobin electrophoresis (to assess presence of sickle cell disease). In addition, a hypercoagulable profile may be performed to evaluate levels of proteins C and S. These proteins often are deficient in the young (<45 yr) stroke patient, who may have no other risk factors for stroke.

Positron emission tomography (PET) and single photon emission computed tomography (SPECT):   To evaluate brain metabolism and blood flow. These tests are performed more commonly in clinical trials in university settings.

Lumbar puncture (LP):   To measure cerebral spinal fluid (CSF) pressures and obtain CSF specimen when infection such as meningitis or neurosyphilis is suspected. It also may be performed when SAH is suspected and CT scan is normal.

EEG: Although not routinely done, it may show slowing or low voltage over the infarct except in lacunar infarcts, where results are usually normal.

COLLABORATIVE MANAGEMENT

Goals of management are to prevent secondary neurologic damage, prevent secondary complications, and promote optimal functional outcome. Early detection *via* accurate neurologic examination and immediate medical or surgical intervention helps prevent stroke extension, increased brain edema, and hydrocephalus. Medical and nursing interventions are guided by the findings derived from the physical examination.

Prevention of stroke extension: Dependent on adequate perfusion of the penumbra, which is the ischemic brain tissue surrounding the initial infarct that is at immediate risk of infarction. Perfusing the penumbra decreases the potential infarct size and optimizes patient outcome. Controlling arterial BP is essential in limiting the infarct size.

BP control is achieved by close monitoring and use of potent vasoactive medications. A "normal" BP may be too low, causing further ischemia and infarct by decreasing cerebral perfusion. Arterial BP should not be lowered abruptly in patients with ACI. At times, maintenance of a somewhat elevated BP may be warranted depending on the underlying vascular and brain pathology. In contrast, with ICH many practitioners believe that an elevated BP should be reduced aggressively. The best approach is unclear, and therefore the treatment of increased BP in ICH necessitates individual consideration.

ICP monitoring and cerebral perfusion pressure (CPP) management: Necessary for patients with increased infarct size, increased edema, and hydrocephalus. Patients with IICP may receive mannitol, which draws water osmotically from healthy brain cells. Careful monitoring of ICP for rebound effect is necessary following mannitol infusion. Serum osmolality needs to be monitored to prevent excessive dehydration. Patients with hydrocephalus often require a ventriculostomy. For more information about ICP monitoring and CPP management, see "Craniocerebral Trauma," p. 131.

Optimizing regulatory functions: To prevent secondary complications (Table 6-9). In general, patients with ischemic strokes should be positioned with the HOB flat to increase cerebral perfusion. HOB should be elevated for patients with hemorrhagic strokes to decrease ICP. Patient response determines the best position.

Rehabilitation: Should begin immediately. Consults to physiatrist, physical therapist, occupational therapist, and speech therapist should be made within the first 24 h.

Pharmacotherapy: No widely accepted regimen for acute stroke. While thrombolytic and neuroprotective agents hold great promise, they remain experimental. At present, pharmacotherapy is aimed at prevention of secondary neurologic damage and recurrent stroke.

Anticoagulation: IV heparin may be indicated for patients with progressing stroke or unstable signs and symptoms of stroke, such as trans-ischemic attacks (TIAs), and for cardioembolic stroke. If long-term anticoagulation is planned, the patient is converted to oral warfarin (Coumadin) therapy.

Antiplatelet therapy: To reduce risk of stroke and decrease frequency of TIAs. The most used agent is aspirin, 30 mg to 1,300 mg daily. Ticlopidine (Ticlid), a new antiplatelet agent, shows an overall risk reduction of nearly 25% for fatal and nonfatal strokes when compared to aspirin (Pryse-Phillips, 1993). A third antiplatelet agent, clopidogrel, is currently being tested for patients at risk for ischemic events (myocardial, cerebrovascular, and peripheral vascular).

Antihypertensives: Frequently used in the stroke population for control and maintenance of optimal BP. Various agents are used, based on the individual's medical history. Long-term therapy is based on the National Heart, Lung, and Blood Institute (NHLBI) algorithm (Figure 6-2). In the acute phase, systolic BP is often elevated and requires careful management. Vasoactive IV medications such as sodium nitroprusside (Nipride) or labetalol (Normodyne) are often used. Hypotension is a concern, especially in the patient with IICP, because with hypotension MAP is decreased. If MAP is decreased in the presence of a normal or elevated ICP, a decrease in CPP results, further compromis-

T A B L E 6 - 9   Maintenance of normal regulatory functions in stroke

Function	Intervention/goal	Rationale
Temperature	Normothermia	To decrease metabolic demands and ICP
Respiratory	O_2, positioning, respiratory therapy	To optimize O_2 delivery to the brain and prevent atelectasis and pneumonia
Cardiac	Monitor dysrhythmias, fluid, electrolytes	To optimize CO to promote perfusion to the brain
GI	H_2-blockers, bowel program	To prevent stress ulcers, constipation
Nutrition	NPO, enteral, long-term diet	NPO to prevent aspiration; diet to promote healing, meet caloric needs; long-term diet: low Na^+, low-fat, weight reduction if needed
GU	Bladder training ASAP	To prevent unnecessary use of Foley catheter, prevent UTI, and avoid embarrassment and possible retention
Musculoskeletal	ROM, positioning, increasing activity as tolerated, sequential compression stockings, mobility beds	To promote proper alignment and prevent contractures and complications of immobility
Skin	Keep clean and dry, pressure relief	To prevent skin breakdown and dependent edema
Communication	Develop appropriate communication techniques; swallow study within 24 h	To prevent aspiration and promote meeting of patient's needs

ing neurologic status. Dopamine or dobutamine may be titrated to keep MAP high enough to maintain CPP >60 mm Hg.

Anticonvulsant therapy: Used for seizures in the acute phase. Generally the patient is given a loading dose of phenytoin (Dilantin) followed by a maintenance dose. Lorazepam (Ativan) or diazepam (Valium) may be used initially, especially if the patient is in status epilepticus (see p. 464).

Sedation: May be necessary for ensuring sleep. A thorough neurologic evaluation to rule out organic causes is indicated for patients who are agitated. Sedation also may be indicated as adjunctive therapy for patients with IICP. Drugs of choice include midazolam (Versed), fentanyl (Sublimaze), or morphine sulfate. Pentobarbitol coma is occasionally used for patients who experience high ICP that does not respond to other forms of therapy.

Life-style modification: diet, exercise, smoking cessation

Inadequate response

↓

Continue life-style modification, add diuretics or beta blockers
(ACE inhibitors, calcium antagonists, alpha$_1$-receptor
blockers, and alpha-beta blockers have not been tested or
shown to reduce morbidity and mortality)

Inadequate response

↓

Increase dosage *or* substitute drug *or* add a second agent

Inadequate response

↓

Add second or third agent and/or diuretic if not already prescribed

Figure 6-2:   The National Heart, Lung, and Blood Institute treatment algorithm for stroke. (From the National High Blood Pressure Education Program, National Institutes of Health, and National Heart, Lung, and Blood Institute: NIH Pub No 93-1088, January 1993.)

Triple H therapy: Hemodilution, hypertension, and hypervolemia are used in some institutions for patients with vasospasm following SAH to improve cerebral perfusion. See "Cerebral Aneurysm and Subarachnoid Hemorrhage," p. 453.
Carotid endarterectomy: Surgical removal of plaque in the obstructed carotid artery to promote blood supply to the brain, which is considered choice treatment for patients with >70% carotid stenosis.
Craniotomy: May be performed for evacuation of a hematoma or for a young ACI patient who has uncontrollable IICP due to massive edema. When this occurs, a craniectomy with a dural incision or temporal lobectomy is considered. In some institutions hematoma evacuation is performed by aspiration through a burr hole.

NURSING DIAGNOSES AND INTERVENTIONS

Decreased adaptive capacity: Intracranial, related to interrupted blood flow secondary to thrombus, embolus, or hemorrhage
Desired outcome: Within 72 h of this diagnosis (or optimally on an ongoing basis), patient has adequate cerebral tissue perfusion as evidenced by no decrease in LOC per NIH stroke scale; no evidence of

deterioration in motor function on the affected side; and no evidence of new or further deterioration of language, cognition, or visual field.

- Assess for neurologic changes qh in the acute phase. Use the NIH stroke scale (see Table 6-8) to record and monitor neurologic changes following stroke.

- If the patient has an ICP monitor, maintain ICP <15 mm Hg and CPP >60 mm Hg. To calculate CPP, see p. 455.

- Position patient to maintain adequate cerebral perfusion. To ensure venous return, avoid extreme rotation or lateral flexion of the neck. Avoid extreme hip flexion to prevent increased intraabdominal pressure, which could result in IICP. When positioning patient from side to side, monitor tolerance to the position change. Keep HOB flat for patients with ischemic infarcts and HOB elevated for those with hemorrhagic infarcts. Bear in mind that each patient will have an individual response to positioning.

- Maintain adequate pulmonary status *via* patent airway, adequate oxygenation (Pao_2 ≥80 mm Hg and O_2 saturation >90%), turning patient as tolerated, and suctioning as needed. Assess breath sounds frequently. Avoid activities or conditions that can increase ICP, including excessive coughing, pulmonary congestion, hypercapnia, and hypoxia.

- Maintain adequate systolic blood pressure (SBP). SBP should not be aggressively reduced. Higher pressures (180-140 mm Hg) are necessary to perfuse the penumbra or area of the brain at risk of infarction. Titration of medications will depend on the patient's individual response.

- Medicate for sedation as prescribed. Monitor patient's response, including the effects of sedation and resulting changes in ICP.

Impaired physical mobility related to decreased motor function of the upper and/or lower extremities and trunk following stroke

Desired outcome: At the time of discharge from ICU, patient exhibits no evidence of complications of immobility such as skin breakdown, contracture formation, pneumonia, or constipation.

- Turn and position patient frequently, as tolerated. See "Wound and Skin Care," Chapter 1, for guidelines to prevent skin breakdown.

- Transfer patient toward unaffected side.

- Teach patient methods for turning and moving using the stronger extremity to move the weaker extremity.

- Position weaker extremities when turning patient to avoid contracture formation, frozen shoulder, or foot drop. See **Risk for disuse syndrome,** p. 80, in "Prolonged Immobility" for guidelines.

- Begin passive ROM within the first 24 h of admission. See **Activity intolerance,** p. 78, in "Prolonged Immobility" for guidelines.

- Obtain PT and OT referral as soon as possible to establish appropriate therapy.

- Have patient cough and deep breathe at scheduled intervals. See "Pneumonia," p. 235, for care of patients at risk for this disorder. Provide percussion and postural drainage for patients for whom coughing and deep breathing are ineffective for mobilizing secretions.

- See **Constipation,** in "Prolonged Immobility," p. 85, and in "Cerebral Aneurysm and Subarachnoid Hemorrhage," p. 458, to treat this condition.

Impaired verbal communication related to aphasia secondary to cerebrovascular insult

Desired outcome: At a minimum of the 24-h period before discharge from ICU, patient demonstrates improved self-expression and relates decreased frustration with communication.

Note: Aphasia is the partial or complete inability to use or comprehend language and symbols and may occur with dominant (left) hemisphere damage. It is not the result of impaired hearing or intelligence. There are many different types of aphasia. *Receptive aphasia* (e.g., Wernicke's, sensory) is characterized by inability to recognize or comprehend spoken words. The patient often is good at responding to nonverbal cues. *Expressive aphasia* (e.g., Broca's, motor) is characterized by difficulty expressing words or naming objects. Gestures, groans, swearing, or nonsense words may be used. Use of a picture or word board may be helpful. Generally the patient has a combination of aphasia types that may vary in severity.

- Evaluate the nature and severity of the patient's aphasia. When doing so, avoid giving nonverbal cues. Assess patient's ability to point or look toward a specific object, follow simple directions, understand yes/no questions, understand complex questions, repeat both simple and complex words, repeat sentences, name objects that are shown, demonstrate or relate the purpose or action of the object, fulfill written requests, write requests, and read. When evaluating patient for aphasia, be aware that patient may be responding to nonverbal cues and may understand less than you think. Document this assessment with simple descriptions and specific examples of the patient's aphasia symptoms. Use it as the basis for a communication plan.

Caution: During your assessment, be alert to dysarthria, a "red flag" that the patient is at risk for aspiration due to ineffective swallowing and gag reflexes. Perform an assessment of the patient's ability to swallow if the muscles of the face, tongue, and gag reflex are involved.

- Obtain a referral to a speech therapist or pathologist as soon as possible for initiation of appropriate therapy. Provide therapist with a list of words that would enhance patient's independence and/or care. In addition, ask for tips that will help improve communication with patient.
- When communicating with the patient, try to reduce distractions in the environment, such as television or others' conversation. Because fatigue affects a person's ability to communicate, try to ensure that patient is well rested.
- Communicate with patient as much as possible. General principles for patients who may not recognize or comprehend the spoken word include: face patient and establish eye contact; speak slowly and clearly; give patient time to process your communication and answer; keep messages short and simple; stay with one clearly defined subject; avoid questions with multiple choices, but rather phrase questions so that they can be answered "yes" or "no"; and use the same words each time you repeat a statement or question (e.g., pill

versus medication, bathroom versus toilet). If patient does not understand after repetition, try different words. Use gestures, facial expressions, and pantomime to supplement and reinforce your message. Give short, simple directions, and repeat as needed to ensure understanding. Use concrete terms (e.g., "water" instead of "fluid," "leg" instead of "limb").

- When helping patients regain use of symbolic language, start with nouns first, and progress to more complex statement as indicated, using verbs, pronouns, and adjectives. For continuity, keep a record at the bedside of words to be used (e.g., "pill" rather than "medication").
- Treat patient as an adult. It is not necessary to raise the volume of your voice unless the patient is hard of hearing. Be respectful.
- When patients have difficulty expressing words or naming objects, encourage them to repeat words after you for practice in verbal expression. Begin with simple words like "yes" or "no" and progress to others like "cup." Progress to more complex statements as indicated. Listen and respond to patient's communication efforts; otherwise patient may give up. Praise accomplishments. Be prepared for labile emotions, because these patients become frustrated and emotional when faced with their impaired speech.
- When improvement is noted, let patient complete your sentence (e.g., "This is a ___"). Keep a list of words patient can say, and add to the list as appropriate. Use this list when forming questions patient can answer. Avoid finishing patient's sentences.
- Patients who have lost the ability to monitor their verbal output may not produce sensible language but may think they are making sense and not understand why others do not comprehend or respond appropriately to them. Avoid labeling patient "belligerent" or "confused" when the problem is aphasia and frustration. Listen for errors in conversation, and provide feedback.
- Patients who have lost the ability to recognize number symbols or relationships will have difficulty understanding time concept or telling time. Avoid instructing patient to "wait 5 minutes," because this may not be meaningful.
- Give practice in receiving word images by pointing to an object and clearly stating its name. Watch signals patient gives you.
- Patients with nondominant (right) hemisphere damage often have no difficulty speaking; however, they may use excessive detail, give irrelevant information, and get off on a tangent. Bring patient back to the subject by saying "Let's go back to what we were talking about."
- Provide a supportive and relaxed environment for those patients who are unable to form words or sentences or speak clearly or appropriately. If patient makes an error, do not criticize patient's effort but rather compliment it by saying "That was a good try." Do not react negatively to patient's emotional displays. Address and acknowledge patient's frustration over the inability to communicate. Maintain a calm and positive attitude. If you do not understand the patient, say so. Ask patient to repeat unclear words, ask for more clues, ask patient to use another word, or have patient point to the object. Observe for nonverbal cues, and anticipate patient's needs. Allow time

to listen if patient speaks slowly. To validate patient's message, repeat or rephrase it aloud.
- Ensure that call light is available and the patient knows how to use it.

ADDITIONAL NURSING DIAGNOSES

Also see nursing diagnoses and interventions in "Nutritional Support," "Prolonged Immobility," "Psychosocial Support," and "Psychosocial Support for the Patient's Family and Significant Others." See "Craniocerebral Trauma" for **Risk for infection,** p. 136.

Meningitis

PATHOPHYSIOLOGY

Meningitis is an inflammation of the brain and spinal cord (the central nervous system [CNS]), which involves the meninges (dura, arachnoid, and pia), invades the brain surface, and damages the cranial nerves. There are several types of meningitis, broadly classified as bacterial (pyogenic), tuberculous, fungal, and aseptic. The first three are discussed here.

Bacterial meningitis: The most common form, it can be associated with a previous or ongoing infection, injury such as open/penetrating skull fracture, basilar and facial skull fracture, shunt occlusion/malfunction, craniotomy, otitis media, sinusitis, and bacteremia (e.g., endocarditis, pneumonia).

Streptococcus pneumoniae (S. pneumoniae), a gram-positive coccus, is the leading cause of adult meningitis in the United States. Pneumococcal meningitis is prevalent in crowded conditions and is spread seasonally (late fall and winter). It follows a recent nasopharyngeal colonization of a virulent pneumococcal strain or upper respiratory tract infection (URI), is seen in the presence of pneumococcal disease, is a complication of conditions associated with CSF leaks, and is more prevalent in immunocompromised persons.

Neisseria meningitidis (N. meningitidis), a gram-negative coccus, is the second leading cause of meningitis in adults. Infection is more likely to occur in patients with complement component deficiencies (e.g., congenital or associated with nephrotic syndrome, hepatic failure, systemic lupus erythematosus, and multiple myeloma).

Haemophilus influenzae (H. influenzae), the most common cause in children, sometimes affects adults as well. Predisposing factors include URIs, hypogammaglobulinemia, diabetes mellitus, alcoholism, asplenia, and head trauma.

Listeria monocytogenes (L. monocytogenes), a gram-positive rod, is being recognized more frequently as a cause of meningitis, especially in immunocompromised patients. Outbreaks have been associated with consumption of contaminated dairy products, including milk and cheese.

Gram-negative species: Escherichia coli, Klebsiella, Proteus, and *Pseudomonas spp.* are gaining increasing importance, especially in the elderly, in the immunocompromised, and in head-injured patients.

Borrelia burgdorferi (B. burgdorferi), the tick-borne spirochete identified as the causative agent in Lyme disease, also has been found to cause meningitis. The disease peaks in late summer and early fall, with highest prevalence in the northeastern United States.

Tuberculous meningitis: *Mycobacterium tuberculosis* infection tends to occur in children where tuberculous presence is high and in elders where tuberculous presence is low. It is difficult to detect on smear or to recover by culture.

Fungal meningitis: The most common fungal infection of the CNS is caused by *Cryptococcus neoformans (C. neoformans),* an opportunistic infection seen in AIDS, with less common infections resulting from other fungi. *C. neoformans* is associated with pigeon excreta and is most likely acquired by inhalation. Most infections occur in individuals with cell-mediated immunity, including corticosteroid therapy, hematologic malignancies, organ transplantation, sarcoidosis, and AIDS.

ASSESSMENT

HISTORY AND RISK FACTORS Should include the time symptoms developed, report of traumatic injury, exposures to disease or organisms, and recent surgical procedures.

CLINICAL PRESENTATION

Streptococcus pneumoniae: The classic presentation is fever, headache, meningismus, and altered mental status that progresses quickly to coma. Nuchal rigidity and Kernig's or Brudzinski's sign are present. Nausea, vomiting, profuse sweats, weakness, myalgia, seizures, and cranial nerve palsies also may be present.

Neisseria meningitidis: Fever, early macular erythematous rash progressing rapidly to petechial and purpuric states, conjunctival petechiae, and aggressive behavior are typical clinical findings. Dysfunctions of cranial nerves VI, VII, and VIII (see Appendix 4) and aphasia, ventriculitis, subdural empyema, cerebral venous thrombosis, and DIC also may occur.

Haemophilus influenzae: The most distinguishing sign is early development of deafness, which can occur within 24-36 h after onset. A morbilliform or petechial rash may be present. Complications include sterile subdural effusions and thrombosis of cerebral veins.

Listeria monocytogenes: Seizures and focal deficits such as ataxia, cranial nerve palsies, and nystagmus are seen early in the course of infection.

Gram-negative species: In elders, fever may be absent or low-grade and headache may not be reported. Meningeal signs may be subtle, but confusion, severe mental changes, and pneumonia commonly are reported. Nuchal rigidity in elders must be differentiated from degenerative changes of the cervical spine.

Borrelia burgdorferi: The clinical presentation of Lyme disease occurs in stages and is heralded by a "bull's eye" rash (erythema migrans) that develops within a few days of the tick bite. During stage one, headache, stiff neck, lethargy, irritability, and changes in mental status, especially memory loss, are observed. Stage two occurs over weeks and months following the tick bite and is characterized by persistent headache, nausea, vomiting, malaise, irritability, cranial nerve deficits, mental status changes, peripheral neuropathies, and myalgias. Arthritic-type symptoms and brain parenchymal changes are observed in the third stage of the disease.

Mycobacterium tuberculosis: Has a slow, chronic course, unlike most bacterial causes of meningitis. Because of the slow onset, neurologic damage may be present even before treatment is sought. Headache, lethargy, confusion, nuchal rigidity, cranial nerve abnormalities, SIADH, weight loss, and night sweats occur. Kernig's and Brudzinski's signs are present, but the chest x-ray may be clear, and purified protein derivative (PPD) may be nonreactive. Residual effects include seizures, mental disturbances, visual disturbances, deafness, and hemiparesis.

Cryptococcus neoformans: Typical symptoms of meningitis occur, but since the infection is subacute, fever and headache may have a subtle pattern lasting weeks. Positive meningeal signs (Table 6-10); alterations in mental status (e.g., hyperactivity, bizarre behavior, emotional lability, and poor judgment); and photophobia may be reported. Seizures are uncommon, but focal neurologic deficits such as cranial nerve III and IV dysfunction, nausea, and vomiting may occur.

PHYSICAL ASSESSMENT   A complete neurologic examination should be performed to establish patient's baseline neurologic function. One or more tests for meningitis usually are positive (see Table 6-10).

DIAGNOSTIC TESTS

CSF analysis: The single most important laboratory test for diagnosing meningitis; CSF is obtained through intraventricular catheter, ventriculostomy and reservoir *via* high cisternal or cervical approach, and lumbar puncture (LP). An LP should not be performed if there is a history of head injury, focal neurologic deficits are present, or papilledema is visualized on funduscopic examination, inasmuch as these signs are associated with IICP (see Table 6-3). Antibiotic therapy should not be delayed if CSF samples cannot be obtained. The CSF is analyzed for cell count with white cell differential, glucose, protein,

---

T A B L E   6 - 1 0   **Positive meningeal signs**

Test/description	Positive findings
Stiff neck sign (nuchal rigidity): Raise patient's head by flexing the neck and attempting to make the patient's chin touch the sternum.	Pain and resistance to neck motion.
Brudzinski's sign: Assess for nuchal rigidity.	Flexion of the hips and knees when the examiner flexes the patient's neck.
Kernig's sign: Flex the patient's leg at the knee and hip when the patient is supine, and then attempt to straighten the leg.	Pain in the lower back and resistance to straightening the leg.

T A B L E   6 - 1 1   **Meningitis: typical CSF finding**

Findings	White cell count	Glucose	Protein
Normal	0-5/mm^3 lymphocytes	40-80 mg/dl	15-50 mg/dl
Bacterial	Predominantly polycytes: 1,000-10,000	<40 mg/dl	100-500 mg/dl
Viral	Predominantly lymphocytes (may see polycytes initially)	Normal	Slightly elevated
Tuberculous	Elevated lymphocytes: 100-400; lymphocyte elevation minimal or absent in immunocompromised patients	<40 mg/dl or 50% of blood sugar drawn simultaneously	100-500 mg/dl; may increase gradually with progression of disease
Fungal	Predominantly elevated lymphocytes	Slightly decreased	Elevated
Lyme disease	Mildly elevated lymphocytes	Normal	Mildly elevated
Aseptic (nonbacterial)	Elevated lymphocytes	Normal	50-100 mg/dl

Gram's stain, acid-fast stain, culture, and sensitivity. See Table 6-11. Other tests of the CSF include:

Counterimmunoelectrophoresis (CIE):   Detects bacterial antigens in the CSF.

Latex agglutination: Detects microbial antigens in the CSF.

Limulus lysate assay: May confirm bacterial infection (gram-negative organisms) even when cultures and Gram's stains are negative.

Enzyme-linked immunosorbent assay (ELISA):   To detect mycobacterial antigens or antimycobacterial antibodies in CSF.

Blood, urine, and sputum cultures: Help identify the infecting organisms.

Serum WBC count: Assesses for presence of infection.

CT scan with contrast and MRI: To rule out hydrocephalus and detect exudate, abscesses, and intracranial pathology, including tumors.

COLLABORATIVE MANAGEMENT

Rapid sterilization of the CSF *via* appropriate pharmacologic therapy (Table 6-12):   Prophylaxis, using appropriate drug therapy for individuals exposed to *N. meningitidis* (rifampin or spiramycin) or *H. influenzae* meningitis, is recommended.

T A B L E   6 - 1 2   **Common drug therapy for the management**
of meningitis

Organism	Treatment choice
Bacterial	
S. pneumoniae (age >50 yr)	cefotaxime or ceftriaxone + dexamethasone, ampicillin (alternative)
	penicillin G (gram positive)
	Alternate: choramphenicol + trimethoprim/sulfamethoxazole (TMP/SMX)
N. meningitidis	cefotaxime or ceftriaxone or penicillin G or ampicillin + dexamethasone
H. influenzae	ampicillin (beta-lactamase negative)
	cefotaxime or ceftriaxone (beta-lactamase positive)
L. monocytogenes	cefotaxime or ceftriaxone or penicillin or ampicillin + dexamethasone
S. aureus	nafcillin or oxacillin (if methicillin resistant, use vancomycin)
Gram-negative species	dependent on identified organism
B. burdorferi	ceftriaxone or penicillin G (alternate)
M. tuberculosis	isoniazid, rifampin, ethambutol, and pyrazinamide
Fungal	
C. neoformans	fluconazole
	amphotericin B with or without flucytosine (alternate)
Aseptic	
Enterovirus	symptomatic treatment
Mumps	symptomatic treatment

Modified from Wispelwey B, Trunkel A, Scheld M: Bacterial meningitis in adults, _Infect Dis Clin North Am_ 4:645-659, 1990.

Adjunctive pharmacologic therapies: Dexamethasone is believed to decrease SAS inflammation by reducing cytokines produced by bacterial products; however, its use is controversial. If given, dexamethasone should be administered 15-20 min before antimicrobial medications and for 4 days. Monoclonal antibodies also have been investigated as therapy because of their ability to decrease inflammation by deactivating bacterial cell surface components and cytokines produced from leukocyte activation.

Nutritional support: Patients who are able should continue oral feeding along with IV therapy. Enteral feeding may be initiated. Parenteral nutrition should be initiated if enteral feeding is contraindicated or not tolerated by the patient.

Anticonvulsant therapy: Initiated if seizures are observed or may be administered prophylactically. Seizures increase the metabolic rate, requiring an increase in cerebral blood flow, which may be detrimental in meningitis associated with cerebral edema and intracranial hypertension.

Maintenance of normothermia: Reduces the risks (increased cerebral blood flow and intracranial pressure) associated with increased metabolic rate. Fever should be controlled by antipyretics such as acetaminophen or use of other cooling measures such as tepid baths or hypothermia treatments.

Infection prevention: According to hospital and CDC guidelines. For droplet contact meningeal microorganisms (e.g., *M. tuberculosis*), Transmission-based Precautions: Droplet can be initiated until effectiveness of antimicrobial treatment is established. See "Infection Prevention and Control," Appendix 8.

Rehabilitation consults: Include PT, OT, and speech and should be initiated as soon as patient is stable to minimize physical and cognitive complications.

Evaluation of need for support services: For patient and significant others, including home health care, support groups, and social services.

NURSING DIAGNOSES AND INTERVENTIONS

Decreased adaptive capacity: Intracranial, related to compromised fluid dynamic mechanisms secondary to brain and spinal cord inflammation

Desired outcomes: Within 72 h of initiation of antimicrobial therapy, patient's ICP returns to normal range as evidenced by orientation to time, place, and person; bilaterally equal and normoreactive pupils; bilaterally equal strength and tone of extremities; absence of cranial nerve palsies; RR 12-20 breaths/min with normal depth and pattern (eupnea); HR 60-100 bpm; BP within patient's normal range; and absence of headache, vomiting, papilledema, and other clinical indicators of IICP. Following instruction, patient verbalizes knowledge of the importance of avoiding Valsalva-like activities.

- Assess neurologic status at least hourly. Monitor pupils, LOC, and motor activity; and perform cranial nerve assessments (see Appendix 4). A decrease in consciousness is an early indicator of IICP and impending herniation. Changes in pupillary size and reaction, a decrease in motor function (i.e., hemiplegia, abnormal posturing), and cranial nerve palsies also may be signs of impending herniation.
- Monitor patient for physical indicators of IICP (see Table 6-3).
- Monitor VS at frequent intervals. Be alert to changes in respiratory pattern, fluctuations in BP and pulse, widening pulse pressure, and slow HR.
- Optimize cerebral perfusion by maintaining a patent airway and delivering oxygen as prescribed. Be sure patient's neck is free of constricting objects such as tracheostomy ties and oxygen tubing.
- Avoid overhydration, which would add to cerebral edema, by ensuring precise delivery of IV fluids at consistent, prescribed rates.
- Ensure timely delivery of medications that are prescribed for the prevention of sudden increases or decreases in BP, HR, or RR.

- Teach patient the importance of avoiding activities that increase ICP: coughing, straining, bending over.
- If patient shows evidence of IICP, implement measures to decrease ICP (see Table 2-5, p. 137).

Pain related to headache, photophobia, and fever secondary to meningeal irritation

Desired outcome: Within 2 h of initiation of therapy, patient's subjective evaluation of discomfort improves, as documented by a pain scale.

- Monitor patient for the presence of pain and discomfort. Devise a pain scale with patient, rating discomfort from 0 (no pain) to 10.
- Monitor temperature q2h and prn. Administer tepid baths or cooling blanket and prescribed antipyretics/antibiotics to keep temperature within prescribed limits.
- Maintain a quiet environment for patient. Overstimulation may increase BP, which can aggravate patient's headache.
- Cluster patient care so that it is administered within a pattern that allows for uninterrupted periods (at least 90 min) of rest.
- Organize visiting hours so that patient can have uninterrupted periods of rest.
- Darken patient's room to minimize the discomfort of photophobia. Provide blindfolds if darkening the room is not possible.
- Administer analgesics as prescribed. Use the pain scale to document the degree of relief obtained.
- See Chapter 1, p. 74, for other pain interventions.

Risk for infection related to potential for cross-contamination secondary to communicable nature of bacterial and aseptic meningitis

Desired outcome: Other patients, staff members, and patient's significant others do not exhibit evidence of having acquired meningitis: diminished LOC, confusion, fever, headache, nuchal rigidity, and other signs (see "Assessment" and "Diagnostic Test" data).

For patients with bacterial meningitis

- Bacterial meningitis is transmitted *via* droplet contact. Provide patient with a private room, if possible, or provide spatial separation of at least 3 ft between patient, other patients, and visitors.
- Initiate Transmission-based Precautions: Droplet upon admission and maintain them for 24 h after start of antimicrobial therapy.
  - □ Ensure that masks are worn by those in close contact with patient.
  - □ As with touching *any* patient secretions or excretions, ensure that gloves are worn during contact with oral secretions.
  - □ Ensure careful handwashing technique after contact with patient and potentially contaminated articles and before coming into contact with another patient.

For patients with viral or nonbacterial meningitis

- Viral meningitis can be transmitted *via* either stool or oral secretions. Follow Standard Precautions:
  - □ Ensure that gowns are worn if soiling of clothing is likely.
  - □ Ensure that gloves are worn for touching infectious material.
  - □ Enforce strict handwashing technique after touching patient or articles that may be contaminated and before caring for another patient.

ADDITIONAL NURSING DIAGNOSES

See "Status Epilepticus" for **Risk for trauma** (oral and musculoskeletal), p. 467. Because these patients are at risk for SIADH, see "Syndrome of Inappropriate Antidiuretic Hormone" for **Risk for injury,** p. 513. Also see appropriate nursing diagnoses and interventions in "Shock," p. 635, inasmuch as these patients are at risk for septic shock. As indicated, see other nursing diagnoses and interventions in "Nutritional Support," p. 12; "Prolonged Immobility," p. 78; "Psychosocial Support," p. 88; and "Psychosocial Support for the Patient's Family and Significant Others," p. 100.

Selected Bibliography

Barnett H et al: *Stroke: pathophysiology, diagnosis, and management,* ed 2, New York, 1992, Churchill Livingstone.

Bell J, Hannon K: Pathophysiology involved in autonomic dysreflexia, *J Neurosci Nurs* 18(2):86-88, 1986.

Bell TE et al: Transcranial Doppler: correlation of blood velocity measurement with clinical status in subarachnoid hemorrhage, *J Neurosci Nurs* 24(4):215-219, 1992.

Brott T et al: Measurements of acute cerebral infarction: a clinical examination scale, *Stroke* 20(7):864-870, 1990.

Farkkila M, Pentilla P: Plasma exchange therapy reduces the nursing care needed in Guillain-Barré syndrome, *J Adv Nurs* 17:672-675, 1992.

Flynn EP: Cerebral vasospasm following intracranial aneurysm rupture: a protocol for detection, *J Neurosci Nurs* 21(6):348-352, 1989.

Hickey JV: Myasthenic crisis: your assessment counts, *RN* 54(4):54-59, 1991.

Hickey JV: *The clinical practice of neurological and neurosurgical nursing,* ed 3, Philadelphia, 1992, Lippincott.

Hummel SK: Cerebral vasospasm: current concepts of pathogenesis and treatment, *J Neurosci Nurs* 21(4):216-225, 1989.

Interqual: The ISD-A review system with adult ISD criteria, August 1992, North Hampton, NH, and Marlboro, MA, Interqual, Inc.

Kaufman HH: *Intracerebral hematomas,* New York, 1992, Raven.

Kim MJ, McFarland GK, McLane AM: *Pocket guide to nursing diagnoses,* ed 6, St Louis, 1995, Mosby.

Lopate G, Pestronk A: Autoimmune myasthenia gravis, *Hosp Pract* 28(1):109-112, 115-117, 121-122, 1993.

MacDonald E: Aneurysmal subarachnoid hemorrhage, *J Neurosci Nurs* 21(5):313-321, 1989.

Manifold SL: Aneurysm SAH: cerebral vasospasm and early repair, *Crit Care Nurse* 10(8):62-71, 1990.

Mocsny N: Cryptococcal meningitis in patients with AIDS, *J Neurosci Nurs* 24(5):265-268, 1992.

Murray DP: Impaired mobility: Guillain-Barré syndrome, *J Neurosci Nurs* 25(2):100-104, 1993.

National High Blood Pressure Education Program, National Institutes of Health, and National Heart, Lung, and Blood Institute: NIH Pub No 93-1088, January 1993.

Pfister SM, Bullas JB: Acute Guillain-Barré syndrome, *Crit Care Nurse* 10(10):68-73, 1990.

Plum F, Posner J: *Diagnosis of stupor and coma,* ed 3, Philadelphia, 1980, Davis.

Pryse-Phillips W: Ticlopidine aspirin stroke study: outcome by vascular distribution of the qualifying event, *J Cerebrovasc Dis* 3(1):49-56, 1993.

Segatore M: Hyponatremia after aneurysmal subarachnoid hemorrhage, *J Neurosci Nurs* 25(2):92-99, 1993.

Seybold ME: Update on myasthenia gravis, *Hosp Med* 27(4):71-72, 77-78, 80, 1991.

Swift CM: Neurologic disorders. In Swearingen PL, editor: *Manual of medical-surgical nursing care: nursing interventions and collaborative management*, ed 3, St Louis, 1994, Mosby.

Weeks D: Washing the blood, *RN* 54(5):60-64, 1991.

Wispelwey B, Tunkel A, Scheld W: Bacterial meningitis in adults, *Infect Dis Clin North Am* 4:645-659, 1990.

Working Group on Status Epilepticus: Treatment of convulsive status epilepticus: recommendations of the Working Group on Status Epilepticus, *JAMA* 270(7):854-859, 1993.

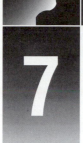

7 ENDOCRINOLOGIC DYSFUNCTIONS

Diabetic ketoacidosis

PATHOPHYSIOLOGY

Diabetic ketoacidosis (DKA) is a life-threatening complication of diabetes mellitus that is characterized by hyperglycemia, dehydration, electrolyte imbalance, ketosis, and acidosis. It occurs most commonly in persons with type I insulin-dependent diabetes mellitus (IDDM) who experience illness, infection, trauma, or surgery. A relative or absolute insulin deficiency prevents the normal utilization of serum glucose and results in cellular starvation despite the abundance of glucose in the serum. The unmet energy requirements of the cells stimulate gluconeogenesis and glycogen conversion in the liver and trigger the release of catabolic stress hormones, which act to elevate the serum glucose even further. The body is forced to break down its fat and protein stores to meet the energy requirements of cell metabolism. The rate of breakdown exceeds the body's ability to use these alternate energy sources, however, and ketone bodies accumulate in the blood. Ketones cause the blood pH level to drop, which results in the potential for profound metabolic ketoacidosis. Hyperglycemia results in increased serum osmolality.

Glucose and ketones not reabsorbed by the renal tubule cause an osmotic diuresis, with losses of sodium, potassium, phosphorus, magnesium, and body water, which can lead to severe dehydration and hypovolemic shock. Despite significant loss of potassium in the urine, the patient initially may present with normal or elevated plasma potassium because of the dramatic shift of potassium out of the cells secondary to insulin deficiency, acidosis, and tissue catabolism. Increased blood viscosity and platelet aggregation can result in thromboembolism. Dehydration also decreases tissue perfusion, and the resulting lactic acid waste products exacerbate the existing acidosis. The lowered pH level stimulates the respiratory center, producing the deep, rapid respirations known as Kussmaul's respirations. The large amount of ketones lends a fruity or acetone odor to the breath. If not treated promptly, elevated serum osmolality, acidosis, and dehydration depress consciousness to the point of coma. Death can result from hypovolemia or profound CNS depression.

ASSESSMENT

HISTORY AND RISK FACTORS Type I (IDDM) diabetes mellitus, recent physical stressor such as illness, infection, trauma, or surgery (most episodes of DKA are precipitated by infection), insufficient exogenous insulin replacement, severe emotional stress, nonadherence to diabetes regimen.

CLINICAL PRESENTATION Recent polyuria, polydipsia, polyphagia, weight loss, weakness, fatigue, nausea, vomiting, and abdominal pain.

PHYSICAL ASSESSMENT Dry and flushed skin, dry mucous membranes, poor skin turgor, hypotension, tachycardia, altered LOC (irritability, lethargy, coma), fruity odor to the breath, Kussmaul's respirations.

ECG AND HEMODYNAMIC FINDINGS ECG may show dysrhythmias associated with hyperkalemia: peaked T waves, widened QRS complex, prolonged PR intervals, flattened-to-absent P wave. After insulin therapy is initiated, hypokalemia is possible (see p. 681).

Note: For additional assessment information, see Table 7-1.

DIAGNOSTIC TESTS
See Table 7-1.

COLLABORATIVE MANAGEMENT

Rehydration: Usually, isotonic saline (0.9%) is administered rapidly (1-2 L during the first hour) to correct the fluid deficit, which is typically 4-6 L but may be even greater. After initial fluid replacement, 0.45% saline is administered to continue the rehydration. Dextrose is added to the IV solution once the blood glucose falls to 250-300 mg/dl to prevent rebound hypoglycemia.

Rapid-acting insulin: A loading dose of regular insulin may be given, followed by either continuous IV insulin infusion, approximately 0.1 U/kg/h, or intermittent IV injections. It is essential that blood glucose be reduced *gradually* to reduce the danger of cerebral edema. The dosage is adjusted on the basis of serial glucose measurements. The insulin drip should be discontinued temporarily if the serum glucose drops to <100 mg/dl, and the physician should be consulted. Be aware that insulin, when added to IV solutions, may be absorbed by the container and plastic tubing. The tubing should be flushed with 100 ml of the insulin solution to ensure maximum absorption before administration.

Restoration of electrolyte balance: Administration of saline restores the body's sodium levels. Potassium is closely monitored and replaced once insulin is administered and potassium returns to the intracellular compartment. Potassium replacement is essential to correct the existing body deficit and prevent severe hypokalemia. Deficits may range from 300-900 mEq and will require days to replace. Phosphate replacement (usually as potassium phosphate) may be indicated if severe depletion has occurred in the presence of prolonged acidosis. Meticulous monitoring of phosphate *and* calcium levels is essential if phosphate replacement is prescribed, because supplemental phosphate may depress plasma calcium levels because of calcium-phosphorus binding (see "Hypophosphatemia," p. 693).

IV bicarbonate: May be prescribed in the presence of severe acidosis (pH <7.2). It is not routinely given in DKA due to the potential for paradoxical cerebral spinal fluid acidosis and hypokalemia. The acidosis of DKA is best corrected by insulin therapy.

Insertion of gastric tube: May be indicated in comatose or obtunded patients when the risk of vomiting and aspiration from gastric distention or paralytic ileus is high.

Treatment of underlying cause: For example, infection is treated with appropriate antibiotics.

NURSING DIAGNOSES AND INTERVENTIONS

Fluid volume deficit related to decreased circulating volume secondary to hyperglycemia and induced osmotic diuresis

Desired outcomes: Within 12 h of initiating treatment, patient is normovolemic as evidenced by BP ≥90/60 mm Hg (or within patient's normal range), MAP ≥70 mm Hg, HR 60-100 bpm, CVP 2-6 mm Hg, PAWP 6-12 mm Hg, balanced I&O, urinary output ≥0.5 ml/kg/h, firm skin turgor, and pink and moist mucous membranes. ECG exhibits normal sinus rhythm.

- Monitor VS q15min until patient's condition is stable for 1 h. Consult physician promptly for the following: HR >120 bpm or BP <90/60 or decreased ≥20 mm Hg from baseline, MAP decreased ≥10 mm Hg from baseline, CVP <2 mm Hg, and PAWP <6 mm Hg.
- Monitor patient for physical indicators of dehydration, such as poor skin turgor, dry mucous membranes, sunken and soft eyeballs, tachycardia, and orthostatic hypotension.
- Measure I&O accurately. Decreasing urinary output may signal diminishing intravascular fluid volume or impending renal failure. Consult physician for urine output <0.5 ml/kg/h for 2 consecutive hours. Weigh patient daily.
- Administer IV fluids as prescribed to ensure adequate rehydration. Be alert to indicators of fluid overload, which can occur as a result of rapid infusion of fluids: jugular vein distention, dyspnea, crackles (rales), CVP >6 mm Hg.
- Monitor results of laboratory tests for abnormalities. Be alert for the development of hypokalemia, a common complication of treatment. Normal range for serum potassium is 3.5-5 mEq/L and for serum sodium is 137-147 mEq/L.
- Monitor patient continuously on cardiac monitor. Observe for ECG changes typical of hyperkalemia or hypokalemia (see "ECG and Hemodynamic Findings," p. 496).
- Observe for clinical manifestations of electrolyte imbalance associated with DKA and its treatment:

  Hypokalemia: ECG changes, muscle weakness, hypotension, anorexia, drowsiness, hypoactive bowel sounds.

T A B L E 7 - 1   Comparison of diabetic ketoacidosis and hyperosmolar hyperglycemic nonketotic syndrome

Criterion	DKA	HHNS
Diabetes type	Usually IDDM (type I)	Usually NIDDM (type II)
Typical age group	Any age	Usually >50 yr
Signs and symptoms	Polyuria, polydipsia, polyphagia, weakness, orthostatic hypotension, lethargy, changes in LOC, fatigue, nausea, vomiting, abdominal pain	Same as DKA, but slower onset and, very commonly, neurologic symptoms predominate
Physical assessment	Dry and flushed skin, poor skin turgor, dry mucous membranes, decreased BP, tachycardia, altered LOC (irritability, lethargy, coma), Kussmaul's respirations, fruity odor to the breath	Same as DKA, but no Kussmaul's respirations or fruity odor to the breath; instead, occurrence of tachypnea with shallow respirations
History and risk factors	Recent stressors such as surgery, trauma, infection, MI; insufficient exogenous insulin; undiagnosed type I diabetes mellitus	Undiagnosed type II diabetes mellitus; recent stressors such as surgery, trauma, pancreatitis, MI, infection; high-caloric enteral or parenteral feedings in a compromised patient; use of diabetogenic drugs (e.g., phenytoin, thiazide diuretics, thyroid preparations, mannitol, corticosteroids, sympathomimetics)
Monitoring parameters	*ECG:* Dysrhythmias associated with hyperkalemia: peaked T waves, widened QRS complex, prolonged PR interval, flattened or absent P wave. Hypokalemia (K^+ <3 mEq/L), which may produce depressed ST segments, flat or inverted T waves, or increased ventricular dysrhythmias	ECG evidence of hypokalemia as listed with DKA *Hemodynamic measurements:* CVP >3 mm Hg below patient's baseline; PADP and PAWP >4 mm Hg below patient's baseline
Diagnostic tests	*Serum glucose:* 200-800 mg/dl	800-2,000 mg/dl
	Serum ketones: elevated	Normal or slightly elevated
	Urine glucose: positive	Positive

Urine acetone: "large"		Negative
Serum osmolality: 300-350 mOsm/L		>350 mOsm/L
Bicarbonate: <15 mEq/L		Normal or slightly decreased if mild acidosis present
Serum pH: <7.2		Normal or mildly acidotic (pH <7.4)
Serum potassium: normal or elevated >5.0 mEq/L initially and then decreased		Normal or <3.5 mEq/L
Serum sodium: elevated, normal, or low		Elevated, normal, or low
Serum Hct: elevated due to osmotic diuresis with hemoconcentration		Elevated due to hemoconcentration
BUN: elevated >20 mg/dl		Elevated
Serum creatinine: >1.5 mg/dl		Elevated
Serum phosphorus, magnesium, chloride: decreased		Decreased
WBC: elevated, even in the absence of infection		Normal unless infection present
Onset	Hours to days	Days to weeks
Mortality rate	<10%	>50% due to age group and complications such as CVA, thrombosis, renal failure

Hyponatremia: Headache, malaise, muscle weakness, abdominal cramps, nausea, seizures, coma.

Hypophosphatemia: Muscle weakness, respiratory failure, decreased oxygen delivery, decreased cardiac function.

Hypomagnesemia: Anorexia, nausea, vomiting, lethargy, weakness, personality changes, tetany, tremor or muscle fasciculations, seizures, confusion progressing to coma.

Risk for infection related to inadequate secondary defenses (suppressed inflammatory response) as a result of protein depletion

Desired outcome: Patient is free of infection as evidenced by normothermia, HR $\leq$100 bpm, BP within patient's normal range, WBC count $\leq$11,000/μl, and negative culture results.

- Assess patient for evidence of infection. Monitor laboratory results for increased WBC count. An initial elevation of WBC count may be a reflection of dehydration and increased adrenocortical secretion.
- Ensure good handwashing technique when caring for patient.
- Because patient is at increased risk of bacterial infection, use of invasive lines should be limited. Peripheral IV sites should be rotated q72h, depending on agency policy. Central lines should be discontinued as soon as feasible and, when in place, should be handled carefully. Schedule dressing changes according to agency policy, and inspect the site(s) for signs of local infection, including erythema, swelling, or purulent drainage. Document the presence of any of these indicators and consult physician accordingly.
- Use meticulous aseptic technique when caring for or inserting indwelling catheters to minimize the risk of bacterial entry *via* these sites. Because of the increased risk of infection, use of indwelling urethral catheter is indicated only when continuous accurate assessment of urine output is essential.
- Provide good skin care to maintain skin integrity. Assess for areas of decreased sensation on the extremities. Use pressure-relief mattress on the bed to help prevent skin breakdown.
- To help prevent pulmonary infection, provide incentive spirometry and encourage its use, along with hourly deep-breathing exercises while patient is awake.

Risk for injury related to altered cerebral function secondary to hyperosmolality, dehydration, cerebral edema associated with DKA, or hypoglycemia

Desired outcome: Patient verbalizes orientation to time, place, and person; normal breath sounds are auscultated over patient's airways; and patient's oral cavity and musculoskeletal system remain intact and free of injury.

- Monitor patient's orientation, LOC, and respiratory status, especially airway patency, at frequent intervals. Keep an appropriate-size oral airway, manual resuscitator and mask, and supplemental oxygen at the bedside.
- Reduce the likelihood of injury due to falls by maintaining bed in lowest position, with side rails up at all times, and using soft restraints as necessary.
- Insert gastric tube in comatose patients, as prescribed, to decrease the likelihood of aspiration. Attach to low intermittent suction, and ensure patency of tube q4h.

- Elevate HOB to 45 degrees to minimize the risk of aspiration.
- Initiate seizure precautions. See **Risk for trauma** (oral or musculo-skeletal) related to seizure activity, p. 467, in "Status Epilepticus."
- Monitor blood glucose qh initially. Consult physician if blood glucose drops faster than 100 mg/dl/h and if it drops to <250-300 mg/dl. Obtain prescription for glucose-containing IV solution accordingly.

Knowledge deficit: New-onset diabetes or misunderstanding of the causes and prevention of DKA

Desired outcome: By the time of discharge from ICU, patient verbalizes understanding of the causes, symptoms, and prevention of DKA and available resources.

- Consider referral to diabetes educator if this is a new-onset diabetes. Provide instructions in simple terms, incorporating patient teaching into patient care routines.
- Explain the relationship of DKA to illness, infection, trauma, and stress. Emphasize the importance of adhering to the entire diabetic regimen concerning meal planning, insulin, exercise, and monitoring.
- Review sick-day guidelines for individuals with diabetes (i.e., need for increased fluid and insulin with illness).
- Alert patient and significant others to hospital and community resources (e.g., dietitian, social worker, local American Diabetes Association [ADA], and support groups).
- Provide address for ADA for pamphlets and magazines related to the disease, its complications, and appropriate treatment: American Diabetes Association, Inc, 18 East 48th St, New York, NY 10017.

ADDITIONAL NURSING DIAGNOSES

See "Hyperosmolar Hyperglycemic Nonketotic Syndrome," p. 503, for **Altered peripheral tissue perfusion.** Also see nursing diagnoses and interventions in "Prolonged Immobility," p. 78; "Psychosocial Support," p. 88; and "Psychosocial Support for the Patient's Family and Significant Others," p. 100.

Hyperosmolar hyperglycemic nonketotic syndrome

PATHOPHYSIOLOGY

Hyperosmolar hyperglycemic nonketotic syndrome (HHNS) is a life-threatening emergency resulting from a relative or actual insulin deficiency that causes severe hyperglycemia. It occurs most commonly in older patients with NIDDM (type II diabetes mellitus), especially in undiagnosed diabetes mellitus. Usually HHNS is precipitated by an acute exacerbation of a chronic disease or a stimulus, such as trauma or infection, that provokes a stress response. The stressor combines with a decreased insulin reserve to initiate the pathophysiologic sequence. Although the body's available insulin is insufficient to control the blood glucose, it usually is adequate to prevent lipolysis and the formation of ketone bodies, thereby avoiding metabolic acidosis. The hyperglycemia of HHNS is more severe than that in DKA, and it results in significant serum hyperosmolality and pronounced osmotic diuresis. Severe dehydration and electrolyte loss occur, and individuals may lose from 15%-25% of their body water. Fluids are pulled from the body cells in response to the hyperosmolality, and significant intracellular dehydration may result. Neurologic deficits frequently occur in response to the severe dehydration and hyperosmolality. The blood becomes more viscous and flow is impeded, increasing the risk of thromboemboli. Increased cardiac workload and decreased renal and cerebral blood flow may result in myocardial infarction, renal failure, and cerebrovascular accident. These severe complications contribute to a mortality rate in excess of 50%.

The dramatic osmotic diuresis that occurs with HHNS results in significant electrolyte depletion. Sodium and potassium levels are variable at diagnosis, although total body deficiencies of both always are present. Phosphorus and magnesium deficiencies also are common.

Unlike DKA, in which acidosis produces severe symptoms that require prompt hospitalization, symptoms of HHNS develop slowly and frequently are nonspecific. The cardinal symptoms of polyuria and polydipsia are the first to appear, but they may be ignored by older adults or their families. Neurologic deficits may be mistaken for senility. Because of the similarity of these symptoms to other disease processes common to this age group, proper diagnosis and treatment may be delayed, allowing progression of pathophysiologic processes.

ASSESSMENT

HISTORY AND RISK FACTORS NIDDM (type II diabetes mellitus); acute exacerbation of a chronic illness, particularly renal or cardiovascular; ingestion of high-caloric enteral or parenteral feedings; stressors, such as trauma or infection, which increase insulin need; use of diabetogenic drugs (e.g., glucocorticoids, some diuretics, phenytoin, thyroid preparations).

CLINICAL PRESENTATION Polyuria, polydipsia, weight loss, weakness, orthostatic hypotension, lethargy, confusion progressing to coma. Neurologic symptoms are common. Although almost all patients present with altered mental status; only 50% are comatose. Seizures are common.

PHYSICAL ASSESSMENT Poor skin turgor, dry mucous membranes, tachycardia, tachypnea with shallow respirations.

ECG AND HEMODYNAMIC FINDINGS Evidence of hypokalemia (increased PVCs, depressed T waves); CVP >3 mm Hg below patient's baseline, PAD pressure >4 mm Hg below patient's baseline, and PAWP >4 mm Hg below patient's baseline.

Note: Because these patients usually are >50 yr old and have preexisting cardiac or pulmonary disorders, hemodynamic factors often cannot be evaluated on the basis of normal values but rather on what is normal or optimal for each individual patient. CVP, PAWP, and PAD pressures therefore should be evaluated in terms of deviations from patient's baseline and concurrent clinical status. See Table 7-1 for a comparison of DKA and HHNS.

DIAGNOSTIC TESTS

See Table 7-1.

COLLABORATIVE MANAGEMENT

Replacement of electrolytes and extracellular fluid volume: Most often, 0.45% saline or isotonic saline is used; potassium phosphate and magnesium supplements are added on the basis of laboratory values. Usually half the estimated water deficit is replaced during the first 12 h and the remainder over the next 24 h. Dextrose will be added to the IV line once the blood glucose falls to 250-300 mg/dl to prevent rebound hypoglycemia.

Rapid-acting insulin: Usually administered in low doses. Because of poor tissue perfusion in these patients, the IV route is preferred. In the majority of cases, continuous drips are used and titrated on the basis of serum glucose levels. In HHNS some insulin secretion occurs, and patients may be extremely sensitive to supplemental doses. Despite severe hyperglycemia, HHNS often requires less insulin to correct it than does DKA. The condition sometimes can be treated with fluid alone.

Insertion of pulmonary artery flow-directed catheter: To assess fluid status on a continuous basis.

Treatment of underlying cause: The most frequent cause is infection, which is treated with appropriate antibiotics.

NURSING DIAGNOSES AND INTERVENTIONS

Altered peripheral tissue perfusion related to interruption of blood flow (thromboembolism) secondary to increased viscosity of blood, increased platelet aggregation and adhesiveness, and patient immobility

Desired outcome: By the time of hospital discharge, patient has adequate perfusion as evidenced by peripheral pulses >2+ on a 0-4+ scale, brisk capillary refill (<2 sec), warm skin, and absence of swelling, bluish discoloration, erythema, and discomfort in the calves and thighs.

- Monitor Hct results. With proper fluid replacement, values should return to normal (40%-54% [male] or 37%-47% [female]) within 24-48 h. Assess for a falling BUN value (<20 mg/dl) as an indicator of improved tissue perfusion and renal function.

- Assess peripheral pulses q2-4h. Consult physician immediately for any decrease in amplitude or absence of pulse(s).

- Be alert to indicators of deep vein thrombosis such as erythema, pain, tenderness, warmth, swelling, bluish discoloration, or prominence of superficial veins in the extremities, especially the lower extremities. Arterial thrombosis may produce cyanosis with delayed capillary refill, mottling, and coolness of the extremity. Report significant findings to physician immediately.

- Assist with or perform ROM exercises to all extremities q4h to increase blood flow to the tissues.

- Apply pneumatic sequential compression stockings or similar devices to the lower extremities as prescribed to aid in the prevention of thrombosis.

Knowledge deficit: New-onset diabetes or causes of HHNS

Desired outcome: Before discharge from ICU, patient verbalizes understanding of the basics of diabetes management and prevention of HHNS.

- Teach patient the causes, prevention, and treatment of HHNS. Allow patient to verbalize fears and feelings about the diagnosis; correct any misconceptions. As needed, explain the disease process of diabetes mellitus and HHNS and the common early symptoms of worsening diabetes, including polyuria, polydipsia, polyphagia, dry and flushed skin, and increased irritability.
- Stress the importance of daily testing of blood glucose levels, or as prescribed, before meals and at bedtime. Explain that blood glucose >250 mg/dl should be reported to physician. As indicated, review testing procedure with patient.
- Explain the importance of taking oral hypoglycemic agents as prescribed. In addition, explain that exogenous insulin may be required during periods of physical and emotional stress and that blood glucose levels should be monitored closely during these times, as well as during illness or injury.
- Describe specific components of the diabetic regimen as appropriate. Review the importance of regular exercise, consistent dietary intake, preventive measures for avoiding infection, and prompt management of minor injuries.
- Describe procedures for obtaining Medic-Alert bracelet or card identifying patient's diagnosis.
- Stress the necessity for continued medical follow-up.
- In addition, provide booklets or pamphlets from the ADA or pharmaceutical companies about diabetes and appropriate treatment. Refer patient and significant others to a diabetes education program, if needed.

ADDITIONAL NURSING DIAGNOSES

See "Diabetic Ketoacidosis" for **Fluid volume deficit,** p. 499; **Risk for infection,** p. 500; and **Risk for injury,** p. 500. For other nursing diagnoses and interventions, see the following, as appropriate: "Psychosocial Support," p. 88; and "Psychosocial Support for the Patient's Family and Significant Others," p. 100.

Diabetes insipidus

PATHOPHYSIOLOGY

Diabetes insipidus (DI) results from a profound deficiency of the antidiuretic hormone (ADH) or decreased renal responsiveness to ADH. It may be caused by a neurogenic dysfunction involving either a deficiency in the synthesis of ADH in the posterior pituitary gland or damage to the hypothalamus, which stimulates its release (central DI). DI also may be nephrogenic in origin secondary to decreased water permeability of the collecting tubules due to decreased ADH effect. DI is frequently temporary, occurring suddenly in response to head injury, major trauma, tumor, or inflammation. In some situations, however, the condition may become permanent. Transient DI typically resolves after approximately 5-7 days. If resolution of the problem does not occur within that time frame, the patient usually progresses to permanent polyuria and polydipsia.

Regardless of the cause, the characteristic feature of DI is the excretion of large quantities of hypotonic urine, frequently 10-12 L/day or more. As a result of the loss of free water, the extracellular fluid volume decreases dramatically, causing plasma osmolality and serum sodium to rise. If individuals are unable to respond adequately to the stimulus of thirst, they face significant risks from extracellular and intracellular dehydration, hypotension, and hypovolemic shock. The increased blood viscosity increases the risk of thromboemboli. Dehydration, decreased cerebral perfusion, and electrolyte imbalance frequently produce neurologic symptoms ranging from confusion, restlessness, and irritability to seizures and coma.

ASSESSMENT
HISTORY AND RISK FACTORS
Central DI: Head injury, especially to the base of the brain; meningitis or encephalitis; brain tumors, especially in the hypothalamus or pituitary region; neoplasms such as leukemia or breast cancer; surgery in the area of the pituitary gland; intracranial hemorrhage; any disorder that causes increased intracranial pressure (IICP); and cerebral hypoxia.
Nephrogenic DI: Congenital disorder, hypercalcemia, hypokalemia, medications (lithium, demeclocycline HCl [Declomycin]).
CLINICAL PRESENTATION Polyuria with dilute urine; extreme thirst.

Note: As much as 5-12 L/day of urine may be excreted, with specific gravity of 1.000-1.005.

PHYSICAL ASSESSMENT Unremarkable in the individual who experiences and can safely satisfy thirst. If fluid intake is inadequate, patients may show signs of dehydration such as poor skin turgor, dry mucous membranes, orthostatic hypotension, hypotension, and tachycardia. Altered LOC may be present if serum hyperosmolality and hypernatremia develop. Altered LOC and neurologic changes also may be related to the precipitating event.
MONITORING PARAMETERS
Urine output: >200 ml/h for 2 consecutive hours or >500 ml/h in the presence of any of the aforementioned risk factors.
CVP: <2 mm Hg.
PAWP: <6 mm Hg.

DIAGNOSTIC TESTS
Urine osmolality: Decreased to <200 mOsm/kg in the presence of disease; may be higher if volume depletion is present.
Specific gravity: <1.007.
Serum osmolality: Increased to >300 mOsm/kg.
Serum sodium: Increased to >147 mEq/L.
Plasma ADH: Decreased in central DI.
Water deprivation test: Preliminary measurements of weight, serum and urine osmolality, and urine specific gravity are obtained. Fluid

intake is prohibited, and the aforementioned values are measured hourly until urine specific gravity exceeds 1.020 and urine osmolality exceeds 800 mOsm/kg (a negative result) or when 5% of body weight is lost or urine specific gravity does not increase for 3 consecutive hours (a positive result). To establish a definite diagnosis of DI, it is necessary also to perform the vasopressin test (see next entry).

Caution: The water deprivation test can take up to 16 h to complete and may produce hypernatremia, severe dehydration, and hypovolemic shock. Patients must be monitored continuously throughout the test. This test may not be necessary for temporary DI in the critical care setting.

Vasopressin test: Vasopressin (exogenous ADH) is administered subcutaneously. Urine specimens are collected q15min for 2 h and evaluated for quantity and osmolality. Urine osmolality generally will rise significantly in response to the ADH unless the DI has a nephrogenic origin, in which case the response may be minimal.

Caution: This test can induce congestive heart failure secondary to fluid overload in susceptible persons.

COLLABORATIVE MANAGEMENT

Rehydration: Hypotonic IV solutions frequently are used to replace free water lost in the urine. Fluid replacement is very rapid until hemodynamic status becomes stabilized, at which time it is then based on urine output.

Exogenous ADH (vasopressin):   Several preparations are available, and dosage is adjusted to patient response. Potential side effects include hypertension, angina, or MI related to its vasoconstrictive effects on blood vessels; abdominal cramping and increased peristalsis from smooth muscle excitation; and water intoxication. Use of desmopressin has become increasingly popular because it produces fewer side effects (Table 7-2).

Thiazide diuretics in combination with a low-sodium, low-protein diet: Major form of therapy for nephrogenic DI. This approach reduces solute excretion and urine production. Chlorpropamide also may be given because it enhances the action of ADH.

Transsphenoidal hypophysectomy: Although not an appropriate treatment for transient DI that occurs after injury or surgery, this surgical approach to the pituitary gland is the treatment of choice for pituitary tumors of all types, whether or not the pituitary gland itself is removed. It produces immediate results, has a low mortality rate, and can be effective in the treatment of tumors that are resistant to radiation therapy.

To enter the sella turcica through the sphenoid process, the upper lip is elevated and an incision is made in the gingiva above the maxilla. Because of the site of the incision, patients are at high risk for postoperative infection, particularly of the brain. To minimize this possibility, antibiotic nasal sprays are used preoperatively, and nasal packing impregnated with an antibiotic ointment is kept in place for 24-72 h after surgery. Complications include pituitary hemorrhage, frontal lobe damage, and hormonal deficiencies after removal of the gland. Tumors most often occur in the anterior pituitary gland; therefore most postoperative hormone deficiencies are caused by a lack of anterior pituitary hormones. In addition, the patient may have IICP due to edema or bleeding in the sella turcica and will return from surgery with bilateral periorbital ecchymosis.

NURSING DIAGNOSES AND INTERVENTIONS

Fluid volume deficit related to failure of regulatory mechanisms (resulting in polyuria) secondary to ADH deficiency or altered ADH action

Desired outcome: Within 12 h of initiating therapy, patient is normovolemic as evidenced by BP 110-120/70-80 mm Hg (or within patient's normal value), CVP ≥ 2 mm Hg, PAWP ≥ 6 mm Hg, HR 60-100 bpm, intake equal to output plus insensible losses, and stable weight.

- Keep careful I&O records. Urine output >200 ml/h for 2 consecutive hours, or 500 ml/h, in the presence of risk factors (see p. 505), should be reported to physician promptly.
- Provide adequate fluids. Keep water pitcher full and within easy reach of patient. Administer hyperosmolar tube feedings or solutions with extreme caution. They can worsen fluid losses through the GI tract by inducing osmotic diarrhea.
- For unconscious patients or those who cannot maintain adequate fluid intake orally, administer IV fluids as prescribed. Usually, a hypotonic solution is administered as follows: 1 ml IV fluid for each 1 ml of urine output. In patients with brain injury, moderate diuresis may be permitted to avoid the need for administering osmotic diuretics. Hypernatremia, if present, must be corrected slowly to prevent cerebral edema, seizures, permanent neurologic damage, or death.
- Administer vasopressin as prescribed; observe for and document effects. Also be alert to side effects of therapy: hypertension, cardiac ischemia, hyponatremia.
- Weigh patient daily, at the same time and using the same scale and garments to prevent error. Consult physician for weight loss >1 kg/ day.
- Monitor for signs of continuing fluid volume deficit: poor skin turgor; dry mucous membranes; rapid and thready pulse; and systolic BP, CVP, or PAWP below patient's baseline.
- Monitor laboratory studies, including serum sodium, serum and urine osmolality, and urine specific gravity; report significant findings to physician. Normal values are as follows: serum sodium 137-147 mEq/L, serum osmolality 275-300 mOsm/kg, urine osmolality 300-900 mOsm/24 h, and urine specific gravity 1.010-1.030. Monitor urine specific gravity qh to evaluate response to therapy. Patients may be allowed to develop hypotonic polyuria between doses of vasopressin to demonstrate persistence of DI when transient or triphasic DI is suspected.

Decreased adaptive capacity: Intracranial, related to interruption of blood flow secondary to cerebral edema or intracranial bleeding after transsphenoidal hypophysectomy

TABLE 7 - 2 Vasopressin preparations

Generic name	Trade name	Onset	Duration	Usual dosage	Advantages/disadvantages	Comments
Nasal						
vasopressin	Pitressin	Within 1 h	4-8 h	5-10 U bid-tid	Action decreased by nasal congestion/discharge or atrophy of nasal mucosa	Administer by spray, cotton pledget, or dropper; used for chronic DI management
desmopressin acetate	DDAVP	Within 1 h	8-20 h	0.1-0.4 ml qd in 1-3 doses (10-40 μg)	See above	See above; stored in refrigerator at 4° C (39.2° F)
lypressin	Diapid	Within 1 h	3-8 h	7-14 μg qid	See above	See above; stored at <40° C (100° F)
Subcutaneous						
vasopressin	Pitressin	½-1 h	2-8 h	0.25-0.5 ml (5-10 U) q3-4h prn increased thirst or increased urine output		Typically used in acute care setting and for emergency management
desmopressin acetate	DDAVP, Stimate	Within ½ h	1½-4 h	0.5-1 ml (2-4 μg) qd in 2 divided doses		Keep refrigerated at 4° C (39.2° F)

		Onset	Duration	Dose	Comments	Storage
Intramuscular vasopressin tannate in oil	Pitressin Tannate in Oil	Within 1-2 h	36-48 h	0.3-1 ml (1.5-5 U) q2-3days for increased thirst or increased urine output	Longer duration of action/slower absorption than SC route; response cumulative over 2-3 days	Stored at 13°-18° C (55°-65° F) Shake well before withdrawing from vial; can warm solution by immersing vial in warm water
vasopressin tannate	Pitressin Tannate	½-1 h	2-8 h	0.25-0.5 ml (5-10 U) q3-4h for increased thirst or increased urine output	Longer duration of action, which makes IM forms more desirable for chronic management	
Intravenous desmopressin acetate	DDAVP	Within ½ h	1½-4 h	0.5-1 ml (2-4 µg) qd in 2 divided doses	Not for home use	Keep refrigerated at 4° C (39.2° F); dilute in 10-50 ml 0.9% NaCl and infuse over 15-30 min

Desired outcomes: Within 24 h after initiating treatment, patient has adequate intracranial adaptive capacity as evidenced by ability to verbalize orientation to time, place, and person; RR 12-20 breaths/min with a normal pattern and depth (eupnea); equal and normoreactive pupils; and bilaterally equal motor strength and tone that are normal for patient. Patient verbalizes understanding of the importance of avoiding Valsalva-type activities.

- Elevate HOB 30 degrees to minimize ICP.
- Perform checks of neurostatus at frequent intervals to assess for signs of IICP, including changes in LOC, respiratory rate or rhythm, and pupillary reflexes (see Table 6-3, p. 449).
- Teach patient to avoid coughing, sneezing, straining, bending, or other Valsalva-type activities because they can increase stress on the operative site, increase ICP, and cause CSF leak. Explain to patient that if coughing or sneezing becomes necessary, it should be done with the mouth open to minimize the increase in ICP. As appropriate, administer cathartics, stool softeners, or antiemetics to minimize straining and nausea.
- If IICP develops, implement the interventions described in Table 2-5, p. 137; see also "Care of the Patient Following Intracranial Surgery," p. 459.

Risk for infection related to inadequate primary defenses secondary to incisional opening into sella turcica

Desired outcome: Patient is free of infection as evidenced by normothermia; verbalization of orientation to time, place, and person; and absence of the indicators of CSF leakage or nuchal rigidity.

- Inspect nasal packing at frequent intervals for frank bleeding or evidence of CSF (nonsanguineous) leak. Using a glucose reagent stick, test all clear drainage for the presence of glucose to determine if it is CSF. Because a CSF leak would signal a serious breach in cranial integrity, elevate the HOB to minimize the chance of bacterial migration into the brain. Consult physician promptly for suspected CSF leaks.
- Be alert to indicators of infection, including elevated temperature, nuchal rigidity, and altered LOC.
- To prevent injury to operative site, which could lead to infection, teach patient to avoid brushing teeth until instructed to do so by physician. Provide mouthwash and sponge-tipped applicators for oral hygiene.
- For additional information, see "Care of the Patient Following Intracranial Surgery," p. 459.

Knowledge deficit: Management of permanent DI; care following transsphenoidal hypophysectomy

Desired outcome: Before discharge from ICU, patient verbalizes understanding of the basics of DI management and care following transsphenoidal hypophysectomy, if appropriate.

- Teach patient appropriate administration of exogenous vasopressin and its side effects.
- Explain the importance of weighing daily at the same time of day and in the same clothing and reporting weight gains or losses to physician.
- Demonstrate the method for accurate measurement of urine specific

gravity and the importance of keeping accurate records of test results.
- Teach the indicators that necessitate medical attention, including signs and symptoms of dehydration and water intoxication.
- Explain the importance of obtaining a Medic-Alert bracelet and ID card.
- Stress the importance of continued medical follow-up.

Care after transsphenoidal hypophysectomy
- Explain the necessity for lifetime exogenous hormone replacement if the anterior posterior gland was removed or damaged.
- If the entire pituitary gland was removed, teach the indicators of hormone replacement excess or deficiency.

Adrenal hormone excess: weight gain, moon face, easy bruising, fatigue, polyuria, polydipsia.

Adrenal hormone deficiency: weight loss, easy fatigability, abdominal pain, excess pigmentation.

Thyroid hormone excess: heat intolerance, irritability, tachycardia, weight loss, diaphoresis.

Thyroid hormone deficiency: bradycardia, cold intolerance, weight gain, slowed mentation.

Androgen replacement deficiency: some degree of sexual dysfunction, ranging from menstrual irregularities to infertility and impotence.
- For patients with permanent need for hormone replacement, explain the method for obtaining a Medic-Alert bracelet and ID card outlining diagnosis and appropriate treatment in the event of an emergency.

ADDITIONAL NURSING DIAGNOSES

See "Diabetic Ketoacidosis" for **Risk for injury,** p. 500. Also see "Hyperosmolar Hyperglycemic Nonketotic Syndrome," p. 503, for **Altered peripheral tissue perfusion.** As appropriate, see the following: "Psychosocial Support," p. 88, and "Psychosocial Support for the Patient's Family and Significant Others," p. 100.

Syndrome of inappropriate antidiuretic hormone

PATHOPHYSIOLOGY

Syndrome of inappropriate antidiuretic hormone (SIADH) is the excessive release of ADH from the pituitary gland. ADH secretion normally occurs in response to (1) increased plasma osmolality, (2) decreased plasma volume, or (3) decreased BP. In SIADH the excess hormone causes severe water retention that expands body fluid volume. This hypotonic expansion of fluid volume dilutes the serum sodium, thereby decreasing serum osmolality. Glomerular filtration increases in response to the fluid volume expansion, and additional sodium is filtered out into the urine. Aldosterone secretion also is suppressed by the increased fluid volume, which adds further to the renal excretion of sodium. The decreased serum osmolality causes water to move into the cells. The resultant water intoxication, cerebral edema, and profound hyponatremia may be life threatening.

SIADH may accompany a wide variety of clinical situations. It can occur as a temporary response to neurologic injury or inflammation, the general stress of surgery, and the stimulation of anesthetic agents. Positive pressure ventilation may promote ADH secretion, and some malignant tumors have demonstrated the capacity to secrete the hormone. The metabolic disruptions of chronic heart, liver, and kidney disease all have demonstrated the potential to disturb the balance of ADH in the body. Certain medications, such as morphine, chlorpropamide, and amitriptyline, may induce SIADH. SIADH also is associated with pulmonary disease such as pneumonia and acute respiratory failure.

ASSESSMENT

HISTORY AND RISK FACTORS Cancer of the lung, pancreas, duodenum, and prostate can secrete a biologically active form of ADH. Other common causes include head trauma, brain tumor, hemorrhage, or infection. Positive pressure ventilation, physiologic stress, chronic metabolic illness, pulmonary disease, and a wide variety of medications all have been linked with SIADH.

CLINICAL PRESENTATION Decreased urine output with inappropriately concentrated urine. Signs of water intoxication may appear, including fatigue, headache, declining LOC, seizures, nausea, and vomiting.

Despite retention of excess water, edema rarely develops. A reduction in the stimulus to the release of aldosterone minimizes fluid volume expansion and edema formation. In addition, retained water expands both the extracellular and intracellular fluid compartments. The primary symptoms of SIADH are neurologic secondary to water movement into the brain cells. The severity of symptoms depends on the degree of cerebral overhydration and how quickly hyponatremia develops.

PHYSICAL ASSESSMENT Weight gain without edema; slightly elevated BP.
MONITORING PARAMETERS CVP >6 mm Hg; PAWP >12 mm Hg in the absence of underlying cardiac or pulmonary disease; and urine output <0.5 ml/kg/h with specific gravity >1.030 in the presence of adequate fluid intake.

DIAGNOSTIC TESTS

Serum sodium level: Decreased to <137 mEq/L.
Plasma osmolality: Decreased to <275 mOsm/kg.
Urine osmolality: Elevated disproportionately in relation to plasma osmolality.
Urine sodium level: Increased to >40 mEq/L.
Urine specific gravity: >1.030.
Plasma ADH level: Elevated in conditions associated with increased production.

COLLABORATIVE MANAGEMENT

Fluid restriction: Based on urine output. Usually fluids are limited to 1,000 ml/day. Once the serum sodium level is normal, fluids may be increased to urine output plus estimated insensible losses.
Isotonic (0.9%) or hypertonic (3%) sodium chloride: May be given if the patient has severe hyponatremia. Supplemental sodium so-

lutions may be administered with IV furosemide (Lasix) or osmotic diuretics, such as mannitol, to promote water excretion.

Lithium or demeclocycline (Declomycin): Inhibits action of ADH on the distal renal tubules to promote water excretion.

Treatment of underlying cause: SIADH associated with surgery, trauma, or drugs usually is temporary and self-limiting. In chronic situations the focus will be on treating the underlying cause, which may include cancer, surgery, radiation, or chemotherapy.

NURSING DIAGNOSES AND INTERVENTIONS

Risk for injury related to hyponatremia, induced alteration in neurologic function, or too-rapid correction of hyponatremia

Desired outcomes: Within 24 h of initiating treatment, patient verbalizes orientation to time, place, and person. CVP, PAWP, and BP are within patient's normal range. Patient remains free of signs of injury.

- Assess LOC, VS, hemodynamic measurements, and I&O hourly; weigh patient daily. Be alert to decreasing LOC; elevated BP, CVP, and PAWP; urine output <0.5 ml/kg/h; and weight gain. Promptly consult physician for significant findings or changes.
- Monitor laboratory results, including those for serum sodium, urine and serum osmolality, and urine specific gravity. Be alert to decreased serum sodium and plasma osmolality, urine osmolality elevated disproportionately in relation to plasma osmolality, and increased urine sodium. Normal values are as follows: urine specific gravity 1.010-1.030, serum sodium 137-147 mEq/L, urine osmolality 300-1090 mOsm/kg, and serum osmolality 275-300 mOsm/kg. Consult physician for significant findings.
- Maintain fluid restriction as prescribed. Explain necessity of this treatment to patient and significant others. Do not keep water or ice chips at the bedside. Ensure precise delivery of fluid administered intravenously by using a monitoring device.
- Elevate HOB no more than 10-20 degrees to promote venous return and thus reduce ADH release. Decreased venous return is a stimulus to the release of ADH.
- Administer demeclocycline, lithium, and furosemide as prescribed; carefully observe and document patient's response.
- Administer hypertonic sodium chloride as prescribed. Rate of administration usually is based on serial serum sodium levels. To minimize the risk of hypernatremia, make sure that specimens for laboratory tests are drawn on time. Monitor patient for evidence of increased fluid volume: increases in CVP, PAWP, and BP. Consult physician promptly for significant findings.
- Institute seizure precautions to prevent injury to the patient in the event of seizure. These include padded side rails, supplemental oxygen, bite block, and oral airway at the bedside, as well as side rails up at all times when staff member is not present.
- Provide bedside care in a calm, unhurried manner to help minimize stress and pain, both of which will increase ADH release.

ADDITIONAL NURSING DIAGNOSES

See "Hyponatremia" for **Altered protection,** p. 679.

Acute adrenal insufficiency

PATHOPHYSIOLOGY

Adrenal insufficiency (decreased production of adrenocortical hormones) occurs as a result of either dysfunction of the adrenal glands (primary) or inadequate stimulation of the adrenal glands by the anterior pituitary (secondary). Conditions associated with primary adrenal insufficiency include autoimmune disease, infection, bilateral adrenal hemorrhage, bilateral adrenalectomy, tumor invasion, and enzymatic deficiencies. A decrease in the production of adrenocortical hormones due to a reduction in functioning adrenal tissue is also termed "Addison's disease." Secondary adrenal insufficiency is associated with exogenous steroid administration and destruction of the pituitary gland by tumors, infarcts, trauma, surgery, or infection.

Acute adrenal insufficiency (addisonian crisis) is a life-threatening condition characterized by severe fluid and electrolyte imbalances related to both mineralocorticoid and glucocorticoid deficiencies. Mineralocorticoid (aldosterone) deficiency results in large urinary losses of sodium and water with the development of hyponatremia and hypovolemia. In addition, hyperkalemia and metabolic acidosis can develop due to decreased urinary excretion of potassium and hydrogen. Glucocorticoid (cortisol) deficiency intensifies the clinical effects of hypovolemia by causing a decrease in vascular tone and decreased vascular response to catecholamines (epinephrine and norepinephrine). Cortisol depletion also may cause hypoglycemia due to the body's inability to maintain blood glucose levels in the fasting state. Severe hypotension, shock, and eventually death will occur without adequate parenteral adrenocortical hormone and fluid replacement. In patients with chronic insufficiency, acute crises may be prevented by tripling replacement hormone doses during periods of stress.

ASSESSMENT

HISTORY AND RISK FACTORS Addisonian crisis may be precipitated by any extreme emotional or physiologic stressor, at which time the need for adrenal hormones is increased dramatically. Patients who take exogenous steroids are also at risk if physiologic demands increase or doses are withdrawn abruptly. Addisonian crisis is also a potential complication of adrenalectomy or hypophysectomy. It also may develop with sepsis and HIV disease.

CLINICAL PRESENTATION Hypotension (particularly postural), tachycardia, confusion, weakness, nausea, abdominal pain, hyperthermia (in some individuals).

PHYSICAL ASSESSMENT Orthostatic hypotension, poor skin turgor, sunken and soft eyeballs, muscle weakness, and weight loss. Patients with primary adrenal insufficiency may have a bronze hue to the skin secondary to excess production of ACTH.

ECG FINDINGS Signs of hyperkalemia: peaked T waves, widening QRS complex, lengthened PR interval, and flattened-to-absent P wave. As hyperkalemia worsens, these signs progress and may result in asystole.

DIAGNOSTIC TESTS

Random serum cortisol levels: Decreased.
Serum sodium levels: Decreased to <137 mEq/L.
Serum aldosterone levels: Depressed in primary Addison's disease.
Serum potassium levels: Increased to >5 mEq/L initially; may decrease dramatically with treatment.
Fasting blood glucose levels: Decreased to <80 mg/dl.

COLLABORATIVE MANAGEMENT

Glucocorticoid replacement: The crisis state requires supraphysiologic doses. An immediate IV bolus of hydrocortisone usually is administered, followed by repeat doses as needed q6-8h or by continuous infusion. Emergency mineralocorticoid replacement (fludrocortisone) usually is unnecessary due to the mineralocorticoid effects of hydrocortisone.
IV fluids: Rapid volume restoration is essential. Initially, D_5NS is the fluid of choice. Typically 1 L of fluid is given in 1 h, followed by an additional 1-2 L over the next 6-8 h as needed. Volume expanders may be used if hypotension persists.
IV glucose: Supplemental glucose usually is included in the IV fluids to correct the hypoglycemia.
Supplemental sodium: Usually provided in the form of normal saline during volume replacement.
Insertion of flow-directed pulmonary artery catheter: To assess volume status on a continuous basis.
Vasopressors: May be used if the patient does not respond to the initial therapy (see Appendix 7). Because these patients have decreased response to catecholamines, vasopressors and inotropic agents will be less effective than they would be in normal individuals.
Treatment of underlying cause.

NURSING DIAGNOSES AND INTERVENTIONS

Fluid volume deficit related to failure of regulatory mechanisms secondary to impaired secretion of aldosterone, causing increased sodium excretion with resultant diuresis
Desired outcome: Within 8 h of initiating treatment, patient is normovolemic as evidenced by BP within patient's normal range; HR 60-100 bpm; RR 12-20 breaths/min with normal pattern and depth (eupnea); CVP 2-6 mm Hg; PAWP 6-12 mm Hg; normal sinus rhythm on ECG; and orientation to time, place, and person.

- Monitor VS and hemodynamic measurements q15min until they have been stable for 1 h. Consult physician promptly for BP <90/60 mm Hg, HR >120 bpm, CVP <2 mm Hg, and PAWP <6 mm Hg.
- Monitor patient at frequent intervals for evidence of hypotension. Measure BP and HR with patient reclining, then sitting. A drop of ≥20 mm Hg or an increase in HR >20 bpm and lasting for more than 3 min after changing position indicates mild to moderate dehydration.
- Administer IV fluids as prescribed to replace extracellular fluid volume. Initially, rapid fluid replacement is essential.
- Maintain accurate I&O records. Weigh patient daily at the same time

of day with the patient wearing the same clothing and using the same scale.

- Monitor patient continuously on cardiac monitor; observe for ECG changes typical of hyperkalemia (see "ECG Findings," p. 514).
- Observe for clinical manifestations of electrolyte imbalance associated with fluid volume deficit as follows:

    Hyperkalemia: lethargy, nausea, hyperactive bowel sounds with diarrhea, numbness or tingling in extremities, muscle weakness.

    Hyponatremia: headache, malaise, muscle weakness, abdominal cramps.
- Monitor laboratory test results for abnormalities. With appropriate treatment, serum sodium levels should rise to normal and serum potassium levels should fall to normal. Normal values are: serum sodium 137-147 mEq/L and serum potassium 3.5-5.0 mEq/L. Promptly consult physician for worsening hyponatremia or hyperkalemia.
- Assess patient's LOC and respiratory status at frequent intervals. Institute safety measures as indicated. Reorient and reassure patient as needed.
- Encourage oral fluid intake as patient's condition stabilizes. Add sodium-rich foods (see Table 10-11, p. 674) as tolerated. Begin oral glucocorticoid replacement therapy as prescribed.

Risk for injury related to potential for acute regulatory dysfunction (cortisol and aldosterone deficiency) secondary to increased psychologic, emotional, or physical stressors with increased hormonal demand and inadequate adrenal reserves

Desired outcome: Patient verbalizes orientation to time, place, and person and has stable weight, urine output <80-125 ml/h, HR 60-100 bpm, BP within patient's normal range, and normothermia.

- Monitor for signs of increasing crisis: urinary output increased from usual amount, changes in LOC, orthostatic hypotension, nausea, vomiting, and tachycardia. Consult physician promptly for any of these findings.
- Provide a quiet environment to reduce external stimuli and stress. Transfer patient to private room, if possible. Keep lights dim and minimize the use of radios or other appliances.
- Monitor patient for hyperthermia. Maintain a cool environmental temperature. As prescribed, use tepid baths, antipyretics, and cooling blankets as needed to reduce body temperature.
- Assist patient with care, and provide 90-min periods of uninterrupted rest as often as possible. Speak softly and reassuringly to patient.
- Limit the number of visitors and the length of time they spend with patient. Caution visitors not to discuss stress-provoking topics with patient but rather to speak softly and reassuringly.
- Maintain strict environmental asepsis and monitor patient carefully for signs of infection. Avoid exposing patient to staff members or visitors with colds or infections.

Knowledge deficit: Prevention of acute adrenal insufficiency in patients with chronic adrenal insufficiency or steroid therapy

Desired outcome: Before discharge from ICU, patient verbalizes understanding of factors that increase the risk of adrenal crisis, how to avoid adrenal crisis, precautions that must be taken, and when to notify physician.

T A B L E   7 - 3   Patient and family education concerning glucocorticoid and mineralocorticoid replacement

---

Glucocorticoids (e.g., cortisone acetate, prednisone)
- Take medication in a diurnal pattern to mimic normal secretion (i.e., two thirds of dose in the morning and one third of dose in the afternoon).
- Take steroids with food to decrease gastric irritation.
- Weigh self regularly and report gains of >2 lb/wk to physician.
- Avoid exposure to infection, and be alert to indicators of infection (e.g., fever, nausea, diarrhea, malaise).
- Contact physician promptly during periods of physical or emotional stress; dosages will require adjustment at these times.
- Indicators of overreplacement: weight gain (moon face, truncal obesity); edema; thin, fragile skin (striae, easy bruising); slow wound healing; chronic fatigue; and emotional lability.
- Indicators of underreplacement: weight loss, hyperpigmentation, skin creases, anorexia, nausea, abdominal discomfort, chronic fatigue, depression, and irritability.

Mineralocorticoids (e.g., fludrocortisone, deoxycorticosterone acetate)
- As prescribed, modify diet with liberal amounts of sodium (see Table 10-11, p. 674), protein, and carbohydrates.
- Weigh self regularly, and report sudden gains or losses >2 lb/wk to physician.
- Contact physician promptly during periods of physical or emotional stress; dosages will require adjustment at these times.
- Indicators of overreplacement: edema, muscle weakness, hypertension.
- Indicators of underreplacement: excessive urination, weight loss, decreased skin turgor.

- Teach patient about prescribed medications, including purpose, dosage, route of administration, and potential side effects (Table 7-3). Medication administration should mimic normal diurnal pattern of plasma cortisol levels (e.g., two thirds in the morning and one third in late afternoon).
- Provide dietary instruction: Dietary sodium and potassium may need to be adjusted on the basis of the patient's clinical condition and drug therapy (see discussions of sodium and potassium in "Fluid and Electrolyte Disturbances," Chapter 10).
- Explain the importance of controlling stress, both emotional and physiologic, which increases adrenal demand. Teach patient to seek medical intervention during times of increased stress (e.g., fever, infection), inasmuch as medication dosages may need to be increased.
- Teach indicators of overreplacement and underreplacement of steroids, which require prompt medical attention (Table 7-3).
- Stress the importance of never abruptly discontinuing use of any steroid preparation. Use must be tapered to avoid precipitation of crisis.
- Remind patient of the importance of continued medical follow-up.

- Explain the procedure for obtaining a Medic-Alert bracelet or card identifying patient's diagnosis.

ADDITIONAL NURSING DIAGNOSES

See "Diabetic Ketoacidosis" for **Risk for infection,** p. 500, and **Risk for injury,** p. 500. See "Hyperosmolar Hyperglycemic Nonketotic Syndrome" for **Altered peripheral tissue perfusion,** p. 503. For other nursing diagnoses and interventions, see "Psychosocial Support," p. 88, and "Psychosocial Support for the Patient's Family and Significant Others," p. 100.

Selected Bibliography

Batcheller J: Disorders of antidiuretic hormone secretion, *AACN Clin Issues* 3(2):370-378, 1992.

Berger W, Keller U: Treatment of diabetic ketoacidosis and nonketotic hyperosmolar diabetic coma, *Baillere's Clin Endocrinol Metab* 6(1):1-22, 1992.

Blevens LS, Wand GS: Diabetes insipidus, *Crit Care Med* 20(1):69-72, 1992.

Brody GM: Diabetic ketoacidosis and hyperosmolar hyperglycemic nonketotic coma, *Top Emerg Med* 14(1):12-22, 1992.

Buonocore CM, Robinson AG: The diagnosis and management of diabetes insipidus during medical emergencies, *Endocrinol Metab Clin North Am* 22(2):411-423, 1993.

Chin R: Adrenal crisis, *Crit Care Clin* 7(1):23-42, 1991.

Epstein CD: Fluid volume deficit for the adrenal crisis patient, *Dimens Crit Care Nurs* 10(4):210-217, 1991.

Epstein CD: Adrenocortical insufficiency in the critically ill patient, *AACN Clinical Issues* 3(3):705-713, 1992.

Fleckman AM: Diabetic ketoacidosis, *Endocrinol Metab Clin North Am* 22(2):181-207, 1993.

Horne MM, Swearingen PL: *Pocket guide to fluids and electrolytes,* ed 2, St Louis, 1993, Mosby.

Horne MM, Heitz UE, Swearingen PL: *Fluid, electrolyte, and acid-base balance: a case study approach,* St Louis, 1991, Mosby.

Interqual: The ISD-A review system with adult ISD criteria, August 1992, North Hampton, NH, and Marlboro, Mass, Interqual, Inc.

Kim MJ, McFarland GK, McLane AM: *Pocket guide to nursing diagnoses,* ed 6, St Louis, 1995, Mosby.

Kovaks L, Robertson GL: Syndrome of inappropriate antidiuresis, *Endocrinol Metab Clin North Am* 21(4):859-875, 1992.

Lee LM, Gumowski J: Adrenocortical insufficiency: a medical emergency, *AACN Clinical Issues* 3(2):319-330, 1992.

Ober KP: Diabetes insipidus, *Crit Care Clin* 7(1):109-125, 1991.

Rose BD: *Clinical physiology of acid-base and electrolyte disorders,* ed 4, New York, 1994, McGraw-Hill.

Seck JR, Dunger DB: Diabetes insipidus: current treatment recommendations, *Drugs* 44(2):216-224, 1992.

Siperstein MD: Diabetic ketoacidosis and hyperosmolar coma, *Endocrinol Metab Clin North Am* 22(2):303-328, 1993.

GASTROINTESTINAL DYSFUNCTIONS

Bleeding esophageal varices

PATHOPHYSIOLOGY

With obstruction of blood flow through the liver, portal venous pressure can rise from a normal of about 7 mm Hg to as high as 20-25 mm Hg. As a result of prolonged increased portal pressure, collateral vessels develop to divert blood from the portal circulation into the systemic circulation. Obstruction of portal flow dilates the smaller veins that normally drain blood from the lower esophagus and stomach into the portal vein. These enlarged and engorged veins that develop beneath the mucosa are known as varices. Rupture of gastroesophageal varices leads to dramatic hematemesis and to hemorrhage, which is exceedingly difficult to control. Blood loss is exacerbated by thrombocytopenia and clotting disorders, which often are found in patients with hepatic disease. Portal hypertension may result in engorgement of vessels in the umbilical, retroperitoneal, and anal areas. Collateral vessels in these sites, however, are less likely to rupture and bleed.

Although any blockage of portal blood as it enters or leaves the liver can elevate portal venous pressure, the most common cause of portal hypertension is intrahepatic blockage of portal blood flow caused by hepatic cirrhosis. When portal venous blood is shunted from the liver by collateral vessels associated with portal hypertension, the liver shrinks in size and has an impaired ability to regenerate or perform normally. Large portosystemic shunts result in complications, including hepatic encephalopathy, septicemia, and metabolic abnormalities. In addition, acute blood loss from variceal bleeding results in hypoxic damage to liver cells and may precipitate complications of hepatic insufficiency such as jaundice, ascites, and encephalopathy. The mortality rate for variceal hemorrhage ranges from 35%-60% and is directly related to the degree of hepatocellular failure.

ASSESSMENT

HISTORY AND RISK FACTORS Recent episode(s) of painless and often sudden hematemesis or melena; excessive ethanol ingestion (averaging >60 g/day); previously diagnosed cirrhosis, hepatitis, intraabdominal or biliary infection; biliary disease; traumatic portal vein injury; congenital liver disease; and tumor invasion. The following events may precipitate bleeding in patients with gastroesophageal varices: (1) insertion of a gastric tube, (2) coagulopathy and/or heparin therapy, (3) mechanical irritants (e.g., rough or unchewed food), (4) Valsalva's maneuver, and (5) vigorous coughing.

CLINICAL PRESENTATION Dramatic hematemesis usually is the first and most common presentation. The average amount of blood lost during a single bleeding episode is 10 U. Melena, with or without hematemesis, is another frequent occurrence. Acute gastritis, peptic ulcer disease, and Mallory-Weiss syndrome (see "Acute Gastrointestinal Bleeding," p. 569) may contribute to the usually massive blood loss, particularly among persons with alcoholic cirrhosis. Rapid blood loss leads initially to thirst and later to dizziness and ultimately hypovolemic shock as the hemorrhage continues.

PHYSICAL ASSESSMENT In the presence of acute blood loss, cool and pale skin and altered mental status are readily apparent. Pale and dry oral mucosa and cracked lips are further evidence of hemorrhage. Yellowing of the skin and sclera is associated with jaundice, which frequently is present. Mild to marked peripheral edema generally develops within hours of bleeding onset. Splenomegaly is commonly associated with portal hypertension. In persons with cirrhosis the liver usually is small and firm. An enlarged and tender liver is associated with hepatic inflammation. Large hemorrhoids may be present on rectal examination, along with stool that contains occult or frank blood. If aspiration of gastric contents has occurred, coarse crackles and rhonchi may be auscultated.

VITAL SIGNS AND HEMODYNAMIC MEASUREMENTS Usually reflect a hypovolemic state (e.g., elevated HR, decreased BP, CVP, PAP, PAWP, CO, and stroke volume and increased SVR). Pulses will be weak and thready. A hyperdynamic cardiovascular state is present in patients. The cardiac output is elevated, peripheral vascular resistance is lowered, pulses are bounding, and the extremities will be warm and flushed. The hyperdynamic state will be more readily apparent in patients who have undergone volume resuscitation and in some patients who have had shunt surgery for portal decompression.

DIAGNOSTIC TESTS

Hematologic tests: Hct and Hgb will be decreased because of acute blood loss and mild anemia associated with hypersplenism. Liver disease and alcoholism may cause an increase in mean corpuscular volume (MCV). When the MCV is increased, the RBC is said to be macrocytic, and thus anemia may be termed macrocytic and normochromic (normal hemoglobin). Platelet and WBC counts may be decreased because of splenic enlargement. PT is prolonged as a result of clotting factor deficiency in patients with hepatocellular disease. The clotting deficiency usually is unresponsive to vitamin K therapy.

Biochemical tests: The severity of liver damage can be estimated by elevations of values in serum total bilirubin, decreases in serum albumin (see "Hepatic Failure," p. 536), and prolongation of PT. The serum ammonia level is elevated as blood is shunted from the liver by collateral vessels and the failing liver is unable to convert ammonia to urea. A large protein load from GI bleeding results in greatly increased ammonia levels if hepatic failure is severe. Dietary protein and blood in the GI tract will increase serum ammonia levels. Antibiotic therapy may decrease the levels.

Note: Blood specimens for serum ammonia should be placed in ice and transported to the laboratory immediately after collection to ensure accuracy of the test.

Blood alcohol: May be tested upon patient's admission to help distinguish acute intoxication from encephalopathy.

Occult blood tests: To test for blood in stool or gastric secretions.

Esophagoscopy: Visualizes the esophagus and stomach directly *via* a fiberoptic esophagoscope. Varices in the esophagus and upper portion of the stomach are identified, and attempts are made to identify the exact source of bleeding. Variceal bleeding may be treated by injection sclerotherapy during the endoscopic procedure (see "Collaborative Management" in the following section). Aspiration and cardiac dysrhythmias are serious complications of the procedure. Endotracheal intubation may be performed before the procedure to protect the airway. See Table 8-1 for nursing implications of esophagoscopy.

T A B L E 8 - 1   Nursing care for the patient undergoing esophagoscopy

---

Before procedure
- Explain procedure to patient and significant others.
- Maintain NPO status for 8 h before procedure.
- Clear stomach of blood and gastric contents immediately before endoscope is passed.
- Verify patency of two large-bore (≥16-gauge) IV catheters.
- Administer sedatives as prescribed. Be aware that dosage usually is reduced if cirrhosis or hepatitis is diagnosed.

During procedure
- Maintain patient in side-lying position to reduce likelihood of aspiration.
- Have pharyngeal and tracheal suction readily available.

After procedure
- Maintain side-lying position until patient is fully alert.
- Note evidence of change in rate of hemorrhage.
- Be alert for immediate complications, such as aspiration pneumonia (evidenced by difficulty breathing, diminished breath sounds, coarse crackles, and rhonchi), cardiac dysrhythmias, and perforation (rare; evidenced by severe retrosternal pain and bleeding).

T A B L E   8 - 2   Nursing care for the patient undergoing angiographic studies

Before procedure
- Explain procedure to patient and significant others.
- Maintain NPO status for 8 h before procedure.
- Verify patency of IV catheter.
- Note allergies to seafood, iodine, and contrast material.
- Administer sedatives as prescribed. Be aware that dosage usually is reduced if cirrhosis or hepatitis is diagnosed.

During procedure
- Assist radiology personnel with positioning and draping patient.
- Monitor VS q15min or more often for evidence of anaphylaxis or hemorrhagic shock.

After procedure
- Check VS q15min initially and q1-2h once patient's condition has stabilized.
- Maintain patient in supine position with affected leg straight.
- Keep pressure dressing and sandbag over puncture site for 6-8 h.
- Evaluate distal pulses and perfusion in affected extremity q1-2h for 8 h. Arterial thrombosis and large hematomas that compromise femoral blood flow may develop as a result of manipulation of the artery and clotting abnormalities associated with liver disease.
- Monitor urine output q1-2h, and report volume <0.5 ml/kg/h.

Angiographic studies: Establish patency of the portal vein and visualize the portosystemic collateral vessels to determine cause and effective treatment for variceal bleeding. Portal venous anatomy must be established before such operations as portal systemic shunt or hepatic transplantation. In patients with previously constructed surgical shunts, patency may be confirmed. See Table 8-2 for nursing implications of angiographic studies.
- The most common procedure is portal venography by indirect angiography. The femoral artery is catheterized, and contrast material is injected into the splenic artery. Contrast material flows through the spleen into the splenic and portal veins.
- Hepatic vein wedge pressure (HVWP) is measured by introducing a balloon catheter into the femoral vein and threading it into a hepatic vein branch. Normal HVWP is 5-6 mm Hg; values of about 20 mm Hg are typical for patients with cirrhosis.
- Direct access to the portal vein may be achieved through transhepatic portography. During this procedure, varices may be obliterated by injection of thrombin or Gelfoam into veins that supply the varices.

Note: Transhepatic portography involves a direct puncture through the liver and has many of the same risks as does liver biopsy. Patients returning from this procedure should be positioned on their right side and monitored closely. (See "Liver Biopsy" in "Hepatic Failure," p. 537).

Barium swallow: Used in nonemergent situations to verify the presence of gastroesophageal varices.

Note: The patient should be on NPO status from midnight until completion of the test. Because of the constipating effects of barium, which can precipitate or enhance hepatic encephalopathy, laxatives or enemas should be given upon patient's return from the procedure.

Liver biopsy: See "Hepatic Failure," p. 537.

COLLABORATIVE MANAGEMENT

Management of gastroesophageal variceal bleeding depends on the underlying cause of portal hypertension, the severity of the bleeding episode, and the previous response to therapy. Every attempt is made to stop the bleeding and preserve liver function. Optimizing liver function is especially important for patients with cirrhosis and underlying hepatocellular disease in order to reduce the risk of disabling encephalopathy.

Fluid resuscitation: Restoration of blood volume is achieved with combinations of isotonic IV solutions, albumin, packed red cells, and fresh-frozen plasma. Until blood products are available, emergency resuscitation with D_5W and albumin, sodium chloride, or Ringer's lactate (RL) is initiated. Excessive saline infusions usually are avoided because sodium is retained and contributes to ascites. RL is not recommended for patients with significant liver dysfunction because the damaged liver may not be able to convert the lactate to bicarbonate. Serum lactate accumulates and contributes to metabolic acidosis. Packed red cells are administered as soon as available to maintain an Hct of 28%-30%. Fresh-frozen plasma is helpful in restoring deficient clotting factors. Platelets are given only if the platelet count is markedly reduced or if spontaneous bleeding from sites other than the varices occurs. Albumin is administered if the patient continues to be hypovolemic despite an Hct in the 28%-30% range or if the patient is hypoalbuminemic. Hydroxyethyl starch (hetastarch) and dextran generally are avoided because these agents may trigger abnormalities in hemostasis. Hemodynamic monitoring of VS, CVP, PAWP, and other parameters is essential to prevent hypovolemic shock while avoiding overtransfusion and associated cardiopulmonary problems. In addition, overtransfusion increases variceal pressure and triggers rebleeding. Serial hematocrit evaluations are necessary to estimate ongoing blood loss and need for RBC replacement.

Vasopressin (Pitressin):   A potent vasoconstrictor that controls variceal hemorrhage by constricting the mesenteric, splenic, and hepatic arteriolar beds, thereby reducing blood flow to the portal vein and lowering portal venous pressure. Vasopressin, 20 U in 100 ml D_5W, is given intravenously over a 20-min period. A continuous IV infusion of 0.1-0.4 U/min is delivered for a prolonged effect. IV nitroglycerin may be given with vasopressin to counter vasopressin-induced cardiac side effects such as vasoconstriction. In addition, portal venous constriction is reduced, thus contributing to the beneficial effects of vasopressin. Close supervision and cardiac monitoring are essential because of the many serious side effects associated with vasopressin (Table 8-3).

T A B L E   8 - 3   Adverse effects of vasopressin

Cardiovascular
  Increased cardiac afterload
  Baroreceptor-mediated bradycardia
  Decreased coronary blood flow
  Impaired cardiac contractility
  Dysrhythmias, including PVC and ventricular tachycardia
  Myocardial ischemia and infarction

Gastrointestinal
  Splanchnic vasoconstriction resulting in bowel ischemia and necrosis
  Increased gut motility resulting in abdominal cramps and diarrhea

Other
  Increased water reabsorption by the kidneys, resulting in antidiuresis and
    water intoxication
  Stimulation of release of plasminogen activator and factor VIII
  Respiratory arrest
  Cerebral hemorrhage

Gastric intubation: A large-lumen gastric tube may be inserted to aspirate blood and clots from the stomach. Frequently, insertion of the tube triggers additional bleeding, and thus this intervention usually is avoided if the source of bleeding is known to be variceal. Lavage with saline or sterile water is helpful in clearing blood from the stomach in order to estimate bleeding or prepare the patient for endoscopy.

Endoscopic sclerotherapy: During endoscopy, varices are injected with a sclerosing solution such as sodium tetradecyl sulfate or morrhuate to contract the varix and stop the bleeding. The sclerosing solution causes inflammation of the varix, venous thrombosis, and eventually scar tissue. Repeated injections strengthen scar tissue in the esophageal wall and lower the risk of recurrent hemorrhage. This treatment is used both to control acute bleeding and to manage long-term bleeding *via* chronic, serial injections. Chronic sclerotherapy limits additional bleeding in many patients, but emergency surgery is necessary if rebleeding becomes uncontrollable. A serious complication of sclerotherapy is esophageal ulceration (see Table 8-4 for other complications). Ulcer prophylaxis with antacids, H_2-receptor blockers, or sucralfate may be initiated.

Esophageal balloon tamponade: Achieves temporary control of variceal hemorrhage *via* inflation of esophageal and gastric balloons until the balloon pressure exceeds variceal pressure and thereby tamponades the bleeding vessels. A multilumen tube (Sengstaken-Blakemore [S-B], Minnesota) is passed through the mouth into the stomach. The gastric balloon is inflated with 250-300 ml of air. The esophageal balloon is inflated to a pressure of 20-45 mm Hg. The gastric balloon is never deflated while the esophageal balloon is inflated. Firm traction is exerted by taping the tube to a firm pad or to the mouth guard of a football helmet, which maintains correct positioning. Complications are numerous and include pharyngeal obstruction with possible asphyxia, as well as mucosal erosion with variceal rupture and

T A B L E 8 - 4   Side effects and complications of esophageal sclerotherapy

Anticipated/mild side effects
Mild restrosternal pain
Transient fever
Diminished breath sounds
Transient dysphagia
Local ulcerations

Serious side effects/complications
Bleeding from remaining varices or ulcers
Stricture formation evidenced by prolonged dysphagia
Perforation evidenced by bleeding, severe substernal pain, or fever
Pulmonary problems, including aspiration pneumonia, pleural effusion, mediastinitis
Bacteremia evidenced by fever, tachycardia, positive blood culture results

---

exsanguination. Esophageal balloon tamponade is useful for control of acute bleeding, but the esophageal balloon should not be inflated for more than 24 h. A high rebleeding rate restricts its use to a preliminary intervention for variceal sclerosis or surgery. (See Table 8-5 for nursing care for the patient with esophageal balloon tamponade.)
Surgical management: Emergency surgery for variceal bleeding is associated with a higher operative mortality rate than elective procedures. It is desirable to control acute bleeding medically and schedule elective surgery at a later time when the patient's condition has stabilized. Portosystemic shunts lower portal pressure by joining the portal vein with the vena cava. The disadvantage of these procedures is total diversion of portal blood flow and consequent disabling encephalopathy in many patients (see "Hepatic Failure" for additional information on portal blood flow and encephalopathy). The distal splenorenal shunt diverts blood from the troublesome varices *via* the short gastric and splenic veins to the renal vein. Portal blood flow to the liver is preserved, and the incidence of encephalopathy is greatly reduced. This procedure is much more difficult to perform and requires a high degree of surgical expertise. Other surgical methods include stapling transection of the lower portion of the esophagus and devascularization procedures. These procedures control hemorrhage, but portal pressure remains high and the risk of recurrent hemorrhage is substantial.

NURSING DIAGNOSES AND INTERVENTIONS

Fluid volume deficit related to active loss of circulating blood volume secondary to variceal bleeding
Desired outcome: Within 12 h of this diagnosis, patient becomes normovolemic as evidenced by MAP >70 mm Hg, HR 60-100 bpm, brisk capillary refill (<2 sec), CVP 2-6 mm Hg, PAWP 6-12 mm Hg, CI $\geq$3 L/min/m^2, urinary output $\geq$0.5 ml/kg/h, and orientation to time, place, and person.
- Administer prescribed fluids at rapid rate (wide open for active, massive bleeding). See "Fluid Resuscitation," p. 523, for types of fluids

---

T A B L E 8 - 5   **Nursing implications for the patient undergoing esophageal balloon tamponade**

Before insertion

Check all lumens for patency.

Inflate all balloons and check for leaks.

Label each lumen to prevent confusion and accidental deflation of gastric balloon after insertion.

Have water-soluble lubricant, manometer, wall suction, large syringe, and traction pad or helmet readily available.

Assist physician with emptying stomach of blood.

Have Yankauer and ET suction equipment at bedside for use in the event of vomiting.

Schedule chest x-ray to confirm tube placement immediately after insertion.

After insertion

Elevate HOB 30-45 degrees to prevent esophageal reflux.

Check tube traction and esophageal balloon pressure q2-4h.

Ensure patency and low, intermittent suction of gastric and nasopharyngeal lumens.

Perform oral care q2-4h.

Ensure that scissors are readily available to transect the tube if respiratory distress occurs.

For additional information, see **Ineffective airway clearance,** p. 528, and **Altered esophageal tissue perfusion,** p. 529.

---

indicated. Minimize IV infusion of sodium-containing solutions, which can contribute to fluid sequestration in the abdomen (ascites) and precipitate hepatorenal syndrome in susceptible patients (see "Hepatic Failure," p. 541).

- Monitor BP q15min, or more frequently in the presence of brisk bleeding. Be alert to decreases in MAP >10 mm Hg less than baseline.
- Monitor HR, ECG, and cardiovascular status q15min or more frequently in the presence of active bleeding or if using vasopressin or similar agents. Be alert to increases in HR, delayed capillary refill, and changes in LOC, which reflect hypovolemia. Be aware that an altered LOC can be caused by encephalopathy as well as by hypovolemia. Anticipate vasopressin-induced reflex bradycardia; consult physician if bradycardia is severe (HR <60 bpm) or compromises tissue perfusion.
- Measure central pressures and thermodilution CO/CI q1-2h, or more frequently if the patient is unstable or receiving vasoactive agents. Be alert to low or decreasing CVP and PAWP. Assess for signs of overaggressive fluid resuscitation, including elevated CVP, PAP, and PAWP and aggravation of variceal bleeding in some patients. Anticipate compensatory increases in CO/CI, with CI usually ≥3. Monitor Svo_2 as available to evaluate adequacy of tissue oxygenation. Evaluate volume status by noting increases or decreases in PAWP values and urinary output.

- Measure urinary output hourly. Be alert to output <0.5 ml/kg/h for 2 consecutive hours. Anticipate decreased urinary output after initial dose of vasopressin. Expect diuresis after vasopressin has been discontinued.
- Monitor for physical indicators of hypovolemia, including cool extremities, capillary refill ≥ 2 sec, absent or decreased amplitude of distal pulses, and change in LOC.
- Measure and record all GI blood losses from hematemesis, hematochezia (red blood through rectum), and melena. Test all stools and gastric contents for occult blood.
- Administer vasopressin as prescribed. Ensure patency of IV catheter. Monitor for serious side effects such as bradycardia, ventricular irritability, chest pain, abdominal cramping, hyponatremia, water intoxication, and oliguria (see Table 8-3). Administer vasopressin concurrently with IV nitroglycerin to reduce adverse cardiovascular effects and improve efficacy. Consult physician and reduce rate of infusion in the presence of serious adverse effects.
- Be alert to adverse side effects of esophageal sclerotherapy: infection, pulmonary complications (i.e., Pao_2 <80 mm Hg, basilar crackles, diminished breath sounds), and esophageal ulceration (i.e., difficulty swallowing, pain, continued bleeding). Anticipate mild retrosternal pain and transient fever after the procedure.
- Avoid use of indwelling gastric tubes for routine gastric drainage because they can irritate varices and prolong or renew bleeding.

Decreased cardiac output related to altered rate or rhythm secondary to myocardial ischemia from prolonged, massive bleeding or vasopressin-induced coronary vasoconstriction; related to decreased preload secondary to acute blood loss; or related to increased afterload secondary to vasoconstrictive effects of shock or vasopressin therapy

Desired outcome: Within 24 h of this diagnosis, patient's cardiac output is adequate as evidenced by normal sinus rhythm on ECG, CI within normal limits or increased (≥ 3 L/min/m^2), MAP >70 mm Hg, and Svo_2 60%-80%.

- Monitor BP, HR, ECG, and PAP (see first four entries under preceding nursing diagnosis, **Fluid volume deficit**).
- Monitor ABG values for evidence of hypoxemia. Be alert to and consult physician for Pao_2 <80 mm Hg. Administer oxygen if its need is indicated by ABG values. Place patient in semi-Fowler's position to optimize oxygenation.
- Monitor Hct; consult physician for values <28-30/100 ml.
- Monitor patient for evidence of myocardial ischemia if Hgb is greatly decreased or if the patient is receiving vasopressin (see eighth entry in preceding nursing diagnosis). Observe ECG for ventricular dysrhythmias and ST-segment changes. Instruct patient to report chest discomfort promptly. Administer PRN nitrates as prescribed.
- Minimize patient's activity during acute bleeding episode in order to reduce myocardial oxygen demands. Explain and encourage adherence to total bed rest regimen. As available monitor Svo_2 to evaluate adequacy of tissue oxygenation (see Table 1-16, p. 38).

- Measure thermodilution CO q1-2h. Be aware that a "normal" CO may be a low value for the patient with a hyperdynamic circulatory state associated with cirrhosis. Maintain CI ≥ 3 L/min/m^2.
- Maintain MAP >70-80 mm Hg (see preceding nursing diagnosis, **Fluid volume deficit**) to promote adequate tissue perfusion. Avoid excessive fluids and hypervolemia, which could increase variceal bleeding.

Ineffective airway clearance related to tracheobronchial obstruction by esophageal balloon device; tracheobronchial obstruction by pharyngeal secretions above the inflated esophageal balloon device; or perceptual/cognitive impairment secondary to encephalopathy

Desired outcome: Within 4 h of this diagnosis, patient's airway becomes clear as evidenced by auscultation of normal breath sounds, absence of adventitious sounds, and RR 12-20 breaths/min with normal depth and pattern (eupnea).

- Position patient in a side-lying position during vomiting episodes unless he or she is *fully* alert and is more comfortable in an upright position.
- As necessary, suction oropharynx with Yankauer or similar suction device to remove blood and secretions.
- Auscultate lung fields during and after vomiting episodes for presence of rhonchi, which can signal aspiration of gastric contents.
- Provide oral care at frequent intervals to assist in mobilizing oropharyngeal secretions. A dilute solution of hydrogen peroxide and normal saline may be helpful in removing dried blood from the teeth and oral mucosa. Use saline to rinse hydrogen peroxide solution from patient's mouth.
- Monitor for early signs of respiratory failure: increasing RR, WOB, and $Paco_2$ and decreasing Spo_2 *via* continuous pulse oximetry and decreasing Pao_2.
- Implement the following interventions for patients with an S-B or similar tube:
  □ Consult physician regarding possibility of ET intubation before S-B tube insertion.
  □ Verify proper tube placement by immediate chest x-ray.
  □ Be certain that oral secretions are suctioned from above the inflated esophageal balloon *via* a proximal tube or an additional lumen in the tube for this purpose. Label proximal tube or lumen with the warning "Do not irrigate."
  □ Ensure patency of gastric and esophageal drainage lumens. Irrigate *gastric* lumen q1-2h, and as necessary, to ensure patency.
  □ Be aware that proximal migration of the esophageal balloon or rupture of the gastric balloon may result in total airway obstruction. Auscultate breath sounds q1-2h. Keep a pair of scissors in an obvious place near the patient at all times in order to cut and immediately deflate all lumens of the S-B tube should respiratory distress occur.
  □ Check security of tape, tube connections, and traction initially and q2h. Firm traction is established by taping the tube to a helmet or a firm, padded retainer. The traction device should be designed

so that it minimizes pressure to facial tissue and prevents tissue necrosis.
  ▫ Document quantity and characteristics of gastric drainage q4h.

Altered esophageal tissue perfusion (or risk for same) related to interruption of venous and arterial blood flow secondary to pressure on esophageal tissue from balloon tamponade; or hypovolemia secondary to variceal hemorrhage

Desired outcomes: Esophageal balloon pressure is maintained within prescribed range (usually 20-45 mm Hg). Patient has no symptoms of esophageal perforation as evidenced by BP within patient's normal range, HR 60-100 bpm, PAP $\geq$20/6, PAWP $\geq$6 mm Hg, SVR $\leq$1,200 dynes/sec/cm^{-5}, CI $\geq$3 L/min/m^2, and absence of sudden substernal or back pain.

• Check the esophageal balloon pressure q2-4h. Maintain pressure within prescribed range (usually 20-45 mm Hg). Release pressure at prescribed intervals.

• Carefully document date and time of balloon inflation and deflation. Tissue necrosis is likely to occur if balloons are left inflated for >24 h.

• After 24 h, assist physician in relieving traction and deflating the esophageal balloon. The tube remains in place with the gastric balloon inflated for the next 24 h, and the patient is closely monitored for rebleeding. If there is no further rebleeding, the gastric balloon is deflated and the tube removed.

• Promptly consult physician for signs of esophageal perforation: sudden epigastric or substernal pain, back pain, shock state.

Impaired swallowing (or risk for same) related to mechanical obstruction secondary to edema or stricture formation after sclerotherapy; or irritated esophageal tissue secondary to sclerotherapy or balloon tamponade

Desired outcome: By the time of discharge from ICU or hospital, patient swallows food and demonstrates ability to pass food through the lower esophagus into the stomach.

• After sclerotherapy treatments, evaluate patient for subjective complaints of difficulty in swallowing or pain during swallowing. Consult physician for significant findings.

• Plan a soft or bland diet, as tolerated by patient, which can be initiated 24 h after sclerotherapy.

• Avoid mechanically or chemically irritating foods.

• Caution patient that certain foods or substances (e.g., alcohol) may cause a burning sensation during the swallowing process due to esophageal mucosal erosion. Instruct patient to avoid mechanical or chemical irritants.

Knowledge deficit: Lack of exposure to health care information or cognitive limitation secondary to hepatic encephalopathy

Desired outcome: Within the 24-h period before hospital discharge, patient states the signs and symptoms of variceal hemorrhage, the importance of medical follow-up, and the necessity of avoiding activities that increase the risk of variceal bleeding.

• Teach patient the signs and symptoms of actual or impending hemorrhage, including nausea, dark stools, lightheadedness, vomiting of

blood, or passing of frank blood in stools. Stress the importance of seeking medical attention promptly if indicators of hemorrhage appear.
- Stress the importance of medical follow-up for management of variceal bleeding, either chronic sclerotherapy or shunt surgery.
- Describe all medications, including drug name, purpose, dosage, schedule, precautions, and potential side effects.
- Caution about the necessity of avoiding heavy lifting, straining, and other activities associated with the Valsalva maneuver.
- Teach the importance of avoiding mechanically irritating foods, such as nuts, corn chips, and unchewed food, and ingestion of nonsteroidal antiinflammatory agents and alcohol, which irritate the esophageal and gastric mucosa.

ADDITIONAL NURSING DIAGNOSES

If portal hypertension is caused by cirrhosis, refer to "Hepatic Failure" for additional nursing diagnoses. For other nursing diagnoses and interventions, see "Psychosocial Support," p. 88, and "Psychosocial Support for the Patient's Family and Significant Others," p. 100.

Hepatic failure

PATHOPHYSIOLOGY

Hepatic failure is loss of the functional capacity of the liver due to extensive hepatocellular damage. The damage may occur slowly, as with cirrhosis, or suddenly, as with acute viral or drug-induced hepatitis. The difference between acute and chronic hepatic failure primarily is the degree and rate of hepatocellular damage and the severity of the portal hypertension.

Cirrhosis: A chronic liver disease associated with widespread tissue necrosis, fibrosis, and nodule formation within the liver. Common causes of cirrhosis include chronic alcohol ingestion; viral hepatitis types B (HBV) and C (HCV) (Table 8-6); prolonged cholestasis; and metabolic disorders. Changes in liver structure due to cirrhosis are irreversible, but compensation of liver function can be achieved if the liver is protected from further damage by cessation of alcohol ingestion or arrest of inflammatory processes.

Acute hepatic failure: Characterized by a sudden and severe liver decompensation due to massive hepatocellular necrosis. Acute hepatic failure may present as the terminal stage of chronic liver disease (e.g., cirrhosis), or it may be the result of an acute process such as viral hepatitis, drug reaction, poisoning, alcoholic hepatitis, or shock, especially severe and prolonged septic shock.

The term "fulminant hepatic failure" (FHF) is used when severe acute hepatic failure with encephalopathy develops in an individual without preexisting liver disease (Kucharski, 1993). FHF develops rarely in persons with viral hepatitis. Hepatitis B, alone or together with hepatitis D, is the most frequent cause of FHF. The frequency of FHF is low in individuals with hepatitis A or C infections. Most cases of viral hepatitis are mild; many are undiagnosed.

Because preexisting liver damage generally is absent in patients with acute hepatic failure, the massive damage is potentially reversible and those who survive the acute episode usually recover completely. Individuals with alcoholic liver disease present a unique set of problems in that they may sustain an acute episode of hepatic failure superimposed on chronic failure due to preexisting cirrhosis.

Jaundice associated with hepatic failure occurs largely due to the inability of the failing liver to metabolize bilirubin. *Metabolic encephalopathy,* with varying alterations in consciousness and mental functioning, is attributed to ammonia toxicity and other metabolic derangements. Increased ICP and cerebral edema are present with acute hepatic failure but usually are not seen in chronic hepatic failure. In patients with cirrhosis, diversion of portal blood flow *via* large collateral vessels contributes to the encephalopathy. *Bleeding tendencies* are caused by inadequate vitamin K absorption, failure of the liver to synthesize clotting factors or clear activated clotting factors, and thrombocytopenia. *Infections,* including sepsis, are common as a result of a generalized state of debilitation and failure of the liver to produce immune-related proteins and filter blood from the intestines. *Circulatory abnormalities* often are present and include a hyperdynamic systemic circulation, with increased cardiac output and decreased vasomotor tone. Circulatory changes in the pulmonary system include dilatation of the pulmonary vasculature and pulmonary arteriovenous shunting with ventilation-perfusion mismatch. In addition, an increased preglomerular vascular resistance reduces glomerular filtration and may result in functional renal failure (hepatorenal syndrome). *Fluid retention* and *ascites* are attributed to several factors, including (1) intrahepatic vascular obstruction with transudation of fluid into the peritoneum, (2) defective albumin synthesis, resulting in decreased colloid osmotic pressure with failure to retain intravascular fluid, and (3) disturbances of various hormones, including renin, aldosterone, and renal prostaglandins, resulting in sodium and water retention. Ascites and edema are associated with chronic and acute hepatic failure, although massive ascites usually is due to cirrhosis. *Metabolic abnormalities* include severe hypoglycemia because of a loss of hepatic glycogen stores and impaired degradation of insulin. Dilutional hyponatremia is caused by secondary hyperaldosteronism. Hypokalemia occurs frequently due to hyperaldosteronism, excessive renal losses prompted by alkalosis, and use of loop diuretics. Hypokalemia increases renal production of ammonia, which contributes to hepatic encephalopathy.

Although prognosis with hepatic failure is difficult to evaluate, the presence of one or more of the following conditions suggests a less-than-favorable outcome: severe prolonged jaundice, persistent ascites, persistently decreased albumin, persistently prolonged prothrombin times, and severe encephalopathy.

ASSESSMENT

HISTORY AND RISK FACTORS Previous hepatic or biliary disease, including cirrhosis, hepatitis, cholecystitis, and metabolic liver disease (e.g., Wilson's disease, alpha-antitrypsin deficiency); excessive alcohol in-

T A B L E 8 - 6   Types and characteristics of viral hepatitis

	Hepatitis A virus	Hepatitis B virus	Hepatitis C virus	Hepatitis D virus	Hepatitis E virus
Likely modes of transmission	Fecal-oral. Food-borne most common; parenteral transmission rare. Most infectious 2 wk before symptoms appear	Contact with blood or serum, sexual contact, perinatal. Often transmitted by chronic carriers. Most infectious before symptoms appear and for 4-6 mo after acute infection	Contact with blood or serum. Perinatal transmission rare unless coexistent HIV infection in mother. Often transmitted by chronic carriers. Most infectious 1-2 wk before symptoms appear and throughout acute infection	Similar to HBV; can cause infection only in presence of HBV. Infectious throughout course of HDV infection	Fecal-oral, food-borne or water-borne routes
Population most often affected	Children; individuals in areas with poor sanitation	Injecting drug users, health care and public safety workers with exposure to blood, clients and staff of institutions for the developmentally disabled, homosexual men, men and women with multiple hetero-	Injecting drug users, recipients of blood products prior to 1991. Potential risk to health care and public safety workers exposed to blood	Infects only individuals with HBV infection. Injecting drug users, hemophiliacs who are recipients of certain blood products, and recipients of multiple blood transfusions	Individuals living in or traveling to parts of Asia, Africa, and Mexico where sanitation is poor

	HAV	HBV	HCV	HDV	HEV
		sexual partners, young children of infected mothers, recipients of certain blood products, hemodialysis patients			
Incubation	2-6 wk	6 wk-6 mo	18-180 days	Variable; not well established	Not well established
Serum markers of acute disease	Antibody to HAV (anti-HAV). IgG class antibody to HAV (IgG anti-HAV) also indicates immunity present	HBsAg, HBeAg, IgM class antibody to HBcAg (IgM anti-HBc)	Only available test is antibody to HCV (anti-HCV), which detects chronic, not acute, cases	Antibody to HDV (anti-HDV)	Not available
Measures for reducing exposure	Handwashing; good personal hygiene; sanitation; Standard Precautions (see Appendix 8)	Handwashing; good personal hygiene; Standard Precautions (see Appendix 8); autoclaving all nondisposable items; avoidance of used needles; careful handling of needles and sharps	As for HBV	As for HBV	As for HAV

Continued

T A B L E   8 - 6   Types and characteristics of viral hepatitis—cont'd

	Hepatitis A virus	Hepatitis B virus	Hepatitis C virus	Hepatitis D virus	Hepatitis E virus
Prophylaxis	Sanitation measures; IG before exposure or 1-2 wk after exposure	Immunization of all health care workers with blood contact, as well as risk groups identified above; HBIG for known exposure to HBsAg-contaminated material; routine immunization of children; condom use; screening of donated blood; protective devices for health care workers	Screening of donated blood; protective devices for health care workers. No vaccine for HCV	Immunization against HBV	Effectiveness of IG manufactured in United States is unknown
Comments	Symptoms usually mild. Rarely causes fulminant hepatic failure	HBsAg persists in carrier state. Chronic hepatitis may develop. Fulminant hepatic failure may ensue	Carrier state and chronic hepatitis may develop. Fulminant hepatic failure may ensue	Increased risk of serious complications (including fulminant hepatic failure) and death. Carrier state and chronic hepatitis may develop	Disease not endemic in United States or Western Europe

CDC, Centers for Disease Control; *HAV*, hepatitis A virus; *HBV*, hepatitis B virus; *HCV*, hepatitis C virus; *HDV*, hepatitis D virus; *HEV*, hepatitis E virus; *IgG*, immunoglobulin G; *IG*, immune globulin; *HBsAg*, hepatitis B surface antigen; *HBeAg*, hepatitis Be antigen; *IgM*, immunoglobulin M; *HBIG*, hepatitis B immune globulin.

gestion; blood transfusion (hepatitis C is the most common transfusion-related hepatitis and is more likely to result in chronic infection than other forms); and exposure to hepatotoxic agents such as halothane, MAO inhibitors, isoniazid, acetaminophen (dose >10 g), and carbon tetrachloride. See Table 8-6 for high-risk populations for each type of hepatitis.

CLINICAL PRESENTATION Neurologic symptoms range from mild confusion to delirium and sometimes deep coma. Jaundice is present in varying degrees, according to the extent of hepatocellular impairment. Urine may be dark because of the presence of bilirubin, and stools may be light because of its absence. Portal hypertension and variceal bleeding (see p. 519) may be present, usually associated with preexisting liver disease. Ascites and edema are common findings. In the later stages of hepatic failure, deep coma, seizures, and decerebrate rigidity are possible.

PHYSICAL ASSESSMENT Jaundice, which usually is present, manifests in the sclera in the early stages and is seen as generalized deep-yellow skin with late or fulminant failure; fluid sequestration noted as edema, ascites, and weight gain; and weight loss and muscle wasting in patients with chronic hepatic failure. Small, bright-red vascular spiders (spider telangiectasis, spider angioma), which frequently are found on the upper portion of the trunk and on the face, neck, and arms of patients with cirrhosis, are notably absent in patients with fulminant hepatic failure. The patient may have a fixed facial expression, slowness of speech and movement, and asterixis (flapping tremor of the hands that occurs with finger extension).

Fetor hepaticus, a sweet fecal odor, may be detected on the patient's breath, especially with severe failure. Multiple ecchymotic areas, purpura, and bleeding of the oral and nasal mucosa are manifestations of clotting abnormalities. Hyperdynamic circulatory changes are manifested by tachycardia, warm extremities, an active precordial impulse, and frequently a soft systolic ejection murmur. Fine crackles may be auscultated if pleural effusion or ascites is present. Cyanosis and nail clubbing may be present in persons with chronic liver disease. These findings are related to pulmonary arteriovenous shunting and ventilation-perfusion mismatch. In chronic liver disease the liver usually is small and hard. Individuals with fulminant failure often have an enlarged, firm liver. The spleen usually is enlarged with chronic failure. Distended abdomen with shifting dullness to percussion and positive fluid wave are present due to ascites. Hydrothorax caused by transdiaphragmatic passage of ascitic fluid into the pleural cavity results in dyspnea, decreased breath sounds, and dullness to percussion on the affected (usually right) side. With severe ascites, hernias are common and the umbilicus frequently is everted. The cardiac apex may be elevated and displaced laterally due to a raised diaphragm. Usually, neck veins are distended as a result of increased RAP caused by increased intrapleural pressures from diaphragmatic elevation. Hormonal changes that result in gynecomastia, testicular atrophy, and scant body hair are common in men with chronic hepatic disease.

VITAL SIGNS AND HEMODYNAMIC MEASUREMENTS Elevated temperature due to infection, normal to bounding pulses, low to normal BP, elevated cardiac output associated with decreased peripheral vascular resistance and expanded total blood volume. In the presence of tense ascites, which increases intraabdominal pressure, patient will exhibit impaired right ventricular filling with decreased stroke volume and decreased cardiac output. With massive variceal hemorrhage or late septic shock, pulses will be diminished and BP will be low, reflecting circulatory collapse.

DIAGNOSTIC TESTS

Virologic markers: Hepatitis A antibody (anti-HAV) is detected in the serum several weeks after the initial infection and continues to be detectable for many years after the infection. The presence of IgM anti-HAV is more helpful diagnostically because it implies a recent infection. The hepatitis B surface antigen (HBsAg) appears about 6 wk after hepatitis B viral infection. The presence of HBsAg for >6 mo is suggestive of a carrier state. The presence of serum IgM or IgG anti-delta markers indicates a coinfection or suprainfection of the delta virus in patients with acute or carrier-state hepatitis B. Antibodies to hepatitis C virus (anti-HCV) are present after infection with HCV. Hepatitis B virus can result in severe acute and chronic infections. Suprainfection with delta virus increases the likelihood for fulminant hepatitis. Hepatitis C infection often becomes chronic.

Serum biochemical tests

Bilirubin levels: Elevated due to failure in hepatocyte metabolism and obstruction in some instances. Very high or persistently elevated levels are considered a poor prognostic sign.

Alkaline phosphatase (ALP) levels: Usually elevated. Isoenzyme of liver origin (ALP_1) is elevated with liver disease. Elevated ALP_2 reflects bone disease.

Alanine aminotransferase (ALT/SGPT):   This enzyme is found primarily in the liver. Elevations are sensitive and specific indicators of liver dysfunction. Usually values >300 IU/L are present with acute hepatic failure.

Aspartate aminotransferase (AST/SGOT):   This enzyme is present in the heart muscle, liver, and skeletal muscle. An AST/ALT ratio >1.0 is present with alcoholic cirrhosis and liver congestion. The ratio is <1.0 with acute hepatitis and viral hepatitis.

Albumin level: Reduced, especially with ascites. Persistently low levels suggest a poor prognosis.

Sodium levels: Normal to low. Sodium is retained but is associated with water retention, which results in normal sodium levels or even a dilutional hyponatremia. Often severe hyponatremia is present in the terminal stage and is associated with tense ascites and hepatorenal syndrome.

Potassium levels: Slightly reduced unless patient has renal insufficiency, which would result in hyperkalemia. Hypokalemic acidosis is common in patients with chronic alcoholic liver disease.

Glucose levels: Hypoglycemia usually is present due to impaired gluconeogenesis and glycogen depletion in patients with severe or terminal liver dysfunction.

BUN levels: May be slightly decreased due to failure of Krebs cycle enzymes in the liver; or elevated due to bleeding or renal insufficiency.

Ammonia levels: Elevation is expected due to inability of the failing liver to convert ammonia to urea and shunting of intestinal blood *via* collateral vessels. GI hemorrhage or an increase in intestinal protein from dietary intake will increase ammonia levels (see "Bleeding Esophageal Varices," p. 521).

Hematologic tests: Liver disease may cause an increase in mean corpuscular volume (MCV). When the MCV is increased, the RBC is said to be macrocytic, and thus the anemia is termed macrocytic and normochromic (normal hemoglobin). With acute variceal hemorrhage a marked decrease in Hgb and Hct will be present. Decreased leukocyte and platelet counts are expected and are due in part to hypersplenism. If infection is present, the leukocyte count may increase to normal levels or be elevated. PT is prolonged and unresponsive to vitamin K therapy.

Liver biopsy: Obtains a specimen of liver for microscopic analysis and diagnosis of cirrhosis, hepatitis, or other liver disease. After local anesthesia is administered and the patient's skin is prepared, a large needle is inserted into the eighth or ninth intercostal space in the midaxillary line. It is critical that patients hold their breath at the end of expiration in order to elevate the liver maximally. Patient movement or failure to sustain expiration can result in puncture through the lung rather than the liver. Type and cross-matching sometimes is performed before the procedure in anticipation of hemorrhagic complications. Percutaneous liver biopsy is contraindicated in patients with markedly prolonged PT or very low platelet counts because of the risk of hemorrhage. In these patients a transvenous biopsy *via* the jugular and hepatic vein may be attempted instead. (See Table 8-7 for nursing care of the patient undergoing liver biopsy.)

EEG: Traces the electrical impulses of the brain to detect or confirm encephalopathy. EEG changes occur very early, usually before behavioral or biochemical alterations.

Psychometric testing: Evaluates for hepatic encephalopathy. A common test is the Reitan number-connection (trail-making) test. The patient's speed and accuracy at connecting a series of numbered circles are evaluated at intervals. A daily handwriting test is an easy check of intellectual deterioration or improvement.

Abdominal paracentesis: Involves the insertion of a catheter or trocar into the abdominal cavity to remove fluids. A small amount of fluid is sent for analysis of protein, electrolytes, WBCs, and culture. Larger amounts of fluid may be drained over several hours if the patient has gross ascites that interferes with cardiopulmonary functioning. Drainage is rarely indicated, because hypovolemia and shock can occur when ascites is drained and then replaced rapidly from the blood, resulting in intravascular depletion. Frequent VS assessment and evaluation of urinary output are indicated. Peritoneal infection is another complication. See **Fluid volume deficit,** p. 543, for nursing implications.

Urinalysis: Gross inspections will reveal dark urine that produces a yellow foam when shaken. Increased urobilinogen and bilirubin will be present. In the presence of ascites, the 24-h urine volume will be decreased and the 24-h sodium value will be reduced (<5 mEq/day in severe cases).

T A B L E   8 - 7   Nursing care of the patient undergoing liver biopsy

---

Before biopsy
  · Explain the procedure to patient and significant others.

During biopsy
  · Assist patient with remaining motionless.
  · Coach patient in sustaining exhalation during puncture (or manually ventilate intubated patient in order to prevent lung inflation during puncture) to avoid pneumothorax.

After biopsy
  · Auscultate breath sounds immediately after the procedure and at 1-2 h intervals for 6-8 h after the procedure to detect pneumothorax or hemothorax (unlikely but serious complications). Diminished sounds on the right side and tachypnea suggest one of these conditions.
  · Position patient on the right side for several hours after the biopsy to tamponade the puncture site.
  · Enforce bed rest for 8-12 h postbiopsy to minimize the risk of hemorrhage from the puncture site.
  · Monitor patient for indicators of peritonitis or intraperitoneal bleeding, which can occur as a result of puncture of blood vessels or major bile duct: severe abdominal pain, abdominal distention and rigidity, rebound tenderness, nausea, vomiting, tachycardia, tachypnea, pallor, decreased BP, and rising temperature.

Liver scan: Imaging by radioisotope, ultrasound, or CT can aid in determining size of the liver and presence of abnormal tissue such as tumors.

COLLABORATIVE MANAGEMENT

Correction of precipitating factors: Hepatic failure may develop in a patient with compensated liver disease if any one of a number of factors disrupts hepatocellular functioning. GI hemorrhage or blood loss from other sources requires prompt detection and immediate volume resuscitation. Hypoxia from any cause can aggravate hepatocellular failure and must be corrected immediately. Acute infections are treated aggressively with appropriate antibiotics. Electrolyte disturbances due to diuretics, diarrhea, or other causes must be corrected promptly. Ethanol and hepatotoxic drugs are eliminated. Sedatives and tranquilizers may contribute to hepatic encephalopathy and should be discontinued.

Fluid and electrolyte management: Unless hyponatremia is profound, sodium-containing fluids are avoided because they contribute to ascites and peripheral edema and may potentiate renal insufficiency. Hypokalemia is common and must be corrected with potassium replacements, because hypokalemic alkalosis can worsen or precipitate encephalopathy. Albumin and D_5W generally are used for fluid resuscitation unless a low Hct level signals the need for packed RBCs. Fresh-frozen plasma may be used if clotting factors are deficient, but infusions of large amounts can lead to hypernatremia. In the patient who is unstable or comatose, CVP or PAP monitoring is initiated to ensure adequate tissue perfusion without fluid overload. A hyperdynamic circulatory state is supported by fluid administration and sympathomimetic agents (e.g., dopamine) as necessary.

Note: Accurate measurements and careful interpretation of hemodynamic parameters are essential because fluid balance is delicate in critically ill patients with hepatic failure; also, hemodynamic measurements can be difficult to interpret due to the hyperdynamic circulatory state. Svo_2 monitoring is helpful in evaluating the adequacy of tissue oxygenation.

Bed rest: Necessary to reduce metabolic demands placed on the liver during normal daily activity. It is strictly enforced until several days to weeks after the patient's condition has stabilized.

Nutritional therapy: A high-calorie, 80-100 g protein diet of high biologic value is indicated for patients without evidence of encephalopathy to ensure tissue repair, inasmuch as the liver is capable of significant regeneration under optimal circumstances. Sodium is moderately restricted, although rigid adherence to a 500-mg or less sodium-restricted diet is necessary in patients with significant ascites. If GI function is impaired and the patient is unable to tolerate enteral feedings, parenteral nutrition is initiated. Total caloric intake should be 2,500-3,000/day.

For the patient with acute hepatic encephalopathy, protein is eliminated totally from the diet until recovery. During recovery, protein is increased gradually, as tolerated, to 40-60 g/day. Use of enteral or parenteral branched-chain amino acid supplements in an attempt to correct the amino acid imbalance that is common among patients with an encephalopathic condition is advocated by some, but their effectiveness is controversial.

Pharmacotherapy: See Table 8-8 for a list of drugs that are hepatotoxic.

Corticosteroids: May be helpful in persons whose liver biopsy results document the presence of some forms of chronic active hepati-

---

T A B L E 8 - 8   Drugs with hepatotoxic potential

acetaminophen	ketoconazole
ampicillin	methotrexate
carbamazepine	methyldopa
carbenicillin	monoamine oxidase (MAO) inhibitors
carbon tetrachloride	nonsteroidal antiinflammatory drugs (NSAIDs)
chloramphenicol	oral contraceptives
chlorpromazine	penicillin
clindamycin	phenytoin
cocaine	propylthiouracil
dantrolene	rifampin
ethanol	salicylates
FUDR (intraarterial)	sulfonamides
halothane	tetracyclines (especially parenteral)
hydrochlorothiazide	valproic acid
isoniazid	

tis. They are not helpful with cirrhosis, and they increase the risk of infection and gastric erosion if used.

Sedatives: Avoided if at all possible because they can precipitate or contribute to encephalopathy. If sedative use is necessary, oxazepam (Serax) is the best choice because it can be eliminated safely by patients with hepatic disease. Other sedatives may be used cautiously and in reduced dosages.

Histamine H_2-receptor antagonists: Prophylactic H_2-receptor antagonists (see Table 8-13) are prescribed to block acid secretion and prevent gastric erosions, which are common in patients with chronic or severe hepatic failure. Ranitidine or famotidine are the preferred agents due to the hepatic side effects of cimetidine.

Sucralfate (Carafate):   Binds to gastric erosions and coats the gastric/duodenal mucosa.

Dextrose: Moderate to severe hypoglycemia can occur because of impaired gluconeogenesis and impaired insulin degradation. Checks of blood sugar levels q8-12h are necessary to detect hypoglycemia. In the event of hypoglycemia, a bolus of 50% dextrose or continual infusion of a 10% solution is indicated.

Protection of health care personnel: Health care workers whose jobs involve potential exposure to blood or other body fluids should be vaccinated with the hepatitis B vaccine. Health care workers must protect themselves from potential infection by frequent handwashing and implementation of appropriate barrier precautions. Gloves must be worn when contact with blood, mucous membranes, or body fluids is possible. Masks, gowns, and eye coverings (goggles or glasses with eye shields) should be used if splashes are possible. Caution must be taken to dispose of needles and sharp instruments carefully.

Management of bleeding complications: Fresh-frozen plasma and platelets are administered to correct defects in clotting factors and thrombocytopenia. Vitamin K may be prescribed to help correct bleeding tendencies. Serious coagulopathies that require specialized component therapy may develop (see "Disseminated Intravascular Coagulation," p. 608).

Management of respiratory failure: Intubation or mechanical ventilation may be indicated in the following instances: impaired gag reflex due to advanced encephalopathy, aspiration of gastric contents, or impairment of ventilation secondary to ascites. Continuous pulse oximetry is used for patients with respiratory failure or those at high risk for same. The need for adequate tissue oxygenation cannot be overemphasized inasmuch as hepatic hypoxia poses a significant contribution to hepatic failure.

Management of ascites

Restriction of fluid intake

Restriction of physical activity: To reduce metabolites that must be handled by the liver and decrease tissue oxygen demands.

Sodium: If ascites causes discomfort, pain, or dyspnea, sodium is limited to <500 mg/day.

Diuretics: If more conservative measures are ineffective in controlling ascites, spironolactone (Aldactone), an aldosterone antagonist with weak diuretic action and potassium conservation, may be used. Another potassium-sparing diuretic, amiloride, may be used as well. If these are ineffective, more potent diuretics such as furosemide (Lasix) or thiazides are added. For severe ascites, mannitol may be added to the regimen. The goal with diuresis is 1 L/day, as estimated by a weight loss of 0.5 kg/day. Too-rapid diuresis may lead to acute hypovolemia, shock, and hepatorenal syndrome.

Paracentesis: Repeated daily removal of 4-6 L/day of ascitic fluid may be attempted as a temporary measure for refractory ascites. Concurrent administration of salt-poor albumin aids in maintaining intravascular volume.

Peritoneal-venous shunt: A shunt system (e.g., LeVeen or Denver) may be placed surgically in patients with refractory or life-threatening ascites. The peritoneal cavity is drained by a long perforated catheter, which is connected to a pressure-sensitive valve. The valve attaches to a subcutaneous catheter that drains into the intrathoracic superior vena cava. The device is designed so that fluid can flow only in one direction—from the peritoneum into the bloodstream. The many complications include fluid overload, infection, disseminated intravascular coagulation (DIC), peritonitis, and shunt occlusion. A rapid increase in intravascular volume may precipitate variceal hemorrhage in susceptible persons. See Table 8-9 and **Fluid volume excess,** p. 544, for nursing implications.

Management of hepatorenal syndrome: The syndrome is characterized by renal failure with normal tubular function in a patient with severe hepatic failure. Often it occurs because of overaggressive diuretic therapy, paracentesis, hemorrhage, diarrhea, or another source of dehydration. Because it is exceedingly difficult to manage, prevention, when possible, is essential. Alleviation of precipitants and conservative measures such as fluid restriction, electrolyte correction, and withdrawal of potentially nephrotoxic drugs (e.g., aminoglycosides) are employed. Ascites is mobilized slowly, and hepatic failure, which is the causative factor, is treated. Generally, sodium-containing solutions are avoided, even in the presence of significant hyponatremia. Renal dialysis seldom is employed because it does not improve survival and can lead to complications such as GI hemorrhage and shock.

Management of encephalopathy

Elimination or correction of precipitating factors: For example, variceal or other hemorrhage, infection, dehydration, electrolyte imbalance, sedative use, dietary protein intake, constipation.

Restriction of physical activity: To reduce metabolites that must be handled by the liver.

Elimination of dietary protein: Reintroduced gradually when symptoms improve.

Early and thorough catharsis by magnesium citrate or enemas (usually tap water):   To remove intestinal contents; are exceedingly helpful in reducing encephalopathy.

Administration of neomycin, a nonabsorbable antibiotic: To reduce intestinal bacteria that produce ammonia. It may be given orally, by gastric tube, or per rectal enema. Because of its nephrotoxic and ototoxic effects, neomycin is used only in acute situations.

Administration of lactulose: To create an environment unfavorable to ammonia-forming intestinal bacteria and cause osmotic

---

T A B L E   8 - 9   Nursing care after peritoneal-venous shunt surgery

---

- Measure urinary output hourly and CVP or PAP q1-2h.
  - □ Anticipate rapid fluid mobilization, as evidenced by increased CVP and urinary output from preoperative values.
  - □ Notify physician of abnormal CVP, PAP, or lack of diuresis. Failure to mobilize ascitic fluid may signal shunt occlusion or failure.
- Administer IV diuretics as prescribed; monitor K^+ levels; and administer K^+ supplements as prescribed.
  - □ Anticipate prescribed K^+ supplements during the first 24 h after surgery.
  - □ Be aware that furosemide (Lasix), which frequently is prescribed, may cause K^+ depletion. Likewise, the anticipated diuresis depletes K^+.
- Instruct and coach patient in the use of incentive spirometer or similar hyperinflation device.
  - □ Devices that create inspiratory resistance and encourage deep inspiration promote negative inspiratory pressure and facilitate flow of ascitic fluid.
- Apply elastic abdominal binder.
  - □ This intervention facilitates the flow of ascitic fluid by increasing the pressure gradient externally.
- Monitor for evidence of variceal bleeding; report evidence of bleeding to physician.
  - □ Expanded blood volume may increase variceal pressure, resulting in bleeding. Bleeding is evidenced by a sudden decrease in Hct (a mild dilutional decrease is anticipated in the immediate postoperative period), unexplained nausea, lightheadedness, dark stools, or hematemesis. (See "Bleeding Esophageal Varices," p. 519.)
- Monitor for evidence of peritonitis, endocarditis, or other infection.
  - □ Infection occurs frequently. Anticipate antibiotic coverage during the immediate postsurgical period. Assess abdominal incision for leakage of peritoneal fluid, which is a common occurrence. Change the dressing immediately if leakage is detected.
- Monitor for evidence of postshunt coagulopathy.
  - □ See **Altered protection,** p. 548, for details.

---

diarrhea. The dose is adjusted to produce 2-3 semiformed stools per day.

ICP monitoring: To detect cerebral edema and guide pharmacologic management (e.g., mannitol and furosemide) and other therapeutic measures, such as positioning, and avoid fluid overload. See discussion in "Craniocerebral Trauma," p. 131.

Management of esophageal varices: See "Bleeding Esophageal Varices," p. 519.

Hepatic transplantation: Indicated for patients with irreversible, progressive liver disease for whom supportive therapy has failed. Transplantation is the only therapy available for FHF and requires a highly skilled team of specialists. Advances in surgical technique, patient selection, critical care management, and immunosuppressive therapy have improved the success rate of liver transplantation to 50%-80% (Kucharski, 1993).

NURSING DIAGNOSES AND INTERVENTIONS

Fluid volume deficit related to decreased intake secondary to medically prescribed restrictions; and decreased circulating volume secondary to hypoalbuminemia, altered hemodynamics, fluid sequestration, and diuretic therapy

Desired outcome: Within 24 h of this diagnosis, patient becomes normovolemic as evidenced by MAP $\geq$70 mm Hg; HR 60-100 bpm; brisk capillary refill ($<$2 sec); distal pulses $>$2+ on a 0-4+ scale; CVP 2-6 mm Hg; PAP 20-30/8-15 mm Hg; PAWP 6-12 mm Hg; CI $\geq$3 L/min/m^2; SVR 900-1,200 dynes/sec/cm^{-5}; urinary output $\geq$0.5 ml/kg/h; and patient oriented to time, place, and person.

- Monitor and document BP hourly, or q15min in the presence of unstable VS. Be alert to MAP decreases $\geq$10 mm Hg from previous measurement.
- Monitor and document HR, ECG, and cardiovascular status hourly, or more frequently in the presence of unstable VS. Be alert to increases in HR suggestive of hypovolemia or circulatory decompensation. Be aware that HR increases also may be caused by fever related to infection or cerebral edema.
- Measure central pressures and thermodilution CO q1-4h. Be alert to low or decreasing CVP, PAWP, and CO. Calculate SVR q4-8h, or more frequently in unstable patients. An elevated HR, decreased PAWP, CO less than baseline, or CI $<$3, along with decreased urinary output, suggests hypovolemia. Because of altered vascular responsiveness, the SVR may not be increased in patients with hypovolemic hepatic failure. Be aware that a "normal" CO value actually may be too low for these patients. A hyperdynamic circulatory state should be supported. Monitor Svo$_2$ as available to evaluate the adequacy of tissue oxygenation.
- Measure and record urinary output hourly. Be alert to output $<$0.5 ml/kg/h for 2 consecutive hours. Estimate volume status and adequacy of cardiovascular function by evaluating BP, HR, CVP, PAP, PAWP, urinary output, amplitude of distal pulses, capillary refill, and LOC. Consider cautious increase in fluid intake (e.g., 50-100 ml/h), and then reevaluate volume status as already described. Use extreme caution in administering potent diuretics, inasmuch as they may precipitate encephalopathy or renal disease by causing rapid diuresis and electrolyte changes. If potent diuretics are necessary, the initial dose should be small in order to evaluate the patient's response.
- Estimate ongoing fluid losses. Measure all drainage from peritoneal or other catheters q2-4h. Weigh patient daily, using the same scale and method. Compare 24-h intake to output, and record the difference. Weight loss should not exceed 0.5 kg/day because more rapid diuresis can lead to intravascular volume depletion and impair renal function.
- Monitor serum albumin, and consult physician if levels are reduced. Administer albumin replacements as prescribed.

Note: If fluid volume deficit is related to variceal hemorrhage, see this nursing diagnosis in "Bleeding Esophageal Varices," p. 525.

Fluid volume excess: Interstitial, related to compromised regulatory mechanisms secondary to acute or chronic hepatic failure

Desired outcomes: Within 48 h of this diagnosis, patient becomes normovolemic as evidenced by CVP 2-6 mm Hg, PAWP 6-12 mm Hg, HR 60-100 bpm, RR 12-20 breaths/min with normal depth and pattern (eupnea), decreasing or stable abdominal girth, and absence of crackles, edema, uncomfortable ascites, and other clinical indicators of fluid volume excess.

- Monitor VS, hemodynamic parameters, and cardiovascular status q1-2h, more frequently if patient is undergoing ultrafiltration therapy, and immediately after peritoneal-venous shunt surgery. Be alert to CVP values >6 mm Hg or PAWP >12 mm Hg. Consult physician for elevated values.
- Monitor patient for evidence of pulmonary edema related to fluid overload. Note presence of dyspnea, orthopnea, basilar crackles that do not clear with coughing, and tachypnea. Consult physician if these signs develop.
- Use minimal amounts of fluids necessary to administer IV medications and maintain IV catheter patency.
- If fluids are restricted, offer mouth care and/or ice chips (included as part of oral fluid measurement).
- Measure and record abdominal girth daily. Be aware that abdominal girth measurements are subject to error and great care is necessary to ensure accurate measurements. Measure at the widest point, and mark this level for subsequent measurement. If tolerated by the patient, measure him or her in the supine position. If the supine position is not possible, measure patient in the same position each time.
- Monitor serum electrolyte levels, especially sodium and potassium, and consult physician for significant deviations from normal. Normal values are serum sodium 137-147 mEq/L and serum potassium 3.5-5 mEq/L.
- Ensure proper functioning of peritoneal-venous shunt in patients after surgery (see Table 8-9).

Altered nutrition: Less than body requirements related to inability to digest food secondary to anorexia, nausea, and medically prescribed dietary restrictions; and decreased absorption of nutrients secondary to decreased intestinal motility, altered portal blood flow, decreased intestinal absorption of vitamins and minerals, and altered protein metabolism

Desired outcomes: Within 3-4 days of this diagnosis, patient has adequate nutrition as evidenced by a state of nitrogen balance found on nitrogen balance studies, thyroxine-binding prealbumin 200-300 μg/ml, and retinol-binding protein 40-50 μg/ml. Blood glucose levels remain within acceptable range (100-160 mg/dl).

- Confer with physician, dietitian, and pharmacist (if parenteral feedings are necessary) to estimate patient's current nutritional and metabolic needs, based on the presence of encephalopathy, chronic hepatic disease, infection, and nutritional status before hospitalization. For general information, see "Nutritional Support," p. 1.
- Provide enteral feedings if possible. In the absence of adequate bowel functioning or with poor oral intake, consult physician regard-

ing administration of parenteral supplements. If insertion of a feeding tube becomes necessary, use caution to minimize the risk of rupturing esophageal varices.

- Note and carefully record oral intake. Note all sources of food (including meals not prepared in the hospital), paying particular attention to foods that contain sodium and significant amounts of protein.
- Administer vitamin supplements as prescribed.
- Encourage supplements brought from home if desired by patient and appropriate for the patient's diet.
- Encourage bed rest to reduce metabolic demands on the liver and to promote hepatic regeneration. Increase patient's activity levels gradually as condition improves and to patient tolerance.
- Monitor blood glucose levels q8h or as prescribed. Consult physician for levels <65 mg/dl. Administer D_{50} or D_{10} as prescribed.
- Monitor patient for clinical indicators of hypoglycemia: altered mentation, irritability, diaphoresis, anxiety, weakness, tachycardia.

Note: Clinical signs of hypoglycemia can be confused with hepatic encephalopathy. Be sure to validate clinical signs with blood glucose levels.

- Be aware that mild elevations in blood sugar are anticipated in some patients, particularly those with chronic liver disease.

Impaired gas exchange related to altered oxygen supply secondary to arteriovenous shunting, ventilation-perfusion mismatch, and diaphragmatic limitation associated with ascites, hydrothorax, or central respiratory depression occurring with encephalopathy

Desired outcome: Within 4 h of this diagnosis, patient has adequate gas exchange as evidenced by Pao_2 ≥80 mm Hg; $Paco_2$ <45 mm Hg; RR 12-20 breaths/min with normal depth and pattern (eupnea); oxygen saturation >92%; and orientation to time, place, and person.

Note: LOC is difficult to evaluate in the presence of moderate to severe hepatic encephalopathy, and thus obtaining a baseline LOC is imperative.

- Monitor and document respiratory rate q1-4h. Note pattern, excursion depth, and effort.
- Administer supplemental oxygen as prescribed to enhance cerebral and hepatic oxygenation.
- Maintain body positions that optimize ventilation. Elevate HOB 30 degrees or higher, depending on patient comfort and hemodynamic status. If patient has unilateral lung problem, position him or her with the unaffected lung dependent. Correlate body position with blood gas and oximetry results.
- Monitor Pao_2, $Paco_2$, and oxygen saturation; consult physician for abnormalities.
- Assess patient q4-8h for indicators of atelectasis (e.g., diminished breath sounds, basilar crackles), hydrothorax (e.g., diminished breath sounds, dullness to percussion), and pulmonary infection (e.g., yellow, greenish, or thick sputum; rhonchi; fever). Consult physician if physical assessment findings suggest respiratory complications.
- Evaluate obtunded patient for presence of the gag reflex. Consult

T A B L E 8 - 1 0 **Factors that contribute to hepatic encephalopathy**

Chronic factors
- Portal-systemic shunting (entry of portal blood into systemic veins without being metabolized by the liver): May occur *via* damaged liver, collateral vessels, or surgically created portacaval anastomosis
- Dietary protein intake
- Intestinal bacteria

Precipitating factors
- Dehydration/electrolyte imbalance: May occur with diuresis, diarrhea, vomiting, or other factors
- Hemorrhage
- Paracentesis
- Surgery
- Excessive alcohol ingestion
- Sedatives/hypnotics
- Infection
- Constipation

Acute hepatocellular damage
- Viral hepatitis
- Alcoholic hepatitis
- Drug/chemical reactions (see Table 8-8)
- Drug overdose

---

physician regarding need for ET intubation if the gag reflex is depressed.

Sensory/perceptual alterations related to endogenous chemical alteration (accumulation of ammonia or other CNS toxins occurring with hepatic dysfunction), therapeutically restricted environment, sleep deprivation, and hypoxia

Desired outcomes: By the time of hospital discharge, patient exhibits stable personality pattern, age-appropriate behavior, intact intellect appropriate for level of education, distinct speech, and coordinated gross and fine motor movements. Handwriting is legible, and psychometric test scores are improved from baseline range.

- Avoid or minimize precipitating factors (Table 8-10).
  □ Check gastric secretions, vomitus, and stools for occult blood. Consult physician promptly if test results are positive for blood or if GI bleeding is obvious.
  □ Evaluate Hct and Hgb for evidence of bleeding. Consult physician for very low values or values that deviate from baseline. Anticipate mild to moderate anemia.
  □ Consult physician promptly for indicators of infection (see **Risk for infection,** p. 547).
  □ Evaluate serum ammonia levels. Report significant elevations from baseline.

Note: Ammonia values vary greatly and do not always correlate directly with encephalopathy. To help ensure accurate results, place specimens for ammonia analysis on ice and transport immediately to laboratory.

- Be alert to potential sources of electrolyte imbalance (e.g., diarrhea, gastric aspiration).
- Avoid use of sedative or tranquilizing agents. If sedatives are necessary, oxazepam (Serax) and antihistamines (e.g., Benadryl) are the safest.
- Avoid use of hepatotoxic drugs (see Table 8-8).
- Correct hypoxemia (see **Impaired gas exchange,** p. 545).
- Evaluate patient for CNS effects such as personality changes, childish behavior, intellectual impairment, slurred speech, ataxia, and asterixis.
- Administer daily handwriting or psychometric tests (if appropriate for patient's LOC) to evaluate mild or subclinical encephalopathy. Report significant deterioration in handwriting or in test scores.
- Consult physician for abnormal EEG reports.
- Eliminate dietary protein in patients with severe encephalopathy. As prescribed, reintroduce protein gradually as tolerated after patient's clinical symptoms improve (i.e., patient becomes more alert and neuromuscular coordination improves). Limit protein to 40-60 g/day in patients with recent or chronic encephalopathy.
- Administer enemas as prescribed to clear the colon of intestinal contents that contribute to encephalopathy. Repeat enemas as necessary to ensure thorough cleansing of the colon.
- Administer neomycin as prescribed to reduce intestinal bacteria, which contribute to the production of cerebral intoxicants. Monitor patient for evidence of ototoxic (i.e., decreased hearing) and nephrotoxic (e.g., urinary output <0.5 ml/kg/h, increased creatinine levels) effects caused by neomycin. Avoid neomycin administration in patients with renal insufficiency.
- Administer lactulose as prescribed to reduce ammonia formation in the intestine. Consult physician to adjust dose to produce two to three semiformed stools daily. Avoid lactulose-related diarrhea because it may cause dangerous dehydration and electrolyte imbalance.
- Protect confused or unconscious patient from injury.
  - Leave side rails up; consider padding them if patient is active. Have call light within patient's reach at all times.
  - Tape all catheters and tubes securely to prevent dislodgment.
- Consider possibility of seizures in the patient with severe encephalopathy; have airway management equipment readily available.
- Minimize unnecessary noise, lights, and other environmental stimuli. For more information, see "Psychosocial Support" for **Sensory/perceptual alterations,** p. 90, and **Sleep pattern disturbance,** p. 91.
- Monitor ICP and cerebral perfusion pressure (CPP). For patients with IICP, position carefully, and avoid fluid overload, hypercarbia, and hypoxemia. Administer mannitol and furosemide (Lasix) as prescribed. Sedation or coma induction may be indicated if cerebral edema does not respond to the above measures.

Risk for infection related to inadequate secondary defenses (impaired reticuloendothelial system phagocytic activity and portal-systemic shunting), multiple invasive procedures, and chronic malnutrition in the individual with cirrhosis

Desired outcome: Patient is free of infection as evidenced by normothermia, HR ≤100 bpm, RR ≤20 breaths/min, negative culture results, WBC count ≤11,000/μl, clear urine, and clear and thin sputum.

- Monitor VS for evidence of infection (e.g., increases in heart and respiratory rates). Check rectal or core temperature q4h for increases. Avoid measuring temperatures rectally in the patient with rectal varices.
- If temperature elevation is sudden, obtain specimens for blood, sputum, and urine cultures, or from other sites as prescribed. Consult physician for positive culture results.
- Monitor CBC count, and consult physician for significant increases in WBC count. Be aware that a normal or mildly elevated leukocyte count may signify infection in patients with hepatic failure inasmuch as patients with chronic liver disease often have leukopenia, with WBC counts as low as 1,500-3,000/μl.
- Evaluate secretions and drainage for evidence of infection (e.g., sputum changes, cloudy urine).
- Evaluate IV, central line, and paracentesis site(s) for evidence of infection (erythema, warmth, unusual drainage). It is normal for a paracentesis puncture site to have a small amount of drainage immediately after the procedure. Prolonged or foul-smelling drainage can signal infection.
- Prevent transmission of infectious agents by washing hands well before and after caring for patient and by wearing gloves when contact with blood or other body substances is possible. Dispose of all needles and other sharp instruments in puncture-resistant, rigid containers. Keep containers in each patient room and in other convenient locations. Avoid recapping and manipulating needles before disposal. Teach significant others and visitors proper handwashing technique. Restrict visitors with evidence of communicable disease.
- Administer antibiotics as prescribed. Use caution and reduced dosage when administering antibiotics (especially aminoglycosides) to patients with low urinary output or renal insufficiency.

Altered protection related to clotting anomaly and thrombocytopenia
Desired outcome: Patient's bleeding, if it occurs, is not prolonged.

- Avoid giving IM injections. If they are necessary, use small-gauge needles and maintain firm pressure over injection sites for several minutes. Avoid massaging IM injection sites.
- Maintain pressure for several minutes over venipuncture sites. Inform laboratory personnel of patient's bleeding tendencies.
- Avoid arterial punctures. If it is necessary to obtain ABG values, consult physician regarding use of an indwelling arterial line. If this is not possible, be certain to maintain pressure for at least 10 min over the arterial puncture site.
- Monitor PT levels and platelet counts daily. Consult physician for significant prolongation of the PT or of significant reduction in the platelet count. Optimal values are PT 11-15 sec and platelet count ≥100,000 μl.
- Assess patient for signs of bleeding. Note oral and nasal mucosal bleeding and ecchymotic areas, and test stools, emesis, urine, and gastric drainage for occult blood. Be alert to prolonged bleeding or

oozing of blood from venipuncture sites and incisions. Consult physician for positive findings.

- Use electric rather than safety razor for patient shaving. Provide soft-bristled toothbrush or sponge-tipped applicator and mouthwash for oral hygiene.
- Avoid indwelling gastric drainage tubes as they may irritate gastric mucosa or varices, causing bleeding to occur.
- Administer fresh-frozen plasma and platelets as prescribed. Monitor carefully for fluid volume overload (see **Fluid volume excess,** p. 544).
- Administer vitamin K as prescribed.
- A postshunt coagulopathy may develop in some patients after peritoneal-venous shunt surgery. Monitor these patients closely (see fifth intervention of this diagnosis).
- If fibrin split products are present in the blood and there is significant thrombocytopenia, the patient may have DIC (see "Disseminated Intravascular Coagulation," p. 608).

Altered renal tissue perfusion related to risk of diminished arterial flow secondary to increased preglomerular vascular resistance (see Table 8-11 for other contributing factors)

Desired outcome: By the time of transfer from ICU, patient has adequate renal perfusion as evidenced by urinary output ≥ 0.5 ml/kg/h.

- Monitor CVP, PAWP, and SV q1-4h to ensure optimal filling pressures (see **Fluid volume deficit,** p. 543). Monitor filling pressures hourly immediately after paracentesis or if patient is dehydrated or hemorrhaging.
- Monitor serum and urine sodium levels. Serum sodium <120 mEq/L and urine sodium <10 mEq/L are associated with the development of hepatorenal syndrome. Consult physician for significant alterations in serum and urine sodium. Normal values are serum sodium 137-147 mEq/L and urine sodium >10 mEq/L.
- Monitor creatinine and potassium values, and consult physician for significant increases. Be aware that BUN level is not an accurate indicator of renal function, especially in the patient with hepatic failure, because alterations in hepatic function can cause decreased levels and GI bleeding results in increased values. Normal serum creatinine is 0.7-1.5 mg/dl, and normal serum potassium is 3.5-5 mEq/L.

T A B L E   8 - 1 1   **Factors that may reduce renal perfusion in persons with chronic liver disease**

Dehydration: Diuresis, vomiting, diarrhea, or inadequate intake

Lactulose therapy: Results in frequent, loose stools (>3-4/day) with dehydration

NSAIDs: Results in renal prostaglandin inhibition and a reduced glomerular filtration rate

Hemorrhage: Results in reduced effective plasma volume

Paracentesis: Causes fluid shifts with a net reduction in effective plasma volume

---

- Minimize infusion of sodium-containing fluids because they contribute to ascites and peripheral edema and may potentiate functional renal failure.
- Avoid administration of nonsteroidal antiinflammatory drugs (NSAIDs).
- For patients receiving lactulose, adjust dosage so that patient has 2-3 soft stools/day.
- For additional information, see nursing diagnoses and interventions in "Acute Renal Failure," p. 397.

Impaired tissue integrity related to chemical irritants (bile salts), impaired mobility, and fluid excess (tissue edema)
Desired outcome: Patient's tissue remains intact; pruritus is relieved or reduced within 12 h of this diagnosis.

- Bathe patient with a nonsoap cleanser such as Cetaphil. Follow baths with unscented lotion, which should be applied while the skin is still moist.
- Use a low-pressure mattress to minimize pressure on fragile tissues.
- Turn and reposition patient at least q2h.
- If patient is confused or obtunded, place his or her hands in soft gloves or mitts to minimize damage from scratching.
- Administer cholestyramine (e.g., Questran) as prescribed to reduce bile acids in the serum and skin and thereby relieve itching. Avoid administration of other oral medications within 2 h of cholestyramine administration because they may bind with it in the intestine and reduce its absorption.

Knowledge deficit: Lack of exposure to health care information or cognitive limitation secondary to hepatic encephalopathy
Desired outcome: Within the 24-h period before hospital discharge, patient states signs and symptoms of early hepatic encephalopathy; the importance of medical follow-up; need to adhere to the prescribed diet; importance of rest; infection control measures; availability of alcohol and drug treatment programs; medication instructions; and signs and symptoms of complications.

- Stress the importance of sufficient rest and adherence to prescribed diet.
- Infection control: If hepatic failure is related to HBV infection, HBV prophylaxis for sexual partners and household contacts with possible blood exposure to HBV (e.g., those who share toothbrushes or razors) should be considered. Prescreening for the presence of HB antibodies is encouraged if it does not delay treatment for more than 14 days after last exposure. A single dose of hepatitis B immune globulin (HBIG) is recommended for sexual contacts and household contacts with possible blood exposure. The HB vaccine series should be initiated for exposures among homosexual men but is optional for heterosexual exposure.
- Inform patient about the availability of alcohol and drug-treatment programs if alcohol- and drug-related hepatic failure has occurred.
- Explain the availability of support groups (i.e., Alcoholics Anonymous, Al-Anon) for patients and family members when hepatic failure is related to chronic alcohol ingestion.
- Caution about the importance of avoiding OTC medications without first consulting physician. Advise patient to confer with physician

regarding use of acetaminophen after hospital discharge for minor aches and pains.

- Provide a list of patient's prescribed medications, including drug name, dosage, purpose, schedule, precautions, and potential side effects.
- Teach the signs and symptoms of infection: fever, unusual drainage from paracentesis or other invasive procedure sites, warmth and erythema surrounding the invasive sites, or abdominal pain. Have patient demonstrate technique for measurement of oral temperature using glass thermometer or type of thermometer used at home.
- Teach the signs and symptoms of unusual bleeding, including prolonged mucosal bleeding, very large or painful bruises, and dark stools. Caution patient that if possible, major dental procedures should be postponed until bleeding times normalize.
- Inform patient about sodium restriction if ascites developed during the course of the illness.
- Advise protein restriction if the patient has residual or chronic encephalopathy. Instruct patient to avoid constipation by increasing bulk in the diet or by using agents prescribed by physician.
- Caution about the necessity of alcohol cessation for at least several months after complete recovery from the acute episode. After full recovery, one or two glasses of beer or wine a day usually are allowed if hepatic failure was not related to alcohol ingestion.
- Instruct patient to perform daily weights and to report weight loss or gain of ≥5 lbs to physician.

ADDITIONAL NURSING DIAGNOSES

As appropriate, see the following for additional nursing diagnoses and interventions: "Nutritional Support," p. 12; "Mechanical Ventilation," p. 24; "Prolonged Immobility" p. 78; "Psychosocial Support," p. 88; and "Psychosocial Support for the Patient's Family and Significant Others," p. 100.

Acute pancreatitis

PATHOPHYSIOLOGY

Pancreatitis is an autodigestive process of pancreatic tissue by its own enzymes. Chronic pancreatitis is an ongoing inflammatory disorder characterized by irreversible damage, causing pain and ultimately loss of function. With acute pancreatitis, elevated pancreatic enzymes and inflammation result in sudden abdominal pain and pancreatic dysfunction. Episodes may recur, but the gland remains normal before and after the attack. Initially, pancreatic ductal flow becomes obstructed, injuring the adjacent acinar cell where pancreatic enzymes are stored in their inactive form. Once acinar cell damage has occurred, enzymes are released and activated, resulting in autodigestion of the organ. Reflux of duodenal or bile content into the ductal system due to structural weaknesses, stone impaction, or sphincter spasm can activate the autodigestive cascade. Other factors, such as endotoxins, ischemia, anoxia, and trauma, are believed to stimulate enzyme secretion and activation (Table 8-12). Edema and vascular insult frequently lead to rupture of the pancreatic ducts and spillage of pancreatic enzymes into the peritoneum, resulting in a chemical peritonitis. Vascular damage causes leakage of fluid from the capillaries. Vasoactive amines, including bradykinin and kallikrein, contribute to capillary leakage and depress myocardial function. The net effect is hypovolemia and cardiovascular failure. Necrosis and hemorrhage are precursors of complete pancreatic dysfunction. Mortality from acute pancreatitis is high, especially in patients with widespread necrosis and hemorrhage.

Complications: Marked depletion of intravascular plasma volume is the result of fluid sequestration into the interstitium and retroperitoneum. Massive, life-threatening hemorrhage from rupture of necrotic tissue results in serious blood volume depletion. Hypoalbuminemia frequently is present and contributes to hypovolemia. Hypotension persists in some patients despite volume repletion. These patients are likely to have decreased vascular tone and other findings associated with a hyperdynamic circulatory state. Edema and increased vascular permeability are additional consequences attributed to vasoactive amines. If hypovolemia is not detected and treated promptly, acute renal failure becomes likely. Mild to severe respiratory failure with hypoxemia is common in acute pancreatitis. Respiratory insufficiency is related to right-to-left vascular shunting within the lung and alveolo-capillary leakage due to circulating proteolytic enzymes and vasoac-

---

T A B L E   8 - 1 2   **Precipitating factors for acute pancreatitis**

Mechanical blockage of pancreatic ducts
- Biliary tract disease (e.g., gallstones)
- Structural abnormalities (e.g., pancreas divisum)

Toxic/metabolic factors
- Alcohol
- Hypertriglyceridemia
- Hypercalcemia (e.g., hyperparathyroidism)

Infection

Trauma
- External
- Surgical
- Iatrogenic

Ischemia
- Prolonged/severe shock
- Vasculitis

Tumors

Drugs
- NSAIDs
- Estrogens
- Corticosteroids
- Thiazides
- Tetracycline
- Sulfonamides

tive amines. In addition, elevation of the diaphragm, atelectasis, and pleural effusion caused by subdiaphragmatic inflammation can compromise ventilation further. Intravascular coagulopathy develops in some patients, which can lead to life-threatening complications such as pulmonary emboli. Hypocalcemia, which is common, is attributed to calcium binding in areas of fat necrosis within the pancreas and small intestine. The formation of pancreatic pseudocysts or abscesses as a result of necrosis and the collection of purulent material within the tissue can lead to rupture, which in turn can cause sepsis. The ensuing circulatory and respiratory failure often leads to death.

ASSESSMENT

HISTORY AND RISK FACTORS Excessive alcohol ingestion; biliary tract disease; high cholesterol levels; use of drugs such as steroids, furosemide, thiazides, NSAIDs; viral infections (especially mumps and hepatitis); open heart surgery; penetrating and blunt injuries to the pancreas. Pregnancy, primary hyperparathyroidism, uremia, and renal transplantation have been implicated as causes because they can lead to ductal stone formation and, as a result, pancreatitis.

CLINICAL PRESENTATION Sudden onset of pain (often after excessive food or alcohol ingestion) lasting 12-48 h, described as mild discomfort to severe distress, and located from the midepigastrium to the RUQ. The pain may radiate to the back. Restlessness may be present as a result of the patient's attempt to find a comfortable position. Nausea and vomiting typically accompany the pain; diarrhea, melena, and hematemesis also may be present. Abdominal tenderness is common. Dyspnea and cyanosis, which are signs of ARDS (see p. 247), may occur as serious complications of acute pancreatitis. With biliary tract disease, jaundice may be present. Grey Turner's sign, a gray-green discoloration of the flank associated with retroperitoneal hemorrhage, is present in about 1% of patients. Urine output decreases as the body attempts to conserve intravascular volume. Hypocalcemia manifests as numbness or tingling in the extremities that can progress to tetany if calcium is severely depleted.

PHYSICAL ASSESSMENT Diminished or absent bowel sounds reflective of GI dysfunction and ileus. Palpation will reveal localized tenderness in the RUQ or diffuse discomfort over the upper portion of the abdomen. Mild to moderate ascites is present and contributes to moderate abdominal distention. Breath sounds may be decreased or absent, suggesting focal atelectasis or pleural effusion. Effusions usually are left sided but can be bilateral. Auscultation of crackles reflects hypoventilation due to pain, early ARDS, or microemboli. In the presence of hemorrhage or severe hypovolemia, the hands will be cool and sweaty, capillary refill will be delayed, and peripheral pulses will be diminished. With severe hypocalcemia, Chvostek's sign (facial twitching following a tap over the facial nerve) or Trousseau's sign (spasm of the hand that occurs when the arm is constricted with a BP cuff) may be elicited.

VITAL SIGNS AND HEMODYNAMIC MEASUREMENTS Increased temperature associated with tachycardia and increased BP. Tachycardia, decreased BP, decreased PAP, and decreased CO are present with hemorrhage, shock, or dehydration. Increase in PVR suggests the presence of ARDS or pulmonary emboli. If systemic inflammation or sepsis is present, CO may be elevated and SVR decreased.

DIAGNOSTIC TESTS

Hematologic studies: Leukocytosis with a WBC count of 11,000-20,000/μl is reflective of the inflammatory process. Hct and Hgb levels vary, depending on the presence of hemorrhage (decreased) or dehydration (increased).

Chemistry studies: Serum amylase level usually is elevated 3-5 times that of normal for the first several days. As damage subsides, the level decreases. Amylase may be normal or even decreased in patients with necrotizing acute pancreatitis because of severe pancreatic damage and decreased amylase secretion. If available, serum lipase levels parallel amylase levels and are more specific for pancreatitis. Generally, urine amylase is elevated for 1-2 wk. The amylase/creatinine clearance ratio usually is elevated with obvious pancreatitis. Hypocalcemia is a frequent finding, and values <8 mg/dl are not uncommon. Because part of the calcium is protein bound, serum levels depend on albumin levels. As serum albumin levels decrease, reductions in serum calcium levels are anticipated. Hyperglycemia and glycosuria are a consequence of glucagon release. Blood glucose values are commonly >200 mg/dl. Persistent elevation of liver enzymes suggests hepatic inflammation due to alcoholic ingestion or viral hepatitis. Increased serum bicarbonate and hypokalemia values reflect metabolic alkalosis, usually due to vomiting or gastric suctioning.

Coagulation studies: Decreases in platelets and fibrinogen will be present. Elevations in circulating levels of fibrin are associated with microthrombi in the pancreas and other tissues.

ABG values: Decreased arterial oxygen tension is a common finding and may be present without other symptoms of pulmonary insufficiency. Early hypoxia produces a mild respiratory alkalosis. Arterial oxygen saturation may be diminished.

ECG: ST-segment depression and T-wave inversion may be seen as a result of the shock state, the severe pain that causes coronary artery spasm, or the effect of trypsin and bradykinins on the myocardium. Hypocalcemia results in widening of the ST segment.

Radiologic procedures: Abdominal x-ray may show dilatation of the bowel and ileus. Chest x-ray findings are helpful in distinguishing effusions from atelectasis and in diagnosing ARDS. Endoscopic retrograde cholangiopancreatography (ERCP) sometimes is helpful after the acute episode in identifying stones or stenosis. However, endoscopic pancreatography (see below) is generally more valuable in detecting abnormalities and is less likely to worsen the course of the disease. Barium studies may reveal displacement of the stomach or duodenum due to edema or pseudocysts.

CT scan: Estimates size of the pancreas; identifies fluid collection, cystic lesions, abscesses, and masses; visualizes biliary tract abnormalities; and monitors inflammatory swelling of the pancreas.

Endoscopic pancreatography: Employed to visualize the opening to the pancreas directly and to observe for swelling, ductal abnormalities, and presence of tumors or stones.

COLLABORATIVE MANAGEMENT

Treatment is more palliative than curative. Efforts are directed at pain relief and resting the pancreas until the autodigestive process subsides.

Analgesia: Narcotic analgesics are administered for relief of severe pain. Continuous or intermittent IV or IM routes are used, depending on the severity of the pain. Many narcotic analgesics, including morphine, fentanyl, and meperidine (Demerol), cause spasm of pancreatic and biliary ducts and may impede ductal flow. Some authorities believe that meperidine is less likely to cause ductal spasm and therefore recommend it for analgesia in patients with pancreatitis. Epidural blockage may be employed for severe pain.

Fluid and electrolyte management: The inflammatory process results in fluid sequestration and extensive intravascular volume loss. Nausea, vomiting, gastric suctioning, and hemorrhage contribute to the hypovolemic state. Colloids and crystalloids are administered to replace volume losses and minimize interstitial edema. Crystalloids alone may be used initially if serum protein levels are adequate. Fluid sequestration in the peritoneum and interstitium continues until the acute phase is arrested; therefore continual volume replacement is essential. If serum potassium and calcium levels are decreased, replacement therapy may be necessary. Because hypercalcemia has been implicated in the genesis of pancreatitis, calcium replacement is prescribed cautiously.

Suppression of pancreatic secretions: Accomplished by withholding oral feedings, including water; aspirating gastric secretions *via* gastric suction; reducing gastric acidity by administering histamine H_2-receptor antagonists (Table 8-13) and antacids; and reducing physical activity. Gastric suction has the additional benefit of relieving abdominal distention and vomiting.

Respiratory support: Pulmonary congestion, pleural effusion, and atelectasis result in respiratory insufficiency. Abdominal distention and retroperitoneal fluid sequestration cause diaphragmatic elevation and

---

T A B L E 8 - 1 3 Histamine H_2-receptor antagonists

Generic name	Trade name	Usual dosage	Comments
cimetidine	Tagamet	800-1,200 mg/day*	Reduces hepatic blood flow; inhibits metabolism of some drugs in the liver
ranitidine	Zantac	150-300 mg/day*	5-12 times more potent than cimetidine; fewer drug interactions than with cimetidine
famotidine	Pepcid	40-120 mg/day*	30-100 times more potent than cimetidine
nizatidine	Axid	150-300 mg/day†	

*PO, IM, or IV administration or continuous IV infusion titrated to gastric pH value.
†Available in oral form only.

ventilatory restriction. Early respiratory failure is detected by a decrease in oxygen tension or oxygen saturation. Frequent or continuous pulse oximetry is performed during the first 2-3 days of therapy to detect early hypoxemia. Oxygen is initiated if hypoxemia is present. If severe pulmonary insufficiency develops, patient requires ET intubation and positive ventilation. If there is evidence of progressive respiratory failure, IV fluids are given cautiously to prevent cardiopulmonary compromise.

Nutritional support: Parenteral feedings that provide nutrients necessary for tissue healing are initiated for patients with severe pancreatitis. High-glucose parenteral regimens compound the hyperglycemia that is commonly present in pancreatitis. For this reason a higher percentage of calories given as fats may be preferable. Use of long-chain fatty acids for patients with acute pancreatitis is controversial because there is concern that fatty-acid administration may exacerbate the pancreatitis. Oral feedings are not indicated during the acute episode because they result in pancreatic inflammation by stimulating glandular secretions. A feeding jejunostomy tube may be inserted to provide enteral feedings for some patients. Feeding tubes are placed orally, percutaneously, or surgically. Low-fat oral feedings are begun after the initial episode subsides and bowel function returns.

Peritoneal lavage: Removes toxic factors present in peritoneal exudate and can result in immediate clinical improvement in many patients with severe pancreatitis. The procedure is similar to peritoneal dialysis. A soft lavage catheter is positioned in the peritoneum, and continual lavage is instituted for 2-7 days, depending on the patient's clinical response. Generally, 2 L of an isotonic, balanced electrolyte solution is infused into the peritoneum over a 15-min period. The solution dwells in the peritoneum for 20-30 min and then is drained into a bedside collection container for 15-20 min. The cycle is repeated hourly. Common lavage additives include potassium, heparin, and a broad-spectrum antibiotic.

Surgical management: In general, nonsurgical management of acute pancreatitis is most effective. Surgical intervention does not improve the patient's condition and increases respiratory complications. Because acute pancreatitis is easily confused with acute abdominal emergencies that require urgent surgery, exploratory laparotomy is necessary for some patients. More aggressive surgical procedures, such as early pancreatic drainage or débridement, remain controversial.

NURSING DIAGNOSES AND INTERVENTIONS

Fluid volume deficit related to active loss secondary to fluid sequestration within the peritoneum and hemorrhage associated with tissue necrosis; and related to insufficient oral intake

Desired outcome: Within 24 h of this diagnosis, patient becomes normovolemic as evidenced by MAP >70 mm Hg, HR 60-100 bpm, normal sinus rhythm on ECG, CVP 2-6 mm Hg, PAWP 6-12 mm Hg, CO ≥4-6 L/min, CI ≥3 L/min/m^2, SVR 900-1,200 dynes/sec/cm^{-5}, PVR 60-100 dynes/sec/cm^{-5}, brisk capillary refill (<2 sec), peripheral pulses >2+ on a 0-4+ scale, urinary output ≥0.5 ml/kg/h, and stable weight.

- Administer crystalloids, colloids, or a combination of both as prescribed.
- Monitor BP q1-4h if losses are due to fluid sequestration, inadequate intake, or slow bleeding. Monitor BP q15min if patient has active blood loss or unstable VS. Be alert to MAP decreases of $\geq$10 mm Hg from previous BP.
- Monitor HR, ECG, and cardiovascular status hourly. Monitor these parameters q15min, or more frequently in the presence of active bleeding or unstable VS. Be alert to increases in HR, which suggest hypovolemia.

Note: Increases in HR also may be due to fever or hypermetabolic state.

- Measure hemodynamic parameters (i.e., CVP, PAWP, and CO) and thermodilution CO q1-4h. Be alert to low or decreasing CVP, PAWP, and CO. Calculate SVR and PVR q4-8h, or more frequently in unstable patients. An elevated HR, decreased PAWP, decreased CO (CI <3 L/min/m^2), and increased SVR suggest hypovolemia. As available, monitor Svo$_2$ to evaluate adequacy of tissue oxygenation. Pulmonary hypertension is anticipated in patients with ARDS. Assess for signs of overaggressive fluid resuscitation (see **Fluid volume excess,** p. 558).
- Measure urinary output hourly. Be alert to output <0.5 ml/kg/h for 2 consecutive hours. Evaluate intravascular volume and cardiovascular function, and increase fluid intake promptly if decreased urinary output is due to hypovolemia and hypoperfusion.
- Monitor for physical indicators of hypovolemia, including cool extremities, delayed capillary refill (>2 sec), and decreased amplitude of or absent distal pulses.
- Estimate ongoing fluid losses. Measure all drainage from tubes, catheters, and drains. Note the frequency of dressing changes due to saturation with fluid or blood. Weigh patient daily, using the same scales and method. Compare 24-h urine output with 24-h fluid intake, and record the difference.
- Evaluate character of all fluid losses. Note color and odor. Be alert to the presence of particulate matter, fibrin, and clots. Test GI aspirate, drainage, and excretions (including stool) for the presence of occult blood.

Decreased cardiac output related to myocardial depression secondary to circulating vasoactive amines or hypocalcemia; or related to decreased preload secondary to hypovolemia

Desired outcome: Within 12 h of this diagnosis, cardiac output becomes adequate as evidenced by CI $\geq$2.5 L/min/m^2, brisk capillary refill (<2 sec), peripheral pulses >2+ on a 0-4+ scale, urinary output $\geq$0.5 ml/kg/h, and warm skin.

- Restore acceptable preload by correcting hypovolemia (see preceding nursing diagnosis, **Fluid volume deficit**).
- Administer inotropic agents as prescribed. Monitor hemodynamic parameters carefully to minimize adverse affects of inotropic therapy (see Appendix 7).
- Provide patient with frequent rest periods. Cluster procedures and

treatments to allow long periods (at least 90 min) of uninterrupted rest.

- Minimize anxiety-producing situations, and assist patient with reducing anxiety (see **Health-seeking behavior,** p. 324, and **Anxiety,** p. 88).

Fluid volume excess related to excessive intake secondary to overaggressive fluid resuscitation and peritoneal lavage

Desired outcome: Within 24 h of this diagnosis, patient becomes normovolemic as evidenced by MAP 70-105 mm Hg, HR 60-100 bpm, RR 12-20 breaths/min with normal pattern and depth (eupnea), CVP 2-6 mm Hg, PAWP 6-12 mm Hg, CI $\geq$2.5 L/min/m^2, and absence of adventitious breath sounds and S$_3$ gallop.

- Evaluate patient q1-4h for clinical indicators of fluid volume excess: dyspnea, orthopnea, increased respiratory rate and effort, S$_3$ gallop, or crackles. Document and report changes and new findings.
- Measure hemodynamic parameters (BP, HR, CVP, PAWP) hourly in patients undergoing peritoneal lavage or in patients with evidence of hypervolemia (i.e., CVP or PAWP increased from baseline or above normal or presence of clinical indicators of fluid volume excess).
- As prescribed, administer inotropic agents to augment myocardial contractility. Evaluate effectiveness by measuring CO and calculating CI q1-2h and by measuring urine output q1-2h. Document and report CI <2.5 L/min/m^2 and urine output <0.5 ml/kg/h for 2 consecutive hours.
- Administer furosemide (Lasix) or other diuretic as prescribed to promote diuresis. Document response to diuretic therapy by noting onset and amount of diuresis.
- Carefully implement peritoneal lavage as prescribed (see "Collaborative Management," p. 556, and Table 8-14).

Pain related to chemical injury to the peritoneum and surrounding tissue secondary to release of pancreatic enzymes

Desired outcomes: Within 2-4 h of this diagnosis, patient's subjective evaluation of discomfort improves, as documented by a pain scale. Ventilation and hemodynamic status are uncompromised as evidenced by MAP 70-105 mm Hg, HR 60-100 bpm, and RR 12-20 breaths/min with normal depth and pattern (eupnea).

- As prescribed, administer IV opiate analgesia before pain becomes severe. Be aware that fentanyl, morphine, meperidine, and other opiate analgesics have been linked with biliary spasm and symptoms of biliary colic.

Note: Opiate analgesics decrease intestinal motility and delay return to normal bowel functioning.

- Pancreatitis can be very painful. Prepare significant others for personality changes and behavioral alterations associated with extreme pain and narcotic analgesia. Family members sometimes misinterpret patient's lethargy or unpleasant disposition and may even blame themselves. Reassure them that these are normal responses.
- Supplement analgesics with nonpharmacologic maneuvers to aid in pain reduction. Modify patient's body position to optimize comfort.

T A B L E 8 - 1 4 **Nursing interventions for the patient undergoing peritoneal lavage for acute pancreatitis**

- Ensure sterile technique throughout all phases of lavage to prevent serious complications caused by infection.
- Warm lavage fluid to patient's body temperature to prevent cramping, hypothermia, and discomfort.
- Measure lavage infusion fluid loss/retention. Document input and output throughout entire procedure. Document and report daily fluid balance, either excess or deficit.
- Turn patient gently from side to side as needed to promote drainage.
- Monitor patient carefully for decrease in ventilatory excursion due to pressure from lavage fluid. Drain fluid and consult physician promptly if signs and symptoms of respiratory distress develop.
- Maintain HOB at 30 degrees or higher.
- Check urine for glucose, and monitor blood glucose levels. Glucose in the lavage fluids can contribute to the glucose intolerance that frequently occurs in patients with pancreatitis. Insulin administration may be required in some instances.
- Note and document characteristics (color, odor, clarity, amount) of lavage return. Document and report changes.

Many patients with abdominal pain find a dorsal recumbent or lateral decubitus bent-knee position most comfortable.

- Because anxiety reduction contributes to pain relief, ensure consistency and promptness in delivering analgesia to relieve patient's anticipation anxiety.
- Patients and family members sometimes are distressed at the health team members' inability to relieve pain. Provide continual reassurance that all possible measures are being implemented.
- Monitor respiratory pattern and LOC closely because both may be depressed by the large amounts of opiate analgesics usually required to control pain.
- Monitor HR and BP q1-4h. Monitor CVP and PAWP q4h or more frequently in unstable patients. Consult physician for significant deviations from baseline. Be aware that opiates cause vasodilatation and can result in serious hypotension, especially in patients with volume depletion.
- Evaluate effectiveness of medication, and consult physician for dose and drug manipulation. If medications are not effective, prepare patient for splanchnic block or other pain-relieving procedure.
- For additional interventions for pain, see Chapter 1, p. 74.

Impaired gas exchange related to alveolar-capillary membrane changes secondary to microatelectasis and pulmonary fluid accumulation

Desired outcome: Within 4 h of this diagnosis, patient has adequate gas exchange as evidenced by Sao_2 ≥92%, Pao_2 ≥80 mm Hg; $Paco_2$ 35-45 mm Hg; RR 12-20 breaths/min with normal depth and pattern (eupnea); patient oriented to time, place, and person; and clear and audible breath sounds.

- Monitor and document respiratory rate q1-4h as indicated. Note pattern, degree of excursion, and whether patient uses accessory muscles of respiration. Consult physician for significant deviations from baseline.
- Auscultate both lung fields q4-8h. Note presence of abnormal (crackles, rhonchi, wheezes) or diminished sounds.
- Be alert to early signs of hypoxia, such as restlessness, agitation, and alterations in mentation.
- Monitor Sao_2 *via* continuous pulse oximetry or ABG values frequently during the first 48 h. Many patients with pancreatitis do not have obvious clinical symptoms of respiratory failure, and a decreased arterial oxygen tension may be the first sign of failure. Consult physician if Pao_2 is <60-70 mm Hg or if oxygen saturation falls below 92%.
- Administer oxygen as prescribed. Check oxygen delivery system at frequent intervals to ensure proper delivery because oxygen is critical to these patients.
- Maintain body position that optimizes ventilation and oxygenation. Elevate HOB 30 degrees or higher, depending on patient's comfort. If pleural effusion or other defect is present on one side, position patient with the unaffected lung dependent to maximize the ventilation-perfusion relationship.
- Avoid overaggressive fluid resuscitation (see **Fluid volume excess,** p. 558).
- See "Adult Respiratory Distress Syndrome," p. 247, for additional information.

Risk for infection related to tissue destruction with resulting necrosis secondary to release of pancreatic enzymes

Desired outcome: Patient remains free of infection as evidenced by core or rectal temperature ≤37.8° C (≤100° F); negative culture results; HR 60-100 bpm; RR 12-20 breaths/min; BP within patient's normal range; CI ≤4 $L/min/m^2$; SVR 900-1,200 $dynes/sec/cm^{-5}$; and orientation to time, place, and person.

- Check rectal or core temperature q4h for increases. Be aware that hypothermia may precede hyperthermia in some patients.
- If there is a sudden elevation in temperature, obtain specimens for culture of blood, sputum, urine, and other sites as prescribed. Monitor culture reports, and report positive findings promptly.
- Evaluate orientation and LOC q2-4h. Document and report significant deviations from baseline.
- Monitor BP, HR, RR, CO, and SVR q1-4h. Be alert to increases in HR and RR associated with temperature elevations. An elevated CO (CI >4 $L/min/m^2$) and decreased SVR (<900 $dynes/sec/cm^{-5}$) suggest systemic inflammatory response or sepsis.
- Administer parenteral antibiotics in a timely fashion. Reschedule antibiotics if a dose is delayed for more than 1 h. Recognize that failure to administer antibiotics on schedule can result in inadequate blood levels and treatment failure. Monitor peak and trough levels for patients receiving aminoglycoside antibiotics. Aminoglycosides are used frequently; therefore monitor patient for hearing loss. Older adults are especially susceptible to the ototoxic and nephrotoxic effects of aminoglycosides. Monitor levels of BUN,

creatinine, and urinary output, which are indicators of renal function.

- Prevent transmission of potentially infectious agents by using good hand-washing technique before and after caring for patient and by disposing of dressings and drainage carefully.

Impaired tissue integrity: GI tract, related to release of chemical irritants into the pancreatic parenchyma and surrounding tissue, including the peritoneum

Desired outcomes: By the time of hospital discharge, patient exhibits no further GI tissue destruction as evidenced by reduction in pain; GI aspirate, stools, drainage, and vomitus negative for blood; and return of bowel sounds and bowel functioning. Gastric pH value remains >5.

- Withhold oral feedings to avoid stimulation of pancreatic enzymes.
- Ensure patency of gastric sump tube to provide continual gastric drainage and prevent pancreatic stimulation. Do not occlude the air vent of double-lumen tube because this may result in vacuum occlusion. Check placement of gastric tube at least q8h, and reposition as necessary.
- Administer antacids and histamine H_2-receptor antagonists (see Table 8-13) as prescribed to decrease gastric and pancreatic secretions and to reduce gastric pH. Monitor gastric pH, and administer antacids to maintain pH value >5.
- Because increased activity can stimulate gastric secretions, limit patient's physical activity during the acute phase.
- Test GI aspirate, drainage, and excretions for the presence of occult blood q12-24h.
- Initiate peritoneal lavage as prescribed (see Table 8-14) to remove irritants from the peritoneum.

Altered nutrition: Less than body requirements related to decreased oral intake secondary to nausea, vomiting, and NPO status; and increased need secondary to tissue destruction or infection

Desired outcome: Patient maintains baseline body weight and demonstrates a state of nitrogen balance on nitrogen studies.

- Collaborate with physician, dietitian, and pharmacist to estimate patient's individual metabolic needs, based on activity level, presence of infection or other stressor, and nutritional status before hospitalization. Develop a plan of care accordingly.
- As prescribed, provide parenteral nutrition during acute phase of pancreatitis. Monitor closely for evidence of hyperglycemia (e.g., Kussmaul's respirations; rapid respirations; fruity acetone breath odor; flushed, dry skin; and deteriorating LOC), which commonly is associated with pancreatitis. Consult physician regarding use of long-chain fatty acids and supplements instead of high-glucose parenteral regimens. Administer insulin as prescribed.
- Administer enteral feedings *via* feeding jejunostomy as prescribed for patients with intestinal peristalsis.
- Monitor bowel sounds q4h. Document and report deviations from baseline. "Hold" oral or jejunostomy feedings if bowel sounds are absent.
- Monitor blood or urine glucose levels q4-8h or as prescribed. Consult physician for blood levels >200 mg/dl.
- Begin low-fat oral feedings when acute episode has subsided and

bowel function has returned. This may take several weeks in some patients.
- For additional detail, see "Nutritional Support," p. 1.

Knowledge deficit: Lack of exposure to health care information
Desired outcome: Within the 24-h period before hospital discharge, patient verbalizes knowledge regarding availability of alcohol rehabilitation programs, prescribed medications, importance of a low-fat diet, indicators of actual or impending GI hemorrhage, indicators of infection, and the importance of seeking medical attention promptly if signs of recurring pancreatitis appear.
- Inform patients whose pancreatitis is caused by excessive alcohol intake about the availability of alcohol rehabilitation programs.
- Teach patient about prescribed medications, including drug name, dosage, purpose, schedule, precautions, and side effects.
- Advise patient about the importance of adhering to a low-fat diet if prescribed.
- Instruct patient about the indicators of actual or impending GI hemorrhage: nausea, vomiting of blood, dark stools, lightheadedness, passage of frank blood in stools.
- Teach the indicators of infection: fever, unusual drainage from surgical incisions or peritoneal lavage site, warmth or erythema surrounding surgical sites, and abdominal pain. Have patient demonstrate oral temperature-taking technique using glass thermometer or type of thermometer that will be used at home.
- Stress the importance of seeking medical attention promptly if signs of recurrent pancreatitis (i.e., pain, change in bowel habits, passing of blood in the stools, or vomiting blood) or infection (see **Risk for infection,** p. 560) appear.

ADDITIONAL NURSING DIAGNOSES

As appropriate, see nursing diagnoses and interventions in the following: "Adult Respiratory Distress Syndrome," p. 250; "Acute Renal Failure," p. 397; "Enterocutaneous Fistulas," p. 580; "Disseminated Intravascular Coagulation," p. 614; and "Sepsis," p. 635. Also see "Prolonged Immobility," p. 78; "Psychosocial Support," p. 88; and "Psychosocial Support for the Patient's Family and Significant Others," p. 100.

Peritonitis

PATHOPHYSIOLOGY

Peritonitis is an inflammation of all or part of the peritoneal cavity, which is caused by diffuse microbial proliferation or chemical irritation from leakage of corrosive gastric or intestinal contents into the peritoneum. Ruptured appendix, perforated peptic ulcer, bowel rupture related to ulcerative colitis or Crohn's disease, pancreatitis, abdominal trauma, and ruptured abdominal abscesses are among the many etiologic factors associated with peritonitis. Indwelling tubes and catheters, such as those used for postoperative drainage and continuous ambulatory peritoneal dialysis (CAPD), are foreign bodies that compromise peritoneal integrity and permit the entry of infective organisms that can trigger peritonitis.

Regardless of the initiating factor, the inflammatory process is similar in every case. The initial reactions, which usually are triggered by histamine release, include hyperemia, edema, and vascular congestion. Fluid shifts from intravascular to interstitial spaces as a result of increased vascular permeability. The circulating blood volume is depleted, and hypovolemic shock may ensue. The transudated fluid contains high levels of fibrinogen and thromboplastin. The fibrinogen is converted to fibrin by the thromboplastin. Under normal conditions the peritoneum has fibrinolytic abilities to stop the fibrin formation. When weakened or injured, however, this ability is hampered and fibrin adhesions form around the damaged area. The fibrin deposits form a barrier that harbors and protects bacteria from the body's defenses, resulting in multiple pockets of infection, which can lead to recurrent infection or septicemia. In most cases the fibrin deposits dissolve, but prolonged or severe inflammation can result in the continuing presence of fibrin, leading to adhesions and potential bowel obstruction.

ASSESSMENT

HISTORY AND RISK FACTORS Inflammatory processes such as diverticulitis, appendicitis, or Crohn's disease; obstructive events in the small bowel and colon; vascular events such as ischemic colitis, mesenteric thrombosis, or embolic phenomena; blunt or penetrating trauma, especially to hollow viscera; severe hepatobiliary disease; and CAPD. General risk factors include those related to poor tissue healing and infection (e.g., advanced age, diabetes, vascular disease, advanced liver disease, malignancy, malnutrition, and debilitation).

CLINICAL PRESENTATION The primary symptom is pain, which may be quite severe, causing the patient to maintain a fetal position and resist any movement that aggravates the pain. Its onset can be sudden or insidious, with the location varying according to the underlying pathology. Fever and restlessness are common findings in many patients. Nausea, vomiting, anorexia, and changes in bowel habits also may be present and are reflective of GI dysfunction.

PHYSICAL ASSESSMENT Auscultation of all four quadrants usually reveals diminished or absent bowel sounds. The complete absence of bowel sounds suggests an ileus, a frequent complication of peritonitis. Palpation of the abdomen elicits tenderness that can be generalized or localized, depending on the nature and extent of infection. Rebound tenderness, guarding, and involuntary rigidity also may be present. Occasionally, mild to moderate ascites is observed, depending on the cause of peritonitis. RR is rapid, and the patient usually has a shallow ventilatory pattern to minimize abdominal movement and pain; as a consequence, breath sounds may be diminished. Fluid shifts and hypovolemia can cause restlessness and confusion due to impaired cerebral perfusion.

VITAL SIGNS AND HEMODYNAMIC MEASUREMENTS Usually, fever is present, accompanied by tachypnea and tachycardia due to increased metabolic demands. During the acute phase the cardiovascular system may be compromised by large fluid shifts from the intravascular space into the abdominal interstitium and peritoneum. This disruption of intravascular volume can lead to hypovolemia with marked tachycardia, hypotension, low CO, decreased PA pressures, and decreased urine output. Depending on disease progression the patient may exhibit signs of septic shock. Endotoxemic vasodilatation is manifested by a low SVR, with an initial increase in HR and CO. This state complicates the initial hypovolemia and may result in a dangerously low MAP, thus impairing renal, cardiac, and cerebral perfusion. See Table 4-17 for a comparison of the hemodynamic profiles for persons with hypovolemic and septic shock.

DIAGNOSTIC TESTS

Hematologic studies: Leukocytosis will be present, with the WBC count usually >20,000/μl. Initially, the Hgb and Hct values may be increased because of hemoconcentration, but they will decrease to baseline levels as normal intravascular volume is restored.

Blood chemistry studies: Depending on the severity of the patient's condition, blood electrolyte levels may be abnormal. If nausea and vomiting are persistent, metabolic alkalosis is expected. This state is reflected by high CO_2 and low Cl^- values. Serum albumin levels often are decreased, especially with bacterial peritonitis. The underlying disease process affects chemistry studies (e.g., patients with pancreatitis usually have elevated amylase levels).

Radiologic procedures: The abdominal x-ray usually reveals dilatation of the large and small bowel, with edema of the small bowel wall. Free air in the abdomen suggests visceral perforation. With CT scanning, abscesses can be visualized and sometimes drained during the procedure, thus avoiding surgery.

Ultrasonography: Useful in locating small amounts of loculated fluid, as well as in differentiating fluid collections in the abdomen.

Diagnostic paracentesis: Abdominal paracentesis involves the insertion of a catheter or trocar into the abdomen to obtain specimens. Sterile saline is infused through the catheter, and the return fluid is analyzed for RBC, WBC, amylase, and bacteria content. If ascites is present, it may not be necessary to infuse saline because fluid can be removed directly for analysis.

COLLABORATIVE MANAGEMENT

Because peritonitis usually is a complication of another condition, the aim of therapy is to treat the underlying disease process. Following are some of the general therapies that apply to the management of peritonitis.

Antimicrobial therapy: Both aerobic and anaerobic organisms are found within the abdomen. Usually a combination of an aminoglycoside such as gentamicin (Garamycin) and vancomycin (Vancocin) is necessary to provide full antimicrobial coverage. Therapeutic levels are drawn to guide therapy. Refer to Table 8-18 for nursing implications for aminoglycoside therapy.

Pain management: The degree of discomfort caused by peritonitis varies greatly. Opiate analgesics are used to ensure patient comfort but are given cautiously to avoid compromise of abdominal and respiratory function. These analgesics usually require frequent administration, with the dose titrated for each individual. Initiation of narcotic analgesia is delayed until the patient's condition has been fully evaluated by a surgeon, inasmuch as important diagnostic clues can be masked.

Fluid and electrolyte management: With bacterial peritonitis a significant intravascular volume depletion may occur. In most cases crystalloids are used initially, unless there is evidence of decreased intravascular proteins, in which event colloids such as albumin are indicated. If peritonitis is complicated by hemorrhage, packed RBCs may be given. Electrolyte replacement, typically potassium, is implemented according to laboratory findings. See "Shock" in Chapter 10 for additional information.

Nutritional therapy: Because of the inflammatory process, GI function is compromised and motility is minimal or absent. An enteric tube is inserted to reduce or prevent distention and promote function. Initially, the patient is placed on NPO status until some GI function is regained. When the resumption of bowel sounds or passing of flatus signals the return of GI motility, enteral nutrition is begun. If the return of gastric motility is delayed for several days, parenteral nutrition may be necessary.

Surgical management: Often necessary, depending on the cause of peritonitis. All intraabdominal foreign material is removed, and nonviable tissue is débrided. Leaky anastomoses are identified and repaired. If present, bowel perforations and obstructions are corrected, and abscesses are drained.

NURSING DIAGNOSES AND INTERVENTIONS

Fluid volume deficit related to active loss secondary to fluid sequestration within the peritoneum

Desired outcome: Within 8 h of this diagnosis, patient becomes normovolemic as evidenced by the following parameters: MAP 70-105 mm Hg; HR 60-100 bpm; normal sinus rhythm on ECG; CVP 2-6 mm Hg; PAWP 6-12 mm Hg; CI 2.5-4 L/min/m^2; urinary output $\geq$0.5 ml/kg/h; warm extremities; peripheral pulses >2+ on a 0-4+ scale; brisk capillary refill (<2 sec); patient oriented to time, place, and person; and stable weight.

- Monitor BP q1-4h, depending on patient stability. Be alert to MAP decreases of $\geq$10 mm Hg from previous BP reading.
- Monitor HR and ECG q1-4h, or more often if VS are unstable. Be alert to increases in HR, which suggest hypovolemia. Usually the ECG will show sinus tachycardia. In the presence of hypokalemia due to prolonged vomiting or gastric suction, ECG may show ventricular ectopy, prominent U wave, and depression of the ST segment.

Note: HR increases also may be due to fever.

- Measure CVP, PAWP, and thermodilution CO q1-4h, depending on patient stability. Be alert to low or decreasing CVP, PAWP, and CO. Calculate SVR q4-8h or more frequently in unstable patients. A decreased CVP and PAWP, decreased CO (CI <2.5 L/min/m^2), and increased SVR (>1,200 dynes/sec/cm^{-5}) suggest hypovolemia.
- Measure urinary output hourly. Be alert to output <0.5 ml/kg/h for 2 consecutive hours, which may signal intravascular volume deple-

tion. Consult physician, and increase fluid intake promptly if decreased urinary output is due to hypovolemia and hypoperfusion.

- Monitor patient for physical indicators of hypovolemia, including cool extremities, capillary refill >2 sec, decreased amplitude of peripheral pulses, and neurologic changes such as restlessness and confusion.
- Estimate ongoing fluid losses. Measure all drainage from tubes, catheters, and drains. Note the frequency of dressing changes due to saturation with fluid or blood. Weigh the patient daily, using the same scales and method. Compare 24-h body fluid output with 24-h fluid intake, and record the difference.

Pain related to biologic or chemical agents causing injury to the peritoneum and intraperitoneal organs

Desired outcomes: Within 2 h of this diagnosis, patient's subjective evaluation of discomfort improves, as documented by a pain scale. Nonverbal indicators of discomfort, such as grimacing, are absent.

- Monitor patient for the presence of discomfort. Devise a pain scale with the patient, such as rating discomfort from 0 (no pain) to 10. Administer analgesics promptly, before pain becomes severe. Consistency and promptness in delivering analgesia also may help to decrease patient's anxiety, which can contribute to the severity of the pain. Rate the degree of pain relief obtained by using the pain scale. Be aware that opiate analgesics decrease GI motility and may delay the return of normal bowel functioning.
- Modify patient's body position to optimize comfort. Many patients with severe abdominal pain find a dorsal recumbent or lateral decubitus bent-knee position more comfortable than other positions.
- Monitor respiratory pattern and LOC hourly because both may be depressed if large amounts of opiates are required to control the pain.
- Monitor HR and BP q1-4h. Monitor CVP and PAWP q4h or more frequently in unstable patients. Consult physician for significant deviations. Be aware that many opiates cause vasodilatation and can result in serious hypotension, especially in patients with volume depletion.
- Evaluate effectiveness of the medication on an ongoing basis. On the basis of the patient's clinical response, discuss dose and drug manipulation with physician.
- Avoid administration of analgesics to newly admitted patients until they have been fully evaluated by a surgeon, because analgesics can mask important diagnostic clues.
- See Chapter 1, p. 74, for additional interventions for patients with pain.

Altered nutrition: Less than body requirements related to decreased intake secondary to impaired GI function

Desired outcome: Patient maintains baseline body weight, and nitrogen studies show a state of nitrogen balance within 5-7 days of this diagnosis.

- Monitor bowel sounds q1-8h; report significant changes (i.e., sudden absence or return).
- Maintain NPO status during the acute phase of peritonitis. Gradually increase oral or enteral intake when gastric motility returns.
- If patient has abdominal distention, measure and document abdomi-

nal girth q8h. Distention can signal complications such as ileus or ascites.
- Administer histamine H$_2$-receptor antagonists, antacids, and sucralfate as prescribed to reduce corrosiveness of gastric acid and prevent complications such as stress ulcers.
- Administer prescribed antiemetic medications as indicated.
- Ensure that gastric, intestinal, and other GI drainage tubes are functioning properly. Evaluate character of the drainage (see Table 2-13, p. 204). Irrigate or reposition tubes as necessary. Patency and proper position of decompression tubes, such as the Miller-Abbott type, are essential for proper functioning.
- For additional information, see "Nutritional Support," p. 1.

Risk for infection related to inadequate primary defenses (traumatized tissue, altered perfusion), tissue destruction, and environmental exposure to pathogens

Desired outcome: Septicemia does not develop as evidenced by HR 60-100 bpm; RR 12-20 breaths/min; SVR 900-1,200 dynes/sec/cm^{-5}; CI 2.5-4 L/min/m^2; normothermia; negative culture results; and orientation to time, place, and person.
- Monitor VS and hemodynamic measurements for evidence of septicemia: increases in HR, RR, and CO (CI >4 L/min/m^2) and a decrease in SVR (<900 dynes/sec/cm^{-5}). Check rectal or core temperature q4h for increases. Be aware that hypothermia may precede hyperthermia in some patients. Also note that older adults and those who are immunocompromised may not demonstrate a fever, even with severe sepsis.
- If the patient has a sudden temperature elevation, obtain culture specimens of blood, sputum, urine, and other sites as prescribed. Monitor culture reports, and report positive findings promptly.
- Administer parenteral antibiotics in a timely fashion. Reschedule antibiotics if a dosage is delayed for more than 1 h. Recognize that failure to administer antibiotics on schedule may result in inadequate drug blood levels and treatment failure. Aminoglycosides are used frequently; therefore monitor patient for hearing loss. Older adults are especially susceptible to the ototoxic effects of aminoglycosides. Check BUN and creatinine levels, and monitor urinary output to ensure that patient has adequate renal function, inasmuch as aminoglycosides are potentially nephrotoxic. Measure peak and trough levels of aminoglycosides, and consult physician for levels that are above or below therapeutic range.
- To minimize microbial growth, facilitate drainage of pus, GI secretions, old blood, necrotic tissue, foreign material such as feces, and other bodily fluids from wounds (Table 2-13, p. 204).
- Evaluate wounds for evidence of infection (e.g., erythema, warmth, swelling, unusual drainage). Culture any unusual drainage (see Table 2-13 for a description of normal drainage).
- Evaluate patient's orientation to time, place, and person and LOC q2-4h. Document and report significant deviations from baseline.
- See discussion of sepsis in "Shock" in Chapter 10 for additional information.

Hyperthermia related to infectious process, increased metabolic rate, and dehydration secondary to peritonitis

---

T A B L E   8 - 1 5   **Interventions that facilitate wound drainage**

- Evaluate and maintain patency of wound drains by suction or sterile irrigation as prescribed. Consult physician in the event of loss of patency or other malfunction of drainage tubes.
- Consult physician about unusual characteristics or changes in wound drainage (see Table 2-13, p. 204).
- Change saturated dressings, using sterile technique.
- Pack open wounds as prescribed, using sterile technique.
- Irrigate wounds as prescribed, using sterile technique.
- Promote débridement of nonviable tissue.
- Turn patient frequently to encourage gravity drainage of secretions.

Desired outcomes: Patient's temperature remains within acceptable limits (36°-38.9° C [97°-102° F]) or returns to acceptable limits within 4-6 h of this diagnosis. An open airway is secured in the event of hyperthermic seizures.
- Monitor rectal or core temperature q2-4h.
- If a hypothermia blanket is required, perform the following interventions:
  - Protect the skin that is in contact with the blanket by placing a sheet between the blanket and patient.
  - Inspect patient's skin q2h for evidence of tissue damage due to local vasoconstriction. Massage patient's skin q2h to promote circulation and minimize tissue damage.
  - Check patient's temperature at frequent intervals to ensure that sudden decreases (along with shivering) do not occur, which could increase metabolic demand.
- If patient has a high fever (i.e., >38.9° C [102° F]), administer tepid baths, which may be helpful in reducing the fever.
- Administer antipyretics as prescribed.
- Keep an appropriate-size oral airway and suction equipment in the patient's room for use in the event of seizure activity.

ADDITIONAL NURSING DIAGNOSES

For other nursing diagnoses and interventions, see the following, as appropriate: "Hemodynamic Monitoring," p. 37; "Prolonged Immobility," p. 78; "Psychosocial Support," p. 88; "Psychosocial Support for the Patient's Family and Significant Others," p. 100; and "Shock," p. 635.

Acute gastrointestinal bleeding

PATHOPHYSIOLOGY

Bleeding can occur at any point along the alimentary tract. The following brief overview presents common GI bleeding sites or occurrences.
Esophagus: Esophageal varices (see p. 519) are the most common cause of massive esophageal hemorrhage. Esophagitis and esophageal

ulcers and tumors also can cause acute bleeding, but they occur less frequently. Maneuvers that increase intraabdominal pressure (e.g., retching, vomiting, straining, coughing) can lead to Mallory-Weiss tear, a laceration at the esophagogastric junction, resulting in massive bleeding.

Stomach and duodenum: The most common causes of hematemesis and melena are duodenal and gastric ulcers, accounting for half of massive upper GI bleeding disorders. Stress ulceration is a common and potentially life-threatening phenomenon in critically ill patients. Stress ulcers, also known as erosive gastritis, tend to be multiple shallow lesions located in the proximal stomach. Cushing's ulceration is a related condition occurring in patients who have sustained serious injury, major surgery, or critical CNS disorders. Curling's ulcers occur in the esophagus, stomach, and duodenum and are associated with deeper mucosal invasion than stress ulcers. Curling's ulcers are seen in patients with major burn injury. They are located in the duodenum and tend to be single deep ulcers. Gastritis, another common cause of GI bleeding, usually occurs as slow, diffuse oozing that is difficult to control. Benign or malignant gastric tumors may initiate severe bleeding episodes, especially tumors located in the vascular system that supplies the GI tract.

Small intestine: This area of the alimentary tract accounts for only a small portion of GI bleeding episodes. Diverticular disease, arteriovenous malformation, intussusception of the small bowel, acute superior mesenteric artery occlusion, and Crohn's disease are some of the possible causes for bleeding.

Large intestine: Arteriovenous malformation of the ascending colon and the cecum is the usual cause of massive colonic bleeding. Inflammatory bowel diseases such as ulcerative colitis and Crohn's disease result in friable intestinal mucosa, which can lead to massive hemorrhage and other serious complications, including bowel obstruction and perforation. In addition, diverticular disease can cause serious, intermittent bleeding episodes. Other causes include benign or malignant neoplasms and congenital malformation such as hemangioma or telangiectasia.

Neighboring organs: Acute pancreatitis (see p. 551) and pancreatic pseudocyst are disorders associated with hemorrhage. Persons with intraabdominal vascular grafts are at risk for the development of aortoenteric fistulas with massive GI hemorrhage.

Systemic organ diseases: Hypoperfusion associated with decreased cardiac output or volume depletion can lead to GI ischemia, resulting in necrosis and hemorrhage. A high incidence of GI bleeding is associated with uremia due to platelet dysfunction. Collagen diseases can result in thrombosis of small vessels in the small intestine, eventually leading to ulceration. Many blood dyscrasias (e.g., disseminated intravascular coagulation [DIC], thrombocytopenia) are associated with hematemesis and melena due to decreased clotting.

Medications: Long-standing use of aspirin, NSAIDs, steroids, or anticoagulants sometimes is associated with serious GI bleeding.

Other trauma: In addition to major abdominal trauma (see p. 196), foreign bodies (e.g., razors, screws, nails) may lacerate gastric or intestinal mucosa, causing bleeding.

ASSESSMENT

HISTORY AND RISK FACTORS Critical illness, especially that caused by major injury, surgery, CNS disorder, or burns; prolonged shock or hypoperfusion; organ failure; excessive alcohol intake, NSAIDs, or steroid ingestion; inflammatory bowel disease; foreign body ingestion; hiatal hernia; hepatic, pancreatic, or biliary tract disease; blood dyscrasias; penetrating or blunt trauma; familial cancer; recent abdominal surgery; and the presence of *Heliobacter pylori*, which is found in >90% of patients with duodenal ulcers and 70% of those with gastric ulcers (Generali, 1994). When multiple risk factors are present, the probability of a significant bleeding episode is greatly increased.

CLINICAL PRESENTATION Varies, depending on the amount of blood lost, rate of bleeding, and its effects on cardiovascular and other body systems. Adults can lose up to 500 ml of blood in 15 min and remain free of associated symptoms. A loss of 1,000 ml in 15 min usually produces tachycardia, hypotension, nausea, weakness, and diaphoresis. Massive hemorrhage generally is defined as loss of >30% of total blood volume, or a bleeding episode that requires transfusion of 6 U of blood in 24 h. Syncope associated with hypotension also may occur. Hematemesis, melena (passage of black, shiny, fetid stools containing blood), and hematochezia (passage of bloody stools) usually are present. Blood can irritate the bowels, thereby increasing transit time and causing diarrhea. Mild to severe pain often is associated with ulcerative or erosive disease. As blood covers and protects the eroded tissue, pain may disappear. Severe hypovolemic shock and decreased cardiac output can lead to ischemia of various organs, especially the brain and kidneys. Alterations in LOC and diminished urinary output will result.

PHYSICAL ASSESSMENT With profuse, active bleeding, a fast assessment can determine if a shock state is present: the presence of tachycardia, hypotension, cool and diaphoretic extremities, decreased peripheral pulses, delayed capillary refill (>2 sec), pallor or cyanosis, restlessness, confusion, decreased urine output, and obvious bleeding. Initially, auscultation of the abdomen may reveal hyperactive bowel sounds due to mucosal irritation by blood, or it may reveal a silent abdomen, which suggests serious complications such as ileus, perforation, or vascular occlusion. Palpation may reveal epigastric tenderness, which is expected in peptic ulceration; or an epigastric mass or enlarged lymph nodes, which indicate gastric malignant disease. Jaundice, vascular spiders, ascites, and hepatosplenomegaly suggest liver disease. A careful digital rectal examination should be performed, along with the testing of vomitus and stool for occult blood. With upper GI bleeding, emesis or gastric aspirate contains obvious whole blood or coffee ground–appearing old blood. Stools usually are black and tarry (melena), with a distinctive fetid odor. With lower GI bleeding, stools may be dark or contain fresh blood. Massive lower GI bleeding is associated with dark red "currant jelly" stools or passing of fresh blood with clots (hematochezia). Bleeding below the level of the duodenum is not associated with hematemesis.

VITAL SIGNS AND HEMODYNAMIC MEASUREMENTS HR and BP are quick indicators of a hypovolemic state. Systolic BP <100 mm Hg with an

HR >100 bpm in a previously normotensive individual signals a 20% or greater reduction in blood volume. In addition, postural VS should be measured. A decrease in systolic BP >10 mm Hg or an increase in HR of 10 bpm indicates a recent blood loss of at least 1,000 ml in the adult. Hemodynamic measurements usually reveal a decreased PAP and CO and an increased SVR. After major abdominal surgery a hyperdynamic state may exist similar to that seen in early septic shock, with an increased CO and decreased SVR (see "Shock" in Chapter 10). RR will be mildly elevated as a response to the diminished oxygen-carrying capacity of the blood. If abdominal pain is present, ventilatory excursion may be limited.

DIAGNOSTIC TESTS

Hematologic tests: Serial Hgb and Hct values will reflect the amount of blood lost. Because the ratio of blood cells to plasma remains unchanged initially, the first Hct value may be near normal. However, the Hct is expected to fall dramatically as volume is restored and extravascular fluid mobilizes into the vascular space. Platelet count rises within 1 h of hemorrhage, and leukocytosis follows.

Chemistry studies: Electrolyte imbalance is not commonly seen in GI bleeding, although excessive vomiting or gastric suction may cause a hypochloremic, hypokalemic state accompanied by a rise in the serum bicarbonate level. Increases in BUN without corresponding creatinine increases occur because of excess intestinal protein from the digestion of RBCs. BUN increases are not seen with bleeding from the colon or the lower portion of the small intestine inasmuch as protein digestion occurs higher in the upper portion. Dehydration and renal insufficiency contribute to an elevated BUN level in affected patients. Plasma protein levels may rise in response to increased hepatic production. Mild hyperglycemia is the result of the body's compensatory response to a stressful stimulus. Hyperbilirubinemia is caused by the breakdown of reabsorbed blood and its pigments. Ammonia levels usually are elevated in patients with hepatic disease.

ABG values: If the shock state is severe, lactic acidosis occurs, reflected by low arterial pH and serum bicarbonate levels and the presence of an anion gap. With a low perfusion state, hypoxemia may be present.

Coagulation studies: Depending on preexisting disease, hypocoagulability may be present. Elevation of fibrinogen levels, fibrin split product (FSP), PT, and PTT may be seen.

12/18-lead ECG: May reflect severe cardiac ischemia as a result of hypoperfusion. Ischemic changes include T-wave depression or inversion.

Esophagogastroduodenoscopy (panendoscopy):   The most accurate means of determining source of upper GI bleeding. The esophagus, stomach, and duodenum are visualized directly with a fiberoptic endoscope, which is passed through the mouth. Lesions in these areas are noted, and attempts are made to identify the exact source of bleeding. The study usually is performed within the first 12 h after the patient's admission. It may be necessary to clear the stomach of blood and clots by lavage before the procedure. Antacids and sucralfate should be withheld until after the procedure because they alter the appearance of the lesions. Electrocautery, laser, and other therapeutic techniques may be employed during this procedure.

Proctosigmoidoscopy: The rectum and sigmoid colon are visualized directly through an endoscope, which is passed through the anus into the lower GI tract. Mucosal bleeding, polyps, hemorrhoids, and other lesions may be seen. Biopsy specimens may be obtained during this procedure.

Radiologic procedures: Flat-plate abdominal x-ray may reveal free air under the diaphragm, which suggests perforation. A chest x-ray is taken to establish baseline pulmonary status. Barium studies usually are reserved for nonemergent situations to verify the presence of tumors or other large GI lesions.

Angiography: If the bleeding is rapid and suspected of being arterial or from a large vein, selective angiography of various GI arterial systems may aid in the visualization of bleeding site(s). If the bleeding site is clearly identified, therapeutic embolization may be attempted during angiography. The catheter may be retained for selective vasopressin infusion. See this discussion under "Diagnostic Tests" in "Bleeding Esophageal Varices," p. 522, and Table 8-2.

COLLABORATIVE MANAGEMENT

Fluid and electrolyte management: Volume replacement in acute GI bleeding must be performed as quickly as possible. Two large-bore IV lines (14 or 16 gauge) are inserted, and rapid fluid resuscitation is initiated. Crystalloid replacement therapy is initiated until dramatic blood loss or differential diagnosis warrants the use of colloids or blood products. In addition to GI blood loss, sequestration of fluid into the peritoneum and interstitium depletes intravascular volume. Packed cells and fresh-frozen plasma should be balanced to provide replacement of cells and clotting components. Generally fresh-frozen plasma is required after 6 U of packed RBCs are infused. All blood components should be warmed to prevent hypothermia. Large transfusions will cause Ca^{2+} to bind with the citrate from the stored blood and deplete free Ca^{2+} levels. In addition, large-volume blood transfusions can lead to coagulopathy disorders. If bleeding is massive, lactated Ringer's solution is the preferred crystalloid volume expander because electrolyte disturbances are minimized. Vasopressors and inotropic agents should be used *only* if tissue perfusion remains compromised despite adequate intravascular volume replacement. Hemodynamic monitoring is essential for continuous evaluation of the patient's volume status, especially in patients >50 yr or those with chronic illnesses such as cardiovascular, pulmonary, renal, or hepatic disease. Overaggressive volume resuscitation results in fluid volume excess with complications of cardiac failure and pulmonary edema. Electrolyte levels are closely monitored, especially in patients with renal or hepatic disease.

Respiratory support: Because of a decrease in the oxygen-carrying capacity of the RBCs in massive blood loss, oxygen therapy by nasal cannula or face mask is initiated. Continuous or frequent pulse oximetry monitoring is recommended in actively bleeding patients to ensure adequate oxygenation. More aggressive ventilatory support may be required for patients with persistent hypoxemia and other evidence of early respiratory failure or impending ARDS (see p. 247).

Nutritional support: As soon as the patient's hemodynamic status stabilizes, nutritional support must be considered. TPN is started for patients whose status is likely to remain NPO for days to weeks. Enteral or oral feedings are started when there is no further evidence of GI hemorrhage and bowel function has returned.

Gastric intubation: Gastric intubation often is necessary, especially with upper GI bleeding. Gastric lavage is performed to clear blood and clots from the stomach and to allow for estimation of ongoing blood loss. A lavage free of blood suggests a lower GI source of bleeding. Gastric intubation is avoided if esophageal varices are the suspected bleeding source because variceal tearing may occur.

Endoscopic electrocoagulation or laser photocoagulation: May be successfully employed in the treatment of bleeding ulcers.

Pharmacotherapy: Gastric alkalinization with antacids, histamine H_2-receptor antagonists, and other agents is effective in preventing and controlling ulceration, but recent evidence suggests that this therapy in critically ill patients is associated with a higher incidence of nosocomial pneumonia. When the acidic environment of the stomach is neutralized, bacterial counts increase. Regurgitation of small amounts of gastric juice is common in intubated patients, and infection occurs if the bacterial count of aspirated juice is elevated. Some clinicians recommend sucralfate therapy over gastric alkalinization because sucralfate does not affect gastric pH. Gastric pH monitoring (see p. 574) can be used to guide therapy.

Antacids: Raise the gastric pH level and decrease the corrosiveness of gastric acid. Antacids should be given as often as required to maintain a gastric pH of 4-5. This may require a continuous gastric infusion or hourly administration. Appropriately dosed antacids will help control pain.

Histamine H_2-receptor antagonists (e.g., famotidine and ranitidine): Block gastric acid and pepsin secretion and are employed in the treatment of erosive and ulcerative disease. Cimetidine usually is avoided in critically ill patients because it reduces hepatic blood flow and inhibits certain liver enzymes, resulting in potential drug interactions with benzodiazepines, calcium channel blockers, labetalol, propranolol, lidocaine, phenytoin, theophylline, and warfarin.

Sucralfate (Carafate):   Oral sucralfate may be prescribed for patients with gastric erosions. The sucralfate combines with gastric acid and forms an adhesive protective coating over damaged mucosa. This drug is not absorbed from the GI tract and frequently leads to constipation.

Misoprostol (Cytotec):   Synthetic prostaglandin E_1 that enhances the body's normal mucosal protective mechanisms and decreases acid secretion. Aspirin and other NSAIDs inhibit natural prostaglandin synthesis, and therefore misoprostol is especially effective for ulceration associated with long-term administration of these drugs.

Omeprazole (Prilosec):   Deactivates the enzyme system that pumps hydrogen ions from the parietal cells, thus inhibiting gastric acid secretion. Omeprazole is highly effective in reducing gastric acid and may completely inhibit gastric acid secretion.

Vasopressin (Pitressin):   Sometimes used for uncontrolled massive bleeding. For additional information on vasopressin, see "Bleeding Esophageal Varices," p. 523.

Gastric pH monitoring: Performed to assess the pH of gastric contents (intraluminal pH) or of gastric mucosal tissue (intramural pH). The goal of therapy is to maintain gastric pH within a given range, usually 4-5. Intraluminal pH is measured by aspirating gastric secretions and testing the aspirate with a pH indicator paper. Some gastric tubes have an electronic pH meter attached to the distal end that permits continuous monitoring of intraluminal pH. A more sophisticated device is the gastrointestinal tonometer and sump tube, which measures gastric mucosal pH. Because the gut is especially vulnerable to ischemia associated with hypoperfusion and septic shock states, the intramural pH is a valuable early predictor of intestinal ischemia, sepsis, and multisystem organ dysfunction.

Surgical management: Many surgical techniques are used, depending on the location and severity of the lesion. Ulcerative disease requires surgery if the lesions continue to bleed despite aggressive medical therapy or if complications such as perforation or obstruction develop. Oversewing of the bleeding vessel usually is followed by an acid-reducing procedure. In the unstable patient, vagotomy and pyloroplasty are performed. Antrectomy or parietal cell vagotomy may be performed in patients who are more stable. A common procedure for duodenal ulcers is gastrojejunostomy (Billroth II procedure). Massive lower GI bleeding is difficult to control and may require aggressive surgical procedures such as a colectomy, with the creation of a permanent ileostomy or internal ileal pouch. If GI bleeding is due to gastroesophageal varices, see "Bleeding Esophageal Varices," p. 525.

NURSING DIAGNOSES AND INTERVENTIONS

Fluid volume deficit related to active loss secondary to hemorrhage from the GI tract

Desired outcome: Within 8 h of this diagnosis, patient becomes normovolemic as evidenced by MAP $\geq$70 mm Hg, HR 60-100 bpm, CVP 2-6 mm Hg, PAWP 6-12 mm Hg, CI $\geq$2.5 L/min/m^2, and urinary output $\geq$0.5 ml/kg/h.

- Monitor BP q15min during episodes of rapid active blood loss or unstable VS. Be alert to MAP decreases of >10 mm Hg from previous reading.
- Monitor postural VS on patient's admission, q4-8h, and more frequently if recurrence of active bleeding is suspected: measure BP and HR with patient in a supine position, followed immediately by measurement of BP and HR with patient in a sitting position (as tolerated). A decrease in systolic BP >10 mm Hg or an increase in HR of 10 bpm with patient in a sitting position suggests a significant intravascular volume deficit, with approximately 15%-20% loss of volume.
- Monitor HR, ECG, and cardiovascular status hourly or more frequently in the presence of active bleeding or unstable VS. Be alert to a sudden increase in HR, which suggests hypovolemia.

Note: Increases in HR may be due to other factors such as pain and anxiety.

- Measure central pressures and thermodilution CO q1-4h. Be alert to low or decreasing CVP, PAWP, and CO. Calculate SVR q4-8h, or more frequently in unstable patients. An elevated HR, decreased PAWP, decreased CO (CI <2.5 L/min/m^2), and increased SVR suggest hypovolemia and the need for volume restoration.
- Replace volume with prescribed fluids (usually a combination of crystalloid and blood products) *via* large-bore IV (18-gauge or larger) catheter.
- Measure urinary output hourly. Be alert to output <0.5 ml/kg/h for 2 consecutive hours. Increase fluid intake if decreased output is due to hypovolemia and hypoperfusion.
- Monitor Hct; consult physician for values <28%-30%.
- Measure and record all GI blood losses from hematemesis, hematochezia, melena.
- Check all stools and gastric contents for occult blood.
- Ensure proper function and patency of gastric tubes. Do not occlude the air vent of double-lumen tubes, because this may result in vacuum occlusion. Confirm placement of gastric tube at least q8h, and reposition as necessary.
- Teach patient signs and symptoms of actual or impending GI hemorrhage: pain, nausea, vomiting of blood, dark stools, lightheadedness, and passage of frank blood in stools. Reinforce the importance of seeking medical attention promptly if signs of bleeding occur.
- Teach patient the importance of avoiding medications/agents with the potential for gastric irritation: aspirin, NSAIDs, ethanol.

Decreased cardiac output related to decreased preload secondary to acute blood loss

Desired outcome: Within 8 h of this diagnosis, cardiac output returns to or approaches normal limits as evidenced by CI ≥2.5 L/min/m^2, MAP ≥70 mm Hg, urinary output ≥0.5 ml/kg/h, normal sinus rhythm on ECG, distal pulses >2+ on a 0-4+ scale, and brisk capillary refill (<2 sec).

- Administer oxygen as prescribed to facilitate maximal oxygen delivery to the tissues.
- Monitor continuous or frequent pulse oximetry and ABG values for hypoxemia. Consult physician if arterial Pao$_2$ is <80 mm Hg or if oxygen saturation falls below 92%.
- Monitor ECG for evidence of myocardial ischemia (i.e., T-wave depression, QT prolongation, ventricular dysrhythmias).
- Monitor for physical indicators of diminished cardiac output, including pallor, cool extremities, capillary refill delayed for >2-3 sec, and decreased or absent amplitude of distal pulses.
- Monitor VS and thermodilution CO, and replace volume as indicated (see the first five entries under **Fluid volume deficit** in preceding nursing diagnosis).
- Monitor urine output hourly; document and report urine output <0.5 ml/kg/h for 2 consecutive hours.

Pain related to chemical or physical injury of GI mucosal surfaces caused by digestive juices and enzymes or tissue trauma

Desired outcomes: Within 2 h of this diagnosis, patient's subjective evaluation of discomfort improves, as documented by a pain scale. Nonverbal indicators of discomfort, such as grimacing, are absent.

- Monitor and document presence of abdominal pain or discomfort. Devise a pain scale with patient, rating discomfort from 0 (no pain) to 10 (severe). Be aware that pain may disappear concomitant with a bleeding episode inasmuch as blood covers and protects eroded tissue.
- Administer gastric alkalizing agents and sucralfate as prescribed to relieve pain due to upper GI disorders.
- Measure gastric pH q2-4h or continuously. If measuring by gastric aspirate, be sure to use a clean syringe and discard the first aspirate to ensure accurate results. Adjust gastric alkalizing therapy to maintain pH of 4-5 or other prescribed range. Avoid excessive alkalization, which has been associated with increased risk of nosocomial pneumonia. As available, use NG tonometer to measure gastric mucosal pH.
- If narcotic analgesics are prescribed for postoperative or severe pain, administer with caution. Many opiate analgesics cause vasodilatation, thereby decreasing preload and afterload. For patients with GI bleeding and markedly reduced preload, opiate administration can result in dramatic hypotension.
- Monitor respiratory rate and depth to avoid opiate-induced respiratory depression.
- Because anxiety reduction contributes to pain relief, ensure consistency and promptness in delivering analgesia.
- Supplement analgesics with nonpharmacologic maneuvers to aid in pain reduction. Modify patient's body position to optimize comfort. Patients who have pain associated with gastric reflux may be more comfortable with HOB elevated, if this position does not compromise hemodynamic status.
- See Chapter 1, p. 74, for additional interventions.

Altered nutrition: Less than body requirements related to inability to ingest or digest food secondary to vomiting, medically prescribed restrictions, or disease process

Desired outcome: Within 7 days of this diagnosis (or by the time of hospital discharge) patient has adequate nutrition as evidenced by stable weight, thyroxine-binding prealbumin 20-30 mg/dl, and a state of nitrogen balance on nitrogen studies.

- Collaborate with physician, dietitian, and pharmacist to estimate patient's individual metabolic needs on the basis of activity level, underlying disease process, and nutritional status before hospitalization.
- Provide parenteral nutrition during acute phase of the bleeding, as prescribed.
- Begin enteral therapy when acute hemorrhagic episode has subsided and bowel function has returned. This may take several weeks in some patients.
- Monitor thyroxine-binding prealbumin, and report decreasing levels.
- Weigh patient daily at the same time of day, using the same scale.

Weight can be a practical indicator of nutritional status if patient's weight changes are interpreted on the basis of the following factors: fluid shifts (edema, diuresis, third spacing), surgical resection, and weight of dressings and equipment.

- For additional information, see "Nutritional Support," p. 1.

Diarrhea related to irritation and increased motility secondary to the presence of blood in the GI tract

Desired outcome: By the time of hospital discharge, patient's stools are normal in consistency and frequency and negative for occult blood.

- Monitor and record the amount, frequency, and character of patient's stools.
- Provide or have bed pan or bedside commode (only for hemodynamically stable patients) readily available.
- Minimize embarrassing odor by removing stool promptly and using room deodorizers.
- Use matter-of-fact approach when assisting patient with frequent bowel elimination. Reassure patient that frequent elimination is a common problem for most patients with GI bleeding.
- Evaluate bowel sounds q4-8h. Anticipate normal to hyperdynamic bowel sounds. Absence of bowel sounds (especially in association with severe pain or abdominal distention) may signal serious complications such as ileus or perforation.
- Monitor serum sodium, potassium, and calcium levels, and consult physician for abnormalities. Normal values are serum sodium 137-147 mEq/L, serum potassium 3.5-5.0 mEq/L, and serum calcium 8.5-10.5 mg/dl.
- Keep patient on NPO status until diarrhea episodes have subsided.

ADDITIONAL NURSING DIAGNOSES

See other nursing diagnoses and interventions, as appropriate: "Hemodynamic Monitoring," p. 37; "Prolonged Immobility," p. 78; "Psychosocial Support," p. 88; and "Psychosocial Support for the Patient's Family and Significant Others," p. 100.

Enterocutaneous fistulas

PATHOPHYSIOLOGY

Enterocutaneous fistulas are formed when trauma, surgery, infection, neoplastic disease, or other pathologic condition results in a gastrointestinal-cutaneous communication. Despite advances in nutritional support and wound management, mortality rates up to 20% have been reported (Lange et al, 1989). High-output proximal small bowel fistulas, which generally are defined as having an output >500 ml/24 h, are the most difficult to manage. Drainage from proximal fistulas is hypertonic; rich in enzymes, electrolytes, and proteins; thin in consistency; and tends to be copious. Losses as high as 2 L/24 h are not uncommon. Extensive skin and tissue breakdown often occurs due to the presence of activated pancreatic enzymes in fistula drainage. Electrolyte and protein loss is great with high-output proximal fistulas.

Drainage from distal sites, such as the ileum and colon, is thick and of less volume than is proximal fistula drainage.

Three factors are associated with mortality in patients with enterocutaneous fistulas: (1) fluid and electrolyte imbalance, (2) malnutrition, and (3) sepsis. Fluid, potassium, sodium, and bicarbonate may be lost in great quantities. Replacement by enteral or parenteral nutrition is complex, and proper balance often is difficult to achieve. Sepsis frequently is associated with bowel fistulization, as either a cause or a result of anastomotic breakdown or due to local wound contamination or inadequate drainage. Hypercatabolism and malnutrition are associated with both sepsis and fistulization, creating a great demand for calories and protein. Aggressive nutritional support and meticulous local wound management are critical to patient survival.

ASSESSMENT

HISTORY AND RISK FACTORS Direct trauma to the GI system, especially to the bowel; infection of surgical wound, drainage tract, or peritoneum; prolonged catabolic state in association with bowel injury, GI neoplasm, GI abscess or severely inflammatory bowel disease; and complex GI surgical procedures, such as lysis of adhesions for intestinal obstruction or complicated intestinal anastomosis.

CLINICAL PRESENTATION Varies, according to cause and location of fistula. Discharge of obvious bile, enteric contents, or gas through a surgical incision is an obvious sign of fistulization, as is a sudden increase in the amount of drainage from a surgical incision or drainage catheter. A change in the nature of drainage from serous or serosanguineous to yellow, green, brown, or foul smelling may indicate a fistula. With pancreatic drainage, a change to milky white suggests a pancreatic fistula. Mental confusion often is present as a result of electrolyte imbalance, dehydration, or early sepsis. Dry mouth, loss of tissue turgor, sunken eyes, and a decreasing urinary output with increasing specific gravity are expected if excessive fluid loss results in dehydration. Erythema, maceration, and edema may be present due to irritating fistula drainage. With persistent fistulization, loss of weight and muscle mass is anticipated because of protein loss and hypercatabolism.

PHYSICAL ASSESSMENT Sunken eyes, poor skin turgor, and dry oral mucosa, which are associated with dehydration; peripheral edema and muscle wasting related to protein loss; diminished or absent bowel sounds if peritonitis or ileus is present; discomfort and guarding on abdominal palpation over an abdominal mass (abscess) or near a drain site or surgical incision; tenderness, erythema, and possibly pain at the incision/fistula site due to irritation from fistula output or infection; and muscle weakness and irregular HR if hypokalemia is present. Other assessment findings related to the underlying disease state (e.g., trauma, neoplasm, infection, pancreatitis) may be present.

VITAL SIGNS AND HEMODYNAMIC MONITORING PARAMETERS Increased temperature and tachycardia due to infection or dehydration; and decreased BP, PAP, and CO if dehydration is present. If early sepsis is present, expect elevated CO and decreased SVR. Oxygen demand is increased and may exceed supply. Svo_2 will fall without aggressive pulmonary and cardiovascular support. The patient will exhibit general hemodynamic instability until fluid balance and infection are controlled.

DIAGNOSTIC TESTS

Radiography: Water-soluble contrast medium may be injected into the suspected fistula (fistulography) to identify the tract. An upper GI series may be indicated if the suspected fistula is proximal. CT scan may be used to identify and direct the drainage of abscesses associated with fistulization.

Biopsy: In patients with neoplastic disease a biopsy specimen of the fistula tract may be obtained to identify the presence of malignancy within the tract.

Culture: Fistula effluent from the stomach, duodenum, biliary tree, and pancreas may be cultured for evidence of infection. Small and large bowel fistulas generally are not cultured due to the expected presence of bacteria.

COLLABORATIVE MANAGEMENT

Nutritional support: With distal small bowel and colonic fistulas, enteral elemental diets may be infused into the proximal small bowel if the patient is capable of proximal absorption. Enteral diets sometimes are used if the fistula is extremely proximal. In these patients the feeding is infused distal to the fistula into the jejunum via a fine, weighted intestinal feeding tube. Enteral feedings are discontinued if fistula output increases after initiation of feedings. Patients with proximal small bowel fistulas, prolonged adynamic ileus, or extensive intraabdominal sepsis usually require TPN. Providing sufficient calories, protein, electrolytes, and fluids for patients with high-output fistulas can be challenging. However, malnutrition in these patients is associated with a very high mortality rate, and the need for nutritional support cannot be overemphasized. Appropriate parenteral nutrition alone may be sufficient therapy to promote spontaneous healing and closure (see "Nutritional Support," p. 1).

Fluid and electrolyte replacement: Balanced salt solutions, usually containing potassium, are administered to maintain fluid and electrolyte balance. Often the amount to be delivered is prescribed in direct relation to fistula output, especially when the output is widely variable. Effluent from each fistula is measured separately for accurate estimation of specific electrolyte and fluid losses. In general, fistulas that are more proximal result in greater fluid, electrolyte, and protein losses than those that are distal.

Local fistula management: Ideally, drainage from each fistula is collected separately to assess individual fistula activity and healing. Individualized systems of gravity or gentle suction drainage and barrier skin protection are devised for each patient. Good local management reduces the incidence of wound-related bacteremias and increases the rate of wound healing.

Antibiotics: Indicated for infection, which frequently is present. Administration of aminoglycosides requires careful monitoring of peak and trough plasma levels to achieve adequate therapeutic results.

Surgery: A large percentage of patients with gastrocutaneous fistulas require surgery. Surgery is indicated in the following instances: (1)
to close fistulas that continue to drain significant amounts despite absence of infection and appropriate nutritional support, (2) to explore
and drain fistula tracts that could not be identified or drained by less
invasive techniques, and (3) if overwhelming sepsis fails to respond
to antibiotics and supportive therapy. In these cases immediate surgery is planned as a life-saving measure. The usual operation to close
persistently draining fistulas is resection with end-to-end anastomosis.
Postoperatively, parenteral nutrition and antibiotic coverage are continued. A gastrostomy usually is created to allow for prolonged intestinal decompression and drainage. The patient is expected to remain
on NPO status for 1-2 wk after surgery, depending on the rate of healing and the return of bowel function.

NURSING DIAGNOSES AND INTERVENTIONS

Impaired tissue integrity related to chemical trauma, infection, or
malnutrition
Desired outcome: Within 72 h of this diagnosis, patient's tissue adjacent to the fistula is free of erythema, excoriation, and edema.
- Assess the extent of the local problem (Table 8-16). Consult physician for signs of extensive damage to the tissue adjacent to the fistula (i.e., severe local erythema, excoriation, edema, or maceration).
- Establish drainage and collection system for each fistula (Table
  8-17). Consult physician regarding use of continuous wound suction device(s).
- Note character, color, odor, and volume of output from each fistula.
  Consult physician for significant changes in any of these indicators.
- If increased fistula output results from oral or enteral feedings, eliminate or modify the feedings as prescribed.
- Consult ostomy nurse or enterostomal therapist for recommendations
  in pouching complex or multiple fistulas.
- See **Altered nutrition,** which follows, and **Risk for infection,** p.
  581, for interventions that optimize nutrition and prevent infection.

Altered nutrition: Less than body requirements related to protein
loss *via* fistula output, disruption of GI tract continuity, or absorptive
disorder

T A B L E   8 - 1 6   **Nursing assessment of the enterocutaneous fistula**

- Evaluate size, shape, and location of the fistula. Reposition or lift skinfolds
  as necessary.
- Identify any potential leakage tracks created by skinfolds or body hollows.
- Examine the condition of adjacent skin and tissue. Note the presence and
  spread of both erythema and excoriation, which suggest leakage tracks.
- Note the consistency and character of fistula output.
- Assess each fistula separately.
- Document all findings and compare them with baseline assessment made at
  the time of initial evaluation.

Desired outcome: By the time of hospital discharge, patient has adequate nutrition as evidenced by food intake that increases to his or her recommended daily allowance and body weight that returns to baseline or within 10% of patient's ideal weight.

- Collaborate with physician, dietitian, and pharmacist to estimate patient's metabolic needs on the basis of activity level, estimated metabolic rate, and baseline nutritional status.
- Monitor for the presence of bowel sounds q8h. If bowel sounds are absent, withhold oral or enteral feedings.
- If fistula output increases in response to enteral feedings, slow the rate of infusion or reduce the strength of the feeding. If the patient tolerates oral feedings but they increase fistula output, increase the frequency of the feedings and decrease the amount consumed at each feeding.
- Be aware that when the entire intestine is not available for normal absorption, elemental feeding formulas (see p. 7) may be more readily absorbed.
- Prepare patient for parenteral feedings if oral/enteral feedings are inadequate for patient's requirements.
- For additional information, see "Nutritional Support," p. 1.

Risk for infection related to inadequate primary defenses (altered integumentary system, disruption in continuity of gastrointestinal system), hypercatabolic state, presence of invasive lines, and protein loss/malnutrition

Desired outcome: Patient remains free of infection as evidenced by core or rectal temperature <37.8° C (100° F); negative culture results;

T A B L E 8 - 1 7   Recommendations for containing fistula drainage

---

- Clean the intact skin surrounding the fistula with a nonirritating antibacterial cleanser.
- Clip body hair (if present) around the fistula.
- Remove pooled drainage from the wound and surrounding area by using sterile absorbent pads or gentle suction. The help of an assistant may be necessary to maintain a dry field during application of the collection device.
- Apply a barrier powder (e.g., karaya or Orahesive) to any excoriated skin. A flexible transparent dressing (e.g., Op-Site) can be used to protect intact skin.
- Use a skin paste (e.g., Stomahesive or karaya) to fill in any grooves surrounding recessed fistulas.
- Apply a sized barrier sheet (e.g., Stomahesive, HolliHesive) to the surrounding skin, being careful not to overlap the fistula.
- Attach a collecting bag to the barrier sheet base. For high-output fistulas, a urostomy bag and collecting system may be necessary. Transparent appliances enable observation of drainage. Devices that have a drainage opening permit emptying and measurement of output.
- Reposition the patient frequently to optimize gravity drainage of fistula output. For example, it sometimes is necessary to use a rotating bed frame or a bed modified with foam blocks to facilitate prone positioning.

T A B L E 8 - 1 8 **Aminoglycoside antibiotics: nursing implications**

- Administer prepared solution over 30-60 min, according to recommendations for specific agent. Too-rapid administration increases the risk of toxicity.
- Reschedule if dosage is delayed >1 h.
- Obtain serum specimen in a timely fashion so that peak and trough levels can be evaluated adequately.
- Monitor patient for evidence of hearing loss.
- Monitor BUN and creatinine levels and urinary output, which are indicators of renal function.
- Be aware that older adults are especially susceptible to ototoxic and nephrotoxic effects of these medications.
- To avoid potential incompatibilities/interactions, administer at separate sites and stagger schedules when penicillin and cephalosporins also are prescribed.

HR 60-100 bpm; RR 12-20 breaths/min; BP within patient's normal range; and orientation to time, place, and person.

- Check rectal or core temperature q4h for increases.
- If there is a sudden elevation in temperature, assess patient for potential sources, noting presence of purulent secretions; erythema around wound, drain, or fistula site; and pain, tenderness, or masses with abdominal palpation. Consult physician for temperature elevation and assessment findings. Obtain specimens for culture of likely sites for infection as prescribed by physician or unit protocol.
- Evaluate orientation and LOC q4h. Document and report significant deviations from baseline values.
- Monitor BP, HR, RR, CO, and SVR q4h. Be alert to increases in HR and RR associated with temperature elevations. As available, monitor Svo_2 continuously or at scheduled intervals. An elevated CO and a decreased SVR suggest early septic shock (see Table 4-17, p. 364, for a complete hemodynamic profile; also see "Shock" in Chapter 10).
- Administer parenteral antibiotics in a timely fashion. Reschedule antibiotics if a dosage is delayed for more than 1 h. Recognize that failure to administer antibiotics on schedule can result in inadequate blood levels and treatment failure. Aminoglycosides are used frequently; administer agents promptly, and monitor patient for potential complications (Table 8-18).
- Optimize gravity drainage of fistula by prone or upright positioning as tolerated by patient.
- Wear gloves when contact with drainage is possible. Prevent transmission of potentially infectious agents by washing hands thoroughly before and after caring for patient and disposing of dressings and drainage carefully.

Fluid volume deficit related to active loss secondary to fistula drainage

Desired outcome: Within 8 h of this diagnosis, patient becomes normovolemic as evidenced by balanced daily I&O, urinary output ≥0.5 ml/kg/h, urine specific gravity 1.010-1.020, moist mucous membranes, good skin turgor, HR ≤100 bpm, CVP 2-6 mm Hg, and PAWP 6-12 mm Hg.

- Evaluate patient's fluid balance by calculating and comparing daily I&O. In patients with high-output fistulas, evaluate total I&O q8h. Record all sources of output, including drainage from each fistula. Replace fistula output with prescribed fluid (usually a balanced salt solution containing potassium) q2-8h.
- Measure urine output q1-4h. Consult physician if urine output is <0.5 ml/kg/h or if the patient has an increasing specific gravity with a decreasing volume of urine.
- Assess and document condition of mucous membranes and skin turgor. Dry membranes and inelastic skin indicate inadequate fluid volume and the need for increase in fluid intake (PO or IV route).
- Measure and evaluate VS, CVP, and PAP (when available) q1-4h, depending on hemodynamic stability. Be alert to increasing HR, decreasing CVP, and decreasing PAP, which indicate inadequate intravascular volume. Encourage increased oral intake (if possible), or consult with physician regarding increase in IV fluid intake.
- Control sources of insensible fluid loss by humidifying oxygen, maintaining comfortable environment, and controlling fever (if present) with antipyretics such as acetaminophen.

Body image disturbance related to biophysical change secondary to presence of external fistula

Desired outcome: By the time of hospital discharge, patient acknowledges body changes as evidenced by viewing fistula and not exhibiting preoccupation with or depersonalization of fistula.

- Evaluate the patient's reaction to the fistula by observing and noting evidence of body image disturbance (see Table 1-41, p. 97).
- Anticipate feelings of shock and repulsion initially. Be aware that the development of an external fistula usually is an unanticipated complication and patients are not emotionally prepared for the disfigurement.
- Anticipate and acknowledge normalcy of feelings of rejection, isolation, and uncleanliness (due to odor and possible presence of feces).
- Offer patient opportunity to view fistula/wound as desired. Use mirrors if necessary.
- Encourage patient and significant others to verbalize feelings regarding fistula/wound.
- If possible, offer the patient an opportunity to participate in wound care. Patient may be able to perform simple tasks, such as holding the bag into which you will deposit the soiled dressing or applying the pouch that collects drainage.
- Convey an accepting attitude toward the patient. Many fistulas that require critical care involve open and infected wounds. If the attending nurse is inexperienced in dressing these complex wounds, another more experienced nurse should be present during the initial dressing change.
- Reassure patient that the fistula is not permanent. Acknowledge that a scar will be visible but the fistula will close with appropriate care.

Altered oral mucous membrane related to prolonged NPO status

Desired outcome: Within 24 h of this diagnosis, patient's oral mucosa is intact, moist, and free of pain and oral lesions.

- Inspect the patient's oral cavity, noting the degree of moisture, inflammation, bleeding, or lesions. Consult physician for open lesions and bleeding.
- Assist patient with brushing teeth with a soft-bristled toothbrush. Irrigate the oral cavity with a solution of 500 ml normal saline and 15 ml sodium bicarbonate. Provide mouth care q4h.
- For patients with altered LOC, massage gums and teeth with saline-moistened sponge-tipped applicator and brush teeth gently if there is no evidence of bleeding. Place patient in a side-lying position, and irrigate the mouth with small amounts of a saline and bicarbonate solution (per second entry). Carefully suction the solution from the oral cavity throughout the procedure with a Yankauer tonsil suction device.
- Keep the lips moist with emollients, such as lanolin or Eucerin cream. Take care to apply emollient to external tissue only. Oil-containing emollients are harmful if aspirated or otherwise introduced into the respiratory tract.

ADDITIONAL NURSING DIAGNOSES

See "Nutritional Support," p. 1, for additional information about the patient with extra nutritional needs. See "Psychosocial Support," p. 88, for psychosocial nursing diagnoses and interventions. Also see nursing diagnoses and interventions related to sepsis under "Shock," p. 635.

Selected Bibliography

Bezzarro ER: Changing perspectives of H_2-antagonists for stress ulcer prophylaxis, *Crit Care Nurs Clin North Am* 5(2):325-331, 1993.

Brown A: Acute pancreatitis: pathophysiology, nursing diagnoses, and collaborative problems, *Focus Crit Care* 18(2):121-130, 1991.

Butler R: Managing the complications of cirrhosis, *Am J Nurs* 94(3):46-49, 1994.

Chernow B, editor: *The pharmacologic approach to the critically ill patient,* ed 3, Baltimore, 1994, Williams & Wilkins.

Covington J: Nursing care of patients with alcoholic liver disease, *Crit Care Nurse* 13(3):47-57, 1993.

Generali J: *Heliobacter pylori* update, *Drug Newsletter* 13(5):39-40, 1994.

Heeg JE, Coleman D: Hepatitis kills, *RN* 55(4):60-67, 1992.

Horne M, Swearingen PL: *Pocket guide to fluids and electrolytes,* ed 2, St Louis, 1993, Mosby.

Interqual: The ISD-A review system with adult ISD criteria, August 1992, North Hampton, NH, and Marlboro, Mass, Interqual, Inc.

Jackson MM, Rymer T: Viral hepatitis: anatomy of a diagnosis, *Am J Nurs* 94(1):43-48, 1994.

Kerber K: The adult with bleeding esophageal varices, *Crit Care Nurs Clin North Am* 5(1):153-162, 1993.

Kim MJ, McFarland GK, McLane AM: *Pocket guide to nursing diagnoses,* ed 6, St Louis, 1995, Mosby.

Krumberger JM: Acute pancreatitis, *Crit Care Nurs Clin North Am* 5(1):169-185, 1993.

Kucharski S: Fulminant hepatic failure, *Crit Care Nurs Clin North Am* 5(1):141-151, 1993.

Lancaster S, Stockbridge J: PV shunts relieve ascites, *RN* 55(8):58-60, 1992.

Lange MP et al: Management of multiple enterocutaneous fistulas, *Heart Lung* 18(4):386-390, 1989.

Martin F: When the liver breaks down, *RN* 55(8):52-57, 1992.

Mullan RJ et al: Guidelines for prevention of transmission of human immuno-deficiency virus and hepatitis B virus to health care and public safety workers, *MMWR* 38(5-6):1, 1989.

Prevost SS, Overle A: Stress ulceration in the critically ill patient, *Crit Care Nurs Clin North Am* 5(1):163-169, 1993.

Sherlock S: *Diseases of the liver and biliary system,* ed 9, Boston, 1992, Blackwell.

Smith SL, Ciferni M: Liver transplantation for acute hepatic failure: a review of clinical experience and management, *Am J Crit Care* 2(2):137-144, 1993.

HEMATOLOGIC DYSFUNCTIONS

The hematologic or hematopoietic system involves the blood, lymph, and components that form and circulate blood and lymph. Blood-forming organs include the bone marrow, thymus gland, liver, spleen, and lymph nodes. Lymph is derived from the interstitial fluid passing into the lymphatic capillaries. The primary functions of the hematologic system are:

Respiratory gas exchange (O_2 and CO_2)
Delivery of nutrients to the body cells
Elimination of wastes from the body cells

In addition, blood also has a role in:

Temperature regulation
Delivery of hormones
Fluid and electrolyte balance
Acid-base balance
Protection from foreign antigens and infectious organisms

Blood is composed of plasma, erythrocytes (red blood cells [RBCs]), leukocytes (white blood cells [WBCs]), and thrombocytes (platelets). Dysfunctions of the hematologic system lead to problems performing the eight functions listed above. Hematologic dysfunctions can be classified as anemias and bleeding and thrombotic disorders.

Profound anemias/hemolytic crisis

PATHOPHYSIOLOGY

Anemia reflects a reduction in total body hemoglobin concentration, potentially caused by hemoglobinopathies (abnormal hemoglobin, including hemoglobin S, which occurs with sickle cell disease), various other hemolytic anemias (e.g., hereditary spherocytosis, G6PD deficiency, pyruvate kinase deficiency, thalassemias [Cooley's or Mediterranean anemia], erythroblastosis fetalis), anemia of renal failure (erythropoieitin deficiency), aplastic anemia (lack of bone marrow production of RBCs related to malignancy, increased IgG antibodies, drugs, or thymoma), megaloblastic anemia (decreased B_{12} or other B vitamins, folic acid, or intrinsic factors; includes pernicious anemia) and anemia related to blood loss/hemorrhage.

As the hemoglobin decreases, the oxygen-carrying capacity of the blood is reduced, resulting in tissue hypoxia unless compensatory mechanisms are adequate to assist the body with oxygen delivery. The anemias discussed above originate from one of three main problems:

- *Acute or chronic blood loss:* Chronic GI bleeding, excessive menstruation, trauma, ruptured blood vessel(s), and other various disorders.
- *Decreased production of erythrocytes:* Iron deficiency, lead poisoning, thalassemias, megaloblastic/pernicious anemia, renal failure, aplastic/hypoplastic anemia.
- *Increased destruction of erythrocytes:* Hemolytic anemias caused by abnormal hemoglobin (hemoglobin S, C, D, E), RBC membrane anomalies (spherocytosis, hemolytic uremic syndrome), physical trauma to blood (extracorporeal "bypass" circulation, balloon counterpulsation, prosthetic heart valves), abnormal RBC-related antibodies (e.g., Tn syndrome, drug-induced hemolysis), and presence of bacterial endotoxins (malaria, clostridia).

Hemolytic crisis

Hemolytic crisis is an acute disorder that frequently accompanies hemolytic anemias. It is characterized by premature pathologic destruction (hemolysis) of RBCs (erythrocytes). As erythrocyte destruction accelerates, there is a decrease in the oxygen-carrying capacity of the blood, which results in a reduction in the amount of oxygen delivered to the tissues. This hypoxic state produces tissue ischemia and can progress to tissue infarction. Hemolytic episodes can be triggered by both emotional and physiologic states, including stress, trauma, surgery, acute infectious processes, and abnormal immune responses.

ASSESSMENT

For anemias

CLINICAL PRESENTATION (CHRONIC INDICATORS) Pallor, melenic or hematochezic stools, fatigue, weight loss, dyspnea on exertion, uremia, sensitivity to cold, intermittent dizziness, excessive menstruation, paresthesias, and history of iron deficiency, folic acid deficiency, B_{12} deficiency.

- *Chronic hemolytic anemia:* Jaundice, renal failure, hematuria, arthritis, increased incidence of gallstones, skin ulcers.

ACUTE INDICATORS Fever, chest pain, congestive heart failure (CHF), confusion, irritability, tachycardia, orthostatic hypotension, dyspnea, tachypnea, frank bleeding.

PHYSICAL ASSESSMENT Inspection may reveal tachypnea, orthopnea, tachycardia, weight loss, altered mental status, spider angiomas, ECG changes, unusual fatigue or weakness, smooth tongue, unusual bleeding (stool, urine, emesis), monoarticular or polyarticular arthritis, and skin ulcers. Palpation may detect bone tenderness (especially sternal), enlargement of the liver and/or spleen, and joint tenderness. Auscultation may reveal crackles associated with CHF.

For hemolytic crisis

RISK FACTORS Individuals with mild or chronic hemolytic anemia may be asymptomatic until they are exposed to a severe stressor, such as an acute infectious process, profound emotional upset, critical illness, surgery, or trauma. With added stress, hemolysis can accelerate to a crisis state wherein patients experience organ congestion from massive amounts of hemolyzed blood cells, precipitating multiple organ dysfunction syndrome (MODS) and shock.

CLINICAL PRESENTATION (ACUTE) Fever; abdominal, chest, joint, and back pain; jaundice; headache; dizziness; palpitations; SOB; hemoglobinuria; lymphadenopathy; splenomegaly; and signs of peripheral nerve damage, including paresthesias, paralysis, chills, and vomiting.

CLINICAL PRESENTATION (CHRONIC) Anemia, pallor, fatigue, dyspnea on exertion, icterus, bone infarctions, monoarticular and polyarticular arthritis, hematuria, renal failure, increased gallstone formation, and skin ulcers.

PHYSICAL ASSESSMENT Depending on severity and duration of the anemia, the patient may exhibit impaired growth and development. Inspection may reveal the presence of jaundice, SOB, monoarticular or polyarticular arthritis, retinal detachment and associated vitreous hemorrhage, and hemiplegia. Palpation may demonstrate splenomegaly, lymphadenopathy, hepatomegaly, or abdominal guarding. Chronic skin ulcers may be seen, particularly in the ankle area.

DIAGNOSTIC TESTS

Red blood cells (RBCs):   Reduced. In hemolytic crisis there will be an increased number of premature RBCs.

Reticulocyte count: RBC precursors; elevated because of increased bone marrow production of RBCs.

Hemoglobin and hematocrit: Decreased.

Morphologic classification of RBCs: Mean corpuscular volume (MCV)
- *Macrocytic:* MCV >100 μ_3
- *Microcytic:* MCV <80 μ_3
- *Normocytic:* MCV 80-100 μ_3

Sickle cell test: Screens for the presence of hemoglobin S, which is indicative of sickle cell anemia.

Hemoglobin electrophoresis: Screens for abnormal hemoglobins often present in hemolytic anemias:
- *Hemoglobin A_1, A_2, and F:* Normally found in the body.
- *Hemoglobin C:* Causes RBCs to sickle.
- *Hemoglobins D and E:* Rarely occur "singly"; sometimes present with sickle cell disease or thalassemias.
- *Hemoglobin H:* Causes premature destruction of RBCs and abnormal binding of O_2 to the RBC.
- *Hemoglobin S:* Most common abnormal hemoglobin, occurring in

10% of the African American population; causes sickle cell disease or seen with sickle cell trait.

Erythrocyte sedimentation rate (ESR):   Elevated in hemolytic anemia, more often than in other anemias.

C_3 proactivator: Increased in hemolytic anemia.

Total iron binding capacity (TIBC):   Normal or reduced, depending on the type of anemia.

Unconjugated bilirubin: Elevated in hemolytic anemia as a result of the liver's inability to process increasing bilirubin released during hemolysis.

Serum lactic dehydrogenase isoenzymes (LDH$_1$ and LDH$_2$):   Elevated in hemolytic anemia because of the release of these enzymes when the RBC is destroyed.

Haptoglobin level: Decreased in hemolytic anemia as a result of increased binding of haptoglobin (a plasma protein) to facilitate removal of increased amounts of hemoglobin from the bloodstream.

Peripheral blood smear: May reveal abnormally shaped RBCs.

Bone marrow aspiration: May reveal abnormally sized, shaped, or amounts of erythrocytes or reticulocytes in various anemias.

Coombs' test: Positive in antibody-mediated/immunologic hemolysis.

Immunoglobulin levels: Frequently elevated with sickle cell disease.

Radiologic examinations/tests
- *X-rays and bone scans:* May reveal increased density or aseptic necrosis of the bones.
- *Liver/spleen scans:* May reveal disease or dysfunction of either organ, which may contribute to anemia.

COLLABORATIVE MANAGEMENT

All anemias

Volume replacement: If patient is hypovolemic, aggressive fluid and/or blood replacement is mandatory to prevent profound hypotension and shock. Fluid challenges/boluses also assist in prevention of deposition of hemolyzed RBCs in the microvasculature.

Transfusions/blood component replacement: Packed RBCs are necessary in the management of profound anemia to assist with elevating the oxygen-carrying capacity of the blood.

Oxygen therapy: To relieve shortness of breath or dyspnea. Methods of oxygen delivery range from nasal cannula to various face masks to mechanical ventilation in severe cases.

Selected anemias

Vitamin B$_{12}$:   Injections or IV infusion is necessary for management of pernicious anemia, a type of megaloblastic anemia caused by failure of the gastric mucosa to absorb vitamin B$_{12}$.

Iron supplements: For iron deficiency states to help increase production of normal-sized RBCs.

Folic acid supplementation: Necessary for RBC production. Supplements of 1 mg/day are used to treat megaloblastic anemia and, theoretically, to prevent hemolytic crisis in patients with hemolytic anemia. It is not effective in all patients with hemolytic anemia.

Epoietin-alfa; erythropoietin, recombinant (Epogen/Procrit): Stimulates production of RBCs in patients with bone marrow hypofunction/lack of production of RBCs, particularly when related to renal failure.

Bone marrow transplantation: Recommended for some patients with sickle cell disease or aplastic anemia to provide a mechanism for regenerating normal RBC production.

Elimination of causative factor: Certain drugs and chemicals, cold temperatures, and stress can worsen many anemias, but most profoundly hemolytic and aplastic anemias. Identifying and removing the causative agent can prevent life-threatening crisis.

Hemolytic anemias only

Red cell exchange therapy for sickle cell crisis: Cytapheresis procedure for patients who are unresponsive to other treatments for sickle cell disease.

Thrombocytapheresis: Cytapheresis procedure for patients experiencing symptoms of excessive thrombosis to reduce platelets rapidly in an attempt to decrease clotting before onset of MODS.

Corticosteroids: Therapy used with limited success in management of hemolytic anemia.

Pain management: Aspirin, acetaminophen, NSAIDs, narcotics, and sedatives may be necessary for relief of pain and anxiety associated with hemolytic anemia, particularly during hemolytic crisis.

Splenectomy: Sometimes recommended for patients suspected of having splenic sequestration crisis related to hemolytic anemia.

Antisickling agents: Some clinical trials currently are underway to evaluate the efficacy of these agents in ablating the sickling phenomenon.

NURSING DIAGNOSES AND INTERVENTIONS

Impaired gas exchange related to lack of RBCs or hemoglobin abnormalities

Desired outcome: Within 48-96 h of onset of treatment, patient has adequate gas exchange as evidenced by HR and RR within 10% of patient's baseline (or HR 60-100 bpm and RR 12-20 breaths/min), Hgb and Hct returned to patient's baseline (or Hgb >12 mg/dl and Hct >37%), oxygen saturation >90%, and BP returned to patient's baseline (or >90 mm Hg systolic within 24 h of initiation of treatment).

- Administer supplemental oxygen as needed, using appropriate device (i.e., nasal cannula, face mask/shield, or mechanical ventilation as necessary).
- Monitor oxygen saturation using pulse oximeter continuously. Consult with physician for persistent values <90% or, if chronically decreased, a sustained drop of >10% of baseline.
- Maintain large-bore (18-gauge) IV catheter(s) in case transfusion or rapid volume expansion is necessary.
- Transfuse with packed cells (RBCs—Table 9-1) as prescribed to facilitate oxygen delivery and assist in volume expansion.
- Describe the purpose of blood product transfusion therapy to the patient and significant others.

T A B L E   9 - 1   Blood and blood products*

Product	Volume	Infusion time	Contents	Possible complications
Whole blood	500 ml/U	2-4 h or <1 h in emergency	All blood components. If fresh, processed with citrate-phosphate-dextrose (CPD)	Hepatitis, transmission of HIV (human immunodeficiency virus), CMV (cytomegalovirus), EBV (Epstein-Barr virus), and other organisms; transfusion reactions: all types
Packed red blood cells	200-250 ml/U	1-4 h or <1 h in emergency	Red blood cells	See whole blood
Fresh-frozen plasma	200-250 ml/U	20 min to thaw; ½ to 1 h or <½ h in emergency	All clotting factors except platelets	See whole blood
Platelets	35-50 ml/U	Direct IV push at 30-50 ml/min. May combine or "pool" several bags into one; given in multiple units	Platelets	Transfusion reaction: febrile or mild allergic; may need to premedicate with acetaminophen (Tylenol) or diphenhydramine HCl (Benadryl); rare instance of septic reaction
Cryoprecipitate	10-20 ml/U	May need 10-30 U unfused at 1 U/min or 10-20 ml/min	Factor VIII; factor XIII and fibrinogen	Small possibility of febrile or mild allergic reaction; rare instance of septic reaction
Granulocytes	300 ml/U	1-2 h; administer slowly for 5 min as test dose	White blood cells (WBC) extracted from 1 U of whole blood	Transfusion reactions: all types; often ineffective in elevating WBC count

Leukocyte-poor and washed, frozen red blood cells	250-300 ml/U	2 h or 1-2 h in emergency	Red cells washed with saline (and possibly irradiated) to remove WBCs and protein from RBCs	Markedly reduced possibility of transfusion reactions: all types
Factor VIII concentrate	10-20 ml/U	May need >10 U infused at 1 U/min	Factor VIII (pooled from possibly thousands of donors)	Small possibility of febrile or mild allergic reaction; rare instance of septic reaction
Factor IX concentrate	20-30 ml/U	May need >10 U infused at 1 U/min	Factor IX (pooled from possibly thousands of donors)	Small possibility of febrile or mild allergic reaction; rare instance of septic reaction
Volume expanders Albumin (5% or 25%) Plasma protein fraction (PPF) Salt-poor albumin	Varies with each product	1 ml/min or as rapidly as tolerated in shock states	Reconstituted from human blood, plasma, or serum	Possible hypervolemia with rapid infusions, particularly with 25% albumin

*Use correct filter with each blood product; most filters can be used to administer 2-4 U; either piggyback or flush products with normal saline solution *only*.

- Evaluate dyspnea and chest pain in sickle cell patients carefully due to the possibility of pulmonary infarction.

Activity intolerance related to anemia/lack of oxygen-carrying capacity of the blood

Desired outcomes: Within 48 h of onset of treatment, patient's activity tolerance improves as evidenced by HR and RR returning to within 10% of baseline (or HR 60-100 bpm and RR 12-20 breaths/min) and BP returning to within 10% patient's baseline (or systolic BP >90% mm Hg). Within 24 h of initiation of treatment patient is able to assist minimally with self-care activities.

- Alternate periods of rest and activity to avoid physically stressing the patient and increasing oxygen demand.
- Reposition patient slowly to evaluate the effects of position change on myocardial and cerebral perfusion.
- Reduce fear, pain, and anxiety to decrease oxygen demand.
- Teach patient to avoid physically and psychologically stressful situations, which can exacerbate symptoms of anemia and precipitate hemolytic crisis in patients with hemolytic anemia.
- Teach patient and significant others to recognize impending hypoxemia: altered mental status, activity intolerance, SOB, chest pain, and weakness.
- Teach patient and significant others about the etiology of the specific anemia that is affecting the patient.
- See this diagnosis in "Prolonged Immobility," p. 78.

Risk for impaired skin integrity related to impaired oxygen transport secondary to chronic anemia

Desired outcome: Patient's skin remains intact during hospitalization.

- Keep extremities warm to promote circulation and help prevent tissue hypoxia.
- Use a bed cradle to reduce pressure of covers on extremities.
- Provide adequate nutrition and nutritional supplements as appropriate. Negative nitrogen state or low serum protein and/or albumin increase the risk for skin breakdown.
- Teach patient the signs of skin breakdown since it can occur at any time with chronic anemia.
- Teach patient about appropriate nutrition as discussed in "Nutritional Support," p. 1.
- Apply appropriate skin-saving dressing (e.g., Duoderm) or initiate aggressive skin care regimen to areas of breakdown.
- For additional interventions, see "Wound and Skin Care," p. 57.

For hemolytic crisis

Altered peripheral, cardiopulmonary, renal, and cerebral tissue perfusion related to interruption of arterial or venous blood flow secondary to microthrombi formation

Desired outcome: Within 24 h of onset of treatment, patient has adequate perfusion as evidenced by warm extremities; pink nail beds; peripheral pulses at least 2+ on a scale of 0-4+ or patient's baseline; capillary refill <2 sec; BP within 10% of patient's normal range or systolic BP >90 mm Hg; HR and RR within 10% of patient's baseline (or HR 60-100 bpm, RR 12-20 breaths/min with a normal depth and pattern ([eupnea]); oxygen saturation >90%; urinary output ≥0.5 ml/kg/h; and patient oriented to time, place, and person.

- Initiate aggressive IV fluid volume replacement as prescribed to prevent deposition of hemolyzed RBCs in the microvasculature.
- Assess extremities for coolness, pallor, and prolonged capillary refill, which are signals of inadequate peripheral perfusion.
- Assess amplitude of peripheral pulses as an indicator of peripheral perfusion. Use Doppler device if unable to palpate pulses.
- Monitor for signs of impending shock, including increased HR and RR, increased restlessness and anxiety, and cool and clammy skin, followed by a decrease in BP.
- Keep lower extremities elevated slightly to promote venous blood flow.
- Monitor for decreased oxygen saturation using continuous pulse oximetry. Consult physician for sustained decreases.
- Monitor ABG values for signs of acidosis (i.e., pH <7.35 and hypercarbia/CO_2 retention [Pa_{CO_2} >45 mm Hg]), indicating hypoperfusion, hypoxemia, and respiratory insufficiency.
- Monitor urinary output for decrease, which can signal decreased renal perfusion. Consult physician for urine output <0.5 ml/kg/h for 2 consecutive hours.
- Monitor neurologic status q2-4h, using the Glasgow Coma Scale (see Appendix 3).
- Teach patient and significant others about hemolytic anemia, including the signs of impending hemolytic crisis, rendering information on the following:
  - *Indicators of impending hemolytic crisis:* Fever, abnormal pain, headache, dizziness, palpitations, paresthesias, and paralysis.
  - *Sensorimotor impairment:* Unsteady gait, paresthesias, blurring of vision, weakness, and paralysis.
  - *Support groups:* Names, phone numbers, and addresses of other persons/groups that can assist with support of people with hemolytic anemias.
  - *Smoking cessation:* Support groups and programs that assist in stopping cigarette smoking to decrease vasoconstriction associated with nicotine intake.
  - *Medications:* Drug name, dosage, frequency, and possible side effects, especially related to steroids: increased appetite, weight gain, "moon face," "buffalo hump," increased possibility of infection, headaches, and increased BP. In addition, discuss the possibility of steroid-induced diabetes mellitus with long-term therapy.
  - *Prevention of infection:* Especially important if patient is on long-term steroid therapy or has had a splenectomy. The patient should obtain an annual flu vaccine; practice good personal hygiene; obtain regular dental check-ups; and get adequate rest, sleep, and relaxation. If a splenectomy has been performed, patients should have a pneumococcal vaccine and wear a Medic-Alert identification bracelet.

Pain related to tissue ischemia secondary to vessel occlusion; or related to inflammation/injury secondary to blood within the joints

Desired outcome: Within 1-2 h of initiating treatment, patient's subjective evaluation of discomfort improves as documented by a pain scale; nonverbal indicators of discomfort are reduced or absent.
- Monitor patient for signs of discomfort, including guarded positioning, muscle spasm, and increases in HR, BP, and RR. Devise a pain scale with patient, rating discomfort from 0 (no pain) to 10.
- Medicate for pain as prescribed, and assess effectiveness of medication on the basis of the pain scale. Confer with physician if pain relief is ineffective; devise an alternate plan for analgesia.
- Consider alternate method of pain control, such as relaxation techniques: guided imagery, controlled breathing, meditation, and playing soft music that is soothing to the patient.
- Use therapeutic/healing touch to relieve pain if practitioner is trained and patient agrees to participate. Or, consult trained practitioner.
- Apply warm compresses to joints to increase circulation and thereby improve tissue oxygenation.
- Apply elastic stockings to promote venous return and enhance circulation.
- Encourage patient to perform isometric or ROM exercises of the extremities to promote circulation.
- Help allay fears by reassuring patient that pain will decrease as the crisis subsides.
- Provide emotional support to patient during the crisis episode. Reassure patient that the crisis is time limited, and enable significant others to be with patient, if possible, during the crisis.
- Teach patient to assess extremities daily for evidence of tissue breakdown or blood sequestration (i.e., swelling, erythema, tenderness) so that early interventions can be implemented in an attempt to prevent severe pain.

Risk for fluid volume deficit or excess related to failure of renal regulatory mechanisms of fluid and electrolyte balance secondary to microthrombi occluding the nephrons

Desired outcome: Patient's volume status returns to normal/baseline as evidenced by urinary output $\geq$0.5 ml/kg/h, stable weight, BP within patient's normal range, HR 60-100 bpm, RR 12-20 breaths/min, good skin turgor, moist mucous membranes, urine specific gravity 1.005-1.025, PAWP 6-12 mm Hg (or patient's baseline), PAD 8-15 mm Hg (or patient's baseline), and CVP 2-6 mm Hg (5-12 cm H_2O).
- Monitor I&O hourly. Consult physician for a urinary output <0.5 ml/kg/h for 2 consecutive hours.
- Evaluate efficacy of volume expansion by closely comparing CVP, PAWP, and PAD. Overzealous volume expansion can lead to congestive heart failure and pulmonary edema with CVP >20%-25% normal values and PAD and/or PAWP >16 mm Hg.
- Administer diuretics as prescribed in the well-hydrated or overhydrated patient with urine output <0.5 ml/kg/h.
- Assess patient for indicators of volume depletion, including poor skin turgor; dry mucous membranes; hypotension; tachycardia; and decreasing urine output, PAWP, PAD, and CVP. As available, check urine specific gravity for increase.
- Monitor electrolytes and serum osmolality. A universal increase in

electrolytes and osmolality is indicative of dehydration. A universal decrease signals fluid overload.

- Assess pH (normal range is 7.35-7.45) before replacing electrolytes, because acidosis and alkalosis alter electrolyte values. Replace potassium cautiously if the patient's pH is outside the normal range.

ADDITIONAL NURSING DIAGNOSES

Uncontrolled bleeding and complications of hemolysis can be terrifying to the patient and significant others, who may fear that the patient may die. See "Psychosocial Support," p. 88, and "Psychosocial Support for the Patient's Family and Significant Others," p. 100, accordingly.

Bleeding and thrombotic disorders

Bleeding can result from qualitative (dysfunctional) or quantitative (lack of) abnormalities of platelets and/or coagulation factors in the plasma. Platelet disorders include heparin-induced thrombocytopenia (HIT), idiopathic thrombocytopenic purpura (ITP), thrombotic thrombocytopenic purpura (TTP), and HELLP syndrome (hemolysis, elevated liver enzymes, and low platelet count). Bone marrow irradiation, hypersplenism, aplastic anemia, vitamin B_{12} or folate deficiencies, metastatic carcinoma, some renal diseases, leukemia, and myeloproliferative disorders also may lead to thrombocytopenia. Platelet destruction may be mediated by either congenital or acquired immunologic or nonimmunologic mechanisms.

Coagulopathies may be caused by liver disease, vitamin K deficiency, pregnancy-induced hypertension associated with HELLP syndrome, or other defects related to blood coagulation factors, such as hemophilia, Von Willebrand's disease, and disseminated intravascular coagulation (DIC). Other disorders that may lead to thromboembolic conditions include roughened surface of vascular endothelium as seen with arteriosclerosis, trauma, infection, or slow/stagnant blood flow through the vessels.

Normal blood coagulation is most often activated as a result of injury to blood vessels, causing the following series of events:

- **Reflex vasoconstriction:** Vascular spasm that decreases blood flow to the site of injury.
- **Platelet aggregation:** Leads to formation of a platelet "plug" to help repair the injury. If the damage to the vessel is small, the "plug" is sufficient to seal the injury. If the "hole" is large, a blood clot is necessary to stop the bleeding.
- **Activation of plasma clotting factors:** Leads to the formation of a fibrin clot. The pathways that initiate clotting factors (see Figure 9-1) include:
  - □ *Intrinsic system:* Initiated by "contact activation" subsequent to an endothelial injury. The problem is "intrinsic" to the circulation or begins with an injury to the blood or circulatory system itself.
  - □ *Extrinsic system:* Initiated by tissue thromboplastin released from injured tissue. The problem is "extrinsic" to the circulation or be-

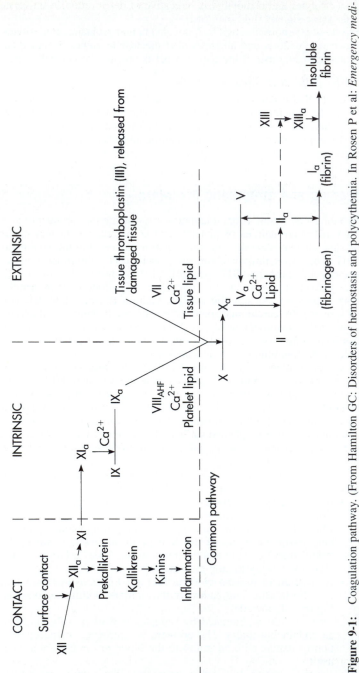

Figure 9-1: Coagulation pathway. (From Hamilton GC: Disorders of hemostasis and polycythemia. In Rosen P et al: *Emergency medicine: concepts and clinical practice*, ed 3, St Louis, 1992, Mosby.)

gins with an injury to tissue rather than within the blood system itself.

▫ *Common pathway:* The "final" part of the coagulation system, which completes the clot formation process begun either by the intrinsic or extrinsic pathway.

▫ *Clot retraction:* Several minutes following its formation, the clot contracts for 30-60 min to express most of the fluid from within the clot. The expressed fluid is called *serum,* for most of the clotting factors have been used/removed by the clot formation process. Serum is unable to clot. The absence of clotting factors differentiates *serum* from *plasma.*

• **Growth of fibrous tissue:** Tissue that completes the organization of the clot within approximately 7-10 days following injury. This process results in permanent closure of the vessel injury.

Both the intrinsic and extrinsic pathways are activated following rupture of a blood vessel. Tissue thromboplastin from the vessel initiates the extrinsic pathway, while contact of factor XII and platelets with the injured vessel wall traumatizes the blood, which initiates the intrinsic pathway. The extrinsic pathway is able to form clots in as little as 15 sec with severe trauma, whereas the intrinsic pathway requires 2-6 min for clot formation.

Heparin-induced thrombocytopenia

PATHOPHYSIOLOGY

Heparin is a widely used anticoagulant that prevents the conversion of fibrinogen to fibrin. Heparin-induced thrombocytopenia (HIT), also called heparin-induced thrombocytopenic thrombosis (HITT) or "white clot syndrome," results when heparin therapy causes either a mild or severe decrease in the number of freely circulating platelets. Platelets in these patients manifest unusual aggregation, which can result in heparin resistance, arterial and venous thrombosis, and subsequent emboli in extreme cases (Figure 9-2). Incidence of HIT ranges from 0-30% in patients receiving SC or IV heparin, with a higher incidence reported with IV use. Bovine (beef-based) heparin has been associated with HIT more frequently than other heparins. Incidence of HIT is not related to the heparin dosage and has been seen in patients receiving low-dose SC heparin, as well as in patients receiving simple heparin "flushes" to maintain patency of IV lines.

There are two types of HIT:

Mild, low morbidity: Generally occurs 1-3 days after initiation of heparin. It may resolve in 5 days after symptoms begin. Platelets may decrease to as low as 100,000/μl or may remain in the low normal range. No treatment is required, and heparin therapy may be continued.

Severe, high morbidity: Generally occurs 4-8 days after initiation of heparin. Symptoms persist until heparin is discontinued. Platelets decrease to <100,000/μl. Thrombosis with subsequent embolization and bleeding are apparent. Complications include pulmonary emboli, myocardial infarction, cerebral infarction, and circulatory impairment

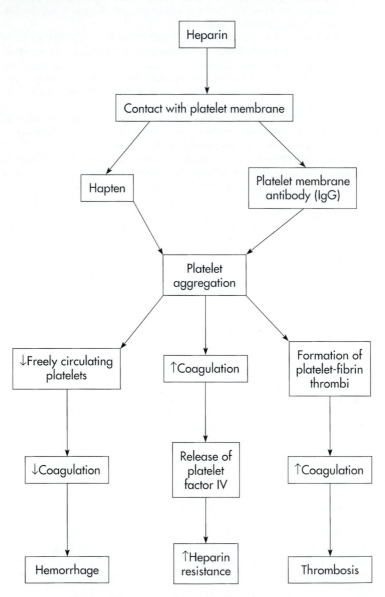

Figure 9-2:   Heparin-induced thrombocytopenia.

resulting in limb amputations. Mortality rate is 29%. Overall, 0.6% of all patients receiving heparin therapy develop thromboembolization. **Heparin must be discontinued immediately** and subsequent complications managed as they occur.

ASSESSMENT

RISK FACTORS Prior drug-induced immunologic thrombocytopenia.

CLINICAL PRESENTATION

Mild, low morbidity: Slight decrease in platelet count without clinical symptoms.

Severe, high morbidity: Hemorrhage, ecchymosis, gingival bleeding, hemoptysis, epistaxis, and possible chest pain, SOB, and "stroke-like" symptoms.

PHYSICAL ASSESSMENT (SEVERE) Presence of petechiae, purpura, bruising from mucosal surfaces or wounds. The patient also may manifest signs of arterial occlusion: cold, pulseless extremities; severe chest pain and/SOB; paresthesias; paralysis; and diminished LOC.

DIAGNOSTIC TESTS

Platelet count: *Mild:* 100,000-150,000/μl; *severe:* <100,000/μl due to severe "clumping" or aggregation of platelets.

Bleeding time: Prolonged if platelets are <100,000/μl.

Platelet antibody screen: Positive findings because of the presence of IgG platelet antibodies.

Coagulation screening (PT, PTT, thromboplastin time):   Normal, inasmuch as the clotting factors that govern these test results are normal.

Fibrinogen: May be low normal or low owing to increased consumption. Normal is 200-400 mg/dl.

Fibrin degradation products: Elevated to $\geq$40 μg/ml because of fibrinolysis of platelet-fibrin thrombi. Normal is <10 μg/ml.

Platelet aggregation: Results will be >100% (or high value of specific laboratory) due to release of platelet membrane antibody.

Heparin-induced platelet aggregation: Reflects abnormal aggregation curve with decrease in the optical density in the aggregometer.

Bone marrow aspiration: Normal or increased number of megakaryocytes (platelet precursors), indicative of normal bone marrow production of platelets.

COLLABORATIVE MANAGEMENT

Heparin therapy: If the platelet count is >100,000/μl and the patient is symptom free, heparin may be continued. Oral anticoagulation should begin immediately, if possible. If the platelet count is <100,000/ μl and the patient develops bleeding or thrombosis, **all heparin should be discontinued immediately, including heparin "flushes."**

Monitoring of heparin therapy: A preheparin platelet count is done to establish baseline values. Daily platelet counts should be done for at least the first 4 days of heparin therapy. Subsequent counts are done q2days. If increasing amounts of heparin are needed to maintain therapeutic levels (i.e., PTT 40-60 sec), heparin resistance should be suspected, which sometimes precedes HIT (see Figure 9-2).

Vena caval filter: If patient experiences thrombosis with decrease or loss of perfusion to an extremity, the physician may consider surgical insertion of a vena caval filter to reduce the risk of pulmonary emboli caused by clot migration from an extremity. See "Pulmonary Emboli," p. 256.

Platelet transfusions: May be initiated following discontinuation of heparin therapy if bleeding fails to subside.

Plasma exchange: In severe cases, 2-3 L plasma is removed and replaced with albumin, crystalloids, or fresh-frozen plasma to assist in decreased bleeding by removing bound heparin from the body.

Alternate anticoagulant: If the patient is in need of further anticoagulation, an alternate medication, such as warfarin sodium (Coumadin), acetylsalicylic acid (aspirin), dipyridamole (Persantine), or dextran should be considered. Streptokinase has been used successfully to manage pulmonary emboli in HIT. Low molecular weight heparin also has been used successfully in many patients.

NURSING DIAGNOSES AND INTERVENTIONS

Altered protection related to decreased platelet count with risk of bleeding and thromboembolization

Desired outcome: Within 24 h of discontinuing heparin therapy, patient exhibits no signs of new bleeding, bruising, or thrombosis as evidenced by HR 60-100 bpm or within 10% of patient's baseline; RR 12-20 breaths/min with normal depth and pattern; systolic BP $\geq$90 mm Hg; and all peripheral pulses at patient's baseline or >2+ on a 0-4+ scale.

- Assess patient at least q2h for signs of bleeding, including hemoptysis, GI bleeding, hematuria, and bleeding from invasive sites or mucous membranes.
- Assess patient at least q2h for signs of thrombosis, including decreased peripheral pulses, altered sensation in extremities (i.e., paresthesias, numbness), pallor, coolness, cyanosis, or capillary refill time >2 sec.
- Avoid IM injections and venous and arterial punctures as much as possible until bleeding time returns to normal.
- Monitor platelet count daily for significant changes. Consult physician for values that remain <150,000/μl or below patient's baseline.
- Assess ECG for heart rate and rhythm, respiratory rate and pattern, and BP for evidence of active bleeding. Be alert to sustained increase in HR and RR or ECG changes, such as ST depression or elevation, since these indicators may precede hypotension.
- Monitor heparin dosage carefully. If increasing doses are required to maintain a therapeutic level (PTT 40-60 sec or 2-2½ times patient's baseline), consult physician for possible heparin resistance, an early indicator of HIT.
- Monitor Hgb and Hct values daily in patients with recent or active bleeding.
- At least q8h assess patient's mental status (orientation to time, place, person, and self) and sensation and strength of movement of extremities.
- Monitor for signs of MODS secondary to thrombosis or prolonged hypotension if patient has hemorrhaged. Be alert for respiratory dis-

tress, chest pain, elevated temperature, decreasing urine output, intolerance of diet or vomiting, abdominal distention, decreasing bowel sounds, and elevated liver enzymes.
- Teach patient and significant others basic pathophysiology of HIT, and instruct them to report this problem to all subsequent health care providers. Teach patient to wear a Medic-Alert bracelet to alert health care providers should patient become unable to speak.

Fluid volume deficit (or risk for same) related to active blood loss
Desired outcome: Patient becomes normovolemic within 24 h of onset of treatment, as evidenced by HR within patient's normal range or 60-100 bpm; RR 12-20 breaths/min with normal depth and pattern; urinary output ≥0.5 ml/kg/h; and absence of abdominal pain/tenderness, back pain, or pain from invasive sites.
- Monitor patient for signs of hypovolemia, including increases in HR and RR, decreases in BP, increased restlessness or fatigue, and decreased urine output.
- Administer supplemental oxygen if patient is actively bleeding.
- Assess for abdominal pain, tenderness, guarding, or back pain, which may signal intraabdominal bleeding.
- Replace lost volume with plasma expanders (albumin, hetastarch [Hespan]), or blood products as indicated. See Table 9-1 for more information.

ADDITIONAL NURSING DIAGNOSES

Uncontrolled bleeding or thrombotic complications can be terrifying for the patient and significant others, who may fear the patient will die. See nursing diagnoses and interventions in "Psychosocial Support," p. 88, and "Psychosocial Support for the Patient's Family and Significant Others," p. 100, accordingly.

Idiopathic thrombocytopenic purpura

PATHOPHYSIOLOGY

Idiopathic thrombocytopenic purpura (ITP) is a disorder characterized by premature platelet destruction, resulting in a decrease in the platelet count to below 100,000/μl. Normal platelet lifespan averages 1-3 wk, whereas in ITP the platelet lifespan averages 1-3 days due to the presence of antiplatelet IgG and IgM antibodies, which destroy platelets in the reticuloendothelial system of the spleen. The coagulopathy is believed to be an autoimmune response and manifests as both an acute and a chronic problem.

Primarily acute ITP is a childhood disease characterized by an abrupt onset of severe thrombocytopenia with evident purpura. Usually it occurs <21 days following a viral infection. At the onset, platelets decrease to <20,000/μl. The chronic form is typically a disease of adults age 20-50 yr, but it has occurred in a small percentage of children and elders. The disease rarely resolves spontaneously and usually is not associated with infection. Women are affected 3 times more often than are men. Petechiae and purpura are commonly seen on the distal upper and lower extremities. Patients may feel symptom free until actual bleeding begins. Intracranial hemorrhage is a potential complication. Platelet counts decrease to as low as 5,000/μl in some patients but may be as high as 75,000/μl in others.

ASSESSMENT

RISK FACTORS In acute ITP there usually is a history of antecedent viral infection occurring about 3 wk before the hemorrhagic episode. The chronic form usually is insidious and sometimes is seen in association with autoimmune hemolytic anemia, HIV disease, hemophilia, Hodgkin's lymphoma, chronic lymphocytic leukemia, systemic lupus erythematosus, sarcoidosis, high-titer anticardiolipin antibodies, and thyrotoxicosis.

CLINICAL PRESENTATION Petechiae, purpura, and prolonged bleeding are commonly seen. Occasionally epistaxis, GI and gingival bleeding, and increased menstrual flow are present. The rarest complication is intracranial hemorrhage, occurring in <1% of patients. Signs of an autoimmune process, such as fever, splenomegaly, or lymphadenopathy, may occur, but since they are not specific to ITP, they require further evaluation.

PHYSICAL ASSESSMENT Presence of petechiae and purpura anywhere on the skin or mucous membrane, most commonly on the distal upper and lower extremities. Ecchymosis is apparent in traumatized areas, along with generalized bruising. Neurologic signs should be monitored closely in acute patients. Joint tenderness and visual (retinal) disturbances may be noted due to bleeding into these areas.

DIAGNOSTIC TESTS

Platelet count: Decreased to 5,000-75,000/μl because of premature destruction. Normal range is 150,000-400,000/μl.

Bleeding time: Prolonged when platelet count is <100,000/μl.

Screening coagulation tests (PT, PTT, thrombin time):   Normal because these tests measure nonplatelet components of the coagulation pathway.

Platelet antibody screen: Positive findings because of the presence of IgG and IgM antiplatelet antibodies.

CBC count with differential: Hgb and Hct may be decreased because of insidious blood loss or simultaneous hemolytic anemia (Evans syndrome); WBC count will be normal unless the ITP is associated with another disease that alters the differential leukocyte count.

Bone marrow aspiration: Biopsy will reveal megakaryocytes (platelet precursors) in normal or increased numbers with a "nonbudding" appearance, possibly indicating defective maturation or failure of platelet production.

Capillary fragility test: Will show >1+, which signals that more than 11 petechiae were present in a 2.5 cm radial area on the skin, following prolonged application of a BP cuff. Normal is 1+ or <10 petechiae.

COLLABORATIVE MANAGEMENT

Platelet transfusions: Platelets are given in cases of life-threatening hemorrhage only. The shortened platelet lifespan renders prophylactic transfusions ineffective.

Glucocorticoid therapy: Adrenocorticosteroids (e.g., prednisone 1-2 mg/kg/day) are effective in increasing the platelet count in 3-14 days following initiation of treatment. Effectiveness is attributed to suppression of phagocytic activity of the macrophage system (particularly the spleen), which increases the lifespan of the antibody-coated platelets. If improvement does not occur within 2-3 wk or excessive doses of steroids are required, splenectomy should be considered. "Normal" responders are able to have steroid dosage tapered over several weeks until platelets reach a sustained value of 50,000/μl.

Splenectomy: Treatment of choice in cases that are refractory to glucocorticoid therapy. The condition stabilizes in 70%-90% of patients who undergo splenectomy. The positive results are attributed to the removal of the site of destruction of the antibody-sensitized platelets.

IV infusions of gammaglobulin: Given 400 mg/kg/day for 5 days, resulting in increased platelet count in 60%-70% of patients. It is less effective in patients with long-standing chronic ITP. The platelet level at initiation of treatment is unrelated to the patient's response. Duration of response may be longest in individuals who achieve the highest initial platelet increases.

Anti-Rh immunoglobulin: Low dose (200-1,000 μg) given IV for 1-5 days has been effective in limited studies. Success of treatment is attributed to sensitization of recipient RBCs, which results in low-grade hemolysis and blockade of the platelet destruction by the reticuloendothelial system.

Immunosuppression: Various immunosuppressive drugs, including azothiaprine, cyclophosphamide, vincristine, and cyclosporine, given alone or in combination with prednisone, have been used successfully in limited situations. A trial of immunosuppression therapy may be indicated in patients who fail to respond to splenectomy or in those who are too unstable to be surgical candidates.

Vinca "alkaloid-loaded" platelets: Transfusions of platelets "loaded" with vinblastine may reduce the phagocytic destruction of platelets in patients who fail to respond to other treatments.

Colchicine: A small percentage of patients refractory to other treatments may improve with 1.2 mg colchicine daily for $\geq$2 wk. The drug has been used successfully in limited studies.

Danazol: 400-800 mg/day has resulted in complete remission or partial improvement in 60%-70% of patients in several studies. Use is controversial as other researchers have reported poor results and many untoward side effects.

Plasmapheresis: Several days of machine-assisted plasma exchange to remove approximately 1.0-1.5 the plasma volume per procedure and replace it with a suitable solution (e.g., colloids, crystalloids, or plasma). Therapy is reserved for patients with life-threatening hemorrhage unresponsive to other measures. It is costly and of marginal benefit.

NURSING DIAGNOSES AND INTERVENTIONS

Altered protection related to decreased platelet count resulting in increased risk of bleeding

Desired outcomes: Within 72 h of onset of treatment, patient exhibits no clinical signs of new bleeding or bruising episodes. Secretions and excretions are negative for blood and VS are within 10% of patient's normal range. Within the 24-h period before discharge from intensive care, patient and significant others verbalize understanding of the indicators of impending bleeding.

- Monitor patient for signs of bleeding, including elevated HR and RR, oozing from invasive sites, bleeding mucous membranes, hematuria, and GI bleeding (i.e., emesis, gastric aspirate, stool with frank or occult blood).
- Avoid IM injections and all unnecessary venous or arterial punctures to minimize oozing from invasive sites.
- Monitor platelet count daily for significant changes. Consult physician for sustained low values (<100,000/μl).
- Avoid administering NSAIDs (e.g., aspirin, ibuprofen). Teach patient to avoid all medications that potentially decrease platelet aggregation, especially aspirin.
- If severe menorrhagia is present, confer with physician regarding need for progestational hormones (e.g., norethindrone acetate, 5-10 mg PO, qd) for suppression of menses. Assess volume of blood loss by weighing perineal pads or tampons.
- During the acute (bleeding) phase of ITP, teach patient to perform oral hygiene using sponge-tipped applicators soaked in water or dilute mouthwash to help prevent gum bleeding.
- Teach patient that it is safer to use an electric razor for shaving, both during and after the bleeding phase of ITP.
- Teach patient and significant others to recognize the signs of impending bleeding, including increased pulse rate, rapid breathing, increased bruising, painful joints, "spitting up" blood, blood in the urine, and tarry stools.

Decreased adaptive capacity: Intracranial (or risk for same), related to potential for intracranial hemorrhage (<1% of patients) secondary to decreased platelet level

Desired outcomes: Throughout the hospitalization, patient remains free of symptoms of intracranial hemorrhage as evidenced by orientation to time, place, and person; normoreactive pupils and reflexes; patient's normal visual acuity, motor strength, and coordination; and absence of headache and other clinical indicators of increased intracranial pressure (IICP).

- Assess patient for initial signs of IICP, including diminished LOC, pupillary responses (unequal or sluggish/absent response to light), visual disturbances, weakness and paralysis, slow HR, and change in respiratory rate and pattern.
- Monitor patient for the presence of headaches, visual disturbances, or motor dysfunction, which are symptoms of IICP.
- If initial signs of IICP are noted, consult physician immediately. Severe intracranial bleeding can lead to herniation. ICP can increase rapidly with severe bleeding, sometimes causing death within 1 h of onset. Signs of impending herniation include unconsciousness, failure to respond to deeply painful stimuli, decorticate or decerebrate posturing, Cushing's triad (bradycardia, increased systolic BP, widening pulse pressure), nonreactive/fixed pupils, unequal pupils, or fixed and dilated pupils. See p. 459 for more information about herniation.

- Consult with physician regarding use of diuretics for occurrence of IICP (see p. 131 for collaborative interventions for IICP).
- Position patient with HOB slightly elevated (30-40 degrees) and neck in neutral position to decrease ICP. For additional interventions for IICP, see Table 2-5, p. 137.
- Teach patient to avoid Valsalva maneuver (e.g., straining at stool or when lifting; forceful and sustained coughing or nose blowing), which could cause intracranial bleeding.
- Teach the importance of avoiding tobacco products (particularly cigarettes) and excessive caffeine, which may cause vasoconstriction. Constricted vessels may prevent platelets from circulating through portions of the capillary network.
- Confer with physician regarding use of stool softeners or cough suppressants, as necessary.

Risk for fluid volume deficit related to active loss secondary to intraabdominal bleeding or postsplenectomy intraabdominal bleeding

Desired outcome: Patient remains normovolemic as evidenced by HR, RR, and BP within 10% of patient's normal range (or HR 60-100 bpm, RR 12-20 breaths/min with normal depth and pattern [eupnea], systolic BP ≥90 mm Hg); urinary output ≥0.5 ml/kg/h; and absence of abdominal pain or tenderness, back pain, and frank bleeding from the splenectomy incision.

- Monitor patient for signs of hypovolemia, including increases in HR and RR, decreases in BP and urinary output, and restlessness and fatigue.
- Administer supplemental oxygen, as necessary, for postoperative status or active bleeding.
- Assess for abdominal pain, tenderness, guarding, or back pain, any of which may signal intraabdominal bleeding.
- Replace lost volume with plasma expanders (albumin, hetastarch [Hespan]) and/or blood products as indicated. See Table 9-1 for information about blood products.
- Inform patient of the importance of wearing a Medic-Alert bracelet and obtaining a pneumococcal vaccination if a splenectomy has been performed.

Pain related to joint inflammation and injury secondary to bleeding into the synovial cavity of the joint(s) or postsplenectomy pain

Desired outcomes: Within 4 h of initiating treatment, patient's subjective evaluation of discomfort improves as documented by a pain scale; nonverbal indicators of discomfort are absent or decreased. HR, RR, and BP are within 10% of patient's baseline.

- Devise a pain scale with patient, rating discomfort from 0 (no pain) to 10. Monitor patient for signs of fatigue and malaise. As appropriate, instruct patient to decrease or eliminate those activities that cause fatigue and malaise.
- Elevate patient's legs to decrease joint pain in the lower extremities. Avoid knee flexion.
- Decrease stress on joints by supporting extremities with pillows, making sure bed is not "gatched" at the knee.
- Teach patient to splint abdomen when coughing postsplenectomy.
- Consult with physician regularly until patient's pain is controlled.

Avoid use of meperidine for pain relief in elders because adverse effects are common.
- Evaluate patient's anxiety level, and provide emotional support to control fear and anxiety. If patient becomes agitated, evaluate potential causes, including hypoxemia, poor pain or anxiety control, fluid and electrolyte imbalance, and alcohol or drug withdrawal, and intervene appropriately.
- See p. 74 for additional pain interventions. Also see "Prolonged Immobility," p. 78, for patients who are unable to move or who have limited movement.

Impaired tissue integrity related to intradermal bleeding
Desired outcome: Within 48 h of initiating treatment, patient has no symptoms of further tissue injury (e.g., bruising, petechiae, or purpura).
- Apply ice pack or manual pressure over sites of intradermal bleeding to promote hemostasis.
- Move/transfer patient carefully and gently to avoid tissue trauma.
- Avoid IM injections and all venous and arterial punctures, which may cause intradermal bleeding. Hold pressure on invasive sites for ≥5 min and subsequently apply a small pressure dressing or collagen-coated adhesive dressing (i.e., "Tipstop") over sites from which needles or IV catheters have been removed.
- Inspect and document appearance of patient's skin q8-12h. Consult physician for new or increased petechiae, purpura, or bruising.
- Explain chronic skin/tissue problems associated with steroids, such as increased vascular fragility, ulceration, "moon face," "buffalo hump," and increased possibility of infections.
- Teach patient the importance of regular check-ups and medical follow-through in managing chronic illness.
- See "Wound and Skin Care," p. 57, for additional interventions.

ADDITIONAL NURSING DIAGNOSES

Uncontrolled bleeding can be terrifying for the patient and significant others, who may fear the patient will die. Refer to nursing diagnoses in "Psychosocial Support," p. 88, and "Psychosocial Support for the Patient's Family and Significant Others," p. 100, for appropriate interventions.

Disseminated intravascular coagulation

PATHOPHYSIOLOGY

Disseminated intravascular coagulation (DIC) is a syndrome characterized by overstimulation of the normal coagulation cascade. DIC is a commonly acquired coagulopathy with the potential to cause both profuse bleeding and widespread thrombosis leading to MODS. Inherent bodily control of bleeding requires a balance between procoagulants and thrombus formation, and anticoagulants, inhibitors, and thrombolysis (Figure 9-1, Table 9-2). The delicate balance may be upset by disease processes (Table 9-3), resulting in a cascade of uncontrolled coagulation and fibrinolysis. The abnormal clotting cascade that develops during DIC is as follows:

T A B L E 9 - 2 Clotting factors: primary actions

Coagulation factor	Thrombin sensitive/promotes vasoconstriction	Vitamin K sensitive	Sites of heparin activity
I Fibrinogen	✔		
II Prothrombin		✔	✔ IIa
III Tissue thromboplastin (tissue factor)			
IV Calcium			
V Proaccelerin (AC globulin [AC-g])	✔		
VI Not assigned			
VII Proconvertin stable factor (prothrombin accelerator)		✔	
VIII Antihemophilic factor A (antihemophilic factor [AHF], antihemophilic globulin AHG])	✔		
IX Antihemophilic factor B (plasma thromboplastin component [PTC], Christmas factor)		✔	✔ IXa
X Stuart-Prower factor (Stuart factor)		✔	✔ Xa
XI Plasma thromboplastin antecedent (antihemophilic factor C)			✔ XIa
XII Hageman factor (contact factor)			
XIII Fibrin stabilizing factor	✔		
Other factors			
Prekallikrein (Fletcher factor)			
High-molecular-weight kininogen (HMWK—Fitzgerald factor)			
Platelets			

- Platelets and coagulation factors are activated by a disease stimulus and are rapidly consumed, particularly factors V and XIII and fibrinogen.
- Thrombin is formed very rapidly, and inherent inhibitors are unable to stop the formation of the vast amounts of thrombin generated. Thrombin directly activates fibrinogen.
- Fibrin is deposited throughout the capillary beds of organs and tissues.
- The fibrinolytic system lyses fibrin and impairs thrombin formation.
- Fibrin degradation products ([FDPs] or fibrin split products

T A B L E 9 - 3 Clinical conditions that can activate disseminated intravascular coagulation

Obstetric	GI disorders	Tissue damage	Infections	Hemolytic processes	Vascular disorders	Miscellaneous
Abruptio placentae	Cirrhosis	Surgery	Viral	Transfusion reaction	Shock	Fat or pulmonary embolism
Toxemia	Hepatic necrosis	Trauma	Bacterial	Acute hemolysis secondary to infection or immunologic disorder	Aneurysm	Snake bite
Amniotic fluid embolism	Pancreatitis	Burns	Rickettsial		Giant hemangioma	Neoplastic disorder
Septic abortion	Peritoneovenous shunts	Prolonged extracorporeal circulation	Protozoal			Acute anoxia
Retained dead fetus	Necrotizing enterocolitis	Transplant rejection	Fungal			
Hydatid mole		Heat stroke				

[FSPs]) result from fibrinolysis, which changes platelet aggregation and inhibits fibrin polymerization. See Figure 9-1 for the normal coagulation pathway.

A predisposing event, such as damage to the vascular endothelium, initiates the clotting cascade. Studies reflect that both the intrinsic and extrinsic pathways are activated initially, resulting in an abnormal acceleration of the clotting process. Thrombocytopenia occurs due to thrombin production and microvascular thrombus formation.

ASSESSMENT

RISK FACTORS Any clinical state or pharmacologic therapy (e.g., chemotherapy) that inhibits the removal of activated clotting factors, FDPs, and thromboplastin by the reticuloendothelial system. DIC may manifest as a profound bleeding/clotting disorder in the *acute* phase or as a less symptomatic *chronic* disorder.

In chronic (compensated) DIC, activation of coagulation and fibrinolysis does not occur rapidly enough to exceed the rate of production of clotting factors or inhibitors. The course of DIC depends on the intensity of the stimulus, coupled with the status of the liver, bone marrow, and vascular endothelium. Bleeding versus thrombosis in DIC is profoundly affected by the underlying disease process.

CLINICAL PRESENTATION *Abrupt onset of bleeding* or oozing of blood from all invasive sites and mucosal surfaces (e.g., oral, nasal, tracheal, gastric, urethral, vaginal, rectal). In addition, the patient may have hematuria, petechiae, stools or gastric aspirate positive for occult blood, pallor, tachycardia, tachypnea, vertigo, hypotension, ecchymoses (e.g., on palate, gums, skin, conjunctivae), petechiae, lethargy, irritability or feeling of "impending doom," and possible back pain and abdominal tenderness.

Abnormal thrombosis may manifest with extremity pain, diminished pulses, oliguria or anuria, diminished or absent bowel sounds, severe chest pain with SOB (indicative of either myocardial infarction or pulmonary embolism), or paresis or paralysis (indicative of cerebral thrombus).

PHYSICAL ASSESSMENT Bleeding from invasive sites and mucosal surfaces, petechiae, ecchymoses, acrocyanosis, bruising, mottling, SOB, tachypnea, possible Grey Turner's sign (flank ecchymosis), purpura, diminished or absent bowel sounds, weakened/absent peripheral pulses, confusion, decreased responsiveness, abdominal tenderness, weakness, ST-segment elevation or depression, and T-wave inversion.

DIAGNOSTIC TESTS

Also see Table 9-4.

Fibrin degradation products or fibrin split products: Increased (>10 μg/ml) because of widespread fibrinolysis, which produces FDPs as the end product of clot lysis. Critical value: >40 μg/ml.

D-dimer assay: Increased to >500 due to increased thrombin and plasmin generation. This is a rapid measurement technique, less sensitive than FDPs, and not recommended as a substitute for FDPs and fibrinogen determinations.

T A B L E 9 - 4   **Blood coagulation screen in disseminated intravascular coagulation**

Parameter	Normal	Acute DIC	Chronic DIC
Fibrinogen	150-400 mg/dl (adult)	Decreased	Normal or increased
Fibrin degradation	<10 μg/ml	Positive (increased)	Positive (increased)
Platelet count	150,000-400,000/μl (adult)	Decreased	Normal or increased
Partial thromboplastin time (PTT, APTT) (also known as activated partial thromboplastin time)	25-35 sec	Increased	Normal
Prothrombin time	11-15 sec	Increased	Normal
Thrombin time	1.5 × control value	Increased	Increased

Fibrinogen levels: May remain normal or decrease in the early acute phase. As the process continues, fibrinogen levels will decrease. Normal range is 150-400 mg/dl.

Partial thromboplastin time (PTT) or activated PTT [APTT]):   Prolonged (>40 sec) due to activation of the intrinsic pathway, causing consumption of coagulation factors. Critical value: >70 sec. In chronic DIC the value may be normal (25-35 sec) or less than normal.

Prothrombin time: Prolonged (>15 sec) because of activation of the extrinsic pathway, causing consumption of the extrinsic clotting factors. Critical value: >40 sec.

Thrombin time: Prolonged (>1.5 times the control value or >2 sec in excess of a 9-13 sec control value) due to rapid conversion of fibrinogen into fibrin.

Antithrombin III (AT-III):   Decreased (<50% of control value using a plasma sample or <80% using functional values) due to rapid consumption of this thrombin inhibitor. The action of AT-III is catalyzed by heparin.

Euglobulin clot lysis time: This test measures fibrinogen activity *via* measurement of plasminogen and plasminogen activator, which assist in prevention of fibrin clot formations. Decreased time is seen with DIC. Normal: lysis in 2-4 h. Critical value: 100% lysis in 1 h.

Platelet count: Decreased (<140,000/μl) due to rapid rate of platelet aggregation to form clots during DIC. Aggregation decreases the freely circulating platelets.

Alpha$_2$-antiplasmin: Decreased due to rapid consumption of same in response to large amounts of plasmin generated. When all alpha$_2$-antiplasmin is depleted, excessive hyperfibrinolysis (massive, rapid clot lysis) occurs.

Protamine sulfate test, fibrin split products: Results are positive (normal: negative), indicative of presence of fibrin strands. It is associated with the formation of excessive amounts of thrombin and secondary fibrinolysis.

Peripheral blood smear: For visualization during microscopic examination of schistocytes and burr cells, which indicate the deposition of fibrin in the small blood vessels.

COLLABORATIVE MANAGEMENT

Treatment of the underlying disease process often corrects the secondary DIC. Other treatments may vary in effectiveness, depending on the underlying disease. Use of heparin and antifibrinolytic agents in DIC is controversial, inasmuch as these agents have not improved survival in DIC and may exacerbate bleeding (heparin) or thrombosis (antifibrinolytic agent). The following treatments have been effective in individual patients.

Treatment of the primary pathology: A primary disease generally promotes the development of DIC. When DIC occurs without apparent cause, the possibility of undiagnosed malignancy (e.g., prostate cancer), a large abdominal aortic aneurysm, a progressive gram-negative bacterial infection, or hepatic cirrhosis should be explored. Idiopathic DIC is extremely rare but has been reported in infants and several adults.

Continuous IV heparin therapy: There are three conditions associated with DIC in which heparin generally is effective:

Underlying malignancy/carcinoma

Acute promyelocytic leukemia (APML)

Purpura fulminans/extreme purpura, often seen with severe sepsis

Low-dose therapy (5-10 U/kg/h) is considered. Heparin binds to antithrombin, which then inhibits proteases involved in both the intrinsic and common coagulation pathways, resulting in a strong anticoagulant effect. Use of higher-dose heparin in DIC is associated with a high risk of bleeding, and greater efficacy has not been documented.

Note: APML patients with DIC often accelerate symptoms of fibrinolysis (declotting) when receiving chemotherapy. If these individuals receive heparin, an antifibrinolytic agent such as epsilon-aminocaproic acid (Amicar) may be added to decrease bleeding.

Antifibrinolytic agents: Epsilon-aminocaproic acid (Amicar) and tranexamic acid (Cyklokapron) are used to inhibit fibrinolysis in patients who are bleeding due to a variety of causes. In DIC patients, these agents should be used with extreme caution as they may convert a bleeding disorder into a thrombotic problem. When used in DIC, these agents are used in combination with heparin to minimize the potential for thrombosis.

Thrombolytic agents: Use of streptokinase, urokinase, and tissue plasminogen activator (TPA) is not indicated for patients with thrombosis, for these agents may facilitate excessive bleeding.

Blood component replacement: Clotting factors and inhibitors are replaced in the form of fresh-frozen plasma. The PT is suggested as the most accurate parameter for guiding plasma replacement. Patients with markedly decreased fibrinogen levels may be given cryoprecipitate, which contains 5-10 times more fibrinogen than plasma. Thrombocytopenia in DIC generally is not severe, and the platelet count usually is >50,000/µl. General replacement therapy guidelines indicate that approximately 10 U of cryoprecipitate should be given for q2-3U of plasma. Platelet transfusions rarely are needed unless the patient has impaired platelet production and profuse bleeding. Antithrombin III concentrate has been used on a limited basis in clinical trials (see Table 9-1).

Red blood cell replacement: Packed RBCs may be administered to increase oxygen-carrying capacity with a hemoglobin value <9 mg/dl or >20% below the patient's baseline if the patient is chronically anemic.

Vitamin K$_1$ (phytonadione) and folate: Patients with DIC are at high risk for deficiency of these substances, and administration of both vitamins is recommended for most patients.

Protease inhibitors: Experimental medications, including gabexate, nafamostat, and transylol, have been used in limited clinical trials.

Vasoactive drugs: If patient becomes severely hypotensive, the following drugs may be considered: amrinone, dobutamine, dopamine, epinephrine, and nitroprusside (see Appendix 7).

NURSING DIAGNOSES AND INTERVENTIONS

Altered protection related to bleeding resulting from overstimulation of the clotting cascade and rapid consumption of clotting factors

Desired outcome: Within 48-72 h of initiation of treatment, patient is free of symptoms of bleeding as evidenced by absence of frank bleeding from invasive sites and mucosal surfaces; secretions and excretions that are negative for blood; absence of large or increasing ecchymoses; decreasing purpura; and HR, RR, and BP within 10% of patient's baseline (or HR 60-100 bpm, RR 12-20 breaths/min, systolic BP >90 mm Hg).

- Discuss bleeding history with patient or significant others as possible, assessing prior incidence of a bleeding problem, gingival bleeding, skin bleeding, hematuria, tarry/bloody stools, muscle bleeding, bleeding into joints, hemoptysis, vomiting of blood, epistaxis, prolonged bleeding from small wounds or following tooth extraction, and unusual or "easy" bruising tendency.
- Question patients who have no previous history of bleeding regarding current medications, including OTC preparations, since many medications promote bleeding (see Table 9-5).
- Monitor coagulation/clotting tests daily. Consult physician for values that exceed normal ranges by 15% (see Table 9-4).
- Monitor closely for increased bleeding, bruising, petechiae, and purpura. Assess for internal bleeding by testing suspicious secretions (i.e., sputum, urine, stool, emesis, and gastric drainage) for the presence of blood.
- Monitor neurologic status (see Glasgow Coma Scale, Appendix 3) q2h by assessing LOC, orientation, pupillary reaction, and movement and strength of extremities. Changes in status can indicate intracranial bleeding.
- Use alcohol-free mouthwash and swabs for oral care to minimize the risk of bleeding from gum injury. Use normal saline solution (NSS) or solution of NSS and sodium bicarbonate (500 ml NSS with

15 ml bicarbonate) to irrigate the oral cavity. Massage gums gently with a sponge-tipped applicator to help remove debris. Do not attempt to remove large clots from the mouth, inasmuch as profuse bleeding may ensue.

- Use electric rather than safety razor for shaving patient.
- Avoid giving unnecessary venipunctures and IM injections.
- If patient undergoes an invasive procedure, manually hold pressure over the insertion site for 3-5 min for IV catheters and 10-15 min for arterial catheters or until bleeding subsides.
- Teach patient the importance of avoiding vitamin K–inhibiting and platelet aggregation–inhibiting medications (Table 9-5), which promote bleeding.

Risk for fluid volume deficit related to bleeding/hemorrhage
Desired outcomes: Patient remains normovolemic as evidenced by HR and RR within patient's baseline (or HR 60-100 bpm and RR 12-20 breaths/min with normal depth and pattern), BP within patient's baseline (or systolic BP >90 mm Hg), warm extremities, distal pulses >2+ on a 0-4+ scale, urinary output ≥0.5 ml/kg/h, and capillary refill <2 sec. Within 24 h of initiating treatment, patient verbalizes orientation to time, place, person, and self.

- Monitor VS at least q2h, noting increases in HR and RR, decreased BP, and decreasing pulse pressure.
- Measure urinary output q2-4h. Consult physician for output <0.5 ml/kg/h.
- Increase frequency of measurement of VS and urine output to at least q30min if patient is bleeding actively. For profuse bleeding, check VS at least q15min. Consider insertion of an arterial line for continuous monitoring of BP.
- Monitor CBC daily for significant alterations in Hct, Hgb, and platelets (Table 9-6).
- Assess patient for signs of impending shock if HR and RR increase or if BP decreases: pallor, diaphoresis, cool extremities, delayed capillary refill, diminished intensity of peripheral pulses, restlessness, agitation, and disorientation.
- Inspect all invasive sites for frank bleeding, including a thorough assessment of all dressings that are covering wounds.
- Maintain at least one 18-gauge or larger IV catheter for use during shock management, at which time rapid infusion of blood products or IV fluids may be necessary. For more information, see ACLS algorithms, Appendix 1.

Altered peripheral, cardiopulmonary, cerebral, and renal tissue perfusion (or risk for same) related to blood loss or presence of microthrombi
Desired outcome: Patient has adequate perfusion as evidenced by peripheral pulses >2+ on a scale of 0-4+; brisk capillary refill (<2 sec); BP within patient's normal range; CVP ≥5 cm H_2O or ≥2 mm Hg; PAWP 6-12 mm Hg; and HR regular and ≤100 bpm. Patient is oriented to time, place, person, and self and has urinary output ≥30 ml/h (0.5 ml/kg/h) and oxygen saturation >90%.

- Assess and document peripheral perfusion q2h, including temperature, sensation, pulses, and movement in extremities. Consult physician for coolness and pallor of extremities, decreased

T A B L E   9 - 5   Medications that may promote bleeding

Medications that inhibit platelets or cause thrombocytopenia			Medications that inhibit vitamin K
Analgesics nonsteroidal antiinflammatory agents (NSAIDs) aspirin acetaminophen antipyrine ibuprofen indomethacin fenoprofen sodium salicylate *Antirheumatic agents* oxyphenbutazone phenylbutazone hydroxychloroquine gold salts *Antimicrobials* ampicillin cephalothin lincomycin methicillin penicillin novobiocin	*Diuretic agents* sulfonamide derivatives acetazolamide chlorpropamide chlorothiazide chlorthalidone clopamide diazoxide furosemide bumetanide hydrochlorothiazide tolbutamide spironolactone mercurial diuretics *Phenothiazines* chlorpromazine promethazine trifluoperazine *Phosphodiesterase inhibitors* caffeine dipyridamole theophyllines	*Other* antihistamines ethanol heparin beta-adrenergic blocking agents general anesthetics local anesthetics chemotherapeutic agents vitamin E estrogens digitoxin cimetidine levodopa propylthiouracil	*Salicylates* aspirin and aspirin combination drugs other salicylates *Coumarins* anisindione dicumarol warfarin *Broad-spectrum antibiotics* sulfonamides triplesulfa sulfadiazine sulfamethizole sulfamethoxazole sulfasalazine sulfisoxazole sulfamethoxazole-trimethoprim clindamycin gentamicin neomycin tobramycin

Medications that inhibit platelets or cause thrombocytopenia		Medications that inhibit vitamin K
Antimicrobials—cont'd	*Prostagladins*	*Broad-spectrum antibiotics—cont'd*
oxytetracycline	I_2	vancomycin
pentamidine	D_2	imipenem
streptomycin	E	cefamandole
sulfonamides (antibiotics)		cefoxitin
sulfamethoxazole	*Sedative-hyponotics*	moxalactam
chloramphenicol	benzodiazepines	*Vitamins*
isoniazid	clonazepam	A
nitrofurantoin	diazepam	E
rifampin		
paraaminosalicylic acid	*Vasodilators*	
trimethoprim	nitroglycerin	
chloroquine	nitroprusside	

T A B L E 9 - 6   Complete blood count values

Parameters	Common measurement value	Population
Red blood cells (RBCs)	4-5.5 million/μl	Adult females
	4.5-6.2 million/μl	Adult males
Hemoglobin (Hgb)	12-16 g/dl	Adult females
	14-18 g/dl	Adult males
Hematocrit (Hct)	37%-47%	Adult females
Mean corpuscular volume (MCV)	83-93 μ^3	Adults
Mean cell hemoglobin (MCH)	26-34 pg	Adults
Mean cell hemoglobin concentration (MCHC)	31%-38%	Adults
White blood cells (WBCs)	4,500-11,000/μl	Adults
Differential white blood cells		
Granulocytes		
Segmented neutrophils (Segs)	54%-62%	Adults
Band neutrophils (Bands)	3%-5%	Adults
Eosinophils (Eos)	1%-3%	Adults
Basophils (Basos)	0-0.75%	Adults
Monocytes (Monos)	3%-7%	Adults
Lymphocytes (Lymphs)	25%-33%	Adults
Platelets	150,000-400,000/μl	Adults

sensation/numbness, localized weakness, and delayed capillary refill.

- Monitor BP and assess for early signs of perfusion deficit at least q2h, including dizziness, confusion, and decreased urinary output.
- Monitor for decreased myocardial or pulmonary perfusion as evidenced by chest pain, ST-segment depression or elevation, T-wave inversion, SOB, dyspnea, and decreased oxygen saturation using continuous pulse oximetry.
- Monitor PAWP frequently, observing for both high and low readings. Decreased pressures are indicative of hypovolemia/hemorrhage. Elevated PAD pressures may signal pulmonary embolus.
- Monitor CO and calculate SVR, PVR, and CI. Anticipate vasoconstriction with hypovolemia. SVR will be elevated >1,400 dynes/sec/cm^{-5}. CO may increase or decrease from normal range of 4-7 L/min, depending on cardiac contractility. PVR will be elevated >240 dynes/sec/cm^{-5} in the presence of pulmonary emboli.

- Monitor GI status by observing tolerance to diet or tube feedings, bowel habits (constipation, diarrhea), character of stool (tarry, bloody), and presence or absence of bowel sounds. Palpate for abdominal tenderness and monitor abdominal girth q8h.

Impaired gas exchange (or risk for same) related to loss of oxygen-carrying capacity through hemorrhage or pulmonary microembolus formation

Desired outcome: Patient's gas exchange is adequate as evidenced by Pao_2 ≥80 mm Hg; $Paco_2$ 35-45 mm Hg; pH 7.35-7.45; RR 12-20 breaths/min with normal depth and pattern (eupnea); oxygen saturation >90%; HR 60-100 bpm; Svo_2 >60%; and orientation to time, place, and person.

- Assess respiratory status q2h, noting rate, rhythm, depth, and regularity of respirations.
- Monitor oxygen saturation *via* pulse oximetry. Consult physician for persistent values ≤90%, which may signal inadequate oxygenation.
- Monitor ABG values, being alert to an increase in $Paco_2$ and decrease in pH, which can signal hypoventilation. Consult physician accordingly.
- If BP is stable, place patient in high Fowler's position or in a comfortable, upright position to promote lung expansion.
- Assess lungs for the presence of bibasilar crackles (rales), which can occur with fluid accumulation.
- Monitor for signs of pulmonary embolus, including sharp, stabbing chest pain; dyspnea; pallor; cyanosis; pupillary dilatation; rapid, irregular pulse; profuse diaphoresis; and anxiety. Assess need for supplemental oxygen and consult physician immediately. Patients with severe pulmonary emboli may require mechanical ventilation. See "Pulmonary Emboli," p. 251.
- Assess patient for changes in sensorium (confusion, lethargy, somnolence), which can indicate either inadequate cerebral oxygenation or carbon dioxide retention (respiratory insufficiency). Notify physician accordingly.

Risk for injury related to blood product administration

Desired outcome: Throughout transfusion and up to 8 h after transfusion, patient does not exhibit signs of a blood transfusion reaction as evidenced by absence of fever and chills; normal appearance of skin (no flushing, rash, lesions); and baseline RR, BP, and HR.

- Check blood to be given with another professional to ensure that the crossmatch report and requisition form match the blood unit information. Verify the following: patient's name and hospital number, blood unit number, blood expiration date, blood group, and blood type.
- When blood products are infusing, check VS q15min for the first h. Check patient frequently throughout the first 15 min of the transfusion to observe for signs of an acute intravascular hemolytic transfusion reaction, including fever, chills, dyspnea, hypotension, flushing, tachycardia, back pain, hematuria, and shock.
- Observe for transfusion reactions throughout the transfusion and dur-

T A B L E 9 - 7   **Acute transfusion reactions**

Type	Symptoms	Time frame
Acute intravascular hemolytic	Fever, chills, dyspnea, tachycardia, hypotension, back pain, flushing, hematuria, shock	Following start of transfusion Within 5-30 min
Acute extravascular hemolytic	Fever, elevated bilirubin, unusually low posttransfusion hematocrit and hemoglobin	Usually within 8 h Delayed: 7-10 days
Allergic (mild)	Rash, hives, pruritus	Within 1 h
Anaphylactic	Dyspnea, shortness of breath, bronchospasms, tachycardia, flushing, hypotension, shock	Within 30 min-1 h
Febrile	Fever, chills	Within 4 h
Hypervolemic	Dyspnea, tachycardia, bibasilar crackles, jugular venous distention, possible hypertension, headache	Within 1-2 h
Septic	Fever, chills, tachycardia, hypotension, vomiting, shock, muscle pain, cardiac arrest	Within 5 min-4 h

ing the 8-h period afterward. If a transfusion reaction (see Table 9-7) occurs, implement the following:

1. If the transfusion is in progress, stop the infusion immediately.
2. Maintain IV access with NSS.
3. Maintain BP with a combination of volume infusion and vasoactive drugs, if indicated. See ACLS algorithms, Appendix 1, accordingly.
4. Monitor HR and ECG for changes. Consult physician and treat symptomatic dysrhythmias as prescribed.
5. Administer diuretics and fluids as prescribed to promote diuresis (urine output approximately 100 ml/h).
6. Obtain blood and urine for a transfusion workup per institutional blood bank protocol.
7. Perform blood cultures if patient exhibits signs of sepsis.

- If an intravascular hemolytic reaction is confirmed, implement the following:
  - Monitor coagulation studies, including PT, PTT, and fibrinogen levels (see Table 9-4).
  - Monitor renal status, noting BUN, creatinine, potassium, and phosphate levels.
  - Monitor laboratory values indicative of hemolysis, including LDH, bilirubin, and haptoglobin.

ADDITIONAL NURSING DIAGNOSES

The uncontrolled bleeding related to DIC can be terrifying to the patient and significant others, who may fear the patient will die. Refer to nursing diagnoses in "Psychosocial Support," p. 88; and "Psychosocial Support for the Patient's Family and Significant Others," p. 100. For patients who manifest activity intolerance, see that nursing diagnosis in "Prolonged Immobility," p. 78.

Selected Bibliography

Aster RH, George RH: Thrombocytopenia due to enhanced platelet destruction by immunologic mechanisms. In Williams WJ et al, editors: *Hematology,* ed 4, New York, 1990, McGraw Hill.

Beaurling-Harbury C, Shade SG: Platelet activation during pain crisis in sickle cell anemia patients, *Am J Hematol* 31(4):237-241, 1989.

Bell WR: Fibrinolytic therapy: indications and management. In Hoffman R et al, editors: *Hematology: basic principles and practice,* New York, 1991, Churchill Livingstone.

Bentler E: The sickle cell diseases and related disorders. In Williams WJ et al, editors: *Hematology,* ed 4, New York, 1990, McGraw Hill.

Chang JE: White clot syndrome associated with heparin-induced thrombocytopenia: a review of 23 cases, *Heart Lung* 16(4):403-407, 1987.

Coller BS, Schneiderman P: Clinical evaluation of hemorrhagic disorders: the bleeding history and differential diagnosis of purpura. In Hoffman R et al, editors: *Hematology: basic principles and practice,* New York, 1991, Churchill Livingstone.

Colman RW et al: *Hemostasis and thrombosis: basic principles and clinical practice,* ed 2, Philadelphia, 1987, Lippincott.

Francis RB: Elevated fibrin D-dimer fragment in sickle cell anemia: evidence for activation of coagulation during the steady state as well as in painful crisis, *Haemostasis* 19(2):105-111, 1989.

George JN, Aster RH: Thrombocytopenia due to enhanced platelet destruction by nonimmunologic mechanisms. In Williams WJ et al, editors: *Hematology,* ed 4, New York, 1990, McGraw-Hill.

Hamilton GC: Disorders of hemostasis and polycythemia. In Rosen P et al, editors: *Emergency medicine: concepts and clinical practice,* ed 3, St Louis, 1992, Mosby.

Harrington L, Hufnagel JM: Heparin-induced thrombocytopenia and thrombosis syndrome: a case study, *Heart Lung* 19(1):93-98, 1990.

Interqual: The ISD-A review system with adult ISD criteria, August 1992, North Hampton, NH, and Marlboro, Mass, Interqual, Inc.

Irvin S: White clot syndrome: a life-threatening complication of heparin therapy, *Focus Crit Care* 17(2):107-110, 1990.

Jennings BM: The hematologic system. In Alspach JG, editor: *Core curriculum for critical care nursing,* ed 4, Philadelphia, 1991, Saunders.

Jones KA et al: Severe HELLP syndrome presenting with acute gum bleeding following toothbrushing at 38 weeks' gestation, *Am J Crit Care* 2(5):395-396, 1993.

Kim MJ, McFarland GK, McLane AM: *Pocket guide to nursing diagnoses,* ed 6, St Louis, 1995, Mosby.

Koenigseder LA, Crane PB, Lucy PW: HELLP: a collaborative challenge for critical care and obstetric nurses, *Am J Crit Care* 2(5):385-392, 1993.

Kotschwar T: Low-molecular-weight heparins: a new class of antithrombotic agents, *Pharmacy and Therapeutics* 34-51, 1994.

Marder VJ: Consumptive thrombohemorrhagic disorders. In Williams WJ et al, editors: *Hematology,* ed 4, New York, 1990, McGraw-Hill.

Nurmohamed MT et al: Low-molecular-weight heparin versus standard heparin in general and orthopedic surgery: a meta-analysis, *Lancet* 340:152-156, 1992.

Santoro SA: Laboratory evaluation of hemostatic disorders. In Hoffman R et al, editors: *Hematology: basic principles and practice,* New York, 1991, Churchill Livingstone.

Sibai BM: The HELLP syndrome (hemolysis, elevated liver enzymes, and low platelets): much ado about nothing? *Am J Obstet Gynecol* 162:311-316, 1990.

Snyder EL: Transfusion reactions. In Hoffman R et al, editors: *Hematology: basic principles and practice,* New York, 1991, Churchill Livingstone.

Steuble BT: Hematologic disorders. In Swearingen PL, editor: *Manual of medical-surgical nursing: nursing interventions and collaborative management,* ed 3, St Louis, 1994, Mosby.

Swearingen PL: *Pocket guide to medical-surgical nursing,* St Louis, 1993, Mosby.

Tollefsen DM: Heparin: basic and clinical pharmacology. In Hoffman R et al, editors: *Hematology: basic principles and practice,* New York, 1991, Churchill Livingstone.

Williams EC, Mosher DF: Disseminated intravascular coagulation. In Hoffman R et al, editors: *Hematology: basic principles and practice,* New York, 1991, Churchill Livingstone.

10 MULTISYSTEM STRESSORS

Shock: septic and anaphylactic

PATHOPHYSIOLOGY

Shock is a multisystem disorder that involves inadequate tissue perfusion and altered metabolism. Inadequate tissue perfusion can be a result of any condition that alters heart function (cardiogenic shock), blood volume (hypovolemic shock), blood pressure, and distribution of blood volume (septic, anaphylactic, and neurogenic shock).

Shock is a very complex clinical syndrome in which tissue perfusion is inadequate to meet tissue demands for oxygen. Inadequate perfusion/oxygenation alters cellular function and eventually impairs organs and body system functioning. Multisystem organ dysfunction syndrome (MODS) is a term used to describe impairment of several systems. Whatever the cause of shock, the condition leads to organ failure and eventually to death unless compensatory mechanisms or medical/nursing interventions reverse the process.

Sepsis and septic shock: Sepsis is an acute systemic clinical syndrome caused by bacteria, viruses, or fungi in the blood, most commonly gram-negative bacilli. It can be described as a continuum from bacteremia to profound septic shock and usually involves multisystem deleterious effects.

In early sepsis a generalized inflammatory response is triggered, causing widespread vasodilatation. The progression to septic shock is believed to be caused by toxins released from the organism involved. The primary toxin, endotoxin, has many effects. Bacterial endotoxin activates the complement, coagulation, and fibrinolytic systems; increases vascular permeability; and triggers the release of vasoactive kinins. A major systemic response is vasodilatation. Kinins, such as bradykinin and serotonin, cause vasodilatation and increase capillary permeability, thereby decreasing systemic vascular resistance and facilitating fluid shifts from intravascular to interstitial spaces. Another response is increased capillary permeability secondary to histamine release, which results in vascular fluid shifts to interstitial spaces. In addition, there is selective blood vessel constriction (e.g., renal, pulmonary, and splanchnic vessels) and vascular occlusion with subsequent sluggish blood flow, systemic pooling, and tissue ischemia. This stage is often referred to as "warm shock" (Table 10-1). It is also associated with increased cardiac contractility and a hyperdynamic cardiac state due to sympathetic nervous system stimulation. As the septic state progresses, the hemodynamics change from vasodilatation to a classic shock presentation, with vasoconstriction and decreased cardiac output. These changes are stimulated by the powerful catecholamines and prostaglandins that are released from ischemic tissues. The stage during which tissue perfusion becomes severely compromised and ischemic cellular damage occurs is termed "cold shock" (Table 10-2). Additionally, fever occurs when the invading microorganisms release pyrogens (e.g., prostaglandins), which affect the thermoregulatory center in the hypothalamus.

The patient with sepsis is at high risk for development of DIC (see p. 608) and ARDS (see p. 247). See Figure 10-1 for a depiction of the pathophysiologic process of sepsis.

Anaphylactic shock: Systemic anaphylactic shock (anaphylaxis) is a potentially life-threatening situation. It is the result of an exaggerated or a hypersensitivity response to an antigen (or allergen). The classic form of anaphylaxis occurs in a sensitized person (i.e., someone who has been exposed previously to the same antigen), usually 1-20 min after introduction of the antigenic substance. The most common substances that cause anaphylaxis are drugs, antibiotic agents, anesthetics, foods, antisera, and blood products.

The hypersensitivity response occurs on the surface of the mast cells, which are located primarily in the lungs, in small blood vessels, and in connective tissue. There the antigen combines with sensitized antibodies from previous exposure (usually IgE type). The antigen also attaches to basophils circulating in the blood. This triggers release of substances from the granules within the cells, including histamine, serotonin, kinins, and eosinophil and neutrophil chemotactic factors. In addition, the antigen-antibody complex activates a cellular process that produces prostaglandins and leukotrienes, which are termed "slow-reacting substances of anaphylaxis" (SRSA). These chemical mediators produce systemic effects that can have deleterious results, including profound shock.

Histamine is the primary mediator in an anaphylactic response. Activation of histamine receptors has many effects, including increased capillary permeability, increased lung secretions, bronchoconstriction, and systemic vasodilatation. The leukotrienes produce bronchoconstriction that is even more severe than that caused by histamine. They also cause venule dilatation and increased permeability. The prostaglandins exaggerate the bronchoconstriction and potentiate the effects of histamine on vascular permeability and lung secretions. Kinins produce vasodilatation and increased vascular permeability. The combined effects of these substances cause respiratory distress and obstruction,

T A B L E   1 0 - 1   Assessment guidelines for the patient with sepsis in the early, hyperdynamic (warm) stage

Clinical indicator	Cause
Cardiovascular	
Increased HR ($\geq$100 bpm)	Sympathetic/autonomic nervous system (SANS) stimulation
Decreased BP (<90 mm Hg systolic)	Vasodilatation
CO >7 L/min; CI >4 L/min/m^2	Hyperdynamic state secondary to SANS stimulation
Svo$_2$ >80%	Decreased utilization of oxygen by cells
PAWP usually <6 mm Hg	Venous dilatation; decreased preload
SVR <900 dynes/sec/cm^{-5}	Vasodilatation
Strong, bounding peripheral pulses	Hyperdynamic cardiovascular system
Respiratory	
Tachypnea (>20 breaths/min) and hyperventilation	Decreases in cerebrospinal fluid pH that stimulate the central respiratory center
Crackles	Interstitial edema occurring with increased vascular permeability
Paco$_2$ <35 mm Hg	Tachypnea and hyperventilation
Dyspnea	Increased respiratory muscle work
Renal	
Decreased urine output (< 0.5 ml/kg/h)	Decreased renal perfusion
Increased specific gravity (1.025-1.035)	Decreased glomerular filtration rate
Cutaneous	
Flushed and warm skin	Vasodilatation
Metabolic	
Increasing body temperature (usually >38.3° C [100.9° F])	Increased metabolic activity; release of pyrogens secondary to invading microorganisms; release of interleukin-I by macrophages
pH <7.35	Metabolic acidosis occurring with accumulation of lactic acid
↑Blood sugar	Release of glucagon; insulin depletion
Neurologic	
Changes in LOC	Decreased cerebral perfusion and brain hypoxia
Fluid	
↑Fluid retention	↑ADH, ↑aldosterone

T A B L E   1 0 - 2   Assessment guidelines for the patient with sepsis in the late (cold) stage

Clinical indicator	Cause
Cardiovascular	
Extreme tachycardia with S_3 sound	Compensatory attempt by sympathetic autonomic nervous system to maintain cardiac output
Profound hypotension	Decreased stroke volume. Diastolic BP may remain high due to vasoconstriction
CO <4 L/min; CI <2.5 L/min/m^2	Failure of compensatory mechanisms
PAWP usually >12 mm Hg	Increased left ventricular end-diastolic pressure (LVEDP) due to increased residual volume from decreased stroke volume
SVR >1,200 dynes/sec/cm^{-5}	Vasoconstriction
Weak or absent peripheral pulses	Decreased peripheral perfusion due to decreased cardiac output
Svo_2 ≤60%	Decreased oxygen binding to hemoglobin due to acidosis
Respiratory	
Decreased respiratory rate (<12 breaths/min) and depth	Failure of compensatory mechanisms (central respiratory center depression)
Crackles, rhonchi, wheezes	Accumulation of lung secretions
Increased Fio_2 required to maintain Pao_2 (may signal development of ARDS)	Ventilation/perfusion mismatch and decreased lung compliance
Increased $Paco_2$ (>45 mm Hg)	Decreased tidal volume

which can lead to respiratory arrest and fluid loss from the vascular space, and vasodilatation can lead to vasogenic shock and end-organ dysfunction due to tissue hypoxia.

Finally, eosinophilic chemotactic factor of anaphylaxis (ECFA) is released. ECFA attracts eosinophils, which work to neutralize mediators such as histamine. However, this response cannot by itself reverse the anaphylaxis. (See Figure 10-2 for a depiction of the pathophysiologic process of anaphylaxis.)

Toxic shock: Toxic shock syndrome is another type of shock believed to be caused by bacterial toxins. The toxins, produced by a strain of *Staphylococcus aureus,* enter the bloodstream from the site of infection, commonly the vagina, by diffusing across the mucous membrane. They are then circulated through the body. These toxins cause massive vasodilatation and eventually the shock state that is common to any cause. Increased awareness, prompt recognition and treatment, and preventive measures all have decreased the incidence of toxic shock syndrome.

T A B L E   1 0 - 2   Assessment guidelines for the patient with sepsis in the late (cold) stage—cont'd

Clinical indicator	Cause
Renal	
Decreased urine output progressing to anuria	Decreased renal perfusion and tubular ischemia
Decreased fractional excretion of sodium	Activation of the aldosterone mechanism and release of antidiuretic hormone, which stimulate retention of sodium and water
Cutaneous	
Cool, pale skin or cyanosis	Sustained vasoconstriction
Metabolic	
Decreasing body temperature	Decreased metabolic activity
Neurologic	
Decreased LOC (e.g., no response to verbal stimuli; deteriorating response to painful stimuli)	Severe hypoxia
Hematologic	
Oozing from previous venipuncture sites	Development of DIC due to stimulation of coagulation process, followed by fibrinolysis
Acid-base status	
pH <7.35; $Paco_2$ ≥45 mm Hg; HCO_3^- ≤22 mEq/L (or less than expected)	Mixed acid-base disorder: respiratory acidosis and metabolic acidosis

ASSESSMENT

For septic shock

HISTORY AND RISK FACTORS Malnutrition, immunosuppression, chronic health problems (e.g., liver or renal disease), or recent traumatic injuries or surgical or invasive procedures; infection due to the following organisms: *Escherichia coli, Klebsiella, Enterobacter, Serratia, Pseudomonas aeruginosa, Streptococcus pneumoniae,* and *Staphylococcus aureus,* as well as viruses and fungi. Underlying diseases or conditions such as splenectomy, injecting drug use, and rheumatic heart disease, predispose the patient to sepsis.

CLINICAL PRESENTATION See Tables 10-1 and 10-2.

For anaphylactic shock

HISTORY AND RISK FACTORS Recent exposure to pharmacologic agents (e.g., penicillin, anesthetics, contrast medium), blood transfusions, or insect bites or stings.

CLINICAL PRESENTATION Dependent on several factors and varies with the portal of antigen entry, the amount absorbed, the rate of absorption, and the degree of hypersensitivity. Dramatic symptoms develop

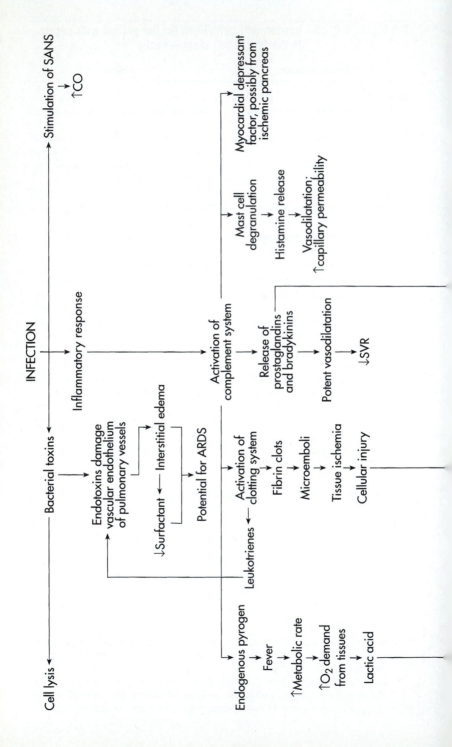

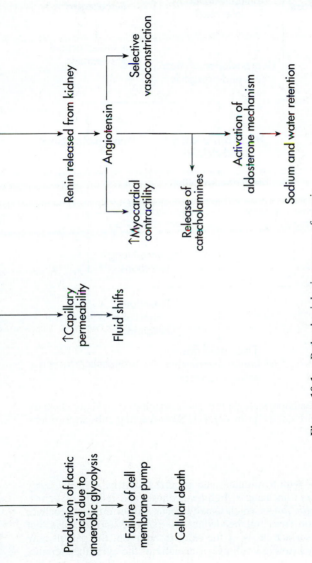

Figure 10-1: Pathophysiologic process of sepsis.

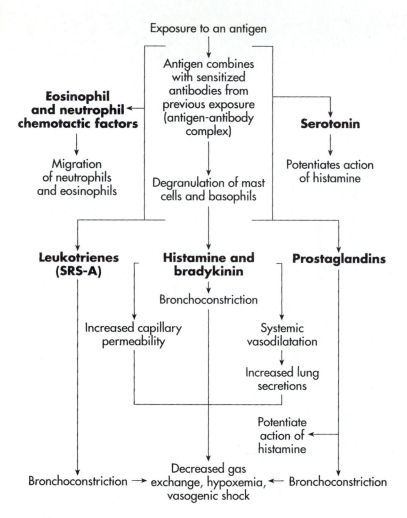

Figure 10-2:   Pathophysiologic process of anaphylaxis. (Major chemical mediators are in boldface print.) *SRS-A*, Slow-reacting substance of anaphylaxis.

rapidly, usually within minutes, and progress swiftly. *General early indicators* include uneasiness, lightheadedness, and itching of palms. *General late indicators* (which usually occur within minutes) include rapid progression from lightheadedness to syncope and urticaria that involves large surface areas of the skin. In addition, the patient may have angioedema (tissue swelling), especially of the eyes, lips, tongue, hands, feet, and genitalia; dyspnea and respiratory distress; and abdominal cramps, diarrhea, and vomiting.

T A B L E 1 0 - 3 Systemic effects of anaphylaxis

System	Effects	Cause
Neurologic	Decreased LOC progressing to coma	Brain hypoxia or cerebral edema occurring with interstitial fluid shifts
Respiratory	Dyspnea progressing to air hunger and complete respiratory obstruction; impaired phonation; noisy breathing; high-pitched, "barking" cough; wheezes, crackles, rhonchi, decreased breath sounds; pulmonary edema (some patients)	Laryngeal edema; bronchoconstriction; increased lung secretions
Cardiovascular	Decreased BP leading to profound hypotension; increased HR; decreased amplitude of peripheral pulses; palpitations (atrial tachycardias, premature atrial beats, premature ventricular beats progressing to ventricular tachycardia or ventricular fibrillation); lymphadenopathy	Systemic vasodilatation; vasogenic shock; decreased cardiac output with decreased circulating volume; reflex increase in HR
Renal	Decreased urine output; incontinence	Decreased renal perfusion; smooth muscle contraction of urinary tract
Gastrointestinal	Nausea, vomiting, diarrhea, abdominal cramping	Smooth muscle contraction of GI tract
Cutaneous	Urticaria; angioedema (hands, lips, face, feet, genitalia); cyanosis; itching; erythema; flushing	Histamine-induced disruption of cutaneous vasculature; increased capillary permeability; decreased oxygen saturation of hemoglobin

Ingestion: Cramping, nausea, and vomiting may precede systemic shock symptoms.
Inhalation: Hoarseness, wheezing, dyspnea.
Allergic: Urticaria or itching at the site of a bee sting or drug injection.
PHYSICAL ASSESSMENT See Table 10-3.
HEMODYNAMIC MEASUREMENTS Decreased arterial BP and MAP due to vasodilatation; decreased CO (<4 L/min) if shock ensues; decreased CI (<2.5 L/min); decreased SVR (<900 dynes/sec/cm^{-5}) because of

vasodilatation; and low PAWP (<6 mm Hg) because of vasodilatation, decreased venous return, and loss of intravascular fluid.

DIAGNOSTIC TESTS

For septic shock

WBC count: Early in septicemia, WBCs will be decreased because of the binding of endotoxins to WBCs. These WBCs then are removed from the circulation. Later in the process, after the immune system becomes active, leukocytosis will occur.

WBC differential: An increase in the number of immature neutrophils (i.e., a shift to the left) occurs because the cells are released into the bloodstream as the body attempts to fight the infection. These cells are called "band neutrophils" or "nonsegmented neutrophils." In addition, monocytes will be increased as an indicator of the initial inflammatory response.

Serum glucose levels: Elevated because of catecholamine-induced hepatic gluconeogenesis and glycogenolysis.

Blood cultures and antibiotic sensitivity testing of isolates: Identify causative organism(s).

Culture and antibiotic sensitivity testing of suspect infection sites (e.g., urine, sputum, blood, IV lines, incisions):   Correlate with blood cultures to identify source(s) of the sepsis.

Abdominal x-ray (flat plate):   To rule out perforated viscus as the cause of the sepsis.

ABG values: Will reflect metabolic acidosis (low HCO_3^-). Early in septicemia a low $Paco_2$ may reflect hyperventilation. As shock progresses, however, respiratory acidosis (retention of CO_2) will occur, and hypoxemia will be present because of respiratory failure.

BUN and creatinine values: Increases reflect decreasing renal perfusion.

Clotting studies: Will demonstrate an increased PT, increased PTT, increased bleeding time, thrombocytopenia, and increased fibrin split products. These results all reflect activation of the clotting cascade and may signal development of DIC.

Liver studies: AST (SGOT), ALT (SGPT), and LDH will be elevated secondary to liver ischemia.

For anaphylactic shock

The diagnosis of anaphylaxis is based on presenting signs and symptoms. There are no specific diagnostic tests for anaphylaxis, and treatment must be initiated before laboratory results are available. IgE levels may confirm allergic origin, and ABG values may be assessed to evaluate respiratory status.

COLLABORATIVE MANAGEMENT

For septic shock

Antibiotic therapy (specific to the causative organism):   Therapy usually is begun immediately after culture specimens are obtained and before sensitivity studies are completed (usually 24-48 h). Empirical treatment depends on the suspected site of infection or acquisition

Community-acquired infections: Usually are gram-positive cocci or gram-negative bacilli. For example, cefazolin or oxacillin and an aminoglycoside may be selected. Ciprofloxacin plus an antipseudomonal penicillin, such as piperacillin, is another frequently used combination.

Caution: Be alert to hypersensitivity reactions to penicillin-type drugs (see p. 643). Aminoglycosides are nephrotoxic and can be dangerous in oliguria because they may cause further damage to renal tubules. When used in combination with cephalosporins, the risk of nephrotoxicity is increased significantly. If renal function is compromised, drug dosage must be adjusted accordingly. Because aminoglycosides are ototoxic as well, the drug should be used with extreme caution in hearing-impaired persons (see Table 8-18).

Hospital-associated infections, including possible **Pseudomonas** *disorders:*   Usually managed with combination antibiotic therapy. Initial treatment may include an aminoglycoside and an antipseudomonal penicillin.
Anaerobes: Clindamycin, penicillin, chloramphenicol, or metronidazole (Flagyl, mainly used for fungal infections), or imipenem/cilastatin (Primaxin).
Hemodynamic monitoring: To guide and evaluate therapy.
Fluid administration: Intravenous volume expansion is implemented to maintain adequate ventricular filling pressures and volume, which become compromised with increased capillary permeability and vasodilatation. Lactated Ringer's solution, normal saline, plasma protein fraction (Plasmanate), albumin, and fresh-frozen plasma are used.
Positive inotropic drugs (e.g., dopamine and dobutamine)**:**   May be given to augment cardiac contractility and cardiac output. In the late stages of sepsis, positive inotropic drugs may be given along with *vasodilators,* such as nitroprusside and nitroglycerin, which decrease preload and afterload by dilating veins and arteries.

Note: Dopamine hydrochloride dosages of 2-5 μg/kg/min will increase renal and mesenteric blood flow. For additional information about inotropic agents and vasodilators, see Appendix, 7.

Vasopressors (e.g., dopamine hydrochloride and norepinephrine)**:** May be administered to reverse vasodilatation and maintain perfusion.

Note: Dopamine hydrochloride dosages >10 μg/kg/min will stimulate the alpha (vasoconstrictor) effects. Norepinephrine often is administered along with phentolamine, which counteracts the local vasoconstrictive effects of norepinephrine. Vasopressors are contraindicated in hypovolemic states. For more information about vasopressors, see Appendix 7.

Intubation and mechanical/positive pressure ventilation: To maintain adequate oxygenation. Positive end-expiratory pressure (PEEP) may be necessary with the development of ARDS.
Sodium bicarbonate: Administered judiciously to correct metabolic acidosis. Dosage is guided by ABG findings so that metabolic alkalosis does not occur.
Nutritional support: Short- and medium-chain fatty acids and branched-chain amino acids are administered to stop protein catabolism. The short- and medium-chain fatty acids are absorbed more readily and metabolized more easily than long-chain fatty acids. They

may be given orally, such as MCT Oil (proprietary name meaning triglycerides of medium-chain fatty acids), or given intravenously (e.g., intralipid solutions). Branched-chain amino acid solutions are used in sepsis because they are metabolized by muscle rather than by the liver and therefore can be used in the presence of organ failure.

Steroids (e.g., dexamethasone 3-6 mg/kg or methylprednisolone sodium 30 mg/kg): Although their use is controversial, steroids may be used to decrease capillary permeability, decrease leukocyte aggregation, decrease formation of microemboli, decrease histamine release, and decrease coagulopathy.

Antipyretic agents, cooled IV fluid, or cooling blanket: To normalize temperature.

Naloxone hydrochloride (Narcan): May be used to reverse some of the vasodilatation effects of sepsis.

Glucose-potassium-insulin (GKI): This combination may be given to increase cardiac performance during sepsis.

For anaphylactic shock

Airway maintenance: May require ET intubation. If laryngeal edema is severe and causes obstruction, a tracheostomy or emergency cricothyroidotomy may be necessary.

Epinephrine: Counteracts the effects of anaphylaxis by increasing myocardial contractility, dilating bronchioles, constricting blood vessels, inhibiting histamine release, and counteracting histamine that already is circulating. Standard dosage is 0.3-0.5 mg (0.3-0.5 ml of a 1:1,000 solution) administered by IM or SC route, although an initial dose of 0.1 mg (0.1 ml of a 1:1,000 solution) may be administered. If given intravenously, which is the route preferred in the presence of shock, 3-5 ml of a 1:10,000 solution usually is diluted in 10 ml normal saline. This initial dosage is followed by IV infusion of 1 μg/min, which may be increased to 4 μg/min as necessary until desired response is achieved.

Supplemental oxygen: May be administered to support oxygen delivery to the tissues. The amount and method of oxygen administration are guided by ABG results, although it usually is initiated at 6 L/min *via* nasal cannula or oxygen mask.

Fluid resuscitation: Crystalloids (e.g., lactated Ringer's solution) or colloids (e.g., albumin and plasma protein fraction [Plasmanate]) to increase intravascular colloid osmotic pressure and retain fluids within the vascular spaces, thus attaining adequate vascular volume. This may require a rapid infusion of 2-3 L.

Vasopressors: Necessary if fluid replacement does not reverse or prevent shock. Drugs such as dopamine hydrochloride, norepinephrine, or epinephrine are titrated for the desired response. Usual dosages: dopamine hydrochloride 5-20 μg/kg/min, norepinephrine 2-8 μg/min, and epinephrine 2-4 μg/min (see Appendix 7).

Antihistamines: Usually given after the patient has been stabilized. Diphenhydramine, for example, may be given IV to relieve urticaria and abdominal cramping. Usual dosage is 20-50 mg.

Aminophylline (theophylline ethylenediamine): May be given by IV drip to stimulate bronchodilatation and relieve bronchospasm. Usual dosage is 2-4 mg/min (0.5 mg/kg).

Corticosteroids: May be given to decrease both capillary permeability and release of chemical mediators. The effect is not immediate.

Military antishock trousers (MAST):   Increase systemic vascular resistance and may improve BP. Use in anaphylaxis is controversial.

Inhaled bronchodilators such as albuterol or terbutaline: May be given for continued bronchospasm.

Glucagon, 1 mg IV bolus: To counteract the effects of beta-blocking drugs. Use is controversial.

ECG monitoring: To detect dysrhythmias.

NURSING DIAGNOSES AND INTERVENTIONS
For septic shock
Fluid volume deficit related to active loss from vascular compartment secondary to increased capillary permeability and shift of intravascular volume into interstitial spaces

Desired outcomes: Within 4 h of initiation of therapy, patient is normovolemic as evidenced by peripheral pulses >2+ on a 0-4+ scale, stable body weight, urine output ≥0.5 ml/kg/h, systolic BP ≥90 mm Hg or within patient's normal range, and absence of edema and adventitious lung sounds. PAWP is 6-12 mm Hg, CO is 4-7 L/min, and SVR is 900-1,200 dynes/sec/cm^{-5}.

- Monitor hemodynamic pressures, particularly PAWP, CO, and SVR. During the early (warm) stage of sepsis, PAWP usually is decreased to <6 mm Hg but will be increased to >12 mm Hg in the late (cold) stage. CO usually is >7 L/min in the early stage and decreased to <4 L/min in the late stage. SVR can be <900 dynes/sec/cm^{-5} in the early stage but usually increases to >1,200 dynes/sec/cm^{-5} in the late stage.
- Administer crystalloid and colloid fluid replacement as prescribed. Often fluid replacement therapy will be given to maintain a PAWP of 6-12 mm Hg. Assess PAWP and lung sounds at frequent intervals during fluid replacement to detect evidence of fluid overload: crackles and increasing PAWP.
- Administer positive inotropic agents as prescribed to maintain adequate cardiac output in the presence of massive vasodilatation.
- Assess fluid volume by monitoring BP and peripheral pulses hourly. Report systolic BP <90 mm Hg (or 20-30 mm Hg less than presepsis level) and decreasing amplitude of peripheral pulses.
- Weigh patient daily; monitor I&O every shift, noting 24-h trends. Report urine output <0.5 ml/kg/h. The patient's weight actually may increase with fluid volume deficit due to shift of intravascular volume into interstitial spaces.
- Monitor specific gravity, being alert to increases >1.030, which indicate a dehydration state, or a fixed specific gravity of 1.010, which may signal inadequate glomerular filtration.
- Assess for interstitial edema as evidenced by pretibial, sacral, ankle, and hand edema, as well as crackles on auscultation of lung fields.
- As prescribed, administer vasopressor agents to help maintain perfusion, and give steroids to decrease capillary permeability.
- Position patient supine with legs elevated to increase venous return and preload.

Decreased cardiac output related to negative inotropic changes in the heart (late stage) secondary to effects of tissue hypoxia
Desired outcome: Within 8 h of initiation of therapy, patient has adequate cardiac output as evidenced by systolic BP ≥90 mm Hg (or within patient's normal range), HR ≤100 bpm, peripheral pulses >2+ on a scale of 0-4+, urine output ≥0.5 ml/kg/h, PAWP ≤12 mm Hg, CO ≥4 L/min, CI ≥2.5 L/min/m², and Svo_2 60%-80%.

- Assess patient for signs of decreased cardiac output: decreasing BP, increasing HR, decreasing amplitude of peripheral pulses, restlessness, decreasing urinary output, and increasing PAWP.
- Administer positive inotropic agents as prescribed to augment cardiac contractility.
- Position patient supine with legs elevated to optimize preload and enhance stroke volume.
- Assess CO at least q4h. Optimally, CO will be ≥4 L/min and CI will be ≥2.5 L/min/m².
- Monitor cardiac rhythm per monitor at frequent intervals. Observe for development of dysrhythmias, such as PVCs, which may occur with hypoxia, and extreme tachycardia, both of which will potentiate a decreased cardiac output.
- Minimize myocardial oxygen demand by assisting patient with ADL and ensuring uninterrupted periods of rest.
- Monitor Svo_2 continuously; report values outside of normal range.

Altered cerebral, renal, and gastrointestinal tissue perfusion related to hypovolemia secondary to vasodilatation (early stage) or interruption of arterial and venous blood flow secondary to vasoconstriction and thrombus obstruction (late stage)
Desired outcomes: Within 24 h of initiating therapy, patient has adequate perfusion as evidenced by orientation to time, place, and person; peripheral pulses >2+ (on a scale of 0-4+); brisk capillary refill (<2 sec); urine output ≥0.5 ml/kg/h; and ≥5 bowel sounds/min. BP is 110-120/70-80 mm Hg (or within patient's normal range); Svo_2 is 60%-80%; SVR is 900-1,200 dynes/sec/$^{cm-5}$; CO is 4-7 L/min; and CI is 2.5-4 L/min/m².

- Assess for changes in LOC as an indicator of decreasing cerebral perfusion.
- Assess for the following signs of decreasing renal perfusion: urine output <0.5 ml/kg/h and increased BUN, serum creatinine, and serum potassium levels. Normal laboratory values are as follows: BUN ≤20 mg/dl; serum creatinine ≤1.5 mg/dl; and serum potassium ≤5 mEq/L. Also be alert to increasing urine specific gravity (normal range for a random urine sample is 1.010-1.020).
- Monitor arterial BP continuously. Be alert to decreased systolic BP, normal or increased diastolic BP, and decreased pulse pressures, which occur in the presence of decreasing perfusion.

Note: Systolic BP will be decreased because of decreased cardiac output, and the diastolic BP may be high secondary to compensatory vasoconstriction.

- Assess peripheral pulses, temperature, color of skin, and capillary refill. With hypoperfusion, pulse amplitude decreases, extremities become cool due to vasoconstriction, skin color becomes pale or mottled because of decreased perfusion, and capillary refill becomes delayed.

- Monitor cellular oxygen consumption (Svo_2) as an indicator of tissue perfusion. With sepsis, cellular oxygen delivery is decreased (precapillary vasoconstriction), and thus cellular oxygen use is decreased. Therefore the mixed venous blood oxygen saturation (Svo_2) will be abnormally high.
- Administer vasoactive drugs as prescribed, and assess SVR and CO during administration to determine the effect of these drugs. Optimally SVR will increase to ≥ 900 dynes/sec/cm^{-5}, CO will be 4-7L/min, and CI will be 2.5-4 L/min/m^2.

Note: Vasoactive drugs probably will include vasopressors (e.g., norepinephrine) early in sepsis and vasodilators (e.g., nitroprusside) late in sepsis. Vasopressors always are accompanied by fluid resuscitation as needed.

- Assess for evidence of decreasing splanchnic (visceral) circulation, including decreased or absent bowel sounds, elevated serum amylase level, and decreased platelet count. Normal values are as follows: serum amylase ≤ 180 Somogyi units/dl; and platelet count $\geq 150,000$ μl.

Impaired gas exchange related to alveolar-capillary membrane changes secondary to interstitial edema, alveolar destruction, and endotoxin release with activation of histamine and kinins

Desired outcome: Within 4 h of initiation of therapy, patient's Pao_2 is ≥ 80 mm Hg; $Paco_2$ is ≤ 45 mm Hg; pH is 7.35-7.45, and the lungs are clear.

- Assess for and maintain a patent airway by assisting patient with coughing or suctioning trachea as necessary.
- Assess all ABG values. Be alert to decreasing Pao_2, increasing $Paco_2$, and acidosis (decreasing pH). Monitor patient for the presence of dyspnea, SOB, and restlessness.
- Listen to breath sounds hourly. The presence of crackles may indicate fluid accumulation.
- If patient exhibits evidence of inadequate gas exchange (e.g., Pao_2 <60 mm Hg on 100% oxygen *via* nonrebreathing mask), prepare for the probability of endotracheal intubation.
- If patient has been placed on mechanical ventilation, monitor inspiratory peak pressures for increasing trends, which may signal decreasing compliance and development of ARDS. Also, assess for and document mode of ventilation, tidal volume, Fio_2, rate of respirations, and level of PEEP. Typically, as ARDS develops, an increasing Fio_2 (>0.50) and increasing levels of PEEP are required to maintain adequate Pao_2 (>60 mm Hg). Consult physician if inspiratory peak pressures increase with each breath or if the following signs of hypoxia occur at the prescribed Fio_2 and level of PEEP: increased HR (≥ 100 bpm), anxiety, cool extremities, change in mentation, or skin color changes (pallor or cyanosis). (See "Mechanical Ventilation," p. 19.)
- Turn patient q2h to maintain optimal ventilation-perfusion ratios and to prevent atelectasis.

- Administer sodium bicarbonate as prescribed to buffer metabolic acidosis. Dosages are determined by level of pH in ABG findings.

Note: Administration of sodium bicarbonate may worsen respiratory acidosis.

Ineffective breathing pattern related to decreased lung expansion secondary to central respiratory depression occurring in late shock
Desired outcome: Within 2 h of treatment/intervention, patient has an effective breathing pattern as evidenced by normal limits of inspiratory-expiratory ratio (1:1-1:2), tidal volume (≥4ml/kg), and maximal inspiratory pressures (≥20 cm H_2O).

- Monitor patient's rate and depth of respirations. Be alert to decreasing rate, depth, and air movement. Ensure that patient demonstrates adequate air movement by noting presence of breath sounds over all lung fields.
- Assist patient into a position for comfort to facilitate respirations. Depending on patient's hemodynamic stability, the optimal position may be having the HOB elevated 15-30 degrees.
- Assess/measure tidal volume and inspiratory force. Be alert to tidal volume <4-5 ml/kg and inspiratory force <20 cm H_2O as indicators of ineffective breathing pattern.
- If patient exhibits respiratory depression/ineffective breathing pattern, prepare for the probability of endotracheal intubation.

Ineffective thermoregulation related to illness with concomitant endotoxin effect on hypothalamic temperature-regulating center
Desired outcome: Within 24 h of initiation of treatment, patient becomes normothermic.

- Monitor patient's temperature continuously or at frequent intervals. Use temperature probe (rectal or tympanic) for continuous monitoring of core temperature. Body temperature can range from 38.3°-40.6° C (101°-105° F) in the early stage of sepsis and can be <35.6° C (96° F) in the late stage. Be alert to shaking chills early in sepsis as temperature increases and to profuse diaphoresis as temperature decreases late in sepsis. The following are weighed for each patient to determine the extent of treatment that should be employed to decrease fever (e.g., acetaminophen):
  - □ Useful effects of a fever: Decreased viral and bacterial replication.
  - □ Harmful effects of a fever: Increased cardiac workload and increased oxygen consumption.
- Administer antimicrobials as prescribed. Observe for untoward effects, including renal toxicity, ototoxicity, allergic reactions, anaphylaxis, pseudomembranous colitis, overgrowth of normal flora, and superimposed infectious processes of the skin, urinary tract, or respiratory tract. Large doses of antibiotics may cause the release of endotoxins from dying bacteria, which may potentiate the progression of septic shock.
- Administer antipyretic agents as prescribed.
- For patients with hyperthermia, use tepid baths, which decrease body temperature by releasing internal heat. Cooled IV fluids also may decrease core temperature. In addition, a cooling blanket may be pre-

scribed to reduce the metabolic rate, thereby decreasing myocardial oxygen demand. Avoid "chilling," which will cause shivering and thus increase myocardial oxygen demand and cardiac workload.

- In the presence of hypothermia, use warm blankets to increase body temperature. Heating devices can damage ischemic cells in peripheral tissues and usually are avoided.

Altered nutrition: Less than body requirements related to increased need secondary to increased metabolic rate

Desired outcome: Within 48 h of initiation of treatment, patient has adequate nutrition as evidenced by stable weight, serum albumin 3.5 g/dl, thyroxine-binding prealbumin 20-30 mg/dl, retinol-binding protein 4-5 mg/dl, urine urea nitrogen 10-20 mg/dl, and a state of nitrogen balance as determined by nitrogen studies.

- Administer nutritional supplements as prescribed.

Note: Standard TPN solutions are not metabolized well in the septic state. Branched-chain amino acid solutions and short- to medium-chain fatty acid solutions may be used (e.g., MCT Oil or Freamine HBC).

- Observe for and document areas of tissue breakdown, which can indicate a negative nitrogen state.
- Monitor laboratory findings for serum albumin, thyroxine-binding prealbumin, retinol-binding protein, and nitrogen studies.
- Assess and record weight and nutritional intake daily. Consult with nutritional services for calorie count.
- If patient is receiving oral feedings, assess for the presence of bowel sounds at least q2h. Paralytic ileus can occur secondary to an ischemic bowel.
- If the patient is receiving continuous gastric tube feedings, assess for residual feeding q2h. Assess for residual before intermittent tube feedings. If residual is ≥100 ml (or 1½ times the hourly rate of infusion), hold the feeding and consult with physician.
- To meet patient's tremendous metabolic demands, provide foods that are high in calories.
- Encourage intake of foods high in protein and carbohydrates.
- For additional information, see "Nutritional Support," p. 1.

For anaphylactic shock

Ineffective airway clearance related to tracheobronchial obstruction secondary to bronchoconstriction and increased secretions associated with histamine response and the presence of leukotrienes and prostaglandins

Desired outcome: Within 2 h of treatment/intervention, patient has adequate airway clearance as evidenced by a state of eupnea and the presence of normal breath sounds in all lung fields.

- Assess patency of airway on a continuing basis. Be alert to decreasing air movement heard on auscultation of the lungs, expiratory wheezing, SOB, and dyspnea, which can progress to "air hunger." Consult physician if assessment reveals signs of airway compromise; prepare for ET intubation if signs are present. Keep suction equipment readily available.

- Administer epinephrine by IV, IM, or SC route, as prescribed. Dosage and route vary. Generally, the following guidelines are used:
  □ IV route if patient is in shock.
  □ Initially, a dosage of 0.1 mg (0.1 ml of 1 : 1,000 solution) diluted in 10 ml normal saline is infused over 5-10 min. The dose may be increased to 0.3-0.5 mg.
  □ After initial dosage, an IV drip of 1 mg of 1 : 1,000 epinephrine in 250 ml 5% dextrose in water is established. Initial infusion usually is 1 μg/min. If given by SC route, the dose is 0.3-0.5 mg (0.3-0.5 ml of a 1 : 1,000 solution) and it is repeated q15-20min as needed.

Note: Patients taking beta-blocking drugs, such as propranolol, may not respond to epinephrine. The use of glucagon to counteract this effect is controversial.

- Auscultate lung fields for presence of wheezes and air movement. As bronchoconstriction and obstruction progress, wheezing may decrease; therefore it is important to listen for air movement as well.
- Prepare for ET intubation if SOB and respiratory distress continue.

Caution: An oral airway provides airway support only as far as the posterior pharynx. If laryngeal edema is present, the oral airway will be ineffective because the obstruction is lower.

- If laryngeal edema prevents intubation, prepare for the possibility of a tracheostomy or cricothyroidotomy.
- If prescribed, administer IV bronchodilators, such as theophylline, to induce bronchodilatation. Usual dosage is 2-4 mg/min. Monitor for side effects such as dysrhythmias.
- Monitor ABG values for evidence of an improving or a worsening condition. Be alert to increasing $Paco_2$ (>50 mm Hg) and decreasing Pao_2 (<60 mm Hg).

Impaired gas exchange related to alveolar-capillary membrane changes secondary to increased capillary permeability associated with histamine response

Desired outcome: Within 2 h of initiation of treatment/intervention, patient has adequate gas exchange as evidenced by eupnea, Pao_2 ≥80 mm Hg, and Spo_2 ≥90.

- Monitor patient for the presence of SOB or dyspnea. Assess ABG values for evidence of an improving or a worsening condition. Be alert to increasing $Paco_2$ (>50 mm Hg) and decreasing Pao_2 (<60 mm Hg).
- Administer oxygen as prescribed.
- Monitor patient with continuous pulse oximetry. Be alert to levels <90.
- Antihistamines, such as diphenhydramine, may be given by IV or IM route to compete with histamine at receptor sites and to control edema in the lungs. Usual dose is 20-50 mg.
- As prescribed, administer glucocorticoids (e.g., hydrocortisone) for

their antiinflammatory effects and potential ability to decrease capillary permeability. Be aware that the effects of glucocorticoids will not be noticed immediately.

- If BP is stable, assist patient to sitting position to enhance gas exchange.
- Remain with patient; encourage slow, deep breathing if possible. Help alleviate patient's anxiety by responding calmly and explaining all procedures before performing them.

Decreased cardiac output related to decreased preload and afterload secondary to release of vasoactive chemical mediators and associated vasodilatation and increased capillary permeability

Desired outcome: Within 4 h of initiation of treatment, patient has adequate cardiac output as evidenced by BP $\geq$90/60 mm Hg, peripheral pulses >2+ on a scale of 0-4+, CO $\geq$4 L/min, CI $\geq$2.5 L/min/m^2, SVR $\geq$900 dynes/sec/cm^{-5}, urinary output $\geq$0.5 ml/kg/h, and normal sinus rhythm on ECG.

- Assess for physical and hemodynamic indicators of decreased cardiac output:
  □ Check apical pulse for irregularity.
  □ Palpate peripheral pulses for decreasing amplitude.
  □ Assess arterial BP for decrease, an indicator of failed compensatory mechanisms.
  □ Calculate SVR. A decrease (<900 dynes/sec/cm^{-5}) is associated with decreased afterload (vasodilatation) and may precipitate decreased CO.
  □ Measure CO if a thermodilution catheter is present.
  □ Calculate CI for a more precise measurement of adequacy of CO. A finding of <2.5 L/min/m^2 usually is associated with hypoperfusion.
- Assess electrical rhythm *via* ECG monitor for dysrhythmias, such as atrial tachycardias, premature ventricular complexes, ventricular tachycardia, and ventricular fibrillation, which may signal hypoxemia or occur as side effects of drugs such as aminophylline or epinephrine.
- Inspect face, lips, hands, feet, and genitalia for edema as an indicator of fluid loss to interstitial spaces. Document edema on a scale of 1+ to 4+.
  1+: A slight depression that disappears quickly
  4+: A deep depression that disappears slowly
- As prescribed, administer epinephrine to decrease capillary permeability, stimulate vasoconstriction, increase systemic vascular resistance, and increase myocardial contractility. Observe for therapeutic effects as evidenced by increased calculated SVR, increased CO/CI, increased arterial BP and MAP, stronger peripheral pulses, warming of extremities, and increased urine output (indicator of increased renal perfusion).
- Administer fluid replacement therapy as prescribed. It may take as much as 2-3 L to attain adequate vascular volume. Volume expanders, such as plasma protein fraction (Plasmanate), albumin, or dextran, may be administered with crystalloid solutions to increase vascular volume.

Note: During fluid resuscitation, assess patient for indicators of fluid volume excess, including crackles with chest auscultation, presence of S_3 heart sounds, and jugular venous distention. If hemodynamic monitoring lines are present, be alert to increasing PAP, PAWP, and RAP.

- Prepare for possible vasopressor infusion to reverse shock state. Possible pharmacologic agents include:
  - *Dopamine hydrochloride:* To increase cardiac contractility and systemic vascular resistance *via* its alpha and beta properties. Usual dosage is 5-20 μg/kg/min.
  - *Norepinephrine:* Alpha-adrenergic stimulator. Initial dosage is 2-8 μg/min and can be increased to achieve the necessary BP.
  - *Methoxamine hydrochloride:* Alpha-adrenergic drug that stimulates intense vasoconstriction.
- If prescribed, apply MAST to increase systemic vascular resistance.

Caution: MAST must be released gradually when no longer needed to prevent precipitous decline in BP.

Altered peripheral, renal, and cerebral tissue perfusion related to hypovolemia secondary to fluid shift from the vascular space to the interstitial space
Desired outcome: Within 4 h of initiation of treatment, patient has adequate perfusion as evidenced by peripheral pulses >2+ (on a scale of 0-4+); brisk capillary refill (<2 sec); urinary output ≥0.5 ml/kg/h); warm, dry skin; and orientation to time, place, and person.
- Palpate peripheral pulses in arms and legs (radial, brachial, dorsalis pedis, posterior tibial), and rate them according to a 0-4+ scale. Report decreased amplitude of pulses.
- Assess capillary refill. Note whether it is brisk (<2 sec) or delayed (>2 sec), which is likely with edema and decreased vascular volume.
- Assess degree of peripheral edema, rating it on a scale of 1+ to 4+.
- Assess color and warmth of extremities; report presence of coolness and pallor.
- Monitor BP at frequent intervals. Be alert to readings >20 mm Hg below patient's normal pressure and other indicators of hypotension, including dizziness, restlessness, altered mentation, and decreased urinary output.
- Observe for indicators of decreased cerebral perfusion such as restlessness, confusion, and decreased LOC.

Note: Changes in LOC may signal either decreased cerebral perfusion (tissue hypoxia) or increasing ICP caused by interstitial swelling from capillary permeability.

- Administer fluid and pharmacologic agents as prescribed (see previous nursing diagnosis).
Impaired skin integrity related to urticaria and angioedema secondary to allergic response
Desired outcomes: Within 4 h of initiation of treatment, patient states that urticaria is controlled. Skin remains intact.

- Assess patient for the presence of urticaria (hives) and itching of hands, feet, neck, and genitalia, which are characteristic of anaphylaxis.
- Administer antihistamines as prescribed to relieve itching.
- Administer epinephrine as prescribed to counteract most of the effects of the hypersensitivity response.
- Discourage patient from scratching the skin. If scratching is unavoidable, teach patient to use pads of fingertips rather than nails.
- Apply cool washcloths or covered ice as a soothing measure to irritated and edematous areas.

Knowledge deficit: Severe hypersensitivity reaction, its causes, and its symptoms

Desired outcome: By the time of discharge from the critical care unit, patient demonstrates increased knowledge of severe hypersensitivity reactions as evidenced by verbalization of potential causative factors, symptoms of allergic reaction, need to inform health care providers of allergies, importance of wearing Medic-Alert identification, and the necessity of informing primary health care provider immediately of any allergic symptoms.

- Provide information about the antigenic agent that caused the anaphylaxis, including ways to avoid it in the future. For example, if the anaphylaxis was caused by penicillin, stress that the patient needs to avoid all penicillin-related drugs and possibly molds because penicillin is made from mold.
- Explain the purpose and necessity of wearing a Medic-Alert identification tag or bracelet to identify the allergy.
- Give information about anaphylaxis emergency treatment kits. Teach patient self-administration technique and the importance of prompt treatment.
- Stress the importance of reporting immediately the symptoms of allergy, including flushing, warmth, itching, anxiety, and hives.
- Explain the importance of identifying and checking all OTC medications for the presence of potential allergens.

ADDITIONAL NURSING DIAGNOSES

Also see nursing diagnoses and interventions in "Hemodynamic Monitoring," p. 37; "Psychosocial Support," p. 88; "Psychosocial Support for the Patient's Family and Significant Others," p. 100; and "Adult Respiratory Distress Syndrome," p. 250. See "Renal Transplantation" for **Knowledge deficit:** Immunosuppressive medications and their side effects, p. 407; **Risk for infection,** p. 409; and **Impaired skin integrity,** p. 409. See "Disseminated Intravascular Coagulation" for **Altered protection,** p. 614, and **Altered tissue perfusion,** p. 617.

Organ rejection

PATHOPHYSIOLOGY

The major problem with all types of organ transplantation is graft rejection. When the body detects the presence of a foreign substance, it mounts the defense of nonspecific inflammation and phagocytosis.

The next level of immune response involves antibody-mediated (humoral) immunity and cell-mediated immunity. Both responses occur in a parallel fashion after exposure to an antigen. *Antibody-mediated immune response* is related to B-lymphocyte activity. When an antigen is encountered, the B lymphocyte enlarges, divides, and differentiates into a plasma cell that produces and secretes antigen-specific immunoglobulins, or antibodies. The formation of this antigen-antibody complex triggers events that augment the nonspecific responses of inflammation and phagocytosis. *Cell-mediated immune response* involves T lymphocytes. A T lymphocyte recognizes a foreign antigen on the surface of the macrophage, binds to the antigen, and enlarges and produces a sensitized clone, which migrates through the body to the site of the antigen. When the sensitized T cell combines with the antigen, chemicals are released that kill foreign cells directly and act to facilitate phagocytosis and the inflammatory response. (See Figure 10-3 for a delineation of this process.)

Because a transplanted organ originates from a donor who is genetically different from the recipient (the exception is a kidney from an identical twin), the organ contains foreign antigens that trigger an immune response in the recipient, which leads to organ rejection. Historically, rejection has been classified as hyperacute, accelerated acute, acute, and chronic (Table 10-4). An untreated

T A B L E   1 0 - 4   **Characteristics of organ rejection by category**

Type of rejection	Characteristics	Outcome
Hyperacute	Described in "Renal Transplantation," p. 404. Occurs immediately Antibody mediated Result of preformed circulatory antibodies	Irreversible and untreatable
Accelerated acute	Occurs 3-5 days posttransplant Antibody mediated Rapid loss of function Fever and oliguria	Irreversible and untreatable
Acute	Primarily T-cell mediated Possible presence of humoral component Occurs weeks, months, or years after transplant	Treatable and reversible; multiple episodes affect long-term graft survival
Chronic	Develops slowly over months to years Probably a combination of cellular- and humoral-mediated processes	Untreatable; eventually leads to graft loss

rejection response results in complete destruction of the organ. Table 10-5 describes the clinical presentation for various types of acute organ rejection.

DIAGNOSIS AND ASSESSMENT OF REJECTION

Biopsy of the transplanted organ provides the means of diagnosing rejection, its severity, and the possibility of response to antirejection therapy. In addition, the following diagnostic tests are performed:

Cardiac

Chest x-ray: Will reveal increased dimension of the heart late in rejection.

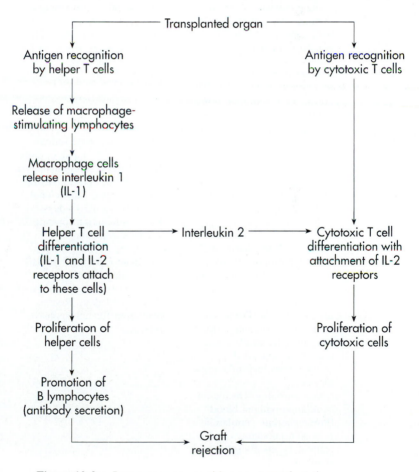

Figure 10-3:   Immune response with organ transplantation.

T A B L E 1 0 - 5   Clinical presentation with acute organ rejection

Organ	Clinical presentation	Treatment options
Heart	Usually seen 10-14 days after transplantation. Indicators include fever, anxiety, lethargy, low back pain, atrial or ventricular dysrhythmias, gallop, pericardial friction rub, jugular venous distention, hypotension, and decreased CO late in rejection	Methylprednisolone sodium succinate (500 mg-1 g) daily for 2-4 days. Antilymphocyte sera (rabbit, horse, or goat) IV for 6-14 days. Monoclonal antibody for 10-14 days. Retransplantation necessary for intractable acute rejection
Liver	Initially seen 4-10 days after transplantation. Indicators include malaise; fever; abdominal discomfort; swollen, hard, tender graft; tachycardia; RUQ or flank pain; cessation of bile flow; change in color of bile from golden to a colorless fluid; jaundice; elevated PT, bilirubin, transaminase, and alkaline phosphatase	Methylprednisolone sodium succinate (500 mg-1 g) daily for 2-4 days. Antilymphocyte sera (rabbit, horse, or goat) IV for 6-14 days. Retransplantation necessary for recurrent, unresponsive rejection
Pancreas	Time of rejection occurrence varies. Difficult to diagnose; patient may have hyperglycemia, pancreatitis, pain over graft. Open biopsy may be necessary to diagnose rejection	Methylprednisolone sodium succinate (250 mg-1 g) daily for 2-4 days. Antilymphocyte sera (rabbit, horse, goat) IV for 6-14 days. Monoclonal antibody for 10-14 days. Retransplantation for unresponsive rejection
Lung	May be expected during the first 21 postoperative days, with increased frequency and severity 6-8 wk after transplantation *Classic rejection:* Decreased lung ventilation and perfusion; alveolar exudate containing desquamated pneumocytes and inflammatory cells *Atypical rejection:* Decreased ventilation without blood flow reduction; ventilation-perfusion imbalances and respiratory insufficiency with shunting *Vascular rejection:* Increased vascular resistance; decreased blood flow to graft	Methylprednisolone sodium succinate (250 mg-1 g) daily for 2-4 days. Antilymphocyte sera (rabbit, horse, goat) IV for 6-14 days. Retransplantation for unresponsive rejection

ECG: Will show presence of atrial and ventricular dysrhythmias and decreased QRS voltage.
CBC count: Will show increased total lymphocyte count.
VS and heart sounds: May reveal decreased stroke volume, cardiac output, cardiac tones, and BP; and presence of S_3 and S_4 sounds, pericardial friction rub, extrasystole, and crackles.

Liver
Serum bilirubin level: Total bilirubin will rise in relation to baseline postoperative level.
Transaminase level: Will increase from baseline; may be markedly elevated early in rejection.
Alkaline phosphatase level: Will increase from baseline.
Prothrombin time: Will be prolonged.
CBC count: May reveal decreased platelet count and increased total lymphocyte count.

Pancreas
Open biopsy is the only means by which a definitive diagnosis can be made.
Fasting and 2-h postprandial plasma glucose: Levels will be increased above normal ranges.
Serum amylase: Levels may be elevated, indicating presence of pancreatitis, an inconsistent marker of rejection.
C peptide (serum and urine): Levels may be decreased.
Pancreas radioisotope flow scan: Determines organ viability. Decreased flow may indicate rejection.

Lung
Transbronchial biopsy is not helpful in detecting rejection; the morbidity risk increases with open biopsy.
Leukocyte and absolute lymphocyte counts: Rise during rejection.
VS and hemodynamics: Can change suddenly with increases in the following: PVR, HR, BP, SVR, and CO.
ABG values: Decrease in Pao_2 and increase in $Paco_2$ occur with rejection.

Renal
See "Renal Transplantation," p. 403.

MECHANISMS OF IMMUNOSUPPRESSIVE AGENTS
The following drugs may be used in various combinations for additive effect in preventing or modifying the rejection response. The goal of therapy is to achieve enough immunosuppression to prevent graft rejection but not so much as to leave the patient in a defenseless state.
Azathioprine (Imuran): Interferes with DNA synthesis and inhibits mitosis of immunologically competent cells. Cell division and proliferation occur in response to antigenic stimulation. Azathioprine affects rapidly replicating cells at an early stage of lymphocyte activation and is believed to block proliferation of helper T cells and cytotoxic T cells. Azathioprine is converted to 6-MP and further metabolized in the liver by xanthine oxidase.

Note: Allopurinol inhibits xanthine oxidase–mediated metabolism and may result in increased activity and toxicity of azathioprine. If allopurinol must be used with azathioprine, the usual dose of azathioprine usually is reduced by one fourth to one third.

Cyclophosphamide (Cytoxan) may be used in place of azathioprine when liver function is compromised.

Corticosteroids: Suppress the production of cytotoxic T lymphocytes from noncytotoxic precursor cells. There is some evidence that steroids prevent the release of interleukin-1 (IL-1) and IL-2. IL-1, released by the macrophages, promotes the differentiation of helper T cells. The release of IL-2 promotes differentiation of cytotoxic cells.

Antilymphocyte sera (antilymphocytic globulin [ALG] or antithymocyte gamma-globulin [ATGAM]):   The antilymphocyte antibodies in the sera are useful in the treatment of steroid-resistant rejection and potent suppressors of cell-mediated immunity. They are directed against many different antigens on the surface of human lymphocytes and affect immunity *via* reduction of T lymphocytes.

Monoclonal antibody (Orthoclone OKT3):   This homologous antibody reacts with and blocks the function of the chemical (T3) complex on the surface of the T lymphocytes. The T3 complex is responsible for the T lymphocyte's identification of a transplanted organ as foreign and attempts to reject it. OKT3 binds to the T3 antigen on the surface of the T cells, enhancing phagocytosis and entrapment of the cells in the spleen and liver. The lymphocytes are removed from the circulation by this process in approximately 10-15 min.

Cyclosporine (Sandimmune):   Inhibits production and release of lymphokines and generation of cytotoxic and plasma cells by blocking the response of cytotoxic T lymphocytes to IL-2. Cyclosporine is metabolized by the cytochrome P-450 enzyme system in the liver. Careful monitoring of cyclosporine drug levels, with concomitant dose adjustments, is necessary when cyclosporine is used with other drugs (Table 10-6).

NURSING DIAGNOSES AND INTERVENTIONS

Anxiety/fear related to threat of change in health status secondary to potential loss of transplanted organ due to rejection

Desired outcomes: Patient expresses anxieties and fears regarding possibility of organ loss and verbalizes accurate information about the signs and symptoms of organ rejection. Within 12 h of this diagnosis, patient's fear and anxiety are controlled as evidenced by BP within patient's normal range, HR ≤ 100 bpm, and RR ≤ 20 breaths/min with normal depth and pattern (eupnea).

- Encourage patient to discuss concerns and fears.
- Assess patient's knowledge about the rejection process and the signs and symptoms that occur.
- Use short, simple sentences to explain patient's current organ function and the signs and symptoms of organ rejection (see Table 10-5).
- Reassure patient that appropriate medications are being given to prevent ongoing rejection. Review medication names, dosage, and action (see p. 650).

T A B L E   1 0 - 6   Cyclosporine (CyA) drug interactions

Drugs causing decreased blood levels of CyA*	Drugs causing increased blood levels of CyA†
carbamazepine	cimetidine
isoniazid	danazol
phenobarbital	diltiazem
phenytoin	erythromycin
rifampin	high-dose corticosteroids
sulfamethoxazole	ketoconazole
trimethoprim	methyltestosterone
	nicardipine
	oral contraceptives
	ranitidine

Note: Careful monitoring of CyA blood levels and adjusting dosage as indicated are necessary when these drugs are used in patients taking cyclosporine.
*Decreased blood levels may precipitate organ rejection.
†Increased blood levels may cause nephrotoxicity.

- Explain to patient that rejection does not necessarily mean organ loss. Under most circumstances, rejection can be reversed.
- Reassure patient that retransplantation is a viable option if organ loss occurs.
- For other interventions related to fear, see this nursing diagnosis, p. 92.

Fluid volume excess (or risk for same) related to compromised regulatory mechanism secondary to diminished organ function associated with rejection episode

Desired outcome: Patient is normovolemic as evidenced by stable weight, urine output ≥0.5 ml/kg/h, BP within patient's normal range, HR 60-100 bpm, RR 12-20 breaths/min with normal depth and pattern (eupnea), and absence of edema, crackles, and other clinical indicators of fluid overload.

- Measure weight daily. Remember that a 1 kg weight gain can signal approximately 1 L of fluid retention.
- Measure I&O q1-2h; note 24-h trends.
- Assess BP, pulse, and respirations q1-2h. Be alert to increased BP, tachycardia, and tachypnea, which are indicators of fluid overload.
- Auscultate for the presence of crackles (rales) and pericardial friction rub at least q8h.
- Assess and document the presence of peripheral, sacral, and periorbital edema on a scale of 0 to 4+.
- Consult physician promptly for any significant findings from the aforementioned assessments.

Powerlessness related to actual and perceived helplessness with controlling organ rejection episodes

Desired outcome: Within 72 h of this diagnosis, patient relates that he or she can control aspects of daily care, as well as assume responsibility for taking medications appropriately and obtaining follow-up care.

- Encourage patient to express feelings of frustration and powerlessness regarding organ rejection.
- Enable and encourage patient to participate in decisions about care routines. Help patient identify areas of the care plan he or she can control, such as timing of morning care or initiating rest periods.
- Reinforce that taking medications appropriately and keeping appointments for follow-up care *are* within patient's control and are significant in the prevention of rejection and organ destruction.
- Solicit comments and opinions from patient. Honor patient's opinions and preferences.
- For other interventions, see this nursing diagnosis, p. 95.

Body image disturbance related to biophysical changes secondary to side effects from immunosuppressive medications

Desired outcome: Within 48-72 h of this diagnosis, patient verbalizes understanding of body changes that may occur with immunosuppression medications, along with interventions that can be made to minimize their effect on body image.

- Identify body changes associated with steroid therapy: profuse diaphoresis, changes in fat distribution, moon face, acne, bruising.
  - Suggest that patient try different brands of deodorants or talcs to help counteract the odor from profuse diaphoresis and wear cotton clothing, which absorbs perspiration.
  - If patient usually wears makeup, suggest that to minimize the effects of facial swelling, patient apply makeup that highlights the eyes.
  - Suggest that patient refrain from wearing prints and stripes, which may increase attention to fat distribution in the trunk area.
  - Advise patient to use facial astringents to keep skin clean and to minimize acne.
  - Suggest that patient wear long sleeves and slacks to cover bruised arms and legs.
- Teach patient about body changes that are associated with cyclosporine: hirsutism, gum hyperplasia.
  - Suggest that female patient use facial depilatories.
  - Teach patient to use a soft-bristled toothbrush and mouthwash for frequent, gentle mouth care.
- For other interventions see this nursing diagnosis, p. 97.

ADDITIONAL NURSING DIAGNOSES

See "Renal Transplantation" for **Knowledge deficit:** Immunosuppressive medications and their side effects, p. 407; **Risk for infection,** p. 409; **Altered oral mucous membrane,** p. 409; and **Impaired skin integrity,** p. 409. For other nursing diagnoses and interventions, see the following, as appropriate: "Prolonged Immobility," p. 78; "Psychosocial Support," p. 88; and "Psychosocial Support for the Patient's Family and Significant Others," p. 100.

Drug overdose

Drug overdose is a widespread problem that affects all ages, races, and socioeconomic levels. There is no one single clinical profile of individuals who overdose with either street, medically prescribed, or over-the-counter (OTC) drugs. Drug overdose can be categorized in several ways, including deleterious reactions to street drugs during a first-time use, chronic abuse of street drugs, chronic abuse of medically prescribed drugs, and overdose experienced by the elderly related to untoward effects of prescribed medications. Overdose may be intentional or nonintentional in all categories.

There is no organ or body system that does not experience some detrimental effect with drug overdose. The type, amount, and route of the drug affect the outcome, prognosis, and physical presentation. The following discussion considers the illicit and medically prescribed drugs commonly involved in drug overdose, the effects of these substances on the body systems, the laboratory tests and collaborative management, and general nursing diagnoses and interventions.

Overview of treatment options

Treatment of drug overdose depends on five factors: the type of drug ingested, the amount, the rate of absorption, the route of administration, and the time span between ingestion and delivery of care. These five factors determine the specific time frames for resolution of the drug's effects. Removal of the orally ingested substance may be accomplished through the following emerging trends in treatment.

Ipecac: Use of this gastric decontamination agent depends on the length of time from ingestion to treatment and on the patient's mental status.

- May be inappropriate in patients who ingested the drug >1 h before seeking treatment. This is especially true with ingestion of drugs in liquid form, because these are rapidly absorbed.
- Contraindicated if patient has altered mental status, because aspiration of gastric contents is a possibility. Commonly ingested agents likely to result in serious alteration of mental status are antihistamines, barbiturates, benzodiazepines, beta-blockers, cyclic antidepressants, ethanol, and opioids.
- May cause bradycardia. In combination with vomiting, this side effect may cause deleterious hemodynamic compromise, particularly if cardiotoxic drugs such as digoxin or cyclic antidepressants are involved.
- Other considerations when assessing the use of ipecac:
  □ Has the patient already vomited?
  □ Has the patient ingested a hydrocarbon or caustic substance?
  □ Is there another oral antidote?
- When ipecac is administered, vomiting should be expected within 20 min. If this does not occur, repeat dose. If ineffective, proceed to gastric lavage.

Activated charcoal: Effectiveness is enhanced when this chemical is mixed with sorbital cathartic, but diminished when food is present in the GI tract. If multidose administration is necessary, provide subsequent doses within 2-6 h. Activated charcoal does not bind with lithium, potassium, potassium chloride, ethanol, or iron.

Gastric lavage: Important adjunct in the treatment of ingested overdose because it results in prompt emptying of gastric contents. It is essential to protect the airway when using this therapy. Lavage should continue until the fluid is clear of fragments, which may take 10-30 min.

ACETAMINOPHEN

Acetaminophen (Tylenol) is one of the drugs most commonly ingested in overdose. Most patients will admit to having taken this medication.

Routes of administration

Oral (most common); rectal per suppository.

Effects on body systems

Cardiovascular: May cause myocardial damage secondary to hepatic damage, which may lead to ischemia and injury (as manifested by chest pain/pressure, nausea, SOB, T-wave inversion and ST-segment elevation on ECG). Cardiac dysrhythmias have been reported.

Respiratory: Bronchospasm (as manifested by increased RR, wheezes, and difficulty breathing) has been reported as a hypersensitivity reaction or as a side effect of N-acetylcysteine. See "Collaborative Management."

Neurologic: Coma and seizures.

Hepatic: Acute ingestion will cause hepatic necrosis, which can lead to hepatic failure. Hypoglycemia, right-sided abdominal pain, and nausea with vomiting may be noted, usually 1-2 days after ingestion.

Renal: Renal tubular necrosis (manifested by oliguria and increased BUN and creatinine values) is seen in some cases but tends to be transient.

Associated findings: Hypophosphatemia, metabolic acidosis, hypothermia, thrombocytopenia, and hemorrhagic pancreatitis.

Diagnostic tests

Serum blood levels for acetaminophen: The first serum blood levels usually are drawn 4 h postingestion, if possible. Subsequent levels are drawn periodically (e.g., q4h) until levels are below the predicted hepatotoxic range.

Additional tests: Serum Na^+, K^+, CO_2, BUN, blood glucose, creatinine, liver enzyme and bilirubin values; PT; coagulation studies; CBC count; protein; amylase; blood gas values; and renal function tests.

Collaborative management

Support of cardiovascular and respiratory systems: Oxygen supplementation. If ABG values indicate a trend toward respiratory failure or if the patient has weak or absent breathing effort, mechanical ventilation is provided. ECGs are monitored serially for evidence of dysrhythmias. Ventricular dysrhythmias are treated with antidysrhythmic agents, and bradyarrhythmias are treated with atropine, dopamine, epinephrine, or a pacemaker.

Removal of acetaminophen from the system: A combination of activated charcoal and N-acetylcysteine (Mycomyst) administered orally or *via* a gastric tube is the preferred treatment. Treatment with these agents is most effective when it is initiated as soon after ingestion as possible but may be effective up to 8-10 h postingestion. These agents bind with acetaminophen until the toxin is passed *via* the GI tract. Lavage also may be initiated to remove the drug or assess the stomach contents for evidence of drug ingestion. Activated charcoal, especially if administered within 1 h of ingestion, is highly effective in absorbing acetaminophen. Ipecac may not be prescribed because the vomiting it induces will delay use of activated charcoal and N-acetylcysteine. Ipecac may be a treatment option if ingestion is recent (e.g., within 1-2 h).

Treatment of nausea and vomiting: Fluid replacement therapy with lactated Ringer's solution or D_5NS; antiemetics, usually promethazine hydrochloride (Phenergan).

Rewarming: A heating blanket is applied if patient has hypothermia.

Treatment of hypoglycemia: Usually with a bolus of D_{50} and continuous infusion of D_5W, based on serum glucose results. Hypoglycemia occurs due to the potent hepatotoxic effects of acetaminophen.

ALCOHOL

Route of administration
Oral.

Effects on body systems
Cardiovascular: Tachycardia, atrial fibrillation, cardiac arrest.
Respiratory: Hypoventilation with acute intoxication; respiratory failure.
Neurologic: Confusion, aggressive behavior, irritability, tremens, hallucinations (especially auditory), memory loss, stupor, coma, seizures related to hypoglycemia, loss of deep tendon reflexes (DTRs).
Renal: May have significant output initially; will demonstrate dehydration with acute intoxication.
Associated findings: Dry oral mucosa, odor of alcohol on breath, hypoglycemia, hypothermia, lactic acidosis, hypokalemia.

Diagnostic tests
Blood alcohol level and urine drug screen are performed, along with serum K^+, Na^+, CO_2, BUN, glucose, and creatinine. In addition, the following may be evaluated: CBC count, liver and renal function studies, and blood gas values.

Collaborative management
Support of cardiovascular and respiratory systems to prevent collapse: Oxygen supplementation; treatment of ventricular dysrhythmias with antidysrhythmic agents; treatment of bradyarrhythmias with atropine.

Fluid/potassium replacement: See discussions, p. 671 and p. 683.

Removal of substance from system: The body can remove alcohol from its system *via* its own metabolic process. Blood alcohol concentration will decrease 20-30 mg/dl/h (legal limit is <100 mg/dl). Coma usually occurs if the level is >300 mg/dl, but this is influenced by each individual's metabolic process and tolerance. In life-threatening intoxication, in which large amounts of alcohol have been absorbed into the system, the liver and kidneys may not be able to break down and excrete the alcohol, and thus hemodialysis (see p. 410) can be of substantial benefit.

Prevention of emesis: Antiemetics are given for nausea and vomiting, and a gastric tube is inserted and maintained at low continuous suction.

Anticipation and treatment of withdrawal: Usually with short-acting benzodiazepines such as oxazepam (Serax) or lorazepam (Ativan). These patients must be medicated with an amount of medication equivalent to their usual 24-h alcohol intake; for example, 60 ml (2 oz) of 80% liquor equals 10 mg diazepam (Valium), 10 mg oxazepam, 30 mg phenobarbital, 25 mg chlordiazepoxide (Librium), or 2 mg lorazepam. Individuals who have been drinking 0.95 L (1 qt) of vodka per day will need 400 mg chlordiazepoxide or 160 mg diazepam. Cautious use of benzodiazepines with long half-lives (refer to Table 10-8) in patients with chronic alcohol consumption is important because of the likelihood of cirrhosis in these individuals. Oxazepam is the drug of choice due to its shorter half-life.

Treatment of hypoglycemia: Usually with a bolus of D_{50} and continuous infusion of D_5W, based on serum glucose results. If thiamine deficiency is suspected, thiamine should be administered before glucose to avoid sudden precipitation of heart failure and worsening neurologic impairment.

Treatment of delirium tremens (DTs):   The most severe progression of withdrawal, which can result in death. Signs and symptoms develop 72-96 h after cessation of drinking and can include disorientation, with loss of touch with reality, delirium, agitation, severe diaphoresis, tachycardia, cardiovascular collapse, and fever. Generally, DTs resolve within 3-5 days. Patients are sedated with benzodiazepines (usually IV diazepam), allowed to rest and sleep, and oriented frequently to reality.

Treatment/prevention of seizures: Because alcohol withdrawal seizures occur during the first 6-48 h after abstinence, benzodiazepines are given to raise the seizure threshold during the withdrawal period. Alcohol withdrawal seizures mandate the use of a heparin lock and IV diazepam (drug of choice) to achieve control over the seizure(s). Additional seizure management should reflect institution protocol. If the patient has a history of a primary seizure disorder, an anticonvulsant agent, such as phenytoin (Dilantin), is indicated.

IM thiamine on admission; supplemental oral thiamine; and multivitamins and multiminerals high in C, B-complex, zinc, and magnesium: Thiamine is given to prevent Wernicke-Korsakoff syndrome (discussed next); multivitamins and multiminerals are given because of the potential for malnutrition related to inadequate food intake and malabsorption caused by alcohol's irritating effect on the GI tract.

Wernicke-Korsakoff syndrome: Caused by thiamine deficiency and manifested by diplopia (the first real diagnostic clue), confusion, excitation, peripheral neuropathy, severe recent memory loss, impaired thought processes, and confabulation. Prophylactic administration of thiamine is recommended.

Caution: Ingestion of carbohydrates, either orally or parenterally, increases the body's demand for thiamine. For patients with a history of chronic alcohol ingestion, administration of thiamine should precede administration of glucose to prevent sudden profound thiamine deficiency and irreversible neurologic impairment.

AMPHETAMINES

Street names
Methamphetamine, speed, crystal, meth, white crosses, ice.

Routes of administration
Oral, IV, IM, smoked.

Effects on body systems
Cardiovascular: Tachycardia, atrial and ventricular dysrhythmias, hypertension, myocardial ischemia and infarction, cardiovascular collapse.

Respiratory: Hyperventilation and respiratory failure related to cardiovascular collapse.

Neurologic: Confusion, aggressive behavior, hyperactivity, convulsions, delusions, irritability, tremens, hallucinations, memory loss, stupor, stroke, coma.

Renal: Renal failure related to dehydration and rhabdomyolysis.

Associated findings: Mydriasis, fasciculations, hyperthermia, thrombocytopenic purpura.

Diagnostic tests
Blood and urine specimens are tested for substances of abuse. In addition to serum K^+, Na^+, CO_2, BUN, glucose, and creatinine, the CBC count and liver and renal studies also are evaluated. Cardiac enzyme levels with isoenzyme fractionations are monitored to evaluate presence and degree of myocardial injury.

Collaborative management
Support of cardiovascular and respiratory systems to prevent collapse: Antidysrhythmic agents, verapamil, and digitalis are given for atrial dysrhythmias. If origin of dysrhythmia is unknown, adenosine triphosphate is administered to convert or diagnose the site of origin. Ischemia is treated with nitrates; myocardial infarction is treated with thrombolytic therapy (see p. 374), PTCA (see p. 271), or CABG (see p. 281).

Removal of substance from the system: For oral ingestion, activated charcoal is administered orally or *via* gastric tube to bind with the ingested substance in the stomach, often followed by gastric lavage. Ipecac is not recommended.

Treatment of hypertension: Usually with antihypertensives, such as nitroprusside (Nipride), which is titrated to decrease BP.

Prevention/treatment of seizures: IV diazepam 0.1-0.2 mg/kg is administered slowly and repeated q5min until sedation is achieved. Haldol can be used *via* the IM route at a dosage of 0.1-0.2 mg/kg.

Treatment of hyperthermia: Cooling blanket, antipyretics.

Treatment of dehydration: Fluid replacement, such as lactated Ringer's solution and D_5NS.

Anticipation and treatment of rhabdomyolysis: Usually treated with sodium bicarbonate, mannitol, or furosemide (Lasix).

BARBITURATES

See Table 10-7.

Street names

Yellow jackets, reds, barbs.

Routes of administration

Oral, IV, IM.

Effects on body systems

Cardiovascular: Hypotension, bradycardia, cardiac arrest.

Respiratory: Respiratory depression leading to hypoventilation, apnea, respiratory failure, and respiratory arrest.

Neurologic: Symptoms may include headache, vertigo, dizziness, lethargy, ataxia, stupor, flaccidity, seizures, absent doll's-eye reflex, coma, loss of DTRs, and nystagmus (see coma scale, which follows).

Renal: Acute renal failure is possible.

Associated findings: Hypothermia, nausea, vomiting. Patient may experience opposite reactions of euphoria and excitability before the normal sedative effects occur. Withdrawal symptoms of tremens and convulsions may occur.

Classification of barbiturate intoxication (McCarron et al, 1982)

Alert: No signs of CNS depression.

Drowsy: CNS depression from alert to stuporous.

T A B L E   1 0 - 7   Common barbiturates

Generic name	Common brand names	Half-life (h)
amobarbital	Amytal	8-42
secobarbital	Seconal	19-34
pentobarbital	Nembutal	15-48
phenobarbital	Luminal and others	24-140
butabarbital	Butisol	34-42
secobarbital/amobarbital	Tuinal	8-42

Drug half-life: Withdrawal symptoms can be correlated with the half-life of the drug that was used. Withdrawal from drugs with shorter half-lives produces intense symptoms that last for shorter periods of time, whereas withdrawal from drugs with longer half-lives produces less intense symptoms that can be prolonged. Moreover, the severity of the withdrawal is directly related to the drug's dosage.

Stuporous: Markedly sedated; responsive to verbal and tactile stimuli.
COMA 1: Responsive to painful but not to verbal and tactile stimuli; no change in respirations or BP.
COMA 2: Unconscious; unresponsive to pain; no change in respirations or BP.
COMA 3: Unresponsive to pain; slow, shallow, or rapid spontaneous respirations; low but adequate BP.
COMA 4: Unresponsive to pain; apnea or inadequate BP or both.

Diagnostic tests

Serum drug screen is analyzed. In addition to serum K^+, Na^+, CO_2, BUN, glucose, and creatinine, the CBC count, ABG values, and liver and renal function studies are evaluated.

Collaborative management

Support of cardiovascular and respiratory systems to prevent collapse: Electrical rhythm is monitored; bradydysrhythmias are treated with atropine, L-dopamine, epinephrine, and possibly isoproterenol, as well as pacing. After fluids are replaced, vasopressor therapy (see Appendix 7), including dopamine and norepinephrine bitartrate (Levophed Bitartrate), may be initiated for hypotension. Mechanical ventilation may be required, depending on the degree of hypoxia and CO_2 retention.
Removal of substance from system: Ipecac to promote vomiting; activated charcoal administered orally or *via* gastric tube to bind with the substance in the stomach; gastric lavage; and hemodialysis, which may be used if patient is in COMA 4 stage.
Prevention/treatment of seizures: Phenytoin or diazepam may be given.
Sedation for withdrawal symptoms: Typically the barbiturate that was ingested is tapered gradually to zero.
Prevention of aspiration: Gastric tube to low suction.
Treatment of nausea and vomiting: Antiemetics, usually IV promethazine hydrochloride.
Treatment of hypothermia: Warming blanket.

BENZODIAZEPINES

See Table 10-8.

Routes of administration

Oral, IM, IV.

Effects on body systems

Cardiovascular: Hypotension and tachycardia.
Respiratory: Respiratory arrest.
Neurologic: Drowsiness, ataxia, slurred speech, coma. Withdrawal may be manifested by seizures.
Renal: Renal failure due to rhabdomyolysis.
Associated findings: Hypothermia.

T A B L E   1 0 - 8   Common benzodiazepines

Generic name	Common brand names	Half-life (h)
chlordiazepoxide	Librium and others	7-28
diazepam	Valium and others	20-90
lorazepam	Ativan	10-20
oxazepam	Serax	3-21
prazepam	Centrax	24-200*
flurazepam	Dalmane	24-100*
chlorazepate	Tranxene, Azene	30-100
temazepam	Restoril	9.5-12.4
clonazepam	Clonopin	18.5-50
alprazolam	Xanax	12-15
halazepam	Paxipam	14

*Includes half-life of major metabolites.
Drug half-life: Withdrawal symptoms can be correlated with the half-life of the drug that was used. Withdrawal from drugs with shorter half-lives produces intense symptoms that last for shorter periods of time, whereas withdrawal from drugs with longer half-lives produces less intense symptoms that can be prolonged. Moreover, the severity of the withdrawal is directly related to the drug's dosage.

Diagnostic tests

Serum and urine drug screens are analyzed. In addition to serum K^+, Na^+, CO_2, BUN, glucose, and creatinine, the CBC count and liver and renal studies are evaluated.

Collaborative management

Support of cardiovascular system to prevent collapse: Electrical rhythm is monitored; tachydysrhythmias are treated with verapamil. Hypotension is treated with fluid replacement, followed by dopamine or norepinephrine bitartrate (Levophed).
Support of respiratory system: Apnea monitoring and mechanical ventilation (see p. 19) may be indicated.
Removal of substance from system: Ipecac to induce vomiting; activated charcoal to bind with the substance in the stomach; gastric lavage.
Prevention of seizures: Administration of phenytoin and diazepam.
Prevention of aspiration: Insertion of gastric tube, which is placed for low intermittent suction.
Identification of rhabdomyolysis: The accumulation of protein in the kidneys, detected by increased BUN, creatinine, and protein values in the urine. Seizure activity and breakdown of muscle cause protein to precipitate in the kidneys, leading to renal failure. Prevention of seizures (see above) is the best treatment for prevention of rhabdomyolysis.
Treatment of hypothermia: Warming blanket if indicated.
Treatment of diazepam overdose: Sedative and respiratory depressant effects may be reversed by flumazenil (Romazicon). Repeat doses may be necessary.

COCAINE

Street names
Crack, rock, freebase, snow.

Routes of administration
Nasal or IV (cocaine, snow); smoked (crack, rock, freebase).

Effects on body systems
Cardiovascular: Hypertension; sinus tachycardia and sinus brady-cardia; ventricular dysrhythmias, such as PVCs, ventricular tachycardia, and ventricular fibrillation; myocardial infarction; congestive heart failure; cardiomyopathy; acute endocarditis; and aortic dissection. Acute intoxication also may result in profound hypotension and shock.

Respiratory: Sharp pleuritic pain, hemoptysis, pneumothorax, bronchospasm, pulmonary edema, and respiratory failure. Both lactic and metabolic acidosis have been associated with cocaine overdose.

Neurologic: The degree of CNS stimulation depends on the route and amount of drug taken, but it can include hyperexcitable state, paranoia, delirium, hallucinations, tremens, and aggression. Mentation may vary from stimulated, euphoric, and excited states to delirium, stupor, and coma. Seizures are common, usually of a tonic-clonic nature, and may last for hours. Initially the individual may seem well coordinated but may deteriorate to tremens and fasciculations. Headache is common.

Renal: Renal failure can occur and has been related to profound hypotension and rhabdomyolysis.

Associated findings: Hyperthermia is common, and rectal temperatures may be elevated to as high as 43° C (109° F). In addition, perforated nasal septum, track marks related to IV use, and mydriasis (dilated pupils) occur.

Indicators of withdrawal: Poor concentration, anergia, anhedonia, bradykinesis, sleep disturbance, decreased libido, intense cocaine craving, depression, and suicidal tendencies.

Indicators of cocaine psychosis: Tactile and visual hallucination and paranoia.

Peak action
Intranasal: 20-60 min
Oral: 60-90 min
IV: 5 min
Smoked: <5 min

Cutting agents
Cutting agents are substances that are used to increase bulk in pure cocaine. These include procaine, phencyclidine (angel dust), amphetamine, quinine, talc, and strychnine. Agents used in the preparation of crack include powdered cocaine, water, baking soda, and lidocaine. Cutting agents can become emboli that shower into cerebral and pulmonary circulation, with subsequent effects.

Diagnostic tests

Assessing blood levels of cocaine usually is of little diagnostic value. Urinalysis provides a quantitative method for identifying the presence of a cocaine metabolite. In addition to serum K^+, Na^+, CO_2, BUN, glucose, and creatinine, the CBC count and renal function studies also are analyzed.

Collaborative management

Support of cardiovascular system to prevent collapse: Electrical rhythm is monitored. Supraventricular tachycardia may be treated with propranolol (Inderal) or verapamil; ventricular dysrhythmias are treated with antidysrhythmics such as lidocaine, procainamide (Pronestyl), and bretylium. Monitor patient's ECG for changes that signal ischemic or infarction pattern. Be alert to T-wave inversion or ST-segment elevation or depression.

Support of respiratory system: Comatose patients are placed on mechanical ventilation (see p. 19).

Identification of route of administration and removal of substance from system if ingested orally: An x-ray of the GI tract may reveal the presence of a cocaine-filled condom. If present, surgery may be performed to remove it. Activated charcoal may be administered to bind with cocaine in the stomach, or a laxative or suppository may be given to facilitate rectal excretion. An approach under investigation to flush cocaine from the system is the administration of IV ammonium chloride.

Treatment of hypotension or hypertension: Antihypertensives or vasopressors as indicated.

Treatment of volume deficiency: IV fluid replacement, such as lactated Ringer's solution or D_5NS.

Prevention/treatment of seizures: Administration of diazepam, phenytoin, or phenobarbital.

Treatment of hyperthermia: Cooling blanket, ice, acetaminophen. Core temperature is monitored for the most accurate measurements.

Prevention of aspiration: Gastric tube is inserted and placed to continuous low suction.

HALLUCINOGENS (ENACTOGENICS)

Common agents

Lysergic acid diethylamide (LSD), mescaline, morning glory seeds, nutmeg, ecstasy.

Routes of administration

Oral, IV, nasal, smoked.

Effects on body systems

Effects will depend on the amount and type of drug ingested.

Respiratory: Apnea, respiratory arrest.

Neurologic: Hallucinations and paranoid behavior patterns, tremors, seizures, coma.

LSD: Description of tasting or hearing colors, mental dissociation.

Mescaline: Sense of being followed by moving geometric shapes.

Ecstasy: Heightened sexual libido.
Associated findings: Hyperthermia and diaphoresis. In addition, visual hallucinations may occur.

Diagnostic tests

Serum plasma is analyzed for the presence of the drug. In addition to serum K^+, Na^+, CO_2, BUN, glucose, and creatinine, the CBC count and liver and renal studies also are evaluated.

Collaborative management

Support of cardiovascular system to prevent collapse.
Removal of substance from system: If orally ingested, ipecac to induce vomiting; activated charcoal administered orally or *via* gastric tube to bind with the substance in the stomach; gastric lavage.
Prevention of seizures: Administration of anticonvulsants such as phenytoin or diazepam.

OPIOIDS

Examples of opioids include codeine, fentanyl, heroin, hydrocodone, hydromorphone hydrochloride (Dilaudid), levorphanol tartrate (Levo-Dromoran), meperidine hydrochloride (Demerol), methadone (Dolophine), morphine, opium, oxycodone hydrochloride (Percocet-5, Tylox), and oxymorphone (Numorphan).

Routes of administration

Oral, IV, IM, smoked.

Effects on body systems

Cardiovascular: Profound hypotension, bradycardia, cardiovascular collapse, sudden death.
Respiratory: Atelectasis, acute pulmonary edema, infiltrates related to aspiration complications, respiratory depression, apnea, hypoventilation, and bronchospasm.
Neurologic: Range from decreased mental alertness to stupor and coma, pinpoint pupils, seizures.
Renal: Renal failure has been associated with profound hypotension and rhabdomyolysis.
Associated findings: Track marks and scarring on arms and in hidden locations of the body, including between the toes and in the vessels underneath the tongue.

Diagnostic tests

Urine sampling for drug detection is the best way to identify the drug. In addition to serum K^+, Na^+, CO_2, BUN, glucose, and creatinine, the CBC count and liver and renal studies also are evaluated.

Collaborative management

Support of cardiovascular system to prevent collapse: Electrical rhythm is monitored; bradyarrhythmias are treated with atropine and pacemaker. Vasopressor therapy is initiated for hypotension after fluids have been replaced.
Removal of drug from system: If oral ingestion is suspected, ip-

ecac is used to induce vomiting; activated charcoal is administered orally or *via* gastric tube to bind with the substance in the stomach.

Reversal of opioid effects: Administration of naloxone hydrochloride (Narcan). After the initial dose of naloxone, the patient must be monitored closely, since additional doses may be required. Respiratory depression and coma may occur when the effects of naloxone wear off and the opiate effects predominate. The half-life of naloxone is 60-90 min, and effects last 2-3 h. If the narcotic effects last longer than the effects of the naloxone, the patient may slip into coma once the naloxone wears off. In this case a continuous naloxone infusion may be considered.

Treatment of drug withdrawal symptoms: Hallucinations are treated with haloperidol (Haldol).

Support of respiratory system: Pulmonary edema is treated with diuretics and restriction of IV fluid intake. An individual whose respiratory system is deteriorating is placed on apnea monitoring or mechanical ventilation (see p. 19).

Prevention of aspiration: Gastric tube is inserted and placed to continuous low suction.

Prevention/treatment of seizure activity: Anticonvulsant therapy, such as phenytoin.

Prevention of rhabdomyolysis: See discussion, p. 658.

PHENCYCLIDINE

Street names
PCP, angel dust, mist.

Routes of administration
Oral, nasal, smoked.

Effects on body systems
Cardiovascular: Hypertension, hypertensive crisis, and tachycardia.
Respiratory: Respiratory depression, respiratory arrest, laryngeal stridor (manifested by crowing sounds), bronchospasm.
Neurologic: Can range from hyperexcitability, hyperreflexia, muscle rigidity, and paranoid and psychotic behavior to stupor, seizures, and coma. Coma state may be accompanied by eyes open in a blank stare, nystagmus, and pinpoint pupils.
Renal: Renal failure precipitated by rhabdomyolysis and myoglobinuria.
Associated findings: Hypothermia or hyperthermia, hypoglycemia.

Diagnostic tests
Blood and urine samples are tested for the presence of the drug. In addition to serum K^+, Na^+, CO_2, BUN, glucose, and creatinine, the CBC count and liver and renal studies also may be evaluated.

Collaborative management
Support of cardiovascular system to prevent collapse: Electrical rhythm is monitored and tachydysrhythmias are treated with verapamil.

Nitroprusside is used for antihypertensive therapy. Nitroglycerin may be given to dilate myocardial vasculature.

Removal of drug from the system: No specific antidote is available, although multiple administrations of charcoal to bind with the ingested substance in the stomach is standard practice. The first dose of charcoal should be accompanied with sorbitol.

Prevention/treatment of seizure activity: Phenytoin and diazepam are given. Diazepam is administered IV at an initial dose of 2-5 mg. This may be repeated q30min until sedation is achieved. Haldol may be given 5-10 mg IV to control psychosis. The effects of Haldol usually occur within 5-10 min of administration.

Respiratory support: Pulmonary edema is treated with diuretics and restriction of IV fluid intake. Persons with hypoxia and deteriorating respiratory integrity are placed on apnea monitoring and potentially on mechanical ventilation.

Prevention of aspiration: Gastric tube is inserted and connected to low suction.

Prevention of rhabdomyolysis: See discussion, p. 658.

Treatment of hypothermia or hyperthermia: Warming or cooling blanket as appropriate.

SALICYLATES

Examples include aspirin, bismuth subsalicylate, fendosal.

Routes of administration

Oral, rectal (suppository).

Effects on body systems

Respiratory: Hyperventilation, hyperpnea, pulmonary edema.

Neurologic: Coma, cerebral edema (manifested by indicators of IICP [see Table 6-3, p. 449]).

Renal: Renal failure secondary to rhabdomyolysis.

Hepatic: Liver dysfunction, hepatitis.

Associated findings: Hyperthermia, bleeding, anemia, thrombocytopenia, hypokalemia, and tinnitus.

Diagnostic tests

Blood plasma is analyzed for the presence and amount of the salicylate and repeated q4-6h. This repetition is helpful, especially if the patient ingested salicylates in a sustained release form. In addition to serum K^+, Na^+, CO_2, BUN, glucose, and creatinine, the CBC count and liver and renal studies also are evaluated.

Collaborative management

Support of cardiovascular system to prevent collapse: Electrical rhythm is monitored. Ventricular dysrhythmias are treated with lidocaine, procainamide hydrochloride (Pronestyl), and bretylium. Bradyarrhythmias are treated with atropine.

Removal of substance from the system: Ipecac to induce vomiting; activated charcoal administered orally or *via* gastric tube to bind with the substance in the stomach; gastric lavage; and hemodialysis, which may be necessary if the substance has been absorbed into the system. Several doses of activated charcoal may be necessary to achieve a 10:1 ratio of charcoal to salicylate.

Fluid replacement: Replace with lactated Ringer's solution or D_5NS 20 ml/kg over 1-2 h. Sodium bicarbonate may be added at a rate of 1 mEq/kg/h to promote forced alkaline diuresis.

Potassium replacement: See discussion, p. 683.

Treatment of hyperthermia: Cooling blanket or applications of ice.

Treatment of cerebral edema: Hyperventilation (*via* mechanical ventilation), mannitol.

Respiratory support: Mechanical ventilation (p. 19) as indicated.

Treatment of pulmonary edema: Nitrates, morphine, diuretics, potassium replacement, IPPB. See discussion, p. 289.

Prevention of aspiration: Insertion of gastric tube, which is then connected to low suction.

Replacement of blood loss: Delivery of blood and blood products.

CYCLIC ANTIDEPRESSANTS

Examples include amitriptyline hydrochloride (Elavil), doxepin hydrochloride (Sinequan), imipramine hydrochloride (Presamine, Tofranil), and trimipramine maleate (Surmontil).

Route of administration
Oral.

Effects on body systems

Cardiovascular: Hypotension, sinus tachycardia, supraventricular tachycardia, ventricular dysrhythmias, conduction defects, myocardial infarction, and cardiopulmonary arrest. Hypertension also has been noted. Monitor for widening of the QRS complex. Progressive widening of this complex signals worsening toxicity.

Respiratory: Respiratory arrest, pulmonary edema, ARDS. Hyperventilation also has been noted.

Neurologic: Coma, seizures, delirium, hallucinations.

Renal: Acute tubular necrosis; renal failure secondary to rhabdomyolysis.

Pancreatic: Pancreatitis.

Associated findings: Hyperthermia or hypothermia.

Diagnostic tests

Blood plasma, urine, and gastric contents are analyzed for the presence and amount of the drug. In addition to serum K^+, Na^+, CO_2, BUN, glucose, and creatinine, the CBC count and liver and renal studies are evaluated. Cardiac enzymes and isoenzyme fractionations are assessed to determine presence and degree of myocardial damage.

Collaborative management

If the patient is symptom free, monitor for a minimum of 6-8 h, noting VS and width of QRS complex.

Support of cardiovascular system to prevent collapse: Electrical rhythm is monitored for at least 6 h to enable assessment for a widening QRS complex, which is a signal of worsening toxicity. Supraventricular tachycardias are treated with verapamil; ventricular dysrhythmias are treated with antidysrhythmics such as lidocaine. Atropine and pacing may be indicated in the presence of symptomatic conduction defects.

Removal of the substance from the system: Activated charcoal is administered *via* gastric tube to bind with the ingested substance in the stomach, facilitating its removal *via* gastric lavage. Ipecac to promote vomiting is not recommended.

Reversal of the effects of the drugs: IV sodium bicarbonate. An alternative approach is to promote a state of respiratory alkalosis by increasing respiratory rate *via* mechanical ventilation.

Prevention/treatment of seizures: Phenytoin and diazepam.

Respiratory support: Mechanical ventilation (see p. 19). Pulmonary edema is treated with nitrates, morphine, diuretics, potassium replacement, and IPPB treatments.

Treatment of hypotension: Fluid replacement, followed by dopamine and norepinephrine bitartrate (Levophed) as indicated.

Treatment of hyperthermia or hypothermia: Cooling or warming blanket as indicated.

Prevention of aspiration: Insertion of gastric tube, which is connected to low suction.

FOR ALL DRUG OVERDOSES
Nursing diagnoses and interventions

Ineffective airway clearance related to presence of tracheobronchial secretions or obstruction or decreased sensorium

Desired outcome: Within 2-24 h of intervention/treatment, patient has a clear airway as evidenced by clear breath sounds over the upper airways and lung fields, RR 12-20 breaths/min with normal depth and pattern (eupnea), Pao_2 ≥80 mm Hg, $Paco_2$ 35-45 mm Hg, pH 7.35-7.45, and Spo_2 ≥92%.

- Assess respiratory function hourly and prn. Be alert to secretions; stridor; gurgling; shallow, irregular, or labored respirations; use of accessory muscles of respiration; restlessness and confusion; and cyanosis (a late sign of respiratory distress).
- Suction oropharynx or *via* ET tube prn.
- Monitor ABG values for evidence of hypoxia (Pao_2 <80 mm Hg) and respiratory acidosis ($Paco_2$ >45 mm Hg and pH <7.35).
- Monitor respiratory patterns; provide continuous apnea monitoring if available.
- If patient has been placed on mechanical ventilation, monitor for indicators of airway obstruction (see "Mechanical Ventilation," p. 19).
- Monitor oxygen saturation continuously. Be alert to values <92%, depending on patient's baseline and clinical presentation.
- Administer and evaluate effects of antiemetics.

Hyperthermia related to overdose of cocaine, hallucinogens, phencyclidine, salicylates, or cyclic antidepressants

Desired outcome: Optimally, within 24-72 h of intervention, patient becomes normothermic.

Note: With massive overdose, temperature regulation may never be achieved.

- Monitor for signs of hyperthermia: temperature >38.3° C (>101° F), pallor, absence of perspiration, and torso that is warm to the touch. If available, provide continuous monitoring of temperature. Otherwise, measure rectal, core, or tympanic temperature hourly and prn.
- Provide and monitor effects of cooling blanket, cooling baths, and ice packs to the axillae and groin.
- Maintain fluid replacement as prescribed. Monitor hydration status and trend of I&O and urine specific gravity (optimal range is 1.010-1.020).
- Monitor neurologic status hourly and prn until stabilized.
- Monitor VS continuously or hourly and prn until stabilized. Be alert to increased BP, HR, and RR.
- Administer and evaluate effects of antipyretic medications.

Risk for fluid volume deficit related to altered intake or excessive losses secondary to vomiting or diaphoresis

Desired outcome: Patient remains normovolemic as evidenced by urine output $\geq$0.5 ml/kg/h, moist mucous membranes, balanced I&O, BP within patient's normal range, HR $\leq$100 bpm, stable weight, urine specific gravity 1.010-1.020, CVP 2-6 mm Hg, and PAWP 6-12 mm Hg.

- Monitor hydration status on an ongoing basis. Be alert to continuing dehydration as evidenced by poor skin turgor, dry mucous membranes, complaints of thirst, weight loss >0.5 kg/day, urine specific gravity >1.020, weak pulse with tachycardia, and postural hypotension.
- Assess for indicators of electrolyte imbalance, in particular presence of hypokalemia. Be alert to irregular pulse, cardiac dysrhythmias, and serum potassium level <3.5 mEq/L.
- Monitor I&O hourly; assess for output elevated out of proportion to intake, bearing in mind the insensible losses.
- Monitor laboratory values, including serum electrolyte levels and serum and urine osmolality. Be alert to BUN values elevated out of proportion to the serum creatinine (indicator of dehydration rather than renal disease), high urine specific gravity, low urine sodium, and rising Hct and serum protein concentration. Optimal values are: serum osmolality 275-300 mOsm/kg, urine osmolality 300-1090 mOsm/kg, BUN 10-20 mg/dl, serum creatinine 0.7-1.5 mg/dl, urine sodium 40-180 mEq/24 h (diet dependent), Hct 37%-47% (female) or 40%-54% (male), and serum protein 6-8.3 g/dl.
- Maintain fluid intake as prescribed; administer prescribed electrolyte supplements.

Sensory/perceptual alterations related to chemical alterations secondary to ingestion of mind-altering drugs

Desired outcome: Within 48 h of intervention, patient verbalizes orientation to time, place, and person.

- Establish and maintain a calm, quiet environment to minimize patient's sensory overload. Dim the lights when possible.
- At frequent intervals, assess patient's orientation to time, place, and person. Reorient as necessary.
- Orient patient to the unit and explain all procedures before performing them. Include significant others in orientation process.

- Do not leave patient alone if he or she is agitated or confused.
- Administer antianxiety agents as prescribed.
- If patient is hallucinating, intervene in the following ways:
  □ Be reassuring. Explain that hallucinations may be very real to patient but that they are not real, that they are caused by the substance patient consumed, and that they will go away eventually.
  □ As appropriate, try to involve family and significant others, because patient may have more trust in them.
  □ Explain that restraints are necessary to prevent harm to patient and others. Reassure patient that restraints will be used only as long as they are needed. As indicated, suggest to patient that you may release one restraint at a time as patient's condition improves.
  □ Tell patient that you will check on him or her at frequent intervals (e.g., q5-10min) or that you will stay at patient's side.

Risk for violence (self-directed) related to mind-altering drugs or depressed state
Desired outcome: Patient remains free of self-inflicted injury.
- If patient's condition is stable, provide auxiliary staff member, such as orderly or nursing assistant, to watch patient when awake.
- Speak with patient in a quiet and calm voice, using short sentences. Limit interventions.
- Administer and evaluate effectiveness of sedation to calm patient.
- Keep all sharp instruments out of patient's room. Follow agency protocol accordingly.
- If necessary, restrain patient. Start with soft restraints but progress to leather restraints if the patient is threatening to self or staff.

ADDITIONAL NURSING DIAGNOSES

See nursing diagnoses and interventions in the following, as appropriate: "Nutritional Support," p. 12; "Mechanical Ventilation," p. 24; "Hemodynamic Monitoring," p. 37; "Prolonged Immobility," p. 78; "Psychosocial Support," p. 88; "Psychosocial Support for the Patient's Family and Significant Others," p. 100; "Adult Respiratory Distress Syndrome," p. 250; "Acute Respiratory Failure," p. 266; "Acute Myocardial Infarction," p. 282; "Congestive Heart Failure/Pulmonary Edema," p. 293; "Cardiomyopathy," p. 298; "Dysrhythmias and Conduction Disturbances," p. 307; "Aortic Aneurysm/Dissection," p. 360; "Acute Renal Failure," p. 397; "Renal Replacement Therapies," p. 418; "Status Epilepticus," p. 467; "Hepatic Failure," p. 543; "Acute Pancreatitis," p. 556; "Fluid and Electrolyte Disturbances," p. 667; and "Acid-Base Imbalances," p. 706. In addition, see "Craniocerebral Trauma" for **Impaired corneal tissue integrity,** p. 138.

Fluid and electrolyte disturbances

The major constituent of the human body is water. The average male adult is approximately 60% water by weight, and the average female adult is 55% water by weight. Typically, body water decreases with both age and increasing body fat. Body water is distributed between two fluid compartments: approximately two thirds is located within the cells (intracellular fluid [ICF]) and the remaining one third is located outside the cells (extracellular fluid [ECF]). The ECF is further divided into interstitial fluid, which surrounds the cells, intravascular fluid, which is contained within blood vessels, and transcellular fluid, the fluid produced by specialized cells (e.g., gastric secretions, cerebrospinal fluid [CSF], and pericardial fluid). The body gains water through oral intake, fluid therapy, and oxidative metabolism. Water is lost from the body *via* the kidneys, GI tract, skin, and lungs.

In addition to water, body fluids contain two types of dissolved substances: electrolytes and nonelectrolytes. *Electrolytes* are substances that dissociate in solution and will conduct an electrical current. They dissociate into positive and negative ions and are measured by their capacity to combine (milliequivalents/liter [mEq/L]) or by the molecular weight in milligrams (millimoles/liter [mmol/L]). *Nonelectrolytes* are substances, such as glucose and urea, that do not dissociate in solution and are measured by weight (milligrams per 100 milliliters, or mg/dl). The body fluid compartments are separated by a semipermeable membrane, which allows movement of these dissolved substances to occur. However, the unique composition of each compartment is maintained (Table 10-9).

The composition and concentration of ECF are regulated by a combination of renal, metabolic, and neurologic functions, providing an optimal bath for the body's cells. Although ECF is altered and then modified as the body reacts with its surrounding environment, ICF remains relatively stable, which is important for maintaining normal cellular function. Composition of ECF is determined by measuring the individual electrolytes and nonelectrolytes. Osmolality (i.e., the number of particles in solution) reflects the concentration. Two important mechanisms for maintaining volume and concentration of ECF are thirst and the release of ADH. ADH is released in response to a reduction in intravascular volume or an increase in extracellular osmolality. It acts on the kidney to increase urine concentration, thereby conserving water. Thirst is stimulated by similar changes in volume and osmolality. Aldosterone is another important regulator of fluid volume. It is released by the adrenal cortex in response to an increased

T A B L E   1 0 - 9   **Primary constituents of body water compartments***

Element	Intravascular	Interstitial	Intracellular (skeletal muscle cell)
Na^+	142 mEq/L	145 mEq/L	12 mEq/L
Cl^-	104 mEq/L	117 mEq/L	4 mEq/L
HCO_3^-	24 mEq/L	27 mEq/L	12 mEq/L
K^+	4.5 mEq/L	4.5 mEq/L	150 mEq/L
HPO_4^{2-}	2 mEq/L	2 mEq/L	40 mEq/L

*This is a partial list. Other constituents include Ca^{2+}, Mg^{2+}, and proteins.

plasma renin level and acts on the kidney to conserve sodium and thus water and to increase potassium and hydrogen excretion. Atrial natriuretic peptide (ANP) is a recently identified hormone believed to be released by the cardiac atria in response to increased atrial stretch. Carotid and renal baroreceptors plus parathyroid hormone levels also may modulate release of ANP during acute volume expansion. ANP acts to reduce blood pressure and vascular volume by increasing excretion of sodium and water by the kidneys, decreasing the release of aldosterone and ADH, and by direct vasodilatation.

Section one: Fluid disturbances

HYPOVOLEMIA

Pathophysiology

Depletion of ECF volume is termed "hypovolemia." It occurs because of abnormal skin, GI, or renal losses; bleeding; decreased intake; or movement of fluid into a nonequilibrating third space. Depending on the type of fluid lost, hypovolemia may be accompanied by acid-base, osmolar, or electrolyte imbalances. Severe ECF volume depletion can lead to hypovolemic shock. Compensatory mechanisms in hypovolemia include increased sympathetic nervous system stimulation (increased heart rate, increased inotropy–cardiac contraction, increased vascular resistance), increased thirst, increased release of ADH, and increased release of aldosterone. Prolonged hypovolemia may lead to the development of acute renal failure.

Hypovolemic shock develops when the intravascular volume decreases to the point that compensatory mechanisms are unable to maintain adequate tissue perfusion and normal cellular function. Altered cellular metabolism results in acidosis, cardiac depression, intravascular coagulation, increased capillary permeability, and release of toxins. If shock is allowed to progress too long without treatment or with inadequate treatment, it may become irreversible, and no amount of intervention will prevent death.

Assessment

HISTORY AND RISK FACTORS

Abnormal GI losses: Vomiting, NG suctioning, diarrhea, intestinal drainage.

Abnormal skin losses: Excessive diaphoresis secondary to fever or exercise; burns.

Abnormal renal losses: Diuretic therapy, diabetes insipidus, renal disease (polyuric forms), adrenal insufficiency, osmotic diuresis (e.g., uncontrolled diabetes mellitus, postdye study).

Third spacing or plasma-to-interstitial fluid shift: Peritonitis, intestinal obstruction, burns, ascites.

Hemorrhage: Major trauma, GI bleeding, obstetric complications.

Altered intake: Coma, fluid deprivation.

CLINICAL PRESENTATION Dizziness, weakness, fatigue, syncope, anorexia, nausea, vomiting, thirst, confusion, constipation.

PHYSICAL ASSESSMENT Decreased BP, especially when standing (orthostatic hypotension); increased HR; decreased urine output; poor skin turgor; dry, furrowed tongue; dry mucous membranes; sunken eyeballs; flat neck veins; increased temperature; and acute weight loss (Table 10-10), except with third spacing.

HEMODYNAMIC MEASUREMENTS Decreased CVP, decreased PAP, decreased CO, decreased MAP, increased SVR.

Diagnostic tests

BUN values: May be elevated due to dehydration, decreased renal perfusion, or decreased renal function. BUN/plasma creatinine ratio of >20:1 suggests hypovolemia.

Hct levels: Elevated with dehydration; decreased in the presence of bleeding, although not initially.

Serum electrolyte levels: Variable, depending on type of fluid lost. Hypokalemia often occurs with abnormal GI or renal losses. Hyperkalemia occurs with adrenal insufficiency. Hypernatremia may be seen with increased insensible or sweat losses and diabetes insipidus. Hyponatremia occurs in most types of hypovolemia due to increased thirst and ADH release, which lead to increased water intake and retention, thus diluting the serum sodium. (See individual electrolyte imbalances, p. 676.)

Serum total CO_2 (also known as CO_2 content):   Decreased with metabolic acidosis and increased with metabolic alkalosis (see "ABG values" on p. 707).

ABG values: Metabolic acidosis (pH <7.35 and HCO_3^- <22 mEq/L) may occur with lower GI losses, shock, or diabetic ketoacidosis. Metabolic alkalosis (pH >7.45 and HCO_3^- >26 mEq/L) may occur with upper GI losses and diuretic therapy.

Urine specific gravity: Increased due to kidneys' attempt to conserve water; may be fixed at approximately 1.010 in the presence of renal disease.

Urine sodium: Demonstrates kidneys' ability to conserve sodium in response to an increased aldosterone level. In the absence of renal disease, osmotic diuresis, or diuretic therapy, value should be <20 mEq/L.

Serum osmolality: Variable, depending on the type of fluid lost and the body's ability to compensate with thirst and ADH.

Urine osmolality: Indicates kidneys' ability to produce a concen-

---

T A B L E   1 0 - 1 0   **Weight loss as an indicator of ECF deficit in the adult**

Acute weight loss	Severity of deficit
2%-5%	Mild
5%-10%	Moderate
10%-15%	Severe
15%-20%	Fatal

trated urine. Level should be increased as the kidneys attempt to conserve water, usually >450 mOsm/kg.

Collaborative management

Restoration of normal fluid volume and correction of acid-base and electrolyte disturbances: The type of fluid replacement depends on the type of fluid lost and the severity of the deficit, serum electrolytes, serum osmolality, and acid-base status. Fluid should be administered at a rate that will induce positive fluid balance (e.g., 50-100 ml *in excess* of the sum of all hourly losses).

Dextrose and water solutions: Provide free water only and will be distributed evenly through both ICF and ECF; used to treat water deficit.

Isotonic saline: Expands ECF only; does not enter ICF. Appropriate for rapid volume replacement in shock.

Blood and albumin: Expand only the intravascular portion of the ECF.

Mixed saline/electrolyte solutions: Provide additional electrolytes (e.g., potassium and calcium) and a buffer (lactate or acetate).

Dextran or hetastarch: Colloid solutions that expand the intravascular portion of the ECF.

Restoration of tissue perfusion (hypovolemic shock): Treatment includes rapid volume replacement with crystalloids. Generally, fluid may be given rapidly as long as cardiac filling pressures and BP remain low. Overaggressive fluid resuscitation in uncontrolled hemorrhage is avoided, because there is an increased risk of secondary hemorrhage as the intravascular hydrostatic pressure increases. The use of colloids (e.g., albumin) to prevent the development of pulmonary edema secondary to rapid volume replacement remains controversial. Blood is administered only as necessary to maintain oxygen-carrying capacity. Hct should not be raised >35%. Vasopressors may be used to augment volume restoration if endotoxic, anaphylactic, or neurogenic shock is also present.

Treatment of underlying cause.

Nursing diagnoses and interventions

Fluid volume deficit related to abnormal loss of body fluids or reduced intake

Desired outcomes: Within 24 h of initiation of fluid therapy, patient becomes normovolemic as evidenced by urine output ≥0.5 ml/kg/h, specific gravity 1.010-1.030, stable weight, no clinical evidence of hypovolemia (e.g., furrowed tongue), BP within patient's normal range, CVP 2-6 mm Hg, PAP 20-30/8-15 mm Hg, CO 4-7 L/min, MAP 70-105 mm Hg, HR 60-100 bpm, and SVR 900-1,200 dynes/sec/cm^{-5}.

- Monitor I&O hourly. Initially, intake should exceed output during therapy. Consult physician for urine output <0.5 ml/kg/h for 2 consecutive hours. Measure urine specific gravity q4h as available. Normal range is 1.010-1.030. Expect it to decrease with therapy.
- Monitor VS and hemodynamic pressures for signs of continued hypovolemia. Be alert to decreased BP, CVP, PAP, CO, and MAP and to increased HR and SVR.

- Place patient who is in shock in a supine position with the legs elevated to 45 degrees to increase venous return. Avoid Trendelenburg position because it causes abdominal viscera to press on the diaphragm, thereby impairing ventilation. Pneumatic antishock garments may be used initially in the treatment of hypovolemic shock.
- Weigh patient daily. Daily weight measurements are the single most important indicator of fluid status, because acute weight changes usually indicate fluid changes. For example, in the individual who is being fed, a decrease in daily weight of 1 kg is equal to the loss of 1 L of fluid. The adult who is not eating or receiving any enteral or parenteral nutrition will lose 0.25 kg of weight daily due to actual loss of body tissue. Weigh patient at the same time of day (preferably before breakfast) on a balanced scale, with patient wearing approximately the same clothing. Document type of scale used (i.e., standing, bed, chair).
- Administer PO and IV fluids as prescribed. Ensure adequate intake, especially in an older adult because of the increased risk of volume depletion in this population. Document response to fluid therapy. Monitor for signs and symptoms of fluid overload or too-rapid fluid administration: crackles (rales), SOB, tachypnea, tachycardia, increased CVP, increased PA pressures, neck vein distention, and edema. Ensure a patent IV access and availability of blood products if needed.
- Monitor patient for hidden fluid losses. For example, measure and document abdominal girth or limb size, if indicated.
- Consult physician for decreases in Hct that may signal bleeding. Remember that Hct will decrease in the dehydrated patient as he or she becomes rehydrated. Decreases in Hct associated with rehydration may be accompanied by decreases in serum sodium and BUN values.
- Hypocalcemia may develop in rapidly transfused patients owing to the citrate in stored blood. Monitor patient for sudden symptoms of hypocalcemia (see p. 688). As prescribed, administer 10 ml calcium chloride or gluconate for every 2 U of blood transfused.

Altered cerebral, renal, and peripheral tissue perfusion related to hypovolemia

Desired outcome: Within 12 h after initiation of therapy, patient has adequate perfusion as evidenced by alertness, warm and dry skin, BP within patient's normal range, HR ≤100 bpm, urinary output ≥0.5 ml/kg/h, and capillary refill <2 sec.

- Monitor for signs of decreased cerebral perfusion: vertigo, syncope, confusion, restlessness, anxiety, agitation, excitability, weakness, nausea, and cool, clammy skin. Consult physician for worsening symptoms. Document response to fluid therapy.
- Protect patients who are confused, dizzy, or weak. Keep side rails up and bed in lowest position with wheels locked. Assist with ambulation in step-down units. Raise patient to sitting or standing positions slowly. Monitor for indicators of orthostatic hypotension: decreased BP, increased HR, dizziness, and diaphoresis. If symptoms occur, return patient to supine position.
- To avoid unnecessary vasodilatation, treat fevers promptly. Cover patient with a light blanket to maintain body temperature.

- Reassure patient and significant others that sensorium changes will improve with therapy.
- Evaluate capillary refill, noting whether it is brisk (<2 sec) or delayed (≥2 sec). Consult physician if refill is delayed.
- Palpate peripheral pulses bilaterally in arms and legs (radial, brachial, dorsalis pedis, and posterior tibial). Use a Doppler ultrasonic device if unable to palpate pulses. Rate pulses on a 0-4+ scale. Consult physician if pulses are absent or barely palpable.

Note: Abnormal pulses also may be caused by a local vascular disorder.

- Consult physician for urinary output <0.5 ml/kg/h for 2 consecutive hours.

Additional nursing diagnoses

For additional nursing diagnoses, see specific medical disorder, electrolyte imbalance, or acid-base disturbance.

HYPERVOLEMIA

Pathophysiology

Expansion of ECF volume is termed "hypervolemia." It occurs in four situations: (1) with excessive retention of sodium and water due to a chronic renal stimulus to conserve sodium and water, (2) with abnormal renal functioning that involves reduced excretion of sodium and water, (3) with excessive administration of IV fluids, or (4) with interstitial-to-plasma fluid shift. Hypervolemia can lead to heart failure and pulmonary edema, especially in the patient with cardiovascular dysfunction.

Assessment

HISTORY AND RISK FACTORS
Retention of sodium and water: Heart failure, hepatic failure, nephrotic syndrome, excessive administration of glucocorticosteroids.
Abnormal renal function: Acute or chronic renal failure with oliguria or anuria.
Excessive administration of IV fluids.
Interstitial-to-plasma fluid shift: Remobilization of fluid after treatment of burns, excessive administration of hypertonic solutions (e.g., mannitol, hypertonic saline) or colloid oncotic solutions (e.g., albumin).
CLINICAL PRESENTATION SOB, orthopnea.
PHYSICAL ASSESSMENT Edema, weight gain, increased BP (decreased BP as the heart fails), bounding pulses, ascites, crackles, rhonchi, wheezes, distended neck veins, moist skin, tachycardia, gallop rhythm.
HEMODYNAMIC MEASUREMENTS Increased CVP, PAP, and PAWP. MAP is increased unless left heart failure is present.

Diagnostic tests

Laboratory findings are variable and usually nonspecific.
Hct levels: Decreased due to hemodilution.
BUN levels: Increased in renal failure.

ABG values: May reveal hypoxemia (decreased Pao_2) and alkalosis (increased pH and decreased $Paco_2$) in the presence of pulmonary edema. Respiratory acidosis (decreased $Paco_2$) may be present in severe pulmonary edema.

Serum sodium and serum osmolality: Will be decreased if hypervolemia occurs as a result of excessive retention of water (e.g., in chronic renal failure).

Urinary sodium: Elevated if the kidney is attempting to excrete excess sodium. Urinary sodium will not be elevated in conditions with secondary hyperaldosteronism (e.g., congestive heart failure, cirrhosis, nephrotic syndrome) because hypervolemia occurs secondary to a chronic stimulus to the release of aldosterone.

Urine specific gravity: Decreased if the kidney is attempting to excrete excess volume. May be fixed at 1.010 in acute renal failure.

Chest x-ray: May reveal signs of pulmonary vascular congestion.

Collaborative management

The goal of therapy is to treat the precipitating problem and return ECF to normal. Treatment may include the following measures.

Restriction of sodium and water: Oral, enteral, or parenteral. Table 10-11 lists some common foods high in sodium.

Diuretics: May be given IV or PO. Loop diuretics (e.g., furosemide) are indicated in severe hypervolemia or renal failure.

Dialysis or continuous arteriovenous hemofiltration: In renal failure or life-threatening fluid overload (see "Renal Replacement Therapies," p. 410).

Note: Also see specific discussions under "Burns," p. 207, "Adult Respiratory Distress Syndrome," p. 247, and "Acute Renal Failure," p. 385.

Nursing diagnoses and interventions

Fluid volume excess related to excessive fluid or sodium intake or compromised regulatory mechanism

Desired outcomes: Within 24 h after initiation of treatment, patient becomes normovolemic as evidenced by absence of edema, BP within patient's normal range, HR 60-100 bpm, CVP 2-6 mm Hg, PAP 20-30/8-15 mm Hg, MAP 70-105 mm Hg, and CO 4-7 L/min.

TABLE 10-11   **Foods high in sodium**

Bouillon	Olives
Celery	Pickles
Cheeses	Preserved meat
Dried fruits	Salad dressings and prepared sauces
Frozen, canned, or packaged foods	Sauerkraut
Monosodium glutamate (MSG)	Snack foods (e.g., crackers, chips, pretzels)
Mustard	Soy sauce

- Monitor I&O hourly. With the exception of oliguric renal failure, urine output should be ≥0.5 ml/kg/h. Measure urine specific gravity q4h. If patient is receiving diuretic therapy, specific gravity should be <1.010-1.020.
- Observe for and document presence of edema (pretibial, sacral, periorbital); rate pitting on a 0-4+ scale.
- Weigh patient daily. Daily weight measurements are the single most important indicator of fluid status. For example, a 2 kg acute weight gain is usually indicative of a 2 L fluid gain. Weigh patient at the same time each day (preferably before breakfast) on a balanced scale, with patient wearing approximately the same clothing. Document type of scale used (i.e., standing, bed, chair).
- Limit oral, enteral, and parenteral sodium intake as prescribed. Be aware that medications may contain sodium (e.g., penicillins, bicarbonate). See Table 10-11 for some foods high in sodium.
- Limit fluids as prescribed. Offer a portion of allotted fluids as ice chips to minimize patient's thirst. Teach patient and significant others the importance of fluid restriction and how to measure fluid volume.
- Provide oral hygiene at frequent intervals to keep oral mucous membrane moist and intact.
- Document response to diuretic therapy (e.g., increased urine output, decreased CVP/PAP, decreased adventitious breath sounds, decreased edema). Many diuretics (e.g., furosemide, thiazides) cause hypokalemia. Observe for indicators of hypokalemia: muscle weakness, dysrhythmias (especially PVCs and ECG changes such as flattened T wave, presence of U waves). See "Hypokalemia," p. 681. Potassium-sparing diuretics (e.g., spironolactone, triamterene) may cause hyperkalemia: weakness, ECG changes (e.g., peaked T wave, prolonged PR interval, widened QRS complex). See "Hyperkalemia," p. 685. Consult physician for significant findings.
- Observe for physical indicators of overcorrection and dangerous volume depletion secondary to therapy: vertigo, weakness, syncope, thirst, confusion, poor skin turgor, flat neck veins, acute weight loss. Monitor VS and hemodynamic parameters for signs of volume depletion occurring with therapy: decreased BP, CVP, PAP, MAP, and CO; increased HR. Consult physician for significant changes or findings.
- Monitor appropriate laboratory tests (e.g., BUN and creatinine in renal failure). Consult physician for abnormal trends.

Impaired gas exchange (or risk for same) related to alveolar-capillary membrane changes secondary to pulmonary vascular congestion occurring with ECF expansion

Desired outcomes: Within 12 h of initiation of treatment, patient has adequate gas exchange as evidenced by RR ≤20 breaths/min with normal depth and pattern (eupnea), HR ≤100 bpm, Pao_2 ≥80 mm Hg, pH 7.35-7.45, $Paco_2$ 35-45 mm Hg, and Spo_2 ≥92%. Patient does not exhibit crackles, gallops, or other clinical indicators of pulmonary edema. PAP is ≤30/15 mm Hg and PAWP is ≤12 mm Hg.

- Acute pulmonary edema is a potentially life-threatening complication of hypervolemia. Monitor patient for indicators of pulmonary edema, including air hunger, anxiety, cough with production of frothy sputum, crackles, rhonchi, tachypnea, tachycardia, gallop rhythm, and elevation of PAP and PAWP. As prescribed, administer diuretics such as furosemide or other medications that reduce venous return to the heart.

- Monitor ABG values for evidence of hypoxemia (decreased Pao_2) and respiratory alkalosis (increased pH and decreased $Paco_2$). As available, monitor Spo_2 for oxygen saturation levels. Administer oxygen as prescribed to maintain Spo_2 at $\geq 92\%$. Increased oxygen requirements may indicate increasing pulmonary vascular congestion.
- Keep patient in semi-Fowler's or position of comfort to minimize dyspnea. Avoid restrictive clothing.

Impaired skin and tissue integrity (or risk for same) related to edema secondary to fluid volume excess

Desired outcome: Patient's skin and tissue remain intact.

- Assess and document circulation to extremities at least each shift. Note color, temperature, capillary refill, and peripheral pulses. Determine whether capillary refill is brisk (<2 sec) or delayed (≥ 2 sec). Palpate peripheral pulses bilaterally in arms and legs (radial, brachial, dorsalis pedis, and posterior tibial). Use Doppler device if unable to palpate pulses. Consult physician if capillary refill is delayed or if pulses are diminished or absent.
- Turn and reposition patient at least q2h to minimize tissue pressure.
- Check tissue areas at risk with each position change (e.g., heels, sacrum, and other areas over bony prominences).
- Use pressure-relief mattress as indicated.
- Support arms and hands on pillows and elevate legs to decrease dependent edema.
- Treat pressure ulcers with occlusive dressings (e.g., Duoderm, Op-Site, Tegaderm) per unit protocol. Consult physician if sores, ulcers, or areas of tissue breakdown are present in patients who are at increased risk for infection (e.g., individuals with diabetes mellitus or renal failure; those who are immunosuppressed).
- Consult a skin/wound care nurse specialist, as available, for advanced tissue breakdown or any alteration in tissue integrity in high-risk patients (e.g., advanced age, debilitation).

Section two: Electrolyte disturbances

SODIUM IMBALANCE

Sodium plays a vital role in maintaining concentration and volume of ECF. It is the main cation of ECF and the major determinant of ECF osmolality. Under normal conditions ECF osmolality can be estimated by doubling the serum sodium value. Sodium imbalances usually are associated with parallel changes in osmolality. Sodium also is important in maintaining irritability and conduction of nerve and muscle tissue and assisting in the maintenance of acid-base balance.

Sodium concentration is maintained *via* regulation of water intake and excretion. If serum sodium concentration is decreased (hyponatremia), the kidneys respond by excreting water. Conversely, if serum sodium concentration is increased (hypernatremia), serum osmolality increases, stimulating the thirst center and causing an increased release of ADH by the posterior pituitary gland. ADH acts on the kidneys to conserve water. The adrenal cortical hormone, aldosterone, is an important regulator of sodium and ECF volume. The release of aldosterone causes the kidneys to conserve sodium and thus water, thereby increasing ECF volume. Because changes in serum sodium levels typically reflect changes in water balance, gains or losses of total body sodium are not necessarily reflected by the serum sodium level. Normal serum sodium is 137-147 mEq/L.

HYPONATREMIA

Pathophysiology

Hyponatremia (serum sodium <137 mEq/L) can occur because of a net gain of water or a loss of sodium-rich fluids that are replaced by water. Clinical indicators and treatment depend on the cause of the hyponatremia and whether it is associated with a normal, decreased, or increased ECF volume. For more information, see "Burns," p. 207; "Congestive Heart Failure," p. 289; "Acute Renal Failure," p. 385; and "Syndrome of Inappropriate Antidiuretic Hormone (SIADH)," p. 511.

Assessment

HISTORY AND RISK FACTORS

Decreased ECF volume

- GI losses: Diarrhea, vomiting, fistulas, NG suction.
- Renal losses: Diuretics, salt-wasting kidney disease, adrenal insufficiency.
- Skin losses: Burns, wound drainage.

Normal/increased ECF volume

- Syndrome of inappropriate antidiuretic hormone (SIADH): Excessive production of antidiuretic hormone.
- Edematous states: Congestive heart failure, cirrhosis, nephrotic syndrome.
- Excessive administration of hypotonic IV fluids or excessively dilute enteral feedings.
- Oliguric renal failure.
- Primary polydipsia.

Note: Hyperlipidemia, hyperproteinemia, and hyperglycemia may cause a pseudohyponatremia. Hyperlipidemia and hyperproteinemia reduce the total percentage of plasma that is water. The sodium-to-water ratio of the plasma does not change, but the amount of sodium in plasma is reduced. With hyperglycemia the osmotic action of the elevated glucose causes a shift of water out of the cells and into the ECF, thus diluting the existing sodium. For every 100 mg/dl that glucose is elevated, sodium is diluted by 1.6 mEq/L.

CLINICAL PRESENTATION Neurologic symptoms usually do not occur until the serum sodium level has dropped to approximately 120-125 mEq/L and are more likely to develop with a sudden decrease than with a gradual decrease. Seizures, coma, and permanent neurologic damage may occur when the plasma sodium level is <115 mEq/L.

Hyponatremia with decreased ECF volume: Irritability, apprehension, dizziness, personality changes, postural hypotension, dry mucous membranes, cold and clammy skin, tremors, seizures, coma.

Hyponatremia with normal or increased ECF volume: Headache, lassitude, apathy, confusion, weakness, edema, weight gain, elevated BP, hyperreflexia, muscle spasms, convulsions, coma.

HEMODYNAMIC MEASUREMENTS

Decreased ECF volume: Evidence of hypovolemia, including decreased CVP, PAP, CO, MAP; increased SVR.

Increased ECF volume: Evidence of hypervolemia, including increased CVP, PAP, MAP.

Diagnostic tests

Serum sodium: Will be <137 mEq/L.

Serum osmolality: Decreased, except in cases of pseudohyponatremia.

Urine specific osmolality: Usually >100 mOsm/kg H_2O but less than the plasma level. In SIADH the urine will be inappropriately concentrated.

Urine sodium: Decreased (usually <20 mEq/L) except in SIADH, salt-wasting kidney disease, and adrenal insufficiency.

Collaborative management

The goals of therapy are to raise the serum sodium at a safe rate, correct any volume abnormality, and treat the underlying cause.

HYPONATREMIA WITH REDUCED ECF VOLUME

Replacement of sodium and fluid losses: Adequate replacement of fluid volume is essential to *turn off* the physiologic stimulus to ADH release and enable the kidneys to restore the balance between sodium and water.

Replacement of other electrolyte losses: For example, potassium, bicarbonate.

IV hypertonic saline: If serum sodium is dangerously low or the patient has extreme symptoms.

HYPONATREMIA WITH EXPANDED ECF VOLUME

Removal or treatment of underlying cause.

Diuretics.

Water restriction: Restricting fluid intake to 1,000 ml/day will establish negative water balance and increase serum sodium levels in most adults.

Note: See "Syndrome of Inappropriate Antidiuretic Hormone," p. 511, for specific treatment.

Nursing diagnoses and interventions

Fluid volume deficit related to active fluid loss, excessive intake of hypotonic solutions, or compromised regulatory mechanisms

Desired outcome: Within 24 h of initiating treatment, patient becomes normovolemic as evidenced by HR 60-100 bpm, RR 12-20

breaths/min, BP within patient's normal range, CVP 2-6 mm Hg, and PAP 20-30/8-15 mm Hg.

- If patient is receiving hypertonic saline, assess carefully for signs of intravascular fluid overload: tachypnea, tachycardia, SOB, crackles (rales), rhonchi, increased CVP, increased PAP, gallop rhythm, and increased BP.
- For other interventions, see "Hypovolemia," p. 671, for **Fluid volume deficit.**

Altered protection related to neurosensory alterations secondary to sodium level <120-125 mEq/L

Desired outcomes: Within 48 h of treatment, patient verbalizes orientation to time, place, and person and does not exhibit signs of physical injury caused by altered sensorium. Serum sodium level increases to >25 mEq/L in the first 48 h after treatment.

- Assess and document LOC, orientation, and neurologic status with each VS check. Reorient patient as necessary. Consult physician for significant changes.
- Inform patient and significant others that altered sensorium is temporary and will improve with treatment.
- Keep side rails up and bed in lowest position with wheels locked.
- Use reality therapy, such as clocks, calendars, and familiar objects; keep these items at the bedside within patient's visual field.
- If seizures are expected, pad side rails and keep an appropriate-size airway at the bedside.
- Monitor serum sodium levels. On average, sodium levels should not increase at a level >0.5 mEq/L/h in patients being treated for symptomatic hyponatremia owing to the risk of neurologic damage. As well, levels should not increase at an average rate of >0.5 mEq/L/h in patients without symptoms. The overall increase during the first 24-48 h of treatment is more important than the individual hourly rate of rise.

HYPERNATREMIA

Pathophysiology

Hypernatremia (serum sodium level >147 mEq/L) may occur with water loss or sodium gain. Because sodium is the major determinant of ECF osmolality, hypernatremia always causes hypertonicity. In turn, hypertonicity causes a shift of water out of the cells, which leads to cellular dehydration and increased extracellular fluid volume.

Assessment

HISTORY AND RISK FACTORS

Sodium gain: IV administration of hypertonic saline or sodium bicarbonate, increased oral intake, primary aldosteronism, saltwater near drowning, drugs such as sodium polystyrene sulfonate (Kayexalate).

Water loss: Increased diaphoresis, respiratory infection, diabetes insipidus, osmotic diuresis (e.g., hyperglycemia).

CLINICAL PRESENTATION Intense thirst, fatigue, restlessness, agitation, coma. Symptoms of hypernatremia occur only in individuals who do not have access to water or who have an altered thirst mechanism (e.g., infants, older adults, those who are comatose).

Note: Symptoms are most likely to develop with a sudden increase in plasma sodium. After approximately 24 h, brain cells adjust to ECF hypertonicity by increasing intracellular osmolality. The exact mechanism by which this occurs is unclear, but it is known that this increased osmolality helps to rehydrate the cells. Thus individuals with chronic hypernatremia may exhibit few symptoms. This adaptive mechanism has great significance in the treatment of hypernatremia. If the plasma sodium is reduced too quickly *via* administration of water, there will be a rapid and dramatic movement of water into the cells due to increased osmolality, which will cause dangerous cerebral edema.

PHYSICAL ASSESSMENT Low-grade fever, flushed skin, peripheral and pulmonary edema (sodium gain); postural hypotension (water loss)—usually mild.
HEMODYNAMIC MEASUREMENT Variable.
Sodium excess: Increased CVP and PAP.
Water loss: Decreased CVP and PAP, although these changes may be minimized by the extracellular shift of fluid that occurs with hypernatremia.

Diagnostic tests
Serum sodium: Will be >147 mEq/L.
Serum osmolality: Increased due to elevated serum sodium.
Urine specific gravity: Increased because of kidneys' attempt to retain water; will be decreased in diabetes insipidus and osmotic diuresis (e.g., hyperglycemia).

Collaborative management
IV or oral water replacement: For water loss. If sodium is >160 mEq/L, IV D_5W or hypotonic saline is given to replace pure water deficit. (See "Diabetes Insipidus," p. 506, for specific treatment.)
Diuretics and oral or IV water replacement: For sodium gain.

Note: Hypernatremia is corrected slowly, over approximately 2 days, to avoid too great a shift of water into brain cells.

Nursing diagnoses and interventions
Altered protection related to neurosensory alterations secondary to primary hypernatremia or cerebral edema occurring with too-rapid correction of hypernatremia
Desired outcomes: Within 48 h after treatment, patient verbalizes orientation to time, place, and person and does not exhibit evidence of injury due to altered sensorium or seizures. Serum sodium level is ≤147 mEq/L.
- Cerebral edema may occur if hypernatremia is corrected too rapidly. Monitor serial serum sodium levels; consult physician for rapid decreases.
- Assess patient for indicators of cerebral edema: lethargy, headache, nausea, vomiting, increased BP, widening pulse pressure, decreased HR, altered sensorium, and seizures.
- Assess and document LOC, orientation, and neurologic status with

each VS check. Reorient patient as necessary. Consult physician for significant changes.
- Inform patient and significant others that altered sensorium is temporary and will improve with treatment.
- Keep side rails up and bed in lowest position with wheels locked.
- Use reality therapy, such as clocks, calendars, and familiar objects; keep these items at the bedside within patient's visual field.
- If seizures are anticipated, pad side rails and keep an airway at the bedside.
- Provide comfort measure to decrease thirst.

Additional nursing diagnoses

See "Hypovolemia," p. 671, for **Fluid volume deficit**; and "Hypervolemia," p. 674, for **Fluid volume excess.**

POTASSIUM IMBALANCE

Potassium is the primary intracellular cation, and thus it plays a vital role in cell metabolism. Because it affects the resting membrane potential of nerve and cardiac cells, abnormal serum potassium levels adversely affect neuromuscular and cardiac function. A relatively small amount of potassium is located within the ECF and is maintained within a narrow range. The vast majority of the body's potassium is located within the cells. Distribution of potassium between ECF and ICF is maintained by the sodium-potassium pump located in the membrane of all body cells and is affected by ECF pH, by glucose and protein metabolism, and by several hormones, including insulin and epinephrine. Acute changes in serum pH are accompanied by reciprocal changes in serum potassium concentration.

The body gains potassium through foods (primarily meats, fruits, and vegetables) and medications. In addition, ECF gains potassium any time there is a breakdown of cells or movement of potassium out of the cell. An elevated serum potassium level usually does not occur unless there is a reduction in renal function. Potassium is lost from the body through the kidneys, GI tract, and skin. Potassium also may be lost from ECF because of an intracellular shift. The kidneys are the primary regulators of potassium balance. Normal serum potassium level is 3.5-5 mEq/L.

Note: Disorders of potassium balance are potentially life threatening because of the effects of altered potassium levels on neuromuscular and cardiac function. Suspected alterations in potassium balance require prompt consultation with physician.

HYPOKALEMIA

Pathophysiology

Hypokalemia (serum potassium level <3.5 mEq/L) occurs because of a loss of potassium from the body or a movement of potassium into the cells.

Note: Changes in serum potassium levels reflect changes in ECF potassium, not necessarily changes in total body levels.

Assessment

HISTORY AND RISK FACTORS

Reduction in total body potassium
- Hyperaldosteronism.
- Diuretic therapy or abnormal urinary losses (e.g., hypomagnesemia).
- Increased GI losses.
- Increased loss through diaphoresis.
- Decreased intake.
- Dialysis.

Note: A poorly balanced or inadequate diet may contribute to, but rarely will cause, hypokalemia because significant amounts of potassium are contained in a variety of foods. Hypokalemia may develop, however, in individuals who are maintained on parenteral fluid therapy with inadequate replacement of potassium or when reduced intake is combined with increased losses.

Intracellular shift
- Increased insulin (e.g., from TPN or treatment of diabetic ketoacidosis [DKA]).
- Acute alkalosis.
- Stress: Any condition causing physical or emotional stress may result in hypokalemia due to increased loss of potassium in the urine secondary to increased release of aldosterone; or an intracellular shift of potassium secondary to increased release of epinephrine.

CLINICAL PRESENTATION Muscle weakness and cramps, soft and flabby muscles, nausea, vomiting, ileus, paresthesias, enhanced digitalis effect.

PHYSICAL ASSESSMENT Decreased bowel sounds, weak and irregular pulse, decreased reflexes, and decreased muscle tone.

ECG FINDINGS Because of the effects of hypokalemia on the shape and slope of the action potential, the heart muscle is slow to return to its fully resting or repolarized state. During this slow return to resting, weak impulses from an irritable myocardium may initiate abnormal beats. Dangerous ventricular tachycardia may develop in severe hypokalemia.

Diagnostic tests

Serum potassium levels: Values will be <3.5 mEq/L.

ABG values: May show metabolic alkalosis (increased pH and HCO_3^-) because hypokalemia usually is associated with this condition. Hypokalemia also may be associated with metabolic acidosis (e.g., DKA, diarrhea, renal tubular acidosis).

ECG findings: ST-segment depression, flattened T wave, presence of U wave, ventricular dysrhythmias. With severe hypokalemia there will be increased amplitude of the P wave, prolonged PR interval, and widening of the QRS complex.

Note: Hypokalemia potentiates the effect of digitalis. ECG may reveal signs of digitalis toxicity in spite of a normal serum digitalis level.

Collaborative management

Treatment of underlying cause.

Replacement of potassium: Accomplished either PO (*via* increased dietary intake or medication) or IV, with the usual dosage 40-80 mEq/L/day in divided doses. IV potassium is necessary if hypokalemia is severe or if the patient is unable to take potassium orally. Potassium is *never* administered by IV push. It *must* be appropriately diluted and administered at rates ≤10-20 mEq/h or in concentrations ≤30-40 mEq/L (when added to IV solutions) unless hypokalemia is severe. Too-rapid an administration can result in life-threatening hyperkalemia. If potassium is administered *via* a peripheral line, the rate of administration may require reduction to prevent irritation of vessels. Patients receiving 10-20 mEq/h should be on a continuous cardiac monitor. The development of peaked T waves suggests the presence of hyperkalemia and requires immediate consultation with a physician. IV potassium may be administered as potassium chloride or potassium phosphate. Table 10-12 lists some foods high in potassium.

Potassium-sparing diuretics: May be given in place of oral potassium supplements.

Nursing diagnoses and interventions

Decreased cardiac output (or risk for same) related to altered conduction secondary to hypokalemia or too-rapid correction of hypokalemia, with resulting hyperkalemia

Desired outcome: Within 2 h of treatment, patient has adequate cardiac conduction as evidenced by normal T-wave configuration and normal sinus rhythm without ectopy on ECG.

• Administer potassium supplement as prescribed. Avoid giving IV po-

---

T A B L E   1 0 - 1 2   Foods high in potassium

Apricots	Mushrooms
Artichokes	Nuts
Avocados	Oranges, orange juice
Bananas	Peanuts
Cantaloupes	Potatoes
Carrots	Prune juice
Cauliflower	Pumpkins
Chocolate	Spinach
Dried beans, peas	Swiss chard
Dried fruit	Sweet potatoes
	Tomatoes, tomato juice, tomato sauce

tassium chloride at a rate faster than recommended, inasmuch as this can lead to life-threatening hyperkalemia. Potassium supplementation for symptomatic hypokalemia usually is given in isotonic saline because D_5W will increase insulin-induced intracellular shift of potassium. Concentrated solutions of potassium may be hung in limited volumes (e.g., 20 mEq in 100 ml of isotonic NaCl), but it should be administered no more rapidly than 40 mEq/h. Concentrated solutions and infusion rates of >10 mEq/h are used only with severe hypokalemia.

Do not add potassium chloride to IV solution containers in the hanging position, because this can cause layering of the medication. Instead, invert the solution container before adding the medication and mix well.

- Be aware that IV potassium chloride can cause local irritation of veins and chemical phlebitis. Assess IV insertion site for erythema, heat, or pain. Alert physician to symptoms. Irritation may be relieved by applying an ice bag, giving mild sedation, or numbing insertion site with a small amount of local anesthetic. Phlebitis may necessitate changing of IV site. Oral supplements may cause GI irritation. Administer with a full glass of water or fruit juice; encourage patient to sip slowly. Consult physician for symptoms of abdominal pain, distention, nausea, or vomiting. Do not switch potassium supplements without physician prescription.
- Monitor I&O hourly. Consult physician for urine output <0.5 ml/kg/h. Unless severe symptoms of hypokalemia are present, potassium supplements should not be given if the patient has an inadequate urine output because hyperkalemia can develop rapidly in patients with oliguria (<15-20 ml/h). Increased urine output increases the risk of hypokalemia.
- Physical indicators of abnormal potassium levels are difficult to identify in the patient who is critically ill. Monitor ECG for signs of continuing hypokalemia (ST-segment depression, flattened T wave, presence of U wave, ventricular dysrhythmias) or hyperkalemia (tall, thin T waves; prolonged PR interval; ST depression; widened QRS complex; loss of P wave), which may develop during potassium replacement.
- Monitor serum potassium levels carefully, especially in individuals at risk for hypokalemia, such as patients taking diuretics or undergoing gastric suction.
- Administer potassium cautiously in patients receiving potassium-sparing diuretics (e.g., spironolactone or triamterene) or ACE inhibitors (e.g., captopril) because of the potential for the development of hyperkalemia.
- Because hypokalemia can potentiate the effects of digitalis, monitor patients receiving digitalis for signs of increased digitalis effect: multifocal or bigeminal PVCs, paroxysmal atrial tachycardia with varying AV block, and other heart blocks.

Ineffective breathing pattern (or risk for same) related to weakness or paralysis of respiratory muscles secondary to sudden *severe* hypokalemia (potassium <2-2.5 mEq/L)

Desired outcome: Within 2 h of treatment, patient has effective

breathing pattern as evidenced by normal respiratory depth and pattern (eupnea) and rate of 12-20 breaths/min.
- If patient is exhibiting signs of worsening hypokalemia, be aware that severe hypokalemia can lead to weakness of respiratory muscles, resulting in shallow respirations and eventually apnea and respiratory arrest. Assess character, rate, and depth of respirations. Consult physician promptly if respirations become rapid and shallow.
- Keep manual resuscitator at patient's bedside if severe hypokalemia is suspected.
- Reposition patient q2h to prevent stasis of secretions; suction airway as needed.
- Encourage deep breathing (and coughing if indicated) q2h in conscious patients.

HYPERKALEMIA

Pathophysiology
Hyperkalemia (serum potassium level >5 mEq/L) occurs because of an increased intake of potassium, a decreased urinary excretion of potassium, or sudden movement of potassium out of the cells.

Note: Changes in serum potassium levels reflect changes in ECF potassium, not necessarily changes in total body levels of potassium.

Assessment
HISTORY AND RISK FACTORS
Inappropriately high intake of potassium: Usually, IV potassium delivery.
Decreased excretion of potassium
- Renal disease, especially acute renal failure.
- Potassium-sparing diuretics, ACE inhibitors.

Movement of potassium out of the cells
- Acidosis.
- Insulin deficiency, particularly in dialysis patients.
- Tissue catabolism (e.g., with fever, sepsis, trauma, surgery).

CLINICAL PRESENTATION Irritability, abdominal cramping, diarrhea, ascending weakness, paresthesias.
PHYSICAL ASSESSMENT Irregular pulse and abdominal distention; cardiac standstill may occur at levels >8.5 mEq/L.

Diagnostic tests
Serum potassium: Will be >5 mEq/L.

Note: Pseudohyperkalemia may occur with mechanical trauma during venipuncture or incorrect handling of the laboratory specimen. It is the result of potassium moving out of the cells during or after the blood specimen has been drawn.

ABG values: May show metabolic acidosis (decreased pH and HCO_3^-) because hyperkalemia often occurs with acidosis.
Diagnostic ECG: Progressive changes include tall, thin T waves;

prolonged PR interval; ST depression; widened QRS complex; loss of P wave. Eventually, QRS complex becomes widened further and cardiac arrest occurs.

Collaborative management

The goal is to treat the underlying cause and return the serum potassium level to normal.

SUBACUTE

Cation exchange resins (e.g., Kayexalate):   Given either orally or *via* retention enema to exchange sodium for potassium in the gut. Oral Kayexalate usually is combined with sorbitol to promote rapid transit through the gut and induce diarrhea and thus increase potassium loss in the bowels. The recommended rectal dose for adults is 30-50 g q6h.

ACUTE

IV calcium gluconate: To counteract the neuromuscular and cardiac effects of hyperkalemia. Serum potassium levels will remain elevated.

IV glucose and insulin: To shift potassium into the cells. This reduces serum potassium temporarily.

Sodium bicarbonate: To shift potassium into the cells. Reduces serum potassium temporarily.

Note: The effects of calcium, glucose and insulin, and sodium bicarbonate are temporary, lasting only a few hours. Usually it is necessary to follow these medications with a therapy that removes potassium from the body (e.g., dialysis or administration of cation exchange resins).

Dialysis: For rapid removal of potassium from the body.

Nursing diagnoses and interventions

Decreased cardiac output (or risk for same) related to electrical factors (ventricular dysrhythmias) secondary to severe hyperkalemia or overcorrection of hyperkalemia, with resulting hypokalemia

Desired outcomes: Within 6 h after initiation of treatment, patient's cardiac output is adequate as evidenced by PAP 20-30/8-15 mm Hg, CVP ≤6 mm Hg, CO 4-7 L/min, HR ≤100 bpm, BP within patient's normal range, and absence of the clinical signs of heart failure or pulmonary edema (e.g., crackles, SOB). ECG shows normal sinus rhythm without ectopy or other electrical disturbances. Serum potassium levels are within normal range (3.5-5 mEq/L).

- Monitor I&O. Consult physician for urine output <0.5 ml/kg/h. Oliguria increases the risk for development of hyperkalemia.
- Monitor for indicators of hyperkalemia (e.g., irritability, anxiety, abdominal cramping, diarrhea, ascending weakness, paresthesias, irregular pulse). Also be alert to indicators of hypokalemia (e.g., muscle weakness and cramps, nausea, vomiting, decreased bowel sounds, paresthesias, weak and irregular pulse) after treatment. Assess for hidden sources of potassium: medications (e.g., potassium penicillin G), banked blood, salt substitute, GI bleeding, or conditions that cause increased catabolism such as infection or trauma.
- Monitor serum potassium levels, especially in patients at risk for hyperkalemia such as persons with renal failure. Consult physician for levels above or below normal range. Monitor other laboratory val-

ues that may affect potassium levels (e.g., BUN, creatinine, ABG values, glucose).

- Physical indicators of abnormal potassium levels are difficult to identify in a patient who is critically ill. Monitor ECG for signs of hypokalemia (ST-segment depression, flattened T waves, presence of U wave, ventricular dysrhythmias), which may result from therapy, or continuing hyperkalemia (tall, thin T waves; prolonged PR interval; ST depression; widened QRS complex; loss of P wave). Consult physician *stat* if ECG changes occur.

- Administer insulin and glucose in the order prescribed. When glucose is administered first, it stimulates endogenous insulin release and may potentiate the potassium, lowering the effect of the exogenous insulin.

- Administer calcium gluconate as prescribed, giving it cautiously in patients receiving digitalis because digitalis toxicity can occur. Do not add calcium gluconate to solutions containing sodium bicarbonate because precipitates may form. For more information about calcium administration, see "Hypocalcemia," p. 689.

- If administering cation exchange resins by enema, encourage patient to retain the solution for at least 30-60 min to ensure therapeutic effects. Administer Kayexalate (without sorbitol) *via* a Foley catheter inserted into the rectum. The balloon is filled with sterile water to keep the catheter in place, and the catheter is clamped. Cleansing enemas are recommended before administration to enhance absorption and afterward to reduce the risk of bowel complications.

CALCIUM IMBALANCE

Calcium, one of the body's most abundant ions, primarily is combined with phosphorus to form the mineral salts of the bones and teeth. In addition, calcium exerts a sedative effect on nerve cells and has important intracellular functions, including development of the cardiac action potential and contraction of muscles. Only 1% of the body's calcium is contained within ECF, yet this concentration is regulated carefully by the hormones parathormone (parathyroid hormone) and calcitonin. Parathormone is released by the parathyroid gland in response to a low serum calcium level. It increases resorption of bone (movement of calcium and phosphorus out of the bone); activates vitamin D, which increases the absorption of calcium from the GI tract; and stimulates the kidneys to conserve calcium and excrete phosphorus. Calcitonin is produced by the thyroid gland when serum calcium levels are elevated. It inhibits bone resorption.

Approximately half of plasma calcium is free, ionized calcium. Slightly less than half is bound to protein, primarily to albumin. The remaining small percentage is complexed (i.e., it is combined with nonprotein anions such as phosphate, citrate, and carbonate). Only the ionized calcium is physiologically important. The percentage of calcium that is ionized is affected by plasma pH and albumin level. Patients with alkalosis may show signs of hypocalcemia because of increased calcium binding. Changes in plasma albumin level will affect total serum calcium level without changing the level of ionized calcium.

HYPOCALCEMIA

Pathophysiology

Symptoms of hypocalcemia may occur because of a reduction of total body calcium or a reduction of the percentage of calcium that is ionized. Total calcium levels may be decreased due to increased calcium loss, reduced intake secondary to altered intestinal absorption, or altered regulation (e.g., hypoparathyroidism). Elevated phosphorus levels and decreased magnesium levels may precipitate hypocalcemia.

Assessment

HISTORY AND RISK FACTORS

Decreased ionized calcium

- Alkalosis.
- Rapid administration of citrated blood. Citrate added to the blood to prevent clotting may bind with calcium, causing hypocalcemia.
- Hemodilution (e.g., occurring with volume replacement with normal saline after massive hemorrhage).

Increased calcium loss in body fluids: As with loop diuretics.

Decreased intestinal absorption

- Decreased intake.
- Impaired vitamin D metabolism.
- Chronic diarrhea.
- After gastrectomy.

Hypoparathyroidism.

Hyperphosphatemia: As in renal failure.

Hypomagnesemia.

Acute pancreatitis.

CLINICAL PRESENTATION Numbness with tingling of fingers and circumoral region, hyperactive reflexes, muscle cramps, tetany, convulsions. Alterations in mental status may include anxiety, depression, and frank psychosis. In chronic hypocalcemia, fractures may be present due to increased bone porosity. Sudden precipitous drops in plasma calcium levels may cause hypotension secondary to vasodilatation and heart failure secondary to decreased myocardial contractility.

PHYSICAL ASSESSMENT

Positive Trousseau's sign: Ischemia-induced carpopedal spasm. It is elicited by applying a BP cuff to the upper arm and inflating it past systolic BP for 2 min.

Positive Chvostek's sign: Unilateral contraction of facial and eyelid muscles. It is elicited by stimulating the facial nerve during percussion of the face just in front of the ear.

ECG CHANGES Prolonged QT interval caused by elongation of ST segment.

Diagnostic tests

Total serum calcium level: Will be <8.5 mg/dl. Serum calcium levels should be evaluated with serum albumin. For every 1 g/dl drop in the serum albumin level, there is a 0.8-1 mg/dl drop in total calcium level. This drop, however, has little impact on the ionized calcium level. Symptomatic hypocalcemia can occur with normal total calcium levels when there is a sudden rise in serum pH.

Ionized serum calcium level: Will be <4.5 mg/dl.

Parathyroid hormone (PTH) level: Decreased levels occur in hypoparathyroidism; increased levels may occur with other causes of hypocalcemia. Normal range is 150-350 pg/ml (varies among laboratories).

Magnesium and phosphorus levels: May be checked to identify potential causes of hypocalcemia.

Collaborative management

Treatment of underlying cause.

Calcium replacement: Hypocalcemia is treated with PO or IV calcium. Tetany is treated with 10-20 ml of 10% calcium gluconate administered intravenously or by continuous drip of 100 ml of 10% calcium gluconate in 1,000 ml D_5W, infused over at least 4 h. Magnesium replacement should be initiated in the individual with magnesium depletion, inasmuch as hypomagnesemia-induced hypocalcemia is often refractory to calcium therapy alone.

Vitamin D therapy (e.g., dihydrotachysterol, calcitriol): To increase calcium absorption from the GI tract.

Aluminum hydroxide antacids: To reduce elevated phosphorus before treating hypocalcemia.

Nursing diagnoses and interventions

Altered protection (risk of tetany and seizures) related to neurosensory alterations secondary to severe hypocalcemia

Desired outcome: Patient does not exhibit evidence of injury caused by complications of severe hypocalcemia.

- Monitor patient for evidence of worsening hypocalcemia: numbness and tingling of fingers and circumoral region, hyperactive reflexes, and muscle cramps. Consult physician promptly if these symptoms develop because they occur before overt tetany. In addition, consult physician if patient has positive Trousseau's or Chvostek's signs because they also signal latent tetany. Monitor total and ionized calcium levels as available.
- Administer IV calcium with caution. IV calcium should not be given faster than 0.5-1 ml/min, inasmuch as rapid administration can cause hypotension. Observe IV insertion site for evidence of infiltration because calcium will slough tissue. Concentrated calcium solutions should be administered through a central line. Do not add calcium to solutions that contain sodium bicarbonate or sodium phosphate because dangerous precipitates will form. Digitalis toxicity may develop in patients taking digitalis because calcium potentiates its effects. Monitor patient for signs and symptoms of hypercalcemia: lethargy, confusion, irritability, nausea, and vomiting.

Note: Always clarify type of IV calcium to be given. Both calcium chloride and calcium gluconate come in 10 ml ampules. One ampule of calcium chloride contains 13.6 mEq of calcium, whereas one ampule of calcium gluconate contains 4.5 mEq of calcium.

- For patients with chronic hypocalcemia, administer oral calcium supplements and vitamin D preparations as prescribed. Administer oral calcium 30 min before meals or at bedtime for maximal absorption. Administer aluminum hydroxide antacids with meals.
- Consult physician if response to calcium therapy is ineffective. Tetany that does not respond to IV calcium may be caused by hypomagnesemia.
- Maintain seizure precautions for patients with symptoms; decrease environmental stimuli.
- Avoid hyperventilation in patients in whom hypocalcemia is suspected. Respiratory alkalosis may precipitate tetany due to increased pH with a reduction in ionized calcium.
- Monitor for calcium loss (e.g., with loop diuretics, renal tubular dysfunction) or conditions that place the patient at risk (e.g., acute pancreatitis).
- Inform patient and significant others that neuropsychiatric symptoms of hypocalcemia will improve with treatment.

Decreased cardiac output related to altered conduction or negative inotropy secondary to hypocalcemia or digitalis toxicity occurring with calcium replacement therapy

Desired outcomes: Within 12 h of initiation of treatment, patient's cardiac output is adequate as evidenced by PAP 20-30/8-15 mm Hg, CVP ≤6 mm Hg, CO 4-7 L/min, HR ≤100, BP within patient's normal range, and absence of the clinical signs of heart failure or pulmonary edema (e.g., crackles, SOB). ECG shows normal sinus rhythm without ectopy or other electrical disturbances.

- Monitor ECG for signs of worsening hypocalcemia (prolonged QT interval) or digitalis toxicity with calcium replacement: multifocal or bigeminal PVCs, paroxysmal atrial tachycardia with varying AV block, and other heart blocks.
- Hypocalcemia may decrease cardiac contractility. Monitor patient for signs of heart failure or pulmonary edema: crackles, rhonchi, SOB, decreased BP, increased HR, increased PAP, or increased CVP.

Ineffective breathing pattern related to laryngeal spasm occurring with severe hypocalcemia

Desired outcome: Within 1 h of initiation of treatment, patient has an effective breathing pattern as evidenced by eupnea, RR 12-20 breaths/min, and absence of the indicators of laryngeal spasm: laryngeal stridor, dyspnea, or crowing.

- Assess patient's respiratory rate, character, and rhythm. Be alert to laryngeal stridor, dyspnea, and crowing, which occur with laryngeal spasm, a life-threatening complication of hypocalcemia.
- Keep an emergency tracheostomy tray at the bedside of all patients with symptoms of hypocalcemia.

HYPERCALCEMIA

Pathophysiology

Symptoms of hypercalcemia can occur because of an increase in total serum calcium or an increase in the percentage of free, ionized calcium. If hypercalcemia is accompanied by a normal or elevated serum phosphorus level, calcium phosphate crystals may precipitate in the serum and deposit throughout the body. Soft tissue calcifications usually occur when the product of the serum calcium and serum phosphorus (i.e., calcium times phosphorus) exceeds 70 mg/dl.

Assessment

HISTORY AND RISK FACTORS The two primary causes of hypercalcemia are hyperparathyroidism, which may be stress-related in the patient in ICU, and malignancy.

Increased intake of calcium: Excessive administration during cardiopulmonary arrest, milk-alkali syndrome.

Increased intestinal absorption: With vitamin D overdose or hyperparathyroidism.

Increased release of calcium from bone: Hyperparathyroidism, malignancies, prolonged immobilization, Paget's disease.

Decreased urinary excretion: Renal failure, medications (e.g., thiazide diuretics), hyperparathyroidism.

Increased ionized calcium: Acidosis.

CLINICAL PRESENTATION Lethargy, weakness, anorexia, nausea, vomiting, polyuria, itching, bone pain, fractures, calculi, constipation, depression, confusion, paresthesias, personality changes, stupor, coma. Cardiovascular effects include hypertension, heart block, digitalis sensitivity, and cardiac arrest.

ECG FINDINGS Shortening of ST segment and QT interval. PR interval is sometimes prolonged. Ventricular dysrhythmias can occur with severe hypercalcemia.

Diagnostic tests

Total serum calcium level: Will be >10.5 mg/dl. Serum calcium level should be evaluated with serum albumin level. For every 1 g/dl drop in serum albumin level, there will be a 0.8-1 mg/dl drop in total calcium.

Ionized calcium level: Will be >5.5 mg/dl.

Parathyroid hormone level: Increased levels occur in primary or secondary hyperparathyroidism.

X-ray findings: May reveal presence of osteoporosis, bone cavitation, or urinary calculi.

Collaborative management

Treatment of underlying cause or contributing factor: For example, antitumor chemotherapy for malignancy or partial parathyroidectomy for hyperparathyroidism; discontinuation of calcium supplements, vitamins A and D, and thiazide diuretics.

IV isotonic saline: Administered rapidly to increase urinary calcium excretion. Concomitant administration of furosemide prevents the development of fluid volume excess and further increases in urinary calcium excretion.

Low-calcium diet and cortisone: To reduce intestinal absorption of calcium. Steroids compete with vitamin D, thereby reducing intestinal absorption of calcium.

Decreased bone resorption: Accomplished *via* increased activity level, indomethacin, or mithramycin. Mithramycin, a cytotoxic antibiotic, acts directly on bone to reduce decalcification and is used primarily to treat hypercalcemia associated with neoplastic disease. Compressional loads (e.g., weight bearing) stimulate bone deposition; thus increased activity decreases bone resorption.

Calcitonin: To reduce bone resorption, increase bone deposition of calcium and phosphorus, and increase urinary calcium and phosphate excretion.

Sodium bicarbonate: To treat acidosis and reduce the percentage of calcium that is ionized.

Gallium nitrate: Inhibits osteoclasts and increases bone calcium. It is used in the treatment of malignancy-induced hypercalcemia.

Etidronate and pamidronate: Bisphosphonates that inhibit bone resorption.

Nursing diagnoses and interventions

Altered protection related to neurosensory alterations secondary to hypercalcemia

Desired outcomes: Within 24-48 h of initiating treatment, patient verbalizes orientation to time, place, and person. Patient does not exhibit evidence of injury due to neurosensory changes.

- Monitor patient for worsening hypercalcemia. Assess and document LOC; patient's orientation to time, place, and person; and neurologic status with each VS check.
- Personality changes, hallucinations, paranoia, and memory loss may occur with hypercalcemia. Inform patient and significant others that altered sensorium is temporary and will improve with treatment. Use reality therapy: clocks, calendars, and familiar objects; keep them at the bedside within patient's visual field.
- Administer fluids and diuretics as prescribed. Evaluate response to therapy. Monitor serum calcium levels and albumin levels. Observe for signs of fluid volume excess with treatment.
- Hypercalcemia causes neuromuscular depression with poor coordination, weakness, and altered gait. Provide a safe environment. Keep side rails up and bed in lowest position with wheels locked. Assist patient with ambulation if it is allowed.
- Because hypercalcemia potentiates the effects of digitalis, monitor patient taking digitalis for signs and symptoms of digitalis toxicity: multifocal or bigeminal PVCs, paroxysmal atrial tachycardia with varying AV block, and other heart blocks.
- Monitor serum electrolyte values for changes in serum calcium as a result of therapy (normal range is 8.5-10.5 mg/dl), potassium (normal range is 3.5-5 mEq/L), and phosphorus (normal range is 2.5-4.5 mg/dl). Consult physician for abnormal values.
- Encourage increased mobility to reduce bone resorption. Ideally patient should be out of bed and up in a chair at least 6 h/day.

Altered urinary elimination related to dysuria, urgency, frequency, and polyuria secondary to administration of diuretics, calcium stone formation, or changes in renal function occurring with hypercalcemia

Desired outcome: Within 24 h of initiation of treatment, patient exhibits voiding pattern and urine characteristics that are normal for patient.

- Monitor I&O hourly. Consult physician for unusual changes in urine volume (e.g., oliguria alternating with polyuria, which may signal urinary tract obstruction, or continuous polyuria). Increased urinary calcium concentrations decrease the kidneys' ability to concentrate the urine, leading to polyuria and potentially to fluid volume deficit. This is a type of nephrogenic diabetes insipidus (see p. 504).

- Because hypercalcemia can impair renal function, monitor patient's renal function carefully: urine output, BUN, creatinine values (see "Acute Renal Failure," p. 385).
- Provide patient with a low-calcium diet, and avoid use of calcium-containing medications (e.g., antacids such as Tums). Encourage intake of fruits (e.g., cranberries, prunes, or plums) that leave an acid ash in the urine. An acidic urine reduces the risk of calcium stone formation. Also increase fluid intake (at least 3 L in nonrestricted patients) to reduce the risk of renal stone formation.
- Assess patient for indicators of kidney stone formation: intermittent pain, nausea, vomiting, hematuria.
- Hypercalcemia leads to an increase in calcium in the urine, which inhibits the kidneys' ability to concentrate urine. This leads to polyuria and potential volume depletion. Be alert to polyuria. Also monitor for signs of volume depletion when giving diuretics: decreased BP, CVP, PAP; increased HR.

PHOSPHORUS IMBALANCE

Phosphorus, the primary anion of the ICF, has a wide variety of vital functions, including formation of energy storing substances (e.g., adenosine triphosphate); formation of red blood cell 2,3-DPG, which facilitates oxygen delivery to the tissues; metabolism of carbohydrates, protein, and fat; and maintenance of acid-base balance. In addition, phosphorus is critical to normal nerve and muscle function and provides structural support to bones and teeth.

Plasma phosphorus levels vary with diet and acid-base balance. Glucose, insulin, or sugar-containing foods cause a temporary drop in phosphorus due to a shift of serum phosphorus into the cells. Alkalosis, particularly respiratory alkalosis, may cause hypophosphatemia as a result of an intracellular shift of phosphorus. Although the exact mechanism for this shift is not fully understood, it may be related to an alkalosis-induced cellular glycolysis, with increased formation of phosphorus-containing metabolic intermediates. Respiratory acidosis may cause a shift of phosphorus out of the cells and contribute to hyperphosphatemia.

The level of ECF phosphate is regulated by a combination of factors, including dietary intake, intestinal absorption, renal excretion, and hormonally regulated bone resorption and deposition. Normal range for serum phosphorus is 2.5-4.5 mg/dl (1.7-2.6 mEq/L).

HYPOPHOSPHATEMIA

Pathophysiology

Hypophosphatemia (serum phosphorus <2.5 mg/dl) may occur due to transient intracellular shifts, increased urinary losses, decreased intestinal absorption, or increased utilization (see "Assessment" in the next section for history and risk factors). Severe phosphorus deficiency also may develop due to a combination of factors in conditions such as chronic alcohol abuse and diabetic ketoacidosis (DKA).

Assessment

HISTORY AND RISK FACTORS

Intracellular shifts: Carbohydrate load, respiratory alkalosis, treatment of DKA.

Increased utilization due to increased tissue repair: TPN with inadequate phosphorus content; recovery from protein-calorie malnutrition.

Increased urinary losses: Hypomagnesemia, ECF volume expansion, hyperparathyroidism, use of thiazide diuretics, diuretic phase of ATN, glucosuria.

Reduced intestinal absorption or increased intestinal loss: Use of phosphorus-binding medications (e.g., aluminum hydroxide antacids such as Amphojel or Alternagel, sucralfate); vomiting and diarrhea; malabsorption disorders such as vitamin D deficiency; prolonged gastric suction.

Dialysis.

Mixed causes: Chronic alcohol abuse, DKA, severe burns, artificially ventilated patients, postsurgery, sepsis.

CLINICAL PRESENTATION Patients may have acute symptoms due to sudden decreases in serum phosphorus, or symptoms may develop gradually owing to chronic PO_4 deficiency. The majority of symptoms are secondary to decreases in ATP and 2,3-DPG.

Acute: Confusion, seizures, coma, chest pain due to poor oxygenation of the myocardium, muscle pain and weakness, increased susceptibility to infection, numbness and tingling of the fingers and circumoral region, incoordination, and respiratory failure.

Chronic: Memory loss, lethargy, weakness, bone pain.

PHYSICAL ASSESSMENT

Acute: Decreased strength as evidenced by difficulty with speaking, weakness of respiratory muscles, and weakening hand grasp. Bruising and bleeding may occur due to platelet dysfunction. Rhabdomyolysis, hemolysis, and myocardial depression may occur in severe hypophosphatemia. Hypoxia may cause an increased RR and metabolic alkalosis because of hyperventilation.

Note: Metabolic alkalosis causes phosphorus to move intracellularly, aggravating the existing hypophosphatemia.

Chronic: Joint stiffness, arthralgia, osteomalacia, cyanosis, and pseudofractures may occur.

HEMODYNAMIC MEASUREMENTS Severely depleted patients may show signs of decreased myocardial function, including increased PAWP, decreased CO, and decreased BP with decreased response to pressor agents.

Diagnostic tests

Serum phosphorus level: Will be <2.5 mg/dl (1.7 mEq/L).
Mild hypophosphatemia: 1-2.5 mg/dl.

Severe hypophosphatemia: <1 mg/dl.
Parathyroid hormone level: Will be elevated in hyperparathyroidism.
Serum magnesium level: May be decreased because of increased urinary excretion of magnesium in hypophosphatemia.
X-ray findings: May reveal skeletal changes of osteomalacia.

Collaborative management

Identification and elimination of the cause: For example, avoiding use of phosphorus-binding antacids (aluminum, magnesium, or calcium gels or antacids); correction of respiratory alkalosis.
Phosphorus supplementation: Mild hypophosphatemia may be treated by increasing intake of foods high in phosphorus (Table 10-13). Mild to moderate hypophosphatemia usually can be treated with oral phosphate supplements such as Neutra-Phos (sodium and potassium phosphate) or Phospho-Soda (sodium phosphate). Administration of IV sodium phosphate or potassium phosphate is necessary in cases of severe hypophosphatemia or when the GI tract is nonfunctional.

Nursing diagnoses and interventions

Altered protection related to neurosensory alterations secondary to hypophosphatemia
Desired outcomes: Within 24 h of initiation of treatment, patient verbalizes orientation to time, place, and person. Patient does not exhibit evidence of injury due to neurosensory changes.
- Monitor serum phosphorus levels in patients at increased risk. Consult physician for decreased levels. Monitor for associated electrolyte and acid-base imbalances: hypokalemia, hypomagnesemia, respiratory alkalosis, and metabolic acidosis.
- Apprehension, confusion, and paresthesias are signals of developing hypophosphatemia. Assess and document LOC, orientation, and neurologic status with each VS check. Reorient patient as necessary. Alert physician to significant changes.
- Inform patient and significant others that altered sensorium is temporary and will improve with treatment.
- Do not administer IV phosphate at a rate greater than that recommended by the manufacturer. Potential complications of IV phos-

---

T A B L E   1 0 - 1 3   Foods high in phosphorus

Dried beans and peas
Eggs and egg products (e.g., eggnog, soufflés)
Fish
Meats, especially organ meats (e.g., brain, liver, kidney)
Milk and milk products (e.g., cheese, ice cream, cottage cheese)
Nuts (e.g., Brazil, peanuts)
Poultry
Seeds (e.g., pumpkin, sesame, sunflower)
Whole grains (e.g., oatmeal, bran, barley)

---

phorus administration include *tetany* as a result of hypocalcemia (serum calcium levels may drop suddenly if serum phosphorus levels increase suddenly; see "Calcium Imbalance," p. 687, for additional information); *soft tissue calcification* (if hyperphosphatemia develops, the calcium and phosphorus in the ECF may combine and form deposits in tissue); and *hypotension,* caused by a too-rapid delivery. When IV phosphorus is administered as potassium phosphate, the infusion rate should not exceed 10 mEq/h. Monitor IV site for signs of infiltration, because potassium phosphate can cause necrosis and sloughing of tissue.
- Keep the side rails up and the bed in its lowest position with wheels locked.
- Use reality therapy, such as clocks, calendars, and familiar objects. Keep these articles at the bedside, within patient's visual field.
- If patient is at risk for seizures, pad the side rails and keep an appropriate-size airway at the bedside.

Impaired gas exchange related to altered oxygen-carrying capacity of the blood secondary to decreased 2,3-DPG

Note: With decreased 2,3-DPG levels, the oxyhemoglobin dissociation curve will shift to the left (i.e., at a given Pao_2 level, more oxygen will be bound to Hgb and less will be available to the tissues).

Desired outcome: Within 12 h of initiation of treatment, patient has adequate gas exchange as evidenced by RR 12-20 breaths/min with normal depth and pattern (eupnea); orientation to time, place, and person; Spo_2 ≥92%; and absence of the indicators of hypoxia (e.g., restlessness, somnolence).
- Assess patient for signs of hypoxia: restlessness, confusion, increased RR, complaints of chest pain, and cyanosis (a late sign).
- Monitor Spo_2 as available. Administer oxygen as prescribed to maintain Spo_2 at ≥92%.

Ineffective breathing pattern related to decreased strength of respiratory muscles secondary to hypophosphatemia
Desired outcome: Within 8 h of initiation of treatment, the nonventilated patient becomes eupneic. Optimally, for the ventilated patient, improved weaning is noted within 24 h of initiation of treatment.
- Monitor rate and depth of respirations in patients with severe hypophosphatemia. Assess for decreased tidal volume or decreased minute ventilation. Consult physician for changes.
- Monitor ABG values for evidence of hypoxemia or hypercapnia. Consult physician for significant changes.
- There is an increased incidence of hypophosphatemia in artificially ventilated patients. Monitor serum phosphate levels in these patients. Hypophosphatemia may contribute to difficulty in weaning patients from ventilators.
- Administer IV phosphorus as prescribed.

Impaired physical mobility related to musculoskeletal impairment (osteomalacia with bone pain and fractures) associated with movement of phosphorus out of the bone secondary to chronic hypophosphatemia; or muscle weakness and acute rhabdomyolysis (breakdown of striated muscle) secondary to severe hypophosphatemia

Desired outcome: Within 24 h of initiation of therapy, patient exhibits ability to move purposefully and has full or baseline ROM and muscle strength.

- Monitor all patients with suspected hypophosphatemia for evidence of decreasing muscle strength. Perform serial assessments of hand grasp strength and clarity of speech. Consult physician for changes.
- Monitor serum phosphorus levels for evidence of worsening hypophosphatemia. Consult physician for changes.
- Assist the patient with ambulation and ADL. Keep personal items within easy reach.
- Encourage intake of foods high in phosphorus (see Table 10-13). Teach patient and significant others the importance of using phosphorus-binding antacids only as prescribed.
- Medicate for pain as prescribed.

Decreased cardiac output related to negative inotropic changes associated with reduced myocardial functioning secondary to severe phosphorus depletion

Desired outcome: Within 12 h of initiation of treatment, patient's cardiac output is adequate as evidenced by CO $\geq$4 L/min, CI $\geq$2.5 L/min/m^2, CVP <6 mm Hg, PAP 20-30/8-15 mm Hg, HR $\leq$100 bpm, BP within patient's normal range, and absence of the clinical signs of heart failure or pulmonary edema.

- Monitor patient for signs of heart failure or pulmonary edema: crackles, rhonchi, SOB, decreased BP, increased HR, increased PAP, or increased CVP.
- Prevent patient from hyperventilating, if possible, inasmuch as metabolic alkalosis will cause an increased movement of phosphorus into the cells, which will negatively affect cardiac output.
- For additional interventions if decreased cardiac output develops, see "Cardiomyopathy," p. 295.

Risk for infection related to inadequate secondary defenses (impaired WBC functioning) secondary to reduced ATP

Desired outcome: Patient is free of infection as evidenced by normothermia and absence of erythema, swelling, warmth, and purulent drainage at invasive sites.

- Monitor temperature q4h for evidence of infection. Obtain cultures of wounds and drainage as prescribed if infection is suspected.
- Use meticulous, aseptic technique when changing dressings or manipulating indwelling lines (e.g., TPN catheters, IV needles).
- Provide oral hygiene and skin care at regular intervals. Intact skin and membranes are the body's first line of defense against infection.

HYPERPHOSPHATEMIA

Pathophysiology

Hyperphosphatemia occurs most often in the presence of renal insufficiency due to the kidneys' decreased ability to excrete excess phosphorus. In addition to renal failure, other causes of hyperphosphatemia include increased intake of phosphates, extracellular shifts (i.e., movement of phosphorus out of the cell and into the ECF), cellular destruction with concomitant release of intracellular phosphorus, and decreased urinary losses that are unrelated to decreased renal function.

As serum phosphorus levels increase, serum calcium levels often drop, which may cause hypocalcemia to develop. Hypocalcemia is most likely to occur in sudden, severe hyperphosphatemia (e.g., after IV administration of phosphates) or when the patient already is prone to hypocalcemia (e.g., with chronic renal failure).

The primary complication of hyperphosphatemia is metastatic calcification (i.e., the precipitation of calcium phosphate in the soft tissue, joints, and arteries). Precipitation of calcium phosphate occurs when the product (calcium times phosphorus) exceeds 70 mg/dl. Chronic hyperphosphatemia in the patient with chronic renal failure may contribute to the development of renal osteodystrophy.

Assessment

HISTORY AND RISK FACTORS
Renal failure: Acute and chronic.
Increased intake: Excessive administration of phosphorus supplements; vitamin D excess with increased GI absorption; excessive use of phosphorus-containing laxatives or enemas; massive transfusion.
Extracellular shift: Respiratory acidosis; diabetic ketoacidosis (before treatment).
Cellular destruction: Neoplastic disease (e.g., leukemia and lymphoma) treated with cytotoxic agents; increased tissue catabolism (breakdown); rhabdomyolysis (breakdown of striated muscle).
Decreased urinary losses: Hypoparathyroidism; volume depletion.
CLINICAL PRESENTATION Anorexia, nausea, vomiting, muscle weakness, hyperreflexia, tetany, tachycardia.

Note: Usually patients experience few symptoms with hyperphosphatemia. The majority of symptoms that do occur relate to the development of hypocalcemia or soft tissue (metastatic) calcifications. Indicators of metastatic calcification include oliguria, corneal haziness, conjunctivitis, irregular heart rate, and papular eruptions.

PHYSICAL ASSESSMENT See "Hypocalcemia," p. 688. In addition, see preceding "Clinical Presentation" for indicators of metastatic calcifications.
ECG CHANGES See "Hypocalcemia," p. 688. Deposition of calcium phosphate in the heart may lead to dysrhythmias and conduction disturbances.

Diagnostic tests

Serum phosphate level: Will be >4.5 mg/dl (2.6 mEq/L).
X-ray: May show skeletal changes of osteodystrophy.
Parathyroid hormone level: Will be decreased in hypoparathyroidism.

Collaborative management

Identification and elimination of the cause.
Use of aluminum, magnesium, or calcium gels or antacids: To bind phosphorus in the gut, thus increasing GI elimination of phosphorus.

Note: Magnesium antacids are avoided in renal failure due to the risk of hypermagnesemia. Serum phosphorus levels may be allowed to remain slightly elevated (4.5-6 mg/dl) in chronic renal failure to ensure adequate levels of 2,3-DPG. This helps to minimize the effects of chronic anemia on oxygen delivery to the tissues.

Dialytic therapy: May be necessary for acute, severe hyperphosphatemia accompanied by symptoms of hypocalcemia. See "Renal Replacement Therapies," p. 410.

Nursing diagnoses and interventions

Knowledge deficit: Purpose of phosphate binders and the importance of reducing GI absorption of phosphorus to control hyperphosphatemia and prevent long-term complications
Desired outcome: Within the 24-h period before discharge from ICU, patient describes the potential complications of uncontrolled hyperphosphatemia and the ways in which they can be prevented.

Note: Because symptoms of hyperphosphatemia may be minimal, prevention of long-term complications relies primarily on adequate patient education.

- Teach patients the purpose of phosphate binders. Stress the need to take binders as prescribed with or after meals to maximize effectiveness.
- Prepare patients for the possibility of constipation as a result of binder use. Encourage use of bulk-building supplements or stool softener if constipation occurs. Phosphate-containing laxatives and enemas must be avoided.
- Phosphate binders are available in liquid or capsule form. Confer with physician regarding an alternate form or brand for individuals who find binders unpalatable or difficult to take. Phosphate binders vary in their aluminum, magnesium, or calcium content, however, and one may not be exchanged for another without first ensuring that the patient is receiving the same amount of elemental aluminum, magnesium, or calcium.
- Encourage patient to avoid or limit foods high in phosphorus (see Table 10-13).
- Review the importance of avoiding phosphorus-containing OTC medications: certain laxatives, enemas, and mixed vitamin-mineral supplements. Instruct the patient and significant others to read the label for the words "phosphorus" and "phosphate."

Risk for injury related to internal factors associated with precipitation of calcium phosphate in the soft tissue (e.g., cornea, lungs, kidney, gastric mucosa, heart, blood vessels) and periarticular region of the large joints (e.g., hips, shoulders, and elbows) or development of hypocalcemic tetany
Desired outcome: Patient does not develop symptoms of physical injury caused by precipitation of calcium phosphate in the soft tissue or joints or hypocalcemic tetany.
- Monitor serum phosphorus and calcium levels. Calculate the calcium-phosphorus product (calcium times phosphorus). Values

≥70 mg/dl are associated with precipitation of calcium phosphate in the soft tissues. Consult physician for abnormal values. Remember that phosphorus values may be kept slightly higher (4-6 mg/dl) to ensure adequate levels of 2,3-DPG in patients with chronic renal failure, thereby minimizing effects of chronic anemia on oxygen delivery to the tissues.

- Avoid vitamin D products and calcium supplements until the serum phosphorus level approaches normal.
- Consult physician if patient develops indicators of metastatic calcification: oliguria, corneal haziness, conjunctivitis, irregular heart rate, and papular eruptions.
- Monitor patient for evidence of increasing hypocalcemia: numbness and tingling of the fingers and circumoral region, hyperactive reflexes, and muscle cramps. Consult physician promptly if these symptoms develop, because they occur before overt tetany. In addition, consult physician if patient shows positive Trousseau's or Chvostek's signs, inasmuch as they signal latent tetany (for a discussion of these signs and for additional information regarding treatment and prevention of hypocalcemia, see p. 688).
- Because hyperphosphatemia can impair renal function, monitor patient's renal function carefully: urine output, BUN, and creatinine values.

MAGNESIUM IMBALANCE

Of the body's magnesium, approximately 60% is located in bone and approximately 1% is located in the ECF. The remaining magnesium is contained within the cells, thereby constituting the second most abundant intracellular cation after potassium. Magnesium is regulated by a combination of factors, including vitamin D–regulated GI absorption and renal excretion.

Because magnesium is a major intracellular ion, it plays a vital role in normal cellular function. Specifically, it activates enzymes involved in the metabolism of carbohydrates and protein, and it triggers the sodium-potassium pump, thus affecting intracellular potassium levels. Magnesium also is important in the transmission of neuromuscular activity, neural transmission within the CNS, and myocardial functioning. Normal serum magnesium level is 1.5-2.5 mEq/L.

HYPOMAGNESEMIA

Pathophysiology

Hypomagnesemia (serum magnesium level <1.5 mEq/L) usually occurs because of decreased GI absorption or increased urinary loss. It also may occur with excessive GI loss (e.g., vomiting, diarrhea) or with prolonged administration of magnesium-free parenteral fluids. Chronic abusers of alcohol (see "History and Risk Factors" in the next section) and patients undergoing critical care are the two most common patient populations. In the critical care setting, hypomagnesemia is associated with increased mortality rates. Dysrhythmias and sudden death increase when decreased magnesium levels occur in combination with myocardial infarction, congestive heart failure, or digitalis toxicity. Hypomagnesemia usually is associated with hypocalcemia and hypokalemia (see "Diagnostic Tests," below, for additional information). Symptoms of hypomagnesemia tend to develop once the serum magnesium level drops below 1 mEq/L. Decreased magnesium intake has been identified as a risk factor for hypertension, cardiac dysrhythmias, ischemic heart disease, and sudden cardiac death.

Assessment

HISTORY AND RISK FACTORS

Chronic alcoholism: The most common cause of hypomagnesemia due to a combination of poor dietary intake, decreased GI absorption, and increased urinary excretion secondary to ethanol effect.

Decreased GI absorption: For example, due to cancer, colitis, pancreatic insufficiency, surgical resection of the GI tract, use of laxatives, diarrhea.

Increased GI loss: Prolonged vomiting or gastric suction.

Administration of low-magnesium or magnesium-free parenteral solutions: Especially with refeeding after starvation.

Hyperaldosteronism: Due to volume expansion.

Diabetic ketoacidosis: A result of movement of magnesium out of the cell and loss in the urine because of osmotic diuresis.

Increased urinary excretion: Resulting from medications such as diuretics, amphotericin, tobramycin, gentamicin, cisplatin, or digoxin or from diuretic phase of ATN.

Protein-calorie malnutrition.

Cardiopulmonary bypass.

CLINICAL PRESENTATION Lethargy, weakness, fatigue, mood changes, hallucinations, confusion, anorexia, nausea, vomiting, paresthesias.

PHYSICAL ASSESSMENT Increased reflexes, tremors, convulsions, tetany, and positive Chvostek's and Trousseau's signs (see p. 688) in part because of accompanying hypocalcemia. Skeletal and respiratory muscle weakness may be present. The patient also may have tachycardia, hypertension, and coronary spasm.

ECG FINDINGS See "Hypokalemia," p. 682; and "Hypocalcemia," p. 688.

Diagnostic tests

Serum magnesium level: <1.5 mEq/L. Hypomagnesemia is the most frequently undiagnosed electrolyte imbalance in hospitalized patients.

Serum albumin level: A decreased albumin level may cause a decreased magnesium level due to a reduction in protein-bound magnesium. The amount of free ionized magnesium may be unchanged. It is the free ionized magnesium that is physiologically important.

Serum potassium level: May be decreased because of failure of the cellular sodium-potassium pump to move potassium into the cell and the accompanying loss of potassium in the urine. This hypokalemia may be resistant to potassium replacement until the magnesium deficit has been corrected.

Serum calcium level: Hypomagnesemia may lead to hypocalcemia due to a reduction in the release and action of parathyroid hormone. Parathyroid hormone is the primary regulator of serum calcium levels.

ECG evaluations: May reflect magnesium, as well as calcium and potassium, deficiencies: tachydysrhythmias, prolonged PR and QT intervals, widening of the QRS complex, ST-segment depression, and flattened T waves. Increased digitalis effect, as evidenced by multifocal or bigeminal PVCs, paroxysmal atrial tachycardia with varying AV block and other heart blocks, also may occur. Dysrhythmias associated with hypomagnesemia include ventricular ectopy, torsade de pointes, and atrial fibrillation.

Collaborative management

Identification and elimination of the cause: For example, ensuring adequate replacement of magnesium in TPN solutions.
IV or IM magnesium sulfate (MgSO₄):   For severe hypomagnesemia or its symptoms.
Oral magnesium: Magnesium-containing antacids (e.g., Mylanta, Maalox, Gelusil, milk of magnesia) may be used. Some foods high in magnesium are listed in Table 10-14.

Nursing diagnoses and interventions

Altered protection related to neurosensory alterations secondary to hypomagnesemia
Desired outcomes: Within 8 h of initiation of treatment, patient verbalizes orientation to time, place, and person. Patient does not exhibit evidence of injury caused by complications of severe hypomagnesemia.
• Monitor serum magnesium levels in patient at risk for hypomagnesemia and its deleterious effects (e.g., those who are alcohol abusers or experiencing congestive heart failure, recent myocardial infarction, or digitalis toxicity). Normal range for serum magnesium is 1.5-2.5 mEq/L. Consult physician for abnormal values.

Note: Symptoms of hypomagnesemia may be mistakenly attributed to delirium tremens of chronic alcoholism. Be especially alert to indicators of magnesium deficit in these patients.

• Administer IV MgSO₄ with caution. Refer to manufacturer's guidelines. Too rapid an administration may lead to dangerous hypermagnesemia, with cardiac or respiratory arrest. Patients receiving IV magnesium should be monitored for decreasing BP, labored respirations, and diminished patellar reflex (knee jerk). An absent patellar

---

T A B L E   1 0 - 1 4   **Foods high in magnesium**

Bananas	Molasses
Chocolate	Nuts and seeds
Coconuts	Oranges
Green, leafy vegetables (e.g., beet greens, collard greens)	Refined sugar
Grapefruits	Seafood
Kelp	Soy flour
Legumes	Wheat bran

reflex is a signal of hyporeflexia due to dangerous hypermagnesemia. Should any of these changes occur, stop the infusion and consult physician *stat* (see "Hypermagnesemia," p. 704). Keep calcium gluconate at the bedside in the event of hypocalcemic tetany or sudden hypermagnesemia.

- For patients with chronic hypomagnesemia, administer oral magnesium supplements as prescribed. All magnesium supplements should be given with caution in patients with reduced renal function because of an increased risk of the development of hypermagnesemia. Caution patient that oral magnesium supplements may cause diarrhea. Administer antidiarrheal medications as needed.
- When it is appropriate, encourage intake of foods high in magnesium (see Table 10-14). For most patients, a normal diet is usually adequate.
- Maintain seizure precautions for patients with symptoms (i.e., those who have hyperreflexia). Decrease environmental stimuli (e.g., keep the room quiet, use subdued lighting).
- For patients in whom hypocalcemia is suspected, caution against hyperventilation. Metabolic alkalosis may precipitate tetany as a result of increased calcium binding.
- Dysphagia may occur in hypomagnesemia. Test the patient's ability to swallow water before giving food or medications.
- Assess and document LOC, orientation, and neurologic status with each VS check. Reorient patient as necessary. Notify physician for significant changes. Inform patient and significant others that altered mood and sensorium are temporary and will improve with treatment.
- See "Hypokalemia," p. 681; "Hypocalcemia," p. 688; and "Hypophosphatemia," p. 693, for nursing care of these disorders.

Note: Because magnesium is necessary for the movement of potassium into the cell, intracellular potassium deficits cannot be corrected until hypomagnesemia has been treated.

Decreased cardiac output related to electrical alterations associated with tachydysrhythmias or digitalis toxicity secondary to hypomagnesemia

Desired outcomes: Within 24 h of initiating treatment, patient's cardiac output is adequate as evidenced by CO ≥4 L/min, CI ≥2.5 L/min/m², normal configurations on ECG, and HR within patient's normal range. Patient exhibits brisk capillary refill (<2 sec) and urinary output ≥0.5 ml/kg/h.

- Monitor heart rate and regularity with each VS check. Consult physician for changes. Be alert to decreased CO and CI.
- Assess ECG for evidence of hypomagnesemia. Consider hypomagnesemia as a cause in patients who develop sudden ventricular dysrhythmias.
- Because hypomagnesemia (and hypokalemia) potentiates the cardiac effects of digitalis, monitor patients taking digitalis for digitalis-induced dysrhythmias. ECG changes may include multifocal or bigeminal PVCs, paroxysmal atrial tachycardia with varying AV block, and other heart blocks.

- Monitor for and report decreased urinary output and delayed capillary refill.

Altered nutrition: Less than body requirements of magnesium related to history of poor intake or anorexia, nausea, and vomiting secondary to hypomagnesemia or starvation

Desired outcome: Within 24 h of resumption of oral feedings, patient receives diet adequate in magnesium.

- Encourage intake of small, frequent meals.
- Teach patient about foods high in magnesium content (see Table 10-14), and encourage intake of these foods during meals.
- Administer antiemetics as prescribed.
- Include patient, significant others, and dietitian in meal planning as appropriate.
- Provide oral hygiene before meals to enhance appetite.
- As with the other major intracellular electrolyte levels, magnesium depletion may develop with refeeding after starvation. Anticipate hypomagnesemia with refeeding, and ensure increased dietary intake or supplementation.
- Consult physician for patients receiving magnesium-free solutions (e.g., TPN) for prolonged periods of time.

HYPERMAGNESEMIA

Pathophysiology

Hypermagnesemia (serum magnesium levels >2.5 mEq/L) occurs almost exclusively in individuals with renal failure who have an increased intake of magnesium (e.g., use of magnesium-containing medications). It also may occur in acute adrenocortical insufficiency (Addison's disease) or in obstetric patients treated with parenteral magnesium for preeclampsia. In rare cases hypermagnesemia occurs because of excessive use of magnesium-containing medications (e.g., antacids, laxatives, enemas). The primary symptoms of hypermagnesemia are the result of depressed peripheral and central neuromuscular transmission. Symptoms usually do not occur until the magnesium level exceeds 4 mEq/L.

Assessment

HISTORY AND RISK FACTORS

Decreased excretion of magnesium: As with renal failure or adrenocortical insufficiency.

Increased intake of magnesium: For example, excessive use of magnesium-containing antacids, enemas, and laxatives or excessive administration of magnesium sulfate (such as in the treatment of hypomagnesemia or preeclampsia).

CLINICAL PRESENTATION Nausea, vomiting, flushing, diaphoresis, sensation of heat, altered mental functioning, drowsiness, coma, and muscular weakness or paralysis. Paralysis of the respiratory muscles may occur when the magnesium level exceeds 10 mEq/L.

PHYSICAL ASSESSMENT Hypotension, soft tissue (metastatic) calcification (see description, p. 698), bradycardia, and decreased deep tendon reflexes. The patellar (knee jerk) reflex is lost once the magnesium level exceeds 8 mEq/L.

HEMODYNAMIC MEASUREMENTS Decreased arterial pressure due to peripheral vasodilatation.

Diagnostic tests

Serum magnesium level: Will be >2.5 mEq/L.

ECG findings: Prolonged QT interval and atrioventricular block may occur in severe hypermagnesemia (levels >12 mEq/L).

Collaborative management

Removal of cause: For example, discontinuing or avoiding use of magnesium-containing medications (Table 10-15) or supplements, especially in patients with decreased renal function.

Diuretics and 0.45% sodium chloride solution: To promote magnesium excretion in patients with adequate renal function.

IV calcium gluconate, 10 ml of a 10% solution: To antagonize the neuromuscular effects of magnesium for patients with potentially lethal hypermagnesemia.

Dialysis with magnesium-free dialysate: For patients with severely decreased renal function.

Nursing diagnoses and interventions

Altered protection related to neurosensory alterations secondary to hypermagnesemia

Desired outcomes: Within 12 h of initiation of treatment, patient verbalizes orientation to time, place, and person. Patient does not exhibit evidence of injury as a result of complications of hypermagnesemia. Patient has no symptoms of soft tissue (metastatic) calcifications: oliguria, corneal haziness, conjunctivitis, irregular heart rate, and papular eruptions.

- Monitor serum magnesium levels in the patient at risk for hypermagnesemia (e.g., those with chronic renal failure). Normal range for serum magnesium levels is 1.5-2.5 mEq/L. Obtain specimens for laboratory analysis as needed.
- Assess and document LOC, orientation, and neurologic status (e.g., hand grasp) with each VS check. Assess patellar (knee jerk) reflex in patients with a moderately elevated magnesium level (>5 mEq/

T A B L E   1 0 - 1 5   Magnesium-containing medications

Antacids

Aludrox	Maalox and Maalox Plus
Camalox	Mylanta and Mylanta-II
Di-Gel	Riopan
Gaviscon	Simeco
Gelusil and Gelusil II	Tempo

Laxatives

Magnesium citrate
Magnesium hydroxide (milk of magnesia, Haley's M-O)
Magnesium sulfate (Epsom salts)
Magnesium-containing mineral supplements

L). With patient lying flat, support the knee in a moderately fixed position and tap the patellar tendon firmly just below the patella. Normally the knee will extend. An absent reflex suggests a magnesium level of ≥ 7 mEq/L. Consult physician for significant changes.

- Reassure patient and significant others that altered mental functioning and muscle strength will improve with treatment.
- Keep side rails up and the bed in its lowest position with the wheels locked.
- Assess patient for the development of soft tissue calcification. Consult physician for significant findings.
- Monitor for cardiopulmonary effects of hypermagnesemia: hypotension, flushing, bradycardia, respiratory depression.

Knowledge deficit: Importance of avoiding excessive or inappropriate use of magnesium-containing medications, especially for patients with chronic renal failure

Desired outcome: Within the 24-h period before discharge from ICU, patient verbalizes the importance of avoiding unusual magnesium intake and identifies potential sources of unwanted magnesium.

- Caution patients with chronic renal failure to review all OTC medications with physician before use.
- Provide a list of common magnesium-containing medications (see Table 10-15).
- Patients with renal failure usually are taking vitamin supplements. Caution these patients to avoid combination vitamin-mineral supplements because they usually contain magnesium.

Acid-base imbalances

For optimal functioning of the cells, metabolic processes maintain a steady balance between acids and bases. Arterial pH is an indirect measurement of hydrogen ion (H^+) concentration and is a reflection of the balance between carbon dioxide (CO_2), an acid regulated by the lungs, and bicarbonate (HCO_3^-), a base regulated by the kidneys. Carbon dioxide, when dissolved in water, becomes carbonic acid (H_2CO_3). Because H_2CO_3 cannot be measured directly, the amount of H_2CO_3 in the blood is reflected by the Pa_{CO_2} (see p. 708). The normal acid-base ratio is $1:20$, representing one part acid (CO_2 [potential H_2CO_3]) to 20 parts base (HCO_3^-). If this balance is altered, derangements in pH occur. If extra acids are present or base is lost and the pH is <7.4, acidosis exists. If extra base is present or there is loss of acid and the pH is >7.4, alkalosis is present.

Section one: Evaluating acid-base balance

Several mechanisms regulate acid-base balance. These mechanisms are exceptionally sensitive to minute changes in pH. Usually the body is able to maintain pH levels without outside intervention, if not at a normal level, at least in a life-sustaining range.

ACID-BASE REGULATION

Buffers

Buffers are present in all body fluids and act immediately (within 1 sec) after an abnormal pH level occurs. They combine with excess acid or base to form substances that do not greatly affect pH. Their effect, however, is limited.

Bicarbonate: The most important buffer of acid, it is present in the largest quantity in body fluids. Its reabsorption, excretion, and generation are regulated by the kidneys.

Phosphate: Aids in the excretion of H^- in the renal tubules.

Ammonium: The kidneys produce an acidic urine by adding H^+ to ammonia (NH_3) to form ammonium (NH_4^+).

Protein: Present in cells, blood, and plasma. Hemoglobin is the most important protein buffer.

Respiratory system

Hydrogen ions (H^+) exert direct action on the respiratory center in the brain as H^+ is released from the chemical reaction of CO_2 (which readily crosses the blood-brain barrier) and H_2O. Acidemia increases alveolar ventilation to 4-5 times the normal level, whereas alkalemia decreases alveolar ventilation to 50%-75% of the normal level. The response occurs quickly—within 1-2 min, during which time the lungs eliminate or retain carbon dioxide in direct relation to arterial pH. Although the respiratory system cannot correct imbalances completely, it is 50%-75% effective.

Renal system

This system regulates acid-base balance by increasing or decreasing bicarbonate (HCO_3^-) concentration in body fluids. This is accomplished through a series of complex reactions that involve H^+ secretion, sodium ion (Na^+) reabsorption, HCO_3^- conservation, and ammonia synthesis for excretion of H^+ in the urine. H^+ secretion is regulated by the amount of carbon dioxide in extracellular fluid: the greater the concentration of carbon dioxide, the greater the amount of H^+ secretion, resulting in an acidic urine. When H^+ is secreted, HCO_3^- is generated by the kidneys, helping to maintain the 1:20 balance of acids and bases. When extracellular fluid is alkalotic, the kidneys conserve H^+ and eliminate HCO_3^-, resulting in alkalotic urine. Although the kidneys' response to an abnormal pH level is slow—several hours to days—they are able to facilitate a near normal pH level because of their ability to excrete large quantities of excess HCO_3^- and H^+ from the body.

Blood gas values

Blood gas analysis usually is based on arterial sampling. Venous values are given as a reference.

Arterial values	**Venous values**
pH: 7.35-7.45	pH: 7.32-7.38
$Paco_2$: 35-45 mm Hg	Pco_2: 42-50 mm Hg
Pao_2: 80-95 mm Hg	Po_2: 40 mm Hg
Saturation: 95%-99%	Saturation: 75%

Continued.

Arterial values—cont'd	Venous values—cont'd
Base excess: $+$ or -1	—
*Serum HCO_3^-: 22-26 mEq/L	Serum HCO_3^-: 23-27 mEq/L

*Although serum bicarbonate is a buffer, it usually is reported as "CO_2 content" or "total CO_2" and not as serum bicarbonate. The serum HCO_3^- concentration usually is obtained separately from ABG analysis and is critical in the determination of acid-base status, although this value may be calculated from $Paco_2$ and pH results *via* the ABG analysis. HCO_3^- values should be obtained with the initial assessment and daily thereafter as indicated.

Arterial blood gas analysis

pH: Measures H^+ concentration and reflects acid-base status of the blood. Values indicate whether arterial pH is normal (7.4), acidic (<7.4), or alkalotic (>7.4). Because of buffers and other compensatory mechanisms, a near-normal pH level does not exclude the possibility of an acid-base disturbance.

$Paco_2$:   Partial pressure of carbon dioxide in the arteries. It is the respiratory component of acid-base regulation and is adjusted by changes in the rate and depth of pulmonary ventilation. Hypercapnia ($Paco_2$ >45 mm Hg) signals alveolar hypoventilation and respiratory acidosis. Alveolar hyperventilation results in hypocapnia ($Paco_2$ <35 mm Hg) and respiratory alkalosis. Respiratory compensation occurs rapidly in metabolic acid-base disturbances. If any abnormality in $Paco_2$ exists, it is important to analyze pH and HCO_3^- parameters to determine if the alteration in $Paco_2$ is the result of a primary respiratory disturbance or a compensatory response to a metabolic acid-base abnormality.

Pao_2:   Partial pressure of oxygen in the arteries. It has no primary role in acid-base regulation if it is within normal limits. The presence of hypoxemia (Pao_2 <80 mm Hg) can lead to anaerobic metabolism, resulting in lactic acid production and metabolic acidosis. There is a normal decline in Pao_2 in the older adult.

Saturation (Sao_2):   Measures the degree to which hemoglobin is saturated by oxygen. It can be affected by changes in temperature, pH, and $Paco_2$. When the Pao_2 falls to <60 mm Hg, there is a large drop in saturation. *Pulse oximetry* (Spo_2) can be used to monitor arterial oxygen saturation and thus determine oxygenation status. This noninvasive monitoring technique frequently is used in critical care areas, operating rooms, and emergency departments. Spo_2 should be correlated with Sao_2 *via* arterial blood gases with the initiation of oximetry. Mixed venous blood gases are drawn intermittently or measured continuously from the distal tip of the pulmonary artery catheter. A blood sample taken from this site ensures complete mixing of blood returned from all parts of the body. Changes in mixed venous oxygen saturation (Svo_2) provide an early indication of perfusion failure or increased tissue demands for oxygen.

Base excess or deficit: Indicates, in general terms, the amount of blood buffer (hemoglobin and plasma bicarbonate) present. Abnormally high values reflect alkalosis; low values reflect acidosis.

Serum bicarbonate: Serum HCO_3^- is the major renal component of acid-base regulation. It is excreted or generated by the kidneys to maintain a normal acid-base environment. Decreased HCO_3^- levels (<22 mEq/L) are indicative of metabolic acidosis (seen infrequently as a compensatory mechanism for respiratory alkalosis); elevated HCO_3^- levels (>26 mEq/L) reflect metabolic alkalosis, occurring either as a primary metabolic disorder or as a compensatory alteration in response to respiratory acidosis.

Step-by-step guide to ABG analysis

A systemic step-by-step analysis is critical to the accurate interpretation of ABG values (Tables 10-16, 10-17, 10-18, and 10-19).

Step 1: Determine if pH is normal. If abnormal, identify whether it is on the acidotic (<7.35) or alkalotic (>7.45) side of normal.

Step 2: Check $Paco_2$ and HCO_3^- to determine which value corresponds to the pH value. For example, if the pH is acidotic, which value most closely reflects acidosis? This determines whether the primary problem is respiratory (involving $Paco_2$) or metabolic (involving HCO_3^-) in nature.

Step 3: If both $Paco_2$ and HCO_3^- are abnormal, the value that deviates the most from normal suggests the primary disturbance responsible for the altered pH. A mixed metabolic-respiratory disturbance or compensatory elements may be present.

Step 4: Check Pao_2 and oxygen saturation to determine whether they are decreased, normal, or increased. Decreased Pao_2 and O_2 saturation can lead to lactic acidosis and may signal the need for increased concentrations of oxygen. Conversely, high Pao_2 may be indicative of the need to decrease delivered concentrations of oxygen.

Arteriovenous oxygen content difference: $C(a-v)o_2$

The difference between the arterial oxygen content and the venous oxygen content reflects the tissue extraction of oxygen. This difference increases when ventricular performance is impaired. Simultaneous analysis of arterial and pulmonary artery blood sampling provides an accurate and reliable index of ventricular function.

T A B L E   1 0 - 1 6   ABG examples of acid-base disorders

	Acidosis			Alkalosis		
	$Paco_2$	pH	HCO_3^-	$Paco_2$	pH	HCO_3^-
Simple						
Respiratory	50	7.15	25	25	7.6	24
Metabolic	38	7.2	15	44	7.54	36
Compensated						
Respiratory	66	7.37	34	25	7.54	21
Metabolic	23	7.28	9	50	7.42	31
Mixed disorder	50	7.2	20	40	7.56	38

TABLE 10-17 Quick assessment guidelines for acid-base imbalances

Acid-base imbalance	pH	Paco$_2$	HCO$_3^-$	Clinical signs and symptoms	Common causes
Acute respiratory acidosis	↓	↑	No change	Tachycardia, tachypnea, diaphoresis, headache, restlessness leading to lethargy and coma, cyanosis, dysrhythmias, hypotension	Acute respiratory failure, cardiopulmonary disease, drug overdose, chest wall trauma, asphyxiation, CNS trauma/lesions, impaired muscles of respiration
Chronic respiratory acidosis (compensated)	↓	↑	↑	No specific symptoms if renal compensation has occurred. Dyspnea and tachypnea with dull headache and weakness when increase in CO$_2$ retention exceeds compensatory ability. Also asterixis, agitation, insomnia, lethargy, and confusion may lead to somnolence and coma	COPD (chronic emphysema, bronchitis, cystic fibrosis); superimposed acute infection of COPD; restrictive lung disease (obesity, such as pickwickian syndrome); neuromuscular abnormalities (amyotrophic lateral sclerosis); and depression of the respiratory center (brain tumor)
Acute respiratory alkalosis	↑	↓	No change (a decrease will occur if condition has been present for hours, providing that renal function is adequate)	Lightheadedness, anxiety, paresthesias (especially of fingers), circumoral numbness	Hyperventilation, salicylate poisoning, hypoxia (e.g., with pneumonia, pulmonary edema, pulmonary thromboembolism), gram-negative sepsis, CNS lesion, decreased lung compliance, inappropriate mechanical ventilation
Chronic respiratory alkalosis	↑	↓	↓	Usually no symptoms but may have increased respiratory rate and depth	Hepatic failure; CNS lesion

Condition				Clinical manifestations	Causes
Acute metabolic acidosis	↓	↓	↓	...ology. May have tachypnea leading to Kussmaul's respirations; changes in LOC (fatigue, confusion, stupor, coma); hypotension; dysrhythmias. With mild to moderate acidosis may have cold and clammy skin. With severe acidosis may have flushed, warm, and dry skin	
Chronic metabolic acidosis	↓	↓ (Not as much as acute type)		Fatigue, anorexia, malaise; symptoms may be related to chronic disease process as well as to acidosis	Chronic renal failure
Acute metabolic alkalosis	↑	↑ (Can be as great as 60)		Muscular weakness and hyporeflexia (due to severe hypokalemia), dysrhythmias, apathy, confusion, and stupor	Volume depletion (chloride depletion) as a result of vomiting, gastric drainage, diuretic use, posthypercapnia; hyperadrenocorticism (e.g., Cushing's syndrome), aldosteronism, severe potassium depletion, excessive alkali intake
Chronic metabolic alkalosis	↑	↑	↑	Usually asymptomatic	Loss of H^+ via GI sources (vomiting, gastric suction, external drainage); via kidneys (potassium-wasting diuretics, hypokalemia); via chronic alkali ingestion (chronic use of antacids containing calcium carbonate); or correction of hypercapnia if Na^+ and K^+ depletion remains uncorrected

↓, Decrease; ↑, increase.

T A B L E   1 0 - 1 8   Acid-base rules: general guidelines

Disturbance	Change in pH	Compensatory response	Results of compensation
Respiratory acidosis			
Acute	pH ↓ 0.08 for every 10 mm Hg ↑ in $Paco_2$	Immediate release of tissue buffers (i.e., HCO_3^-)	1 mEq/L ↑ in HCO_3^- from patient's baseline for every 10 mm Hg ↑ in $Paco_2$
Chronic	Depends on renal compensation; often near normal	↑ renal reabsorption of HCO_3^-; ↑ excretion of H^+ clinically evident after 8 h; maximal effect 3-5 days	3.5 mEq/L ↑ in HCO_3^- for every 10 mm Hg ↑ in $Paco_2$
Respiratory alkalosis			
Acute	pH ↑ 0.08 for every 10 mm Hg ↓ in $Paco_2$	Immediate release of tissue buffers	2 mEq/L ↓ in HCO_3^- from patient's baseline for every 10 mm Hg ↑ in $Paco_2$
Chronic	pH can be returned to normal if renal function is adequate	↓ renal reabsorption of HCO_3^-	Maximal renal compensation causes HCO_3^- to ↓ 5 mEq/L for every 10 mm Hg ↓ in $Paco_2$; maximal effect can take 7-9 days and may normalize pH

Continued.

Section two: Caring for adults with acid-base imbalances

ACUTE RESPIRATORY ACIDOSIS

Pathophysiology

Respiratory acidosis (hypercapnia) occurs secondary to alveolar hypoventilation and results in an elevated $Paco_2$. $Paco_2$ derangements are direct reflections of the degree of ventilatory function or dysfunction. The degree to which the increased $Paco_2$ alters the pH depends on the rapidity of onset and the body's ability to compensate through the blood buffer and renal systems. The acidemia may develop rapidly because of the delay (hours to days) before renal compensation occurs. Acute rises in $Paco_2$ precipitate a rise in extracellular HCO_3^- (primarily hemoglobin and proteins) even before renal compensation occurs,

T A B L E   1 0 - 1 8   Acid-base rules: general guidelines—cont'd

Metabolic acidosis

Acute	pH ↓ 0.15 for every 10 mEq/L ↓ in HCO_3^-	Hyperventilation occurs immediately	1.2 mm Hg ↓ in Pa_{CO_2} for every 1 mEq/L ↓ in HCO_3^-
Chronic	pH same as it would be if no respiratory compensation were present	Hyperventilation	Effects of hyperventilation ↓ over 1-2 days because ↓ in Pa_{CO_2} causes a further ↓ in renal reabsorption of HCO_3^-

Metabolic alkalosis

Acute	pH ↑ 0.15 for every 10 mEq/L ↑ in HCO_3^-	Hypoventilation occurs immediately	0.7 mm Hg ↑ in Pa_{CO_2} for every 1 mEq/L ↑ in HCO_3^-
Chronic	pH same as it would be if respiratory compensation were present	Hypoventilation	Effects of hypoventilation last for only a few days because ↑ in Pa_{CO_2} causes ↑ renal excretion of H^+ and ↑ serum HCO_3^-

↓, Decrease; ↑, increase.

but the extracellular rise is not sufficient to maintain a normal pH in the presence of an elevated Pa_{CO_2}. The most common causes of acute respiratory acidosis are sudden respiratory failure from a depressed respiratory center (drugs or cerebral injury) or a catastrophic event, such as cardiac arrest.

Assessment

HISTORY AND RISK FACTORS
Acute respiratory disease.
Overdose of drugs: Oversedation with drugs that cause respiratory center depression.
Chest wall trauma: Flail chest, pneumothorax.
CNS trauma/lesions: Can lead to depression of respiratory center.
Asphyxiation: Mechanical obstruction, anaphylaxis.
Impaired respiratory muscles: Can occur with hypokalemia, hyperkalemia, poliomyelitis, Guillain-Barré syndrome.
Iatrogenic: Inappropriate mechanical ventilation (increased dead space, insufficient rate or volume); high Fi_{O_2} in the presence of chronic CO_2 retention.

T A B L E   1 0 - 1 9   Review of basic evaluation criteria with simple
acid-base disturbances

Acid-base disturbance	pH	Paco$_2$	HCO$_3$$^-$
Respiratory acidosis	↓	↑ Primary disorder	↑ Compensatory change
Respiratory alkalosis	↑	↓ Primary disorder	↓ Compensatory change
Metabolic acidosis	↓	↓ Compensatory change	↓ Primary disorder
Metabolic alkalosis	↑	↑ Compensatory change	↑ Primary disorder

CLINICAL PRESENTATION Dyspnea, nausea, vomiting, headache, fine tremors, asterixis, and restlessness and confusion leading to lethargy and coma. The restlessness and confusion are early signs that may be subtle but are very important indicators.

PHYSICAL ASSESSMENT Increased heart and respiratory rates, hypotension, and diaphoresis. Severe hypercapnia may cause cerebral vasodilatation, resulting in increased intracranial pressure (IICP). Another finding may be dilated conjunctival and facial blood vessels.

MONITORING PARAMETERS Presence of ventricular dysrhythmias; IICP.

Diagnostic tests

ABG analysis: Aids in diagnosis and determination of severity of respiratory acidosis. Paco$_2$ will be >45 mm Hg and pH will be <7.35. If the patient is breathing room air, hypoxemia always will be present to some degree with increased Paco$_2$.

Serum bicarbonate: Initially, HCO$_3$$^-$ values will be normal (22-26 mEq/L) unless a mixed disorder is present.

Serum electrolyte levels: Usually not altered; depend on cause of respiratory acidosis.

Chest x-ray: Determines presence of underlying respiratory disease.

Drug screen: Determines presence and quantity of drug if patient is suspected of taking an overdose.

Collaborative management

Restoration of effective alveolar ventilation: Accomplished by supporting respiratory function. If Paco$_2$ is >50-60 mm Hg, Pao$_2$ is ≤50 mm Hg, and clinical signs of ventilatory failure (e.g., such as confusion and lethargy) are present, the patient usually requires intubation and mechanical ventilation. Generally, use of bicarbonate is avoided because of the risk of alkalosis when the respiratory disturbance has been corrected. Although a life-threatening pH must be corrected to an acceptable level promptly, a normal pH is not the immediate goal.

Treatment of underlying disorder.

Nursing diagnoses and interventions

Nursing diagnoses and interventions are specific to the pathophysiologic process. See appropriate section(s) in this and other chapters for diagnoses such as **Impaired gas exchange, Ineffective airway clearance,** and **Activity intolerance.**

CHRONIC RESPIRATORY ACIDOSIS (COMPENSATED)

Pathophysiology

This disorder occurs in pulmonary diseases in which effective alveolar ventilation is decreased and a ventilation-perfusion mismatch is present. Over time the amount of CO_2 eliminated is less than the amount generated, and thus $Paco_2$ levels increase. Chronic hypercapnia occurs with chronic obstructive pulmonary disorders (e.g., chronic emphysema and bronchitis and cystic fibrosis), restrictive disorders (e.g., pickwickian syndrome), neuromuscular abnormalities (amyotrophic lateral sclerosis), and respiratory center depression (e.g., brain tumor). In patients with a chronic lung disease, a nearly normal pH can be seen if renal function is normal, even if the $Paco_2$ is as high as 60 mm Hg. Chronic compensatory metabolic alkalosis (serum HCO_3^- >26 mEq/L) occurs and maintains an acceptable acid-base environment, which results in compensated respiratory acidosis and a near normal pH level. Patients with chronic lung disease can experience acute rises in $Paco_2$ secondary to superimposed disease states such as pneumonia. If the chronic compensatory mechanisms in place (e.g., elevated HCO_3^-) are inadequate to meet the sudden increase in $Paco_2$, decompensation may occur with a resultant decrease in pH.

Assessment

HISTORY AND RISK FACTORS
COPD: Predominantly emphysema and bronchitis; cystic fibrosis.
Extreme obesity: Pickwickian syndrome.
Acute respiratory infection in a patient with COPD.
Exposure to pulmonary toxins: Occupational risk; pollution.
CLINICAL PRESENTATION If the $Paco_2$ does not exceed the body's ability to compensate, no specific findings will be noted. If $Paco_2$ rises rapidly, the following may occur: dyspnea, asterixis, agitation, and insomnia progressing to somnolence and coma. The progression of symptoms may be subtle. Therefore, thorough assessment and evaluation are important.
PHYSICAL ASSESSMENT Tachypnea, cyanosis (depending on the underlying disorder). Severe hypercapnia ($Paco_2$ >70 mm Hg) may cause cerebral vasodilatation resulting in increased ICP, papilledema, and dilated conjunctival and facial blood vessels. Depending on the underlying pathophysiologic process, edema may be present secondary to right ventricular failure.
MONITORING PARAMETERS Supraventricular tachycardia and ventricular tachycardia are common if an acute exacerbation is present.

Diagnostic tests

ABG values: Provide data necessary for determining the diagnosis and severity of respiratory acidosis. Although the $Paco_2$ will be elevated, the pH level will be near normal, although on the acidic (low) side of normal except in patients who are also experiencing an acute pulmonary disorder superimposed on chronic hypercapnia (e.g., pneumonia). If the $Paco_2$ has increased abruptly from baseline value, a pH value lower than normal may be seen.

Serum electrolyte levels: Serum HCO_3^- is especially helpful in determining the level of metabolic compensation that has occurred (i.e., HCO_3^- increased with a near normal pH value if fully compensated). This information is particularly useful in identifying "mixed" acid-base disturbances because the HCO_3^- is expected to be elevated in chronic respiratory acidosis. If the HCO_3^- is normal or low, this could be diagnostic of a second pathologic process (e.g., metabolic acidosis) concurrent with the first.

Chest x-ray: Determines extent of underlying pulmonary disease and identifies further pathologic changes that may be responsible for acute exacerbation (e.g., pneumonia).

ECG: Isoelectric P wave and an isoelectric QRS complex in lead I in a middle-aged or older adult suggest chronic bronchitis or emphysema.

Sputum culture: Determines presence of pathogens causing an acute exacerbation of a chronic pulmonary disease (e.g., pneumonia) present in a patient with COPD.

Collaborative management

Oxygen therapy: Used cautiously in patients with chronic CO_2 retention for whom hypoxemia, rather than hypercapnia, stimulates ventilation. Patient may require intubation and mechanical ventilation for stupor and coma precipitated by oxygen if the drive to breathe is eliminated by high concentrations of oxygen. Continuous pulse oximetry may be used for close monitoring of oxygen delivery and to help ensure maintenance of oxygen saturation within acceptable range (e.g., 90%-92%).

Pharmacotherapy: Bronchodilators and antibiotics, as indicated. Narcotics and sedatives can depress the respiratory center and are avoided unless intubation and mechanical ventilation are in place.

IV fluids: Maintain adequate hydration for mobilizing pulmonary secretions.

Chest physiotherapy: Aids in expectoration of sputum. Includes postural drainage if hypersecretions are present. Assess patient closely during this procedure because it may be poorly tolerated, especially the postural drainage component.

Nursing diagnoses and interventions

Impaired gas exchange related to alveolar-capillary membrane changes secondary to pulmonary tissue destruction

Desired outcome: Within 24 h of initiation of treatment, patient has adequate gas exchange as evidenced by $Paco_2$, pH, and Sao_2 normal or within 10% of patient's baseline.

- Monitor serial ABG results to assess patient's response to therapy. Consult physician for significant findings: increasing $Paco_2$ and decreasing pH, Pao_2, and Sao_2 values.
- Monitor oxygen saturation *via* pulse oximetry (Spo_2). Compare Spo_2 with Sao_2 values to assess reliability. Watch Spo_2 closely, especially when changing Fio_2 or to evaluate patient's response to treatment (e.g., repositioning, chest physiotherapy).

- Assess and document patient's respiratory status: respiratory rate and rhythm, exertional effort, and breath sounds. Compare pretreatment findings to posttreatment (e.g., oxygen therapy, physiotherapy, or medications) findings for evidence of improvement.
- Assess and document patient's LOC. If $Paco_2$ increases, be alert to subtle, progressive changes in mental status. A common progression is agitation→insomnia→somnolence→coma. To avoid a comatose state caused by rising CO_2 levels, always evaluate the "arousability" of a patient with elevated $Paco_2$ who appears to be sleeping. Consult physician if patient is difficult to arouse.
- Ensure appropriate delivery of prescribed oxygen therapy. Assess patient's respiratory status after every change in Fio_2. Patients with chronic CO_2 retention may be very sensitive to increases in Fio_2, resulting in depressed ventilatory drive. If patient requires mechanical ventilation, be aware of the importance of maintaining the compensated acid-base status. If the $Paco_2$ is rapidly decreased by excessive mechanical ventilation, a severe metabolic alkalosis (posthypercapnic metabolic alkalosis) could develop. The sudden onset of metabolic alkalosis may lead to hypocalcemia, which can result in tetany (see "Hypocalcemia," p. 688). Severe alkalosis also can precipitate cardiac dysrhythmias.
- Assess for presence of bowel sounds and monitor for GI distention, which can impede movement of the diaphragm and restrict ventilatory effort further.
- In patient without intubation, encourage use of pursed-lip breathing (inhalation through nose, with slow exhalation through pursed lips), which helps airways to remain open and allows for better air excursion. Optimally, this technique will diminish air entrapment in the lungs and make respiratory effort more efficient.

ACUTE RESPIRATORY ALKALOSIS (HYPOCAPNIA)

Pathophysiology

Respiratory alkalosis occurs as a result of an increase in the rate of alveolar ventilation (alveolar hyperventilation). It is defined as $Paco_2$ <35 mm Hg. Acute alveolar hyperventilation most frequently results from anxiety and is commonly referred to as "hyperventilation syndrome." In addition, numerous physiologic disorders that cause hypoxemia (e.g., pneumonia, pulmonary edema, pulmonary emboli) can cause acute hypocapnia. If the underlying condition worsens, respiratory acidosis can occur as the exchange of CO_2 is impaired. Because CO_2 is 20 times more diffusible than O_2 across the alveolar membrane, hypoxemia is the first abnormality noted in many pulmonary diseases. Hypocapnia will result in increased pH. The rise in pH is modified to a small degree by intracellular buffering. To compensate for increased CO_2 loss and the resultant base excess, hydrogen ions are released from tissue buffers, which in turn lowers the plasma HCO_3^- concentration. Renal compensation for the respiratory alkalosis is not clinically apparent for hours; maximal compensation is not seen for days. Acute respiratory alkalosis can progress to chronic respiratory alkalosis if it persists for >6 h and renal compensation occurs.

Assessment

HISTORY AND RISK FACTORS

Anxiety: Patient is often unaware of hyperventilation.

Acute hypoxemia: Pulmonary disorders (e.g., pneumonia, pulmonary edema, and pulmonary thromboembolism) and extremely high altitudes (e.g., >6,500 ft) may result in hypoxemia, which stimulates the ventilatory effort, causing respiratory alkalosis.

Hypermetabolic states: Fever; sepsis, especially gram-negative–induced septicemia.

Salicylate intoxication.

Excessive mechanical ventilation: Increased tidal volume or RR.

CNS trauma: That which results in damage to respiratory center.

CLINICAL PRESENTATION Lightheadedness, anxiety, paresthesias (especially of the fingers), circumoral numbness. In extreme alkalosis, confusion, tetany, syncope, and seizures may occur.

PHYSICAL ASSESSMENT Increased rate and depth of respirations.

MONITORING PARAMETERS Cardiac dysrhythmias.

Diagnostic tests

ABG values: $Paco_2$ <35 mm Hg and pH >7.45 will be present. A decreased Pao_2, along with the clinical picture (e.g., pneumonia, pulmonary edema, and pulmonary embolism), may help diagnose cause of the respiratory alkalosis.

Serum electrolyte levels: HCO_3^- will be decreased 2 mEq/L for each 10 mm Hg drop in $Paco_2$ as a result of H^+ release from nonbicarbonate buffers and tissues (not from renal compensation).

- *Sodium and potassium* may be decreased slightly (potassium will shift from the extracellular space to the intracellular space in exchange for H^+).
- *Serum calcium* may be decreased because of increased calcium and bicarbonate binding. Signs of hypocalcemia include muscle cramps, hyperactive reflexes, carpal spasm, tetany, and convulsions.
- *Serum phosphorus* may decrease (<2.5 mg/dl), especially with salicylate intoxication and sepsis, because the alkalosis causes increased uptake of phosphorus by the cells. No symptoms occur and treatment usually is not required unless a preexisting phosphorus deficit is present.

ECG: Detects cardiac dysrhythmias, which may occur with alkalosis.

Collaborative management

Treatment of underlying disorder.

Reassurance or sedation: If anxiety is the cause of decreased $Paco_2$. If symptoms are severe, it may be necessary for patient to rebreathe exhaled air *via* a paper bag.

Oxygen therapy: If hypoxemia is the causative factor.

Adjustments to mechanical ventilators: Settings are checked and adjustments made to ventilatory parameters in response to ABG results that signal hypocapnia. Respiratory rate and/or volume are decreased and dead space is added, if necessary, by attaching extra tubing to the mechanical ventilator circuitry.

Pharmacotherapy: Sedatives and tranquilizers may be given for anxiety-induced respiratory alkalosis.

Nursing diagnoses and interventions

Ineffective breathing pattern related to anxiety

Desired outcome: Within 4 h of initiating treatment, patient's breathing pattern is effective as evidenced by a state of eupnea, $Paco_2$ $\geq$35 mm Hg, and pH $\leq$7.45.

- To help alleviate anxiety, reassure patient that a staff member will remain with him or her.
- Encourage patient to breathe slowly. Pace patient's breathing pattern by having him or her mimic your own breathing pattern.
- Monitor patient's cardiac rhythm. Consult physician for new or increased dysrhythmias. With acute respiratory alkalosis, even a modest alkalosis can precipitate dysrhythmias in a patient with a preexisting heart disease who is also taking inotropic drugs (see Appendix 7). In part, this is caused by the hypokalemia that occurs with alkalosis.
- Administer sedatives or tranquilizers as prescribed. Assess and document effectiveness.
- Have patient rebreathe into a paper bag as indicated.
- Ensure that patient rests undisturbed after his or her breathing pattern has stabilized. Hyperventilation can result in fatigue.

Note: Hyperventilation may lead to hypocalcemic tetany despite a normal or near normal calcium level due to increased binding of calcium.

CHRONIC RESPIRATORY ALKALOSIS

Pathophysiology

Chronic respiratory alkalosis is a state of chronic hypocapnia caused by stimulation of the respiratory center. The decreased $Paco_2$ stimulates the renal compensatory response and results in a proportionate decrease in plasma bicarbonate until a new, steady state is reached. Maximal renal compensatory response requires several days to occur and can result in a normal or near normal pH. Chronic respiratory alkalosis is not commonly seen in acutely ill patients, but when present it can signal a poor prognosis.

Assessment

HISTORY AND RISK FACTORS

Cerebral disease: Tumor, encephalitis, cerebrovascular accident.

Chronic hepatic insufficiency: A sustained respiratory alkalosis with this diagnosis has a poor prognosis.

Restrictive lung diseases: Interstitial pulmonary fibrosis. Respiratory alkalosis continues throughout the course of the disease. A normal $Paco_2$ followed by increased $Paco_2$ occurs in the terminal stage of the disease.

Pregnancy.

Chronic hypoxia: Adaptation to high altitude, cyanotic heart disease, lung disease resulting in decreased compliance (e.g., fibrosis).

CLINICAL PRESENTATION Individuals with chronic respiratory alkalosis usually are free of symptoms.

PHYSICAL ASSESSMENT Increased respiratory rate and depth.

Diagnostic tests

ABG values: $Paco_2$ will be <35 mm Hg, with a nearly normal or normal pH; Pao_2 may be decreased if hypoxemia is the causative factor.

Serum electrolyte levels: Probably will be normal, with the exception of plasma HCO_3^-, which will decrease as renal compensation occurs.

Phosphate levels: Hypophosphatemia (as low as 0.5 mg/dl) may be seen with intense hyperventilation. Alkalosis causes increased uptake of phosphate by the cells.

Collaborative management

Treatment of underlying cause.

Oxygen therapy: If hypoxemia is present and identified as causative factor in respiratory alkalosis.

Nursing diagnoses and interventions

Nursing diagnoses and interventions are specific to the pathophysiologic process. See appropriate medical disorders and nursing diagnoses in this and other chapters.

ACUTE METABOLIC ACIDOSIS

Pathophysiology

Metabolic acidosis is caused by a primary decrease in plasma bicarbonate, as reflected by a serum HCO_3^- of <22 mEq/L with a pH <7.4. The decrease in serum HCO_3^- is caused by one of the following mechanisms: (1) increase in the concentration of H^+ in the form of nonvolatile acids (e.g., ketoacidosis associated with diabetes and alcoholism, lactic acidosis), (2) loss of alkali (e.g., severe diarrhea, intestinal malabsorption), and (3) decreased acid excretion by the kidneys (e.g., acute and chronic renal failure). The decrease in pH stimulates respirations. Attempts to compensate occur rapidly, as manifested by lowering of the $Paco_2$, which may be reduced to as much as 10-15 mm Hg. The most important mechanism for ridding the body of excess H^+ is the increase in acid excretion by the kidneys. Nonvolatile acids, however, may accumulate more rapidly than they can be neutralized by the body's buffers, compensated for by the respiratory system, or excreted by the kidneys.

Assessment

HISTORY AND RISK FACTORS

Ketoacidosis: Diabetes mellitus, alcoholism, starvation.

Lactic acidosis: Respiratory or circulatory failure, drugs and toxins, hereditary disorders, septic shock. Lactic acidosis can be associated with other disease states, such as leukemia, pancreatitis, bacterial infection, and uncontrolled diabetes mellitus.

Renal disease: Acute renal failure, renal tubular acidosis.
Poisonings and drug toxicity: Salicylates, methanol, ethylene glycol, ammonium chloride.
Loss of alkali: Draining wounds (e.g., pancreatic fistulas), diarrhea, ureterostomy.

CLINICAL PRESENTATION Findings vary, depending on underlying disease states and the severity of the acid-base disturbance and speed with which it developed. There may be changes in LOC that range from fatigue and confusion to stupor and coma.

PHYSICAL ASSESSMENT Tachycardia (until pH <7, then bradycardia), decreased BP, tachypnea leading to alveolar hyperventilation (Kussmaul's respirations), dysrhythmias, and shock state. With mild to moderate acidosis the skin will be cold and clammy, while with severe acidosis it will be flushed, warm, and dry. Mild metabolic acidosis (HCO_3^- 15-18 mEq/L) may result in no symptoms, while with a pH <7.2, symptoms will develop.

MONITORING PARAMETERS A waveform suggestive of hyperkalemia (prolonged P-R interval, widened QRS, and peaked T waves) may occur.

Diagnostic tests

ABG values: Determine pH (usually <7.35) and degree of respiratory compensation as reflected by $Paco_2$, which usually is <35 mm Hg.
Serum bicarbonate: Determines presence of metabolic acidosis (HCO_3^- <22 mEq/L).
Serum electrolyte levels: Elevated potassium ($K^+ > 5$ mEq/L) may be present as the H^+ moves into the cells to be buffered and the K^+ moves out of the cells to maintain electroneutrality. Hyperkalemia related to metabolic acidosis occurs most frequently in renal failure. If the K^+ is normal or low in the presence of metabolic acidosis, this signals low body stores of K^+.

To help identify the cause of metabolic acidosis, an analysis of serum electrolytes to detect anion gap may be helpful. Anion gap reflects unmeasurable anions present in plasma and is calculated by subtracting the sum of chloride and sodium bicarbonate from plasma sodium concentration

$$Anion\ gap = Na^+ - (Cl^- + HCO_3^-)$$

Normal anion gap is 12 (+ or − 2) mEq/L. Normal anion gap acidosis results from direct loss of HCO_3^- (e.g., diarrhea, renal tubular acidosis, pancreatic fistulas) or the addition of chloride-containing acids (e.g., ammonium chloride, hydrochloric acid), some hyperalimentation fluids, and oral calcium chloride. An increased anion gap acidosis >12-14 mEq/L results from accumulation of nonvolatile acids (acids from lactic acidosis, diabetes ketoacidosis, renal failure, and salicylate and methanol toxicity).
ECG: Detects dysrhythmias, which may be caused by acidosis or hyperkalemia. Changes seen with hyperkalemia include peaked T waves, depressed ST segment, decreased size of R waves, decrease or

absence of P waves, and widened QRS complex. Ventricular fibrillation also may occur with metabolic acidosis.

Collaborative management

Sodium bicarbonate (NaHCO$_3$):   May be indicated when arterial pH is $\leq$7.2. The usual mode of delivery is IV drip: 2-3 ampules (44.5 mEq/ampule) in 1,000 ml D$_5$W, although NaHCO$_3$ may be given IV push in emergencies. Concentration depends on severity of the acidosis and presence of any serum sodium disorders. NaHCO$_3$ must be given very cautiously to avoid metabolic alkalosis and pulmonary edema as a result of the sodium load.

Potassium replacement: Usually, hyperkalemia is present, but a potassium deficit can occur. If a potassium deficit exists (K$^+$ <3.5), it must be corrected before NaHCO$_3$ is administered, because when the acidosis is corrected, the potassium shifts back to intracellular spaces. This shift in K$^+$ could result in serum hypokalemia with serious consequences, such as cardiac irritability with fatal dysrhythmias and generalized muscle weakness. See "Hypokalemia," p. 681, for more information.

Mechanical ventilation: If mechanical ventilation is required on the basis of ABG results and clinical signs, it is important that the patient's compensatory hyperventilation be allowed to continue in order to prevent acidosis from becoming more severe. Therefore the respiratory rate on the ventilator should not be set lower than the rate at which patient has been breathing spontaneously, and the tidal volume should be large enough to maintain compensatory hyperventilation until the underlying disorder can be resolved.

Treatment of underlying disorder

Diabetic ketoacidosis: Insulin and fluids. If acidosis is severe (with a pH of <7.1 or HCO$_3$$^-$ 6-8 mEq/L), judicious administration of NaHCO$_3$ may be necessary.

Alcoholism-related ketoacidosis: Glucose and saline.

Diarrhea: Usually occurs in association with other fluid and electrolyte disturbances; correction addresses concurrent imbalances.

Acute renal failure: Hemodialysis or peritoneal dialysis to maintain an adequate level of plasma HCO$_3$$^-$.

Renal tubular acidosis: May require modest amounts (<100 mEq/ day) of bicarbonate.

Poisoning and drug toxicity: Treatment depends on drug ingested or infused. Hemodialysis or peritoneal dialysis may be necessary.

Lactic acidosis: Correction of underlying disorder. Mortality associated with lactic acidosis is high. Treatment with NaHCO$_3$ is only transiently helpful.

Nursing diagnoses and interventions

Nursing diagnoses and interventions are specific to the pathophysiologic process. See **Altered oral mucous membrane** in other sections of this text. Also see nursing diagnoses and interventions in "Mechanical Ventilation," p. 24; "Psychosocial Support," p. 88; "Psychosocial Support for the Patient's Family and Significant Others," p. 100; "Acute Renal Failure," p. 397; and "Diabetic Ketoacidosis," p. 499.

CHRONIC METABOLIC ACIDOSIS

Pathophysiology

Most often metabolic acidosis is seen with chronic renal failure in which the kidneys' ability to excrete acids (endogenous and exogenous) is exceeded by acid production and ingestion. The acidosis usually is mild in the initial stage, with HCO_3^- 18-22 mEq/L and a pH of 7.35. Treatment is indicated when serum HCO_3^- levels reach 15 mEq/L. Respiratory compensation occurs but only to a limited degree. A modest decrease in $Paco_2$ will be noted on ABG values.

Assessment

HISTORY AND RISK FACTORS Chronic renal failure, renal tubular acidosis, loss of alkaline fluid (e.g., with diarrhea or pancreatic or biliary drainage) for >3-5 days.

CLINICAL PRESENTATION Usually the process leading to chronic metabolic acidosis is gradual and the patient is symptom free until serum HCO_3^- is $\leq$15 mEq/L. Fatigue, malaise, and anorexia may be present in relation to the underlying disease.

Diagnostic tests

ABG values: $Paco_2$ will be <35 mm Hg; pH will be <7.35.
Serum bicarbonate: Will be <22 mEq/L (usually 18-21 mEq/L). With severe acidosis, it will be <15 mEq/L.
Serum electrolyte levels: Serum calcium level is checked before treatment of acidosis is initiated to prevent tetany induced by hypocalcemia (caused by a decrease in ionized calcium). Serum phosphorus level is evaluated to determine presence of hyperphosphatemia, a common complication of chronic renal failure. Serum potassium level should be monitored after acidosis has been corrected to detect hypokalemia, inasmuch as potassium shifts back into the cells after correction of the acidosis.

Collaborative management

Alkalizing agents: For serum HCO_3^- levels <15 mEq/L, oral alkalis are administered ($NaHCO_3$ tablets or sodium citrate and citric acid oral solution [Shohl's solution]). They are used cautiously to prevent fluid overload and tetany caused by hypocalcemia.

Caution: Be alert to the possibility of pulmonary edema if bicarbonate is administered parenterally to patients with renal insufficiency or cardiovascular disorders.

Oral phosphates: Given if hypophosphatemia is present (not common with chronic renal failure) but may result from overuse of phosphate binders given to treat hyperphosphatemia.
Hemodialysis or peritoneal dialysis: If indicated by chronic renal failure or other disease processes (see p. 410).

Nursing diagnoses and interventions

Nursing diagnoses and interventions are specific to the underlying pathophysiologic process. See other sections of this text, particularly Chapter 5.

ACUTE METABOLIC ALKALOSIS

Pathophysiology

Acute metabolic alkalosis results in an elevated serum HCO_3^- (up to 45-50 mEq/L) as a result of H^+ loss or excess alkali intake. A compensatory increase in $Paco_2$ (up to 50-60 mm Hg) will be seen. Respiratory compensation is limited because of hypoxemia, which develops as a result of decreased alveolar ventilation. The major causes of this disturbance are loss of gastric acid from vomiting or gastric suction, diuretic therapy, posthypercapnic alkalosis (which occurs when chronic CO_2 retention is corrected rapidly), and excessive $NaHCO_3$ administration (i.e., overcorrection of a metabolic acidosis). Even when the causative factors have been removed, the alkalosis will be maintained until volume and electrolyte disturbances that are contributing to the alkalosis have been corrected. Severe alkalosis (pH >7.6) is associated with high morbidity and mortality. The body can tolerate a greater degree of acidosis than alkalosis.

Assessment

HISTORY AND RISK FACTORS
Clinical circumstances associated with volume/chloride depletion: Vomiting or gastric drainage; cystic fibrosis in hot weather when excessive chloride and sodium losses are not replaced.
Diuretic use: Usually a mild metabolic alkalosis will occur with diuretic use. The alkalosis will be more severe if using a potent diuretic (i.e., furosemide), especially in patients on sodium-restricted diets.
Posthypercapnic alkalosis: May occur after rapid correction of chronic hypercapnia.
Excessive alkali intake: May be iatrogenic from overcorrection of metabolic acidosis (frequently seen during CPR).
CLINICAL PRESENTATION Muscular weakness, neuromuscular instability, and hyporeflexia because of accompanying hypokalemia. Decrease in GI tract motility may result in an ileus. Severe alkalosis can result in apathy, confusion, and stupor. Seizures may occur.
PHYSICAL ASSESSMENT Decreased respiratory rate and depth, periods of apnea, tachycardia (atrial or ventricular).
MONITORING PARAMETERS Atrial-ventricular dysrhythmias as a result of cardiac irritability secondary to hypokalemia; prolonged QT interval.

Diagnostic tests

ABG values: Determine severity of alkalosis and response to therapy.
Serum bicarbonate levels: Values will be elevated to >26 mEq/L.
Serum electrolyte levels: Usually, serum potassium will be low (<4 mEq/L) as will serum chloride (<95 mEq/L).
Urinalysis: Urine chloride levels can help identify the cause of the metabolic alkalosis. Urine chloride level will be <15 mEq/L if hypo-

volemia and hypochloremia are present and >20 mEq/L with excess retained HCO_3^-. This test is not reliable if diuretics are used within the previous 12 h.

ECG findings: To assess for dysrhythmias, especially if profound hypokalemia or alkalosis is present.

Collaborative management

Management will depend on the underlying disorder. Mild or moderate metabolic alkalosis usually does not require specific therapeutic interventions.

Saline infusion: Normal saline infusion may correct volume (chloride) deficit in patients with gastric alkalosis because of gastric losses. Metabolic alkalosis is difficult to correct if hypovolemia and chloride deficit are not corrected.

Potassium chloride (KCl):   Indicated for patients with low potassium levels. KCl is preferred over other potassium salts because chloride losses can be replaced simultaneously.

Sodium and potassium chloride: Effective for posthypercapnic alkalosis, which occurs when chronic CO_2 retention is corrected rapidly (e.g., *via* mechanical ventilation). If adequate amounts of chloride and potassium are not available, renal excretion of excess HCO_3^- is impaired and metabolic alkalosis continues.

Cautious IV administration of isotonic hydrochloride solution, ammonium chloride, or arginine hydrochloride: May be warranted if severe metabolic alkalosis (pH >7.6 and HCO_3^- >40-45 mEq/L) exists, especially if chloride or potassium salts are contraindicated. The medication is delivered *via* continuous IV infusion at a slow rate, with frequent monitoring of IV insertion site for signs of infiltration. Ammonium chloride and arginine hydrochloride may be dangerous to patients with renal or hepatic failure.

Nursing diagnoses and interventions

Nursing diagnoses and interventions are specific to the underlying pathophysiologic process. See Chapter 5, particularly.

CHRONIC METABOLIC ALKALOSIS

Pathophysiology

Chronic metabolic alkalosis results in a pH >7.45 and HCO_3^- >26 mEq/L. Pa_{CO_2} will be elevated (>45 mm Hg) to compensate for the loss of H^+ or excess serum HCO_3^-. There are three clinical situations in which this can occur: (1) abnormalities in the kidneys' excretion of HCO_3^- related to a mineralocorticoid effect, (2) loss of H^+ through the GI tract, and (3) long-term diuretic therapy, especially the thiazides and furosemide.

Assessment

HISTORY AND RISK FACTORS

Diuretic use: Thiazide diuretics cause a loss of chloride, potassium, and hydrogen ions. Massive depletion of potassium stores with loss of up to 1,000 mEq, which is one third of total body potassium, may occur, causing profound hypokalemia (K^+ ≤ 2.0 mEq/L).

Hyperadrenocorticism: Cushing's syndrome, primary aldosteronism. This is not a chloride deficit but a chronic loss of potassium, which can lead to total body depletion of potassium with profound hypokalemia (K^+ $\leq$2.0 mEq/L).

Chronic vomiting or chronic GI losses through GI suction.

Milk-alkali syndrome: An infrequent cause of metabolic alkalosis.

Hypercalcemic nephropathy and alkalosis: Develop as a result of excessive intake of absorbable alkali (antacids containing calcium carbonate).

CLINICAL PRESENTATION Patient may be free of symptoms. With severe potassium depletion and profound alkalosis, patient may experience weakness, neuromuscular instability, and decrease in GI tract motility, which can result in ileus.

MONITORING PARAMETERS Frequent PVCs or U waves with hypokalemia and alkalosis.

Diagnostic tests

ABG values: Determine severity of acid-base imbalance. $Paco_2$ will be increased (>45 mm Hg), and pH will be >7.4.

Serum bicarbonate levels: Will be >26 mEq/L.

Serum electrolyte levels: Usually potassium will be profoundly low (may be $\leq$2 mEq/L). Chloride may be <95 mEq/L. Magnesium may be <1.5 mEq/L in both renal system abnormalities.

Collaborative management

The goal is to correct the underlying acid-base disorder *via* the following interventions.

Fluid management: If volume depletion exists, normal saline infusions are given.

Potassium replacement: If a chloride deficit also is present, KCl is the drug of choice. If a chloride deficit does not exist, other potassium salts are acceptable.

IV potassium: If the patient is undergoing cardiac monitoring, up to 20 mEq/h of KCl is given for serious hypokalemia. Concentrated doses of KCl (>40 mEq/L) require administration through a central venous line because of blood vessel irritation.

Oral potassium: Tastes very unpleasant; 15 mEq/glass is all most patients can tolerate, with a maximum daily dose of 60-80 mEq. Slow-release potassium tablets are an acceptable form of KCl. All forms of KCl may be irritating to gastric mucosa.

Dietary: Normal diet contains 3 g or 75 mEq of potassium, but not in the form of KCl. Dietary supplementation of potassium is not effective if a concurrent chloride deficit is also present.

Potassium-sparing diuretics: May be added to treatment if thiazide diuretics are the cause of hypokalemia and metabolic alkalosis.

Identify and correct cause of hyperadrenocorticism.

Nursing diagnoses and interventions

Nursing diagnoses and interventions are specific to the underlying pathophysiologic process. See Chapter 5 for examples.

Selected Bibliography

Ahrens T, Rutherford K: *Essentials of oxygenation: implications for clinical practice,* Boston, 1993, Jones & Bartlett.

Bickell WH: Are victims of injury sometimes victimized by attempts at fluid resuscitation? *Ann Emerg Med* 22(2):225-226, 1993.

Boxer MB: Anaphylaxis without cause, *Emerg Med* 25(1):20-22, 27, 30, 1993.

Burdick J, Racusen L, Solez K: *Kidney transplant rejection: diagnosis and treatment,* ed 2, New York, 1992, Dekker.

Carpenter K: Oxygen transport in the blood, *Crit Care Nurse* 11(9):20-31, 1991.

Chamberlain J et al: Use of activated charcoal in a simulated poisoning with acetaminophen: a new loading dose for N-acetylcysteine? *Ann Emerg Med* 22(9):1398-1402, 1993.

Cogan MG: *Fluid and electrolytes: physiology and pathophysiology,* Norwalk, Conn, 1991, Appleton & Lange.

Cullen L: Interventions related to fluid and electrolyte balance, *Nurs Clin North Am* 27(2):569-597, 1992.

Dixon AC: New therapeutic strategies in sepsis and septic shock, *Asepsis* 14(1):2-11, 1992.

Fein AM: Sepsis and acute lung injury, *Emerg Med* 22(15):81-82, 85-87, 1990.

Flye M: *Principles of organ transplantation,* Philadelphia, 1989, Saunders.

Foster MT: Septicemia, *Hosp Pract* 28(suppl 5):43-47, 1991.

Hazinski MF: Epidemiology, pathophysiology, and clinical presentation of gram-negative sepsis, *Am J Crit Care* 2(3):224-237, 1993.

Herfindal ET, Gourley DR, Hart LL: *Clinical pharmacy and therapeutics,* Baltimore, 1992, Williams & Wilkins.

Hollingsworth HM: Anaphylaxis, *Emerg Med* 24(12):142, 145-148, 1992.

Horne M, Jansen PR: Renal-urinary disorders. In Swearingen PL, editor: *Manual of medical-surgical nursing care: nursing interventions and collaborative management,* ed 3, St Louis, 1994, Mosby.

Horne M, Swearingen PL: *Pocket guide to fluid, electrolyte, and acid-base balance,* ed 2, St Louis, 1993, Mosby.

Horne M, Heitz UE, Swearingen PL: *Fluid, electrolyte, and acid-base balance: a case study approach,* St Louis, 1991, Mosby.

Imm A, Carlson RW: Fluid resuscitation in circulatory shock, *Crit Care Clin* 9(2):313-333, 1993.

Innerarity SA: Hyperkalemic emergencies, *Crit Care Nurs Q* 14(4):32-39, 1992.

Interqual: The ISD-A review system with adult ISD criteria, August 1992, North Hampton, NH, and Marlboro, Mass, Interqual, Inc.

Keough V, McNamara P: Case review: a 27-year-old with tricyclic overdose, *J Emerg Nurs* 19(5):382-384, 1993.

Kim MJ, McFarland GK, McLane AM: *Pocket guide to nursing diagnoses,* ed 6, St Louis, 1995, Mosby.

Klein DM: Advances in immunotherapy of sepsis, *Dimens Crit Care Nurs* 11(2):75-89, 1992.

Ljutic D, Rumboldt Z: Should glucose be administered before, with, or after insulin, in the management of hyperkalemia? *Ren Fail* 15(1):73-76, 1993.

Lowenstein J: *Acid and basics,* New York, 1993, Oxford University Press.

Markenson D, Greenberg M: Cyclic antidepressant overdose: mechanism to management, *Emerg Med* 25(11):49-56, 1993.

McCarron MM et al: Short-acting barbiturate overdose, *JAMA* 248(1):55-61, 1982.

McConnell EA: Myths and facts about septic shock, *Nurs* 22(7):26, 1992.

Meyer I: Sodium polystyrene sulfonate: a cation exchange resin used in treating hyperkalemia, *ANNA J* 20(1):93-95, 1993.

Narins RG, Emmett M: Simple and mixed acid-base disorders: a practical approach, *Medicine* 59(3):161-187, 1980.

Robins EV: Burn shock, *Crit Care Nurs Clin North Am* 2(2):299-307, 1990.

Rose B: *Clinical physiology of acid-base and electrolyte disorders,* ed 4, New York, 1994, McGraw-Hill.

Sigardson-Poor K, Haggerty L: *Nursing care of the transplant recipient,* Philadelphia, 1990, Saunders.

Workman ML: Magnesium and phosphorus: the neglected electrolytes, *AACN Clin Issues* 3(3):655-663, 1992.

Wrenn K, Rodewald L, Dockstader L: Potential misuse of ipecac, *Ann Emerg Med* 22(9):1408-1412, 1993.

1

THE AMERICAN HEART ASSOCIATION'S ADVANCED CARDIAC LIFE SUPPORT (ACLS) ALGORITHMS

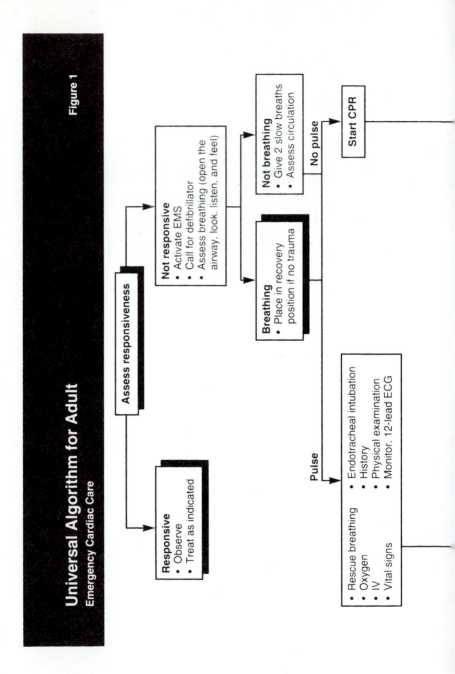

Universal Algorithm for Adult
Emergency Cardiac Care

Figure 1

Assess responsiveness

Responsive
- Observe
- Treat as indicated

Not responsive
- Activate EMS
- Call for defibrillator
- Assess breathing (open the airway. look. listen, and feel)

Breathing
- Place in recovery position if no trauma

Not breathing
- Give 2 slow breaths
- Assess circulation

Pulse
- Rescue breathing
- Oxygen
- IV
- Vital signs
- Endotracheal intubation
- History
- Physical examination
- Monitor. 12-lead ECG

No pulse

Start CPR

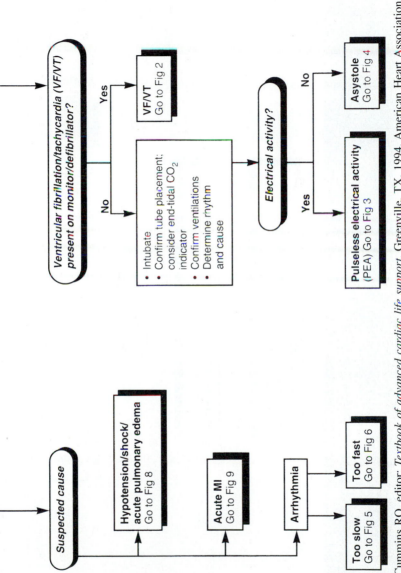

From Cummins RO, editor: *Textbook of advanced cardiac life support*, Greenville, TX, 1994, American Heart Association.

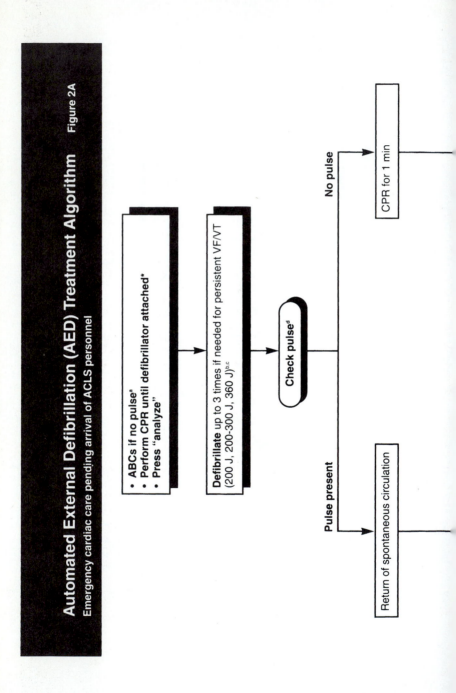

Automated External Defibrillation (AED) Treatment Algorithm   Figure 2A

Emergency cardiac care pending arrival of ACLS personnel

- **ABCs if no pulse**[a]
- **Perform CPR until defibrillator attached***
- **Press "analyze"**

Defibrillate up to 3 times if needed for persistent VF/VT (200 J, 200-300 J, 360 J)[b,c]

Check pulse[d]

Pulse present

Return of spontaneous circulation

No pulse

CPR for 1 min

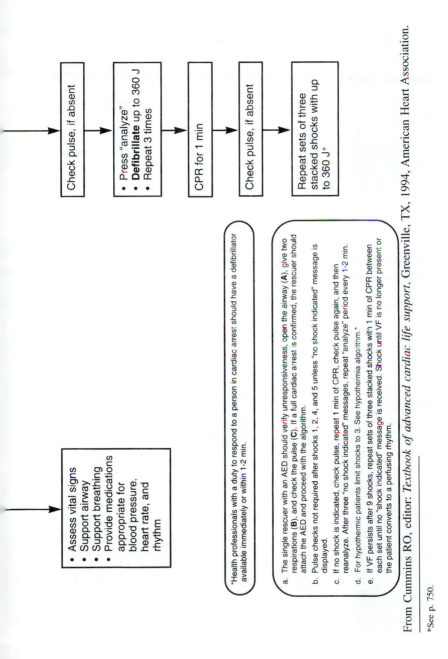

Check pulse, if absent

- Press "analyze"
- **Defibrillate** up to 360 J
- Repeat 3 times

CPR for 1 min

Check pulse, if absent

Repeat sets of three stacked shocks with up to 360 J[e]

- Assess vital signs
- Support airway
- Support breathing
- Provide medications appropriate for blood pressure, heart rate, and rhythm

*Health professionals with a duty to respond to a person in cardiac arrest should have a defibrillator available immediately or within 1-2 min.

a. The single rescuer with an AED should verify unresponsiveness, open the airway (**A**), give two respirations (**B**), and check the pulse (**C**). If a full cardiac arrest is confirmed, the rescuer should attach the AED and proceed with the algorithm.

b. Pulse checks not required after shocks 1, 2, 4, and 5 unless "no shock indicated" message is displayed.

c. If no shock is indicated, check pulse, repeat 1 min of CPR, check pulse again, and then reanalyze. After three "no shock indicated" messages, repeat "analyze" period every 1-2 min.

d. For hypothermic patients limit shocks to 3. See hypothermia algorithm.*

e. If VF persists after 9 shocks, repeat sets of three stacked shocks with 1 min of CPR between each set until no "shock indicated" message is received. Shock until VF is no longer present or the patient converts to a perfusing rhythm.

From Cummins RO, editor: *Textbook of advanced cardiac life support*, Greenville, TX, 1994, American Heart Association.

*See p. 750.

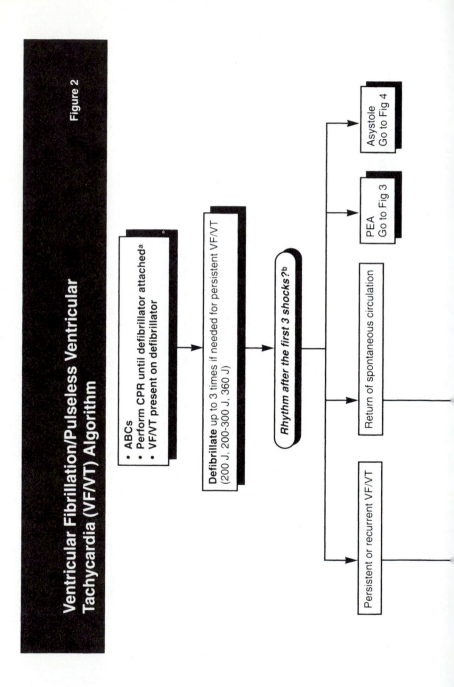

Figure 2

Ventricular Fibrillation/Pulseless Ventricular Tachycardia (VF/VT) Algorithm

- ABCs
- Perform CPR until defibrillator attached[a]
- VF/VT present on defibrillator

Defibrillate up to 3 times if needed for persistent VF/VT (200 J, 200-300 J, 360 J)

Rhythm after the first 3 shocks?[b]

Persistent or recurrent VF/VT

Return of spontaneous circulation

PEA
Go to Fig 3

Asystole
Go to Fig 4

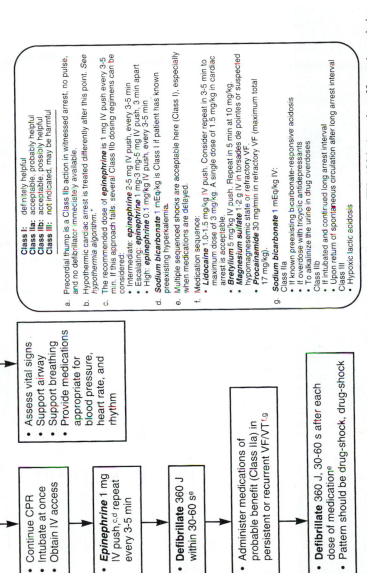

- Assess vital signs
- Support airway
- Support breathing
- Provide medications appropriate for blood pressure, heart rate, and rhythm

- Continue CPR
- Intubate at once
- Obtain IV access

- *Epinephrine* 1 mg IV push,[c,d] repeat every 3-5 min

- **Defibrillate** 360 J within 30-60 s[e]

- Administer medications of probable benefit (Class IIa) in persistent or recurrent VF/VT[f,g]

- **Defibrillate** 360 J, 30-60 s after each dose of medication[e]
- Pattern should be drug-shock, drug-shock

Class I: definitely helpful
Class IIa: acceptable, probably helpful
Class IIb: acceptable, possibly helpful
Class III: not indicated, may be harmful

a. Precordial thump is a Class IIb action in witnessed arrest, no pulse, and no defibrillator immediately available.

b. Hypothermic cardiac arrest is treated differently after this point. *See hypothermia algorithm.*

c. The recommended dose of *epinephrine* is 1 mg IV push every 3-5 min. If this approach fails several Class IIb dosing regimens can be considered:
  - Intermediate: *epinephrine* 2-5 mg IV push, every 3-5 min
  - Escalating: *epinephrine* 1 mg-3 mg-5 mg IV push, 3 min apart
  - High: *epinephrine* 0.1 mg/kg IV push, every 3-5 min

d. **Sodium bicarbonate** 1 mEq/kg is Class I if patient has known preexisting hyperkalemia.

e. Multiple sequenced shocks are acceptable here (Class I), especially when medications are delayed.

f. Medication sequence:
  - **Lidocaine** 1.0-1.5 mg/kg IV push. Consider repeat in 3-5 min to maximum dose of 3 mg/kg. A single dose of 1.5 mg/kg in cardiac arrest is acceptable.
  - **Bretylium** 5 mg/kg IV push. Repeat in 5 min at 10 mg/kg.
  - **Magnesium sulfate** 1-2 g IV in torsades de pointes or suspected hypomagnesemic state or refractory VF.
  - **Procainamide** 30 mg/min in refractory VF (maximum total 17 mg/kg).

g. **Sodium bicarbonate** 1 mEq/kg IV:
  Class IIa
  - If known preexisting bicarbonate-responsive acidosis
  - If overdose with tricyclic antidepressants
  - To alkalinize the urine in drug overdoses
  Class IIb
  - If intubated and continued long arrest interval
  - Upon return of spontaneous circulation after long arrest interval
  Class III
  - Hypoxic lactic acidosis

From Cummins RO, editor: *Textbook of advanced cardiac life support*, Greenville, TX, 1994, American Heart Association.

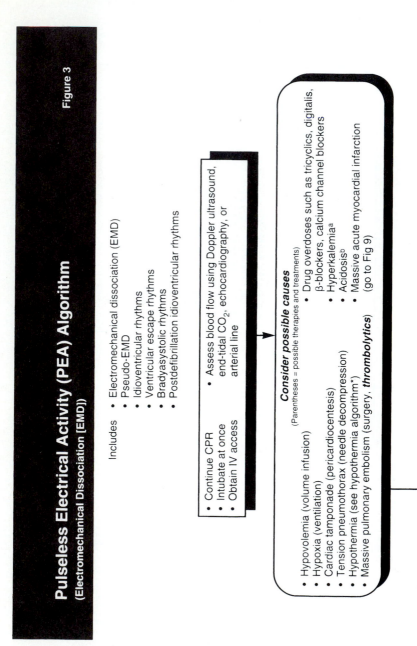

Pulseless Electrical Activity (PEA) Algorithm
(Electromechanical Dissociation [EMD])

Figure 3

Includes
- Electromechanical dissociation (EMD)
- Pseudo-EMD
- Idioventricular rhythms
- Ventricular escape rhythms
- Bradyasystolic rhythms
- Postdefibrillation idioventricular rhythms

- Continue CPR
- Intubate at once
- Obtain IV access

- Assess blood flow using Doppler ultrasound, end-tidal CO_2, echocardiography, or arterial line

Consider possible causes
(Parentheses = possible therapies and treatments)

- Hypovolemia (volume infusion)
- Hypoxia (ventilation)
- Cardiac tamponade (pericardiocentesis)
- Tension pneumothorax (needle decompression)
- Hypothermia (see hypothermia algorithm*)
- Massive pulmonary embolism (surgery, *thrombolytics*)

- Drug overdoses such as tricyclics, digitalis, β-blockers, calcium channel blockers
- Hyperkalemia[a]
- Acidosis[b]
- Massive acute myocardial infarction (go to Fig 9)

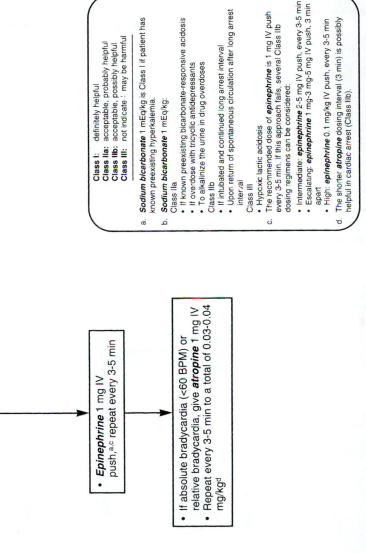

- *Epinephrine* 1 mg IV push,[a,c] repeat every 3-5 min

- If absolute bradycardia (<60 BPM) or relative bradycardia, give *atropine* 1 mg IV
- Repeat every 3-5 min to a total of 0.03-0.04 mg/kg[d]

Class I: definitely helpful
Class IIa: acceptable, probably helpful
Class IIb: acceptable, possibly helpful
Class III: not indicated; may be harmful

a. *Sodium bicarbonate* 1 mEq/kg is Class I if patient has known preexisting hyperkalemia.

b. *Sodium bicarbonate* 1 mEq/kg:
   Class IIa
   - If known preexisting bicarbonate-responsive acidosis
   - If overdose with tricyclic antidepressants
   - To alkalinize the urine in drug overdoses
   Class IIb
   - If intubated and continued long arrest interval
   - Upon return of spontaneous circulation after long arrest interval
   Class III
   - Hypoxic lactic acidosis

c. The recommended dose of *epinephrine* is 1 mg IV push every 3-5 min. If this approach fails, several Class IIb dosing regimens can be considered:
   - Intermediate: *epinephrine* 2-5 mg IV push, every 3-5 min
   - Escalating: *epinephrine* 1 mg-3 mg-5 mg IV push, 3 min apart
   - High: *epinephrine* 0.1 mg/kg IV push, every 3-5 min

d. The shorter *atropine* dosing interval (3 min) is possibly helpful in cardiac arrest (Class IIb).

From Cummins RO, editor: *Textbook of advanced cardiac life support*, Greenville, TX, 1994, American Heart Association.

*See p. 750.

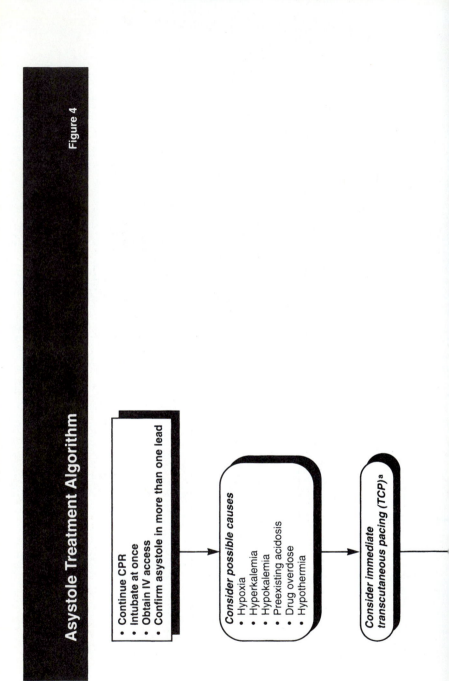

Asystole Treatment Algorithm

- **Continue CPR**
- **Intubate at once**
- **Obtain IV access**
- **Confirm asystole in more than one lead**

Consider possible causes
- Hypoxia
- Hyperkalemia
- Hypokalemia
- Preexisting acidosis
- Drug overdose
- Hypothermia

Consider immediate transcutaneous pacing (TCP)[a]

Figure 4

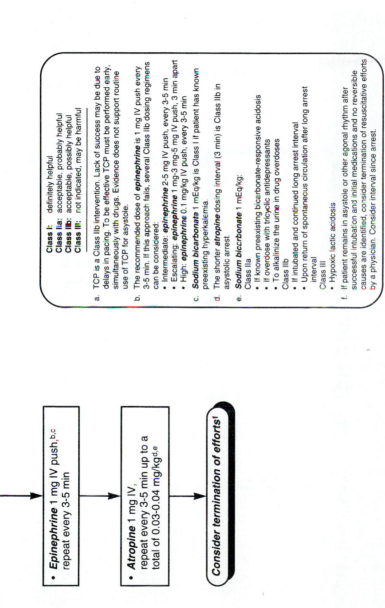

Class I: definitely helpful
Class IIa: acceptable, probably helpful
Class IIb: acceptable, possibly helpful
Class III: not indicated, may be harmful

a. TCP is a Class IIb intervention. Lack of success may be due to delays in pacing. To be effective TCP must be performed early, simultaneously with drugs. Evidence does not support routine use of TCP for asystole.

b. The recommended dose of *epinephrine* is 1 mg IV push every 3-5 min. If this approach fails, several Class IIb dosing regimens can be considered:
   • Intermediate: *epinephrine* 2-5 mg IV push, every 3-5 min
   • Escalating: *epinephrine* 1 mg-3 mg-5 mg IV push, 3 min apart
   • High: *epinephrine* 0.1 mg/kg IV push, every 3-5 min

c. *Sodium bicarbonate* 1 mEq/kg is Class I if patient has known preexisting hyperkalemia.

d. The shorter *atropine* dosing interval (3 min) is Class IIb in asystolic arrest.

e. *Sodium bicarbonate* 1 mEq/kg:
   Class IIa
   • If known preexisting bicarbonate-responsive acidosis
   • If overdose with tricyclic antidepressants
   • To alkalinize the urine in drug overdoses
   Class IIb
   • If intubated and continued long arrest interval
   • Upon return of spontaneous circulation after long arrest interval
   Class III
   • Hypoxic lactic acidosis

f. If patient remains in asystole or other agonal rhythm after successful intubation and initial medications and no reversible causes are identified, consider termination of resuscitative efforts by a physician. Consider interval since arrest.

• *Epinephrine* 1 mg IV push,[b,c] repeat every 3-5 min

• *Atropine* 1 mg IV, repeat every 3-5 min up to a total of 0.03-0.04 mg/kg[d,e]

Consider termination of efforts[f]

From Cummins RO, editor: *Textbook of advanced cardiac life support*, Greenville, TX, 1994, American Heart Association.

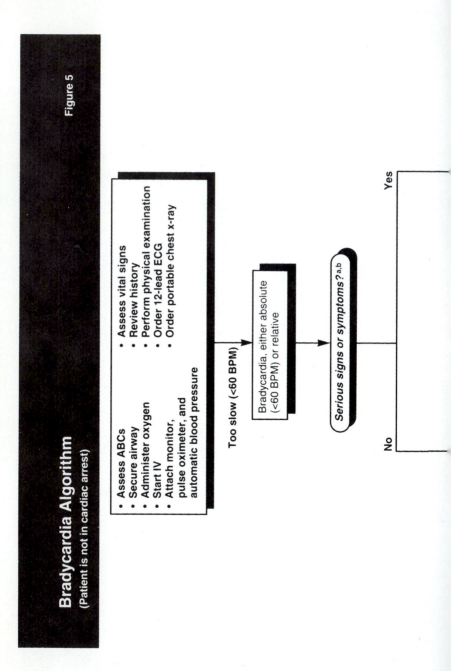

Bradycardia Algorithm
(Patient is not in cardiac arrest)

- Assess ABCs
- Secure airway
- Administer oxygen
- Start IV
- Attach monitor, pulse oximeter, and automatic blood pressure
- Assess vital signs
- Review history
- Perform physical examination
- Order 12-lead ECG
- Order portable chest x-ray

Too slow (<60 BPM)

Bradycardia, either absolute (<60 BPM) or relative

Serious signs or symptoms? [a,b]

No   Yes

Figure 5

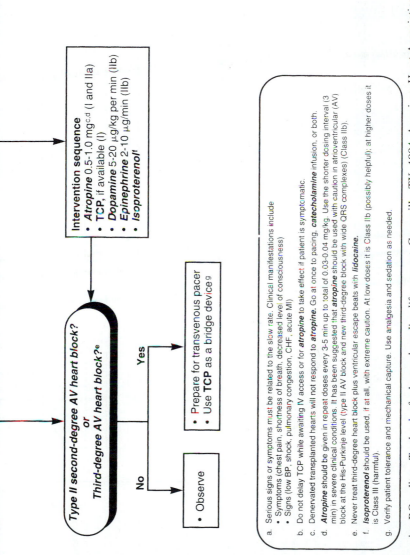

Type II second-degree AV heart block?
or
Third-degree AV heart block?[e]

Intervention sequence
- *Atropine* 0.5-1.0 mg[c,d] (I and IIa)
- **TCP**, if available (I)
- *Dopamine* 5-20 µg/kg per min (IIb)
- *Epinephrine* 2-10 µg/min (IIb)
- *Isoproterenol*[f]

No

- Observe

Yes

- Prepare for transvenous pacer
- Use **TCP** as a bridge device[g]

a. Serious signs or symptoms must be related to the slow rate. Clinical manifestations include
   - Symptoms (chest pain, shortness of breath, decreased level of consciousness)
   - Signs (low BP, shock, pulmonary congestion, CHF, acute MI)

b. Do not delay TCP while awaiting IV access or for *atropine* to take effect if patient is symptomatic.

c. Denervated transplanted hearts will not respond to *atropine*. Go at once to pacing, *catecholamine* infusion, or both.

d. *Atropine* should be given in repeat doses every 3-5 min up to total of 0.03-0.04 mg/kg. Use the shorter dosing interval (3 min) in severe clinical conditions. It has been suggested that *atropine* should be used with caution in atrioventricular (AV) block at the His-Purkinje level (type II AV block and new third-degree block with wide QRS complexes) (Class IIb).

e. Never treat third-degree heart block plus ventricular escape beats with *lidocaine*.

f. *Isoproterenol* should be used, if at all, with extreme caution. At low doses it is Class IIb (possibly helpful); at higher doses it is Class III (harmful).

g. Verify patient tolerance and mechanical capture. Use analgesia and sedation as needed.

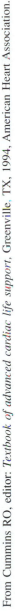

From Cummins RO, editor: *Textbook of advanced cardiac life support*, Greenville, TX, 1994, American Heart Association.

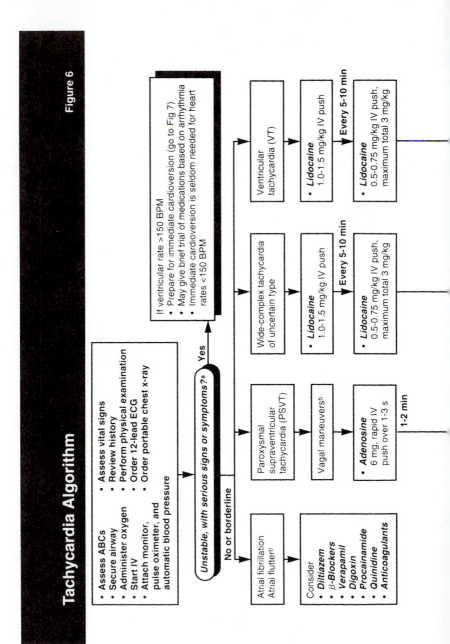

Tachycardia Algorithm

Figure 6

- Assess ABCs
- Secure airway
- Administer oxygen
- Start IV
- Attach monitor, pulse oximeter, and automatic blood pressure
- Assess vital signs
- Review history
- Perform physical examination
- Order 12-lead ECG
- Order portable chest x-ray

Unstable, with serious signs or symptoms?[a]

No or borderline

Yes

If ventricular rate >150 BPM
- Prepare for immediate cardioversion (go to Fig 7)
- May give brief trial of medications based on arrhythmia
- Immediate cardioversion is seldom needed for heart rates <150 BPM

Atrial fibrillation Atrial flutter[b]

Consider
- *Diltiazem*
- *β-Blockers*
- *Verapamil*
- *Digoxin*
- *Procainamide*
- *Quinidine*
- *Anticoagulants*

Paroxysmal supraventricular tachycardia (PSVT)

Vagal maneuvers[b]

- *Adenosine* 6 mg, rapid IV push over 1-3 s

1-2 min

Wide-complex tachycardia of uncertain type

- *Lidocaine* 1.0-1.5 mg/kg IV push

Every 5-10 min

- *Lidocaine* 0.5-0.75 mg/kg IV push, maximum total 3 mg/kg

Ventricular tachycardia (VT)

- *Lidocaine* 1.0-1.5 mg/kg IV push

Every 5-10 min

- *Lidocaine* 0.5-0.75 mg/kg IV push, maximum total 3 mg/kg

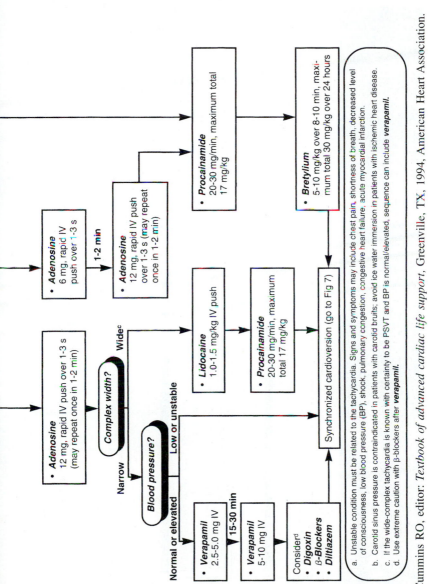

Adenosine
12 mg, rapid IV push over 1-3 s
(may repeat once in 1-2 min)

Complex width?

Narrow

Wide[c]

Blood pressure?

Normal or elevated

Low or unstable

Adenosine
6 mg, rapid IV
push over 1-3 s

1-2 min

Adenosine
12 mg, rapid IV push
over 1-3 s (may repeat
once in 1-2 min)

Lidocaine
1.0-1.5 mg/kg IV push

Procainamide
20-30 mg/min, maximum
total 17 mg/kg

Procainamide
20-30 mg/min, maximum total
17 mg/kg

Bretylium
5-10 mg/kg over 8-10 min, maximum total 30 mg/kg over 24 hours

Synchronized cardioversion (go to Fig 7)

Verapamil
2.5-5.0 mg IV

15-30 min

Verapamil
5-10 mg IV

Consider[d]
• **Digoxin**
• **β-Blockers**
• **Diltiazem**

a. Unstable condition must be related to the tachycardia. Signs and symptoms may include chest pain, shortness of breath, decreased level
    of consciousness, low blood pressure (BP), shock, pulmonary congestion, congestive heart failure, acute myocardial infarction.
b. Carotid sinus pressure is contraindicated in patients with carotid bruits; avoid ice water immersion in patients with ischemic heart disease.
c. If the wide-complex tachycardia is known with certainty to be PSVT and BP is normal/elevated, sequence can include *verapamil*.
d. Use extreme caution with β-blockers after *verapamil*.

From Cummins RO, editor: *Textbook of advanced cardiac life support*, Greenville, TX, 1994, American Heart Association.

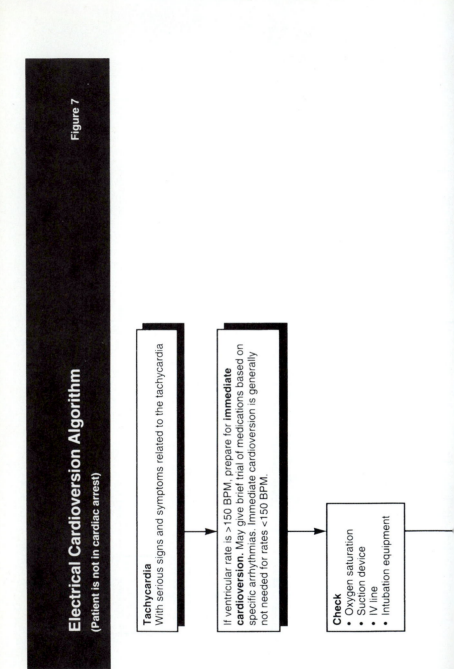

Electrical Cardioversion Algorithm
(Patient is not in cardiac arrest)

Tachycardia
With serious signs and symptoms related to the tachycardia

If ventricular rate is >150 BPM, prepare for **immediate cardioversion.** May give brief trial of medications based on specific arrhythmias. Immediate cardioversion is generally not needed for rates <150 BPM.

Check
- Oxygen saturation
- Suction device
- IV line
- Intubation equipment

Figure 7

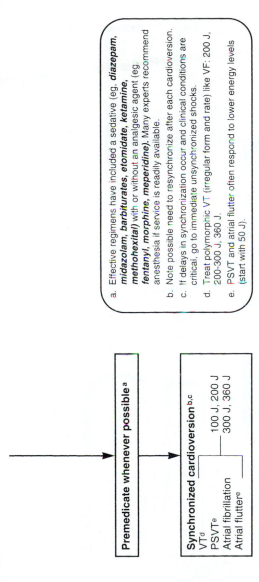

Premedicate whenever possible[a]

Synchronized cardioversion[b,c]

VT[d]	— 100 J, 200 J
PSVT[e]	300 J, 360 J
Atrial fibrillation	
Atrial flutter[e]	

a. Effective regimens have included a sedative (eg, *diazepam, midazolam, barbiturates, etomidate, ketamine, methohexital*) with or without an analgesic agent (eg, *fentanyl, morphine, meperidine*). Many experts recommend anesthesia if service is readily available.

b. Note possible need to resynchronize after each cardioversion.

c. If delays in synchronization occur and clinical conditions are critical, go to immediate unsynchronized shocks.

d. Treat polymorphic VT (irregular form and rate) like VF: 200 J, 200-300 J, 360 J.

e. PSVT and atrial flutter often respond to lower energy levels (start with 50 J).

From Cummins RO, editor: *Textbook of advanced cardiac life support*, Greenville, TX, 1994, American Heart Association.

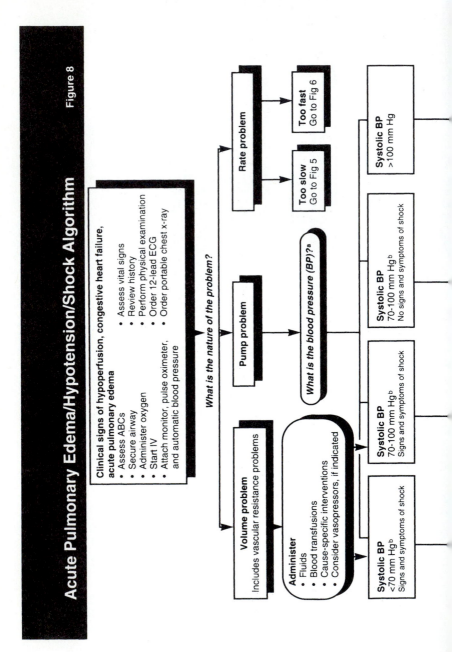

Acute Pulmonary Edema/Hypotension/Shock Algorithm

Figure 8

Clinical signs of hypoperfusion, congestive heart failure, acute pulmonary edema
- Assess ABCs
- Secure airway
- Administer oxygen
- Start IV
- Attach monitor, pulse oximeter, and automatic blood pressure
- Assess vital signs
- Review history
- Perform physical examination
- Order 12-lead ECG
- Order portable chest x-ray

What is the nature of the problem?

Volume problem
Includes vascular resistance problems

Pump problem

Rate problem

Too slow
Go to Fig 5

Too fast
Go to Fig 6

Administer
- Fluids
- Blood transfusions
- Cause-specific interventions
- Consider vasopressors, if indicated

What is the blood pressure (BP)? [a]

Systolic BP
<70 mm Hg [b]
Signs and symptoms of shock

Systolic BP
70-100 mm Hg [b]
Signs and symptoms of shock

Systolic BP
70-100 mm Hg [b]
No signs and symptoms of shock

Systolic BP
>100 mm Hg

Consider
- **Norepinephrine**
  0.5-30 µg/min IV or
- **Dopamine**
  5-20 µg/kg per min

- **Dopamine**[c]
  2.5-20 µg/kg per min IV
  (Add **norepinephrine** if **dopamine** is >20 µg/kg per min)

- **Dobutamine**[d,e]
  2-20 µg/kg per min IV

- **Nitroglycerin** start 10-20 µg/min IV
  (use if ischemia persists and BP remains elevated. Titrate to effect)
  and/or
- **Nitroprusside** 0.1-5.0 µg/kg per min IV

Consider
further actions, especially if the patient is in acute pulmonary edema

First-line actions
- **Furosemide** IV 0.5-1.0 mg/kg
- **Morphine** IV 1-3 mg
- **Nitroglycerin** SL
- **Oxygen**/intubate PRN

Second-line actions
- **Nitroglycerin** IV if BP >100 mm Hg
- **Nitroprusside** IV if BP >100 mm Hg
- **Dopamine** if BP <100 mm Hg
- **Dobutamine** if BP >100 mm Hg
- Positive end-expiratory pressure (PEEP)
- Continuous positive airway pressure (CPAP)

Third-line actions
- **Amrinone** 0.75 mg/kg then 5-15 µg/kg per min (if other drugs fail)
- **Aminophylline** 5 mg/kg (if wheezing)
- **Thrombolytic** therapy (if not in shock)
- **Digoxin** (if atrial fibrillation, supraventricular tachycardias)
- Angioplasty (if drugs fail)
- Intra-aortic balloon pump (bridge to surgery)
- Surgical interventions (valves, coronary artery bypass grafts, heart transplant)

a. Base management after this point on invasive hemodynamic monitoring if possible. Guidelines presume clinical signs of hypoperfusion.
b. Fluid bolus of 250-500 mL normal saline should be tried. If no response, consider sympathomimetics.
c. Move to **dopamine** and stop **norepinephrine** when BP improves. Avoid **dopamine** (consider **dobutamine**) if no signs of hypoperfusion.
d. Add **dopamine** (and avoid **dobutamine**) if systolic BP drops below 90 mm Hg.
e. Start with **nitroglycerin** if initial blood pressures are in this range.

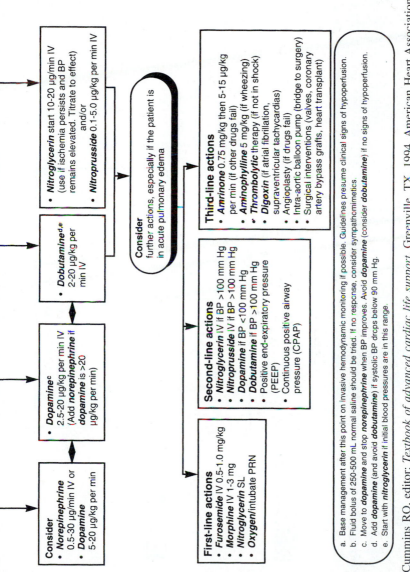

From Cummins RO, editor: *Textbook of advanced cardiac life support*, Greenville, TX, 1994, American Heart Association.

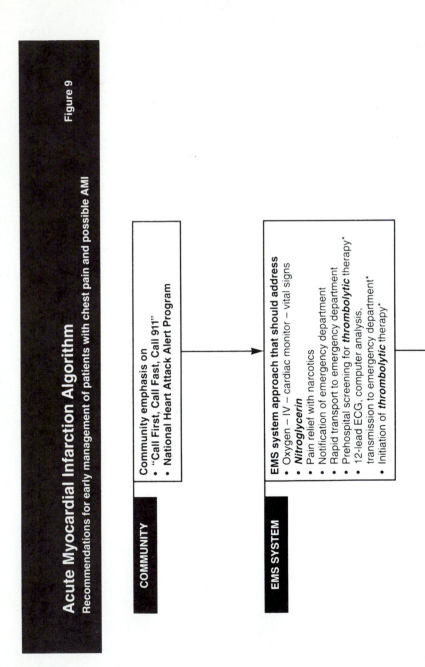

Acute Myocardial Infarction Algorithm
Recommendations for early management of patients with chest pain and possible AMI

Figure 9

COMMUNITY

Community emphasis on
- "Call First, Call Fast, Call 911"
- National Heart Attack Alert Program

EMS SYSTEM

EMS system approach that should address
- Oxygen – IV – cardiac monitor – vital signs
- *Nitroglycerin*
- Pain relief with narcotics
- Notification of emergency department
- Rapid transport to emergency department
- Prehospital screening for *thrombolytic* therapy*
- 12-lead ECG, computer analysis, transmission to emergency department*
- Initiation of *thrombolytic* therapy*

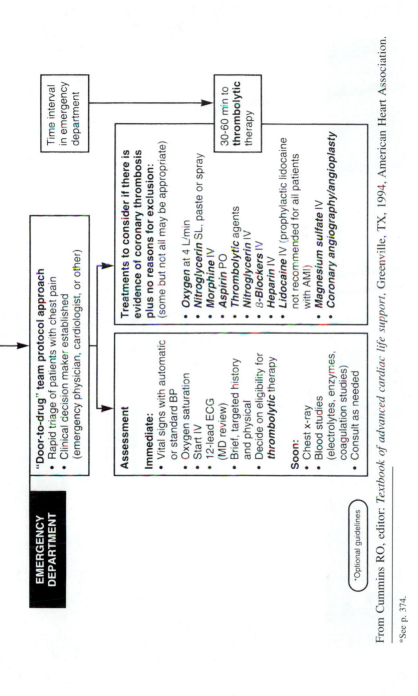

EMERGENCY DEPARTMENT

Time interval in emergency department

"Door-to-drug" team protocol approach
- Rapid triage of patients with chest pain
- Clinical decision maker established (emergency physician, cardiologist, or other)

30-60 min to **thrombolytic** therapy

Assessment

Immediate:
- Vital signs with automatic or standard BP
- Oxygen saturation
- Start IV
- 12-lead ECG (MD review)
- Brief, targeted history and physical
- Decide on eligibility for *thrombolytic* therapy

Soon:
- Chest x-ray
- Blood studies (electrolytes, enzymes, coagulation studies)
- Consult as needed

Treatments to consider if there is evidence of coronary thrombosis plus no reasons for exclusion:
(some but not all may be appropriate)
- *Oxygen* at 4 L/min
- *Nitroglycerin* SL, paste or spray
- *Morphine* IV
- *Aspirin* PO
- *Thrombolytic* agents
- *Nitroglycerin* IV
- *β-Blockers* IV
- *Heparin* IV
- *Lidocaine* IV (prophylactic lidocaine not recommended for all patients with AMI)
- *Magnesium sulfate* IV
- *Coronary angiography/angioplasty*

*Optional guidelines

From Cummins RO, editor: *Textbook of advanced cardiac life support*, Greenville, TX, 1994, American Heart Association.

*See p. 374.

Hypothermia Algorithm

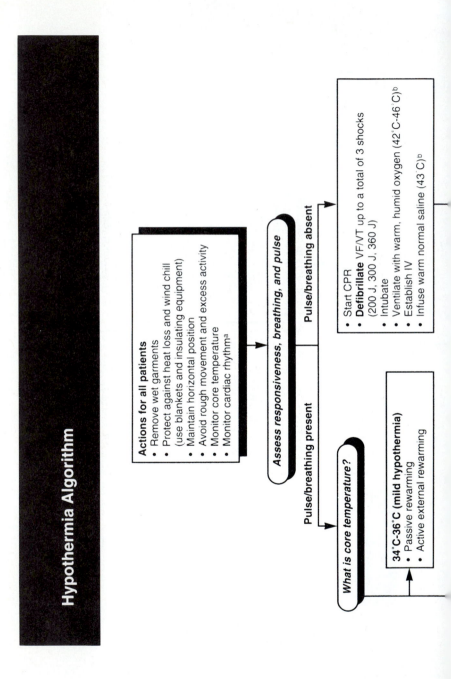

Actions for all patients
- Remove wet garments
- Protect against heat loss and wind chill (use blankets and insulating equipment)
- Maintain horizontal position
- Avoid rough movement and excess activity
- Monitor core temperature
- Monitor cardiac rhythm[a]

Assess responsiveness, breathing, and pulse

Pulse/breathing present

Pulse/breathing absent

What is core temperature?

34°C-36°C (mild hypothermia)
- Passive rewarming
- Active external rewarming

- Start CPR
- **Defibrillate** VF/VT up to a total of 3 shocks (200 J, 300 J, 360 J)
- Intubate
- Ventilate with warm, humid oxygen (42°C-46°C)[b]
- Establish IV
- Infuse warm normal saline (43°C)[b]

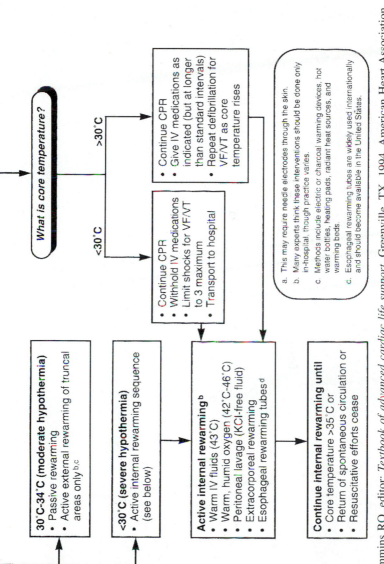

What is core temperature?

<30°C

- Continue CPR
- Withhold IV medications
- Limit shocks for VF/VT to 3 maximum
- Transport to hospital

>30°C

- Continue CPR
- Give IV medications as indicated (but at longer than standard intervals)
- Repeat defibrillation for VF/VT as core temperature rises

a. This may require needle electrodes through the skin.

b. Many experts think these interventions should be done only in-hospital, though practice varies.

c. Methods include electric or charcoal warming devices, hot water bottles, heating pads, radiant heat sources, and warming beds.

d. Esophageal rewarming tubes are widely used internationally and should become available in the United States.

30°C-34°C (moderate hypothermia)
- Passive rewarming
- Active external rewarming of truncal areas only [b,c]

<30°C (severe hypothermia)
- Active internal rewarming sequence (see below)

Active internal rewarming [b]
- Warm IV fluids (43°C)
- Warm, humid oxygen (42°C-46°C)
- Peritoneal lavage (KCl-free fluid)
- Extracorporeal rewarming
- Esophageal rewarming tubes [d]

Continue internal rewarming until
- Core temperature >35°C or
- Return of spontaneous circulation or
- Resuscitative efforts cease

From Cummins RO, editor: *Textbook of advanced cardiac life support*, Greenville, TX, 1994, American Heart Association.

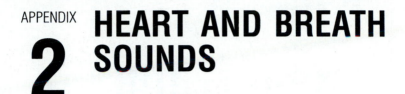

APPENDIX **2** **HEART AND BREATH SOUNDS**

Assessing heart sounds

Sound	Auscultation site	Timing	Pitch	Clinical occurrence	End-piece/patient position
S_1 (M_1 T_1)	Apex	Beginning of systole	High	Closing of mitral and tricuspid valves; normal sound	Diaphragm/patient supine
S_1 split	Apex	Beginning of systole	High	Ventricles contracting at different times due to electrical or mechanical problems (e.g., a longer time span between M_1 T_1 caused by right bundle-branch heart block, or reversal [T_1, M_1] caused by mitral stenosis)	Same as S_1
S_2 (A_2 P_2)	A_2 at second ICS, RSB; P_2 at second ICS, LSB	End of systole	High	Closing of aortic and pulmonic valves; normal sound	Diaphragm/patient supine
S_2 physiologic split	Second ICS, LSB	End of systole	High	Accentuated by inspiration; disappears on expiration. Sound that corresponds with the respiratory cycle due to normal delay in closure of pulmonic valve during inspiration. It is accentuated during exercise or in individuals with thin chest walls; heard most often in children and young adults	Same as S_2
S_2 persistent (wide) split	Second ICS, LSB	End of systole	High	Heard throughout the respiratory cycle; caused by late closure of pulmonic valve or early closure of aortic valve. Occurs in atrial septal defect, right ventricular failure, pulmonic stenosis, hypertension, or right bundle-branch heart block	Same as S_2

S$_2$ paradoxic (reversed) split (P$_2$ A$_2$)	Second ICS, LSB	End of systole	High	Because of delayed left ventricular systole, the aortic valve closes after the pulmonic valve rather than before it. (Normally during expiration the two sounds merge.) Causes may include left bundle-branch heart block, aortic stenosis, severe left ventricular failure, MI, and severe hypertension	Same as S$_2$
S$_2$ fixed split	Second ICS, LSB	End of systole	High	Heard with equal intensity during inspiration and expiration due to split of pulmonic and aortic components, which are unaffected by blood volume or respiratory changes. May be heard in pulmonary stenosis or atrial septal defect	Same as S$_2$
S$_3$ (ventricular gallop)	Apex	Early diastole just after S$_2$	Dull, low	Early and rapid filling of ventricle, as in early ventricular failure, CHF. Common in children, during last trimester of pregnancy, and possibly in healthy adults >50 yr of age	Bell/patient in left lateral or supine position
S$_4$ (atrial gallop)	Apex	Late in diastole just before S$_1$	Low	Atrium filling against increased resistance of stiff ventricle, as in CHF, coronary artery disease, cardiomyopathy, pulmonary artery hypertension, ventricular failure. May be normal in infants, children, and athletes	Same as S$_3$

ICS, Intercostal space; *LSB*, left sternal border; *RSB*, right sternal border.

Commonly occurring heart murmurs

Type	Timing	Pitch	Quality	Auscultation site	Radiation
Pulmonic stenosis	Systolic ejection	Medium-high	Harsh	Second ICS, LSB	Toward left shoulder, back
Aortic stenosis	Midsystolic	Medium-high	Harsh	Second ICS, RSB	Toward carotid arteries
Ventricular septal defect	Late systolic	High	Blowing	Fourth ICS, LSB	Toward RSB
Mitral insufficiency	Holosystolic	High	Blowing	Fifth-sixth ICS, left MCL	Toward left axilla
Tricuspid insufficiency	Holosystolic	High	Blowing	Fourth ICS, LSB	Toward apex
Aortic insufficiency	Early diastolic	High	Blowing	Second ICS, RSB	Toward sternum
Pulmonary insufficiency	Early diastolic	High	Blowing	Second ICS, LSB	Toward sternum
Mitral stenosis	Mid-late diastolic	Low	Rumbling	Fifth ICS, left MCL	Usually none
Tricuspid stenosis	Mid-late diastolic	Low	Rumbling	Fourth ICS, LSB	Usually none

ICS, Intercostal space; *LSB*, left sternal border; *MCL*, midclavicular line; *RSB*, right sternal border.

Assessing normal breath sounds

Type	Normal site	Duration	Characteristics
Vesicular	Peripheral lung	I > E	Soft and swishing sounds. Abnormal when heard over the large airways
Bronchial	Trachea and bronchi	E > I	Louder, coarser, and of longer duration than vesicular. Abnormal if heard over peripheral lung
Bronchovesicular	Sternal border of major bronchi	E = I	Moderate in pitch and intensity. Abnormal if heard over peripheral lung

I, Inspiration; *E,* expiration.

Assessing adventitious breath sounds

Type	Waveform	Characteristics	Possible clinical condition
Coarse crackle		Discontinuous, explosive, interrupted. Loud; low in pitch	Pulmonary edema; pneumonia in resolution stage
Fine crackle		Discontinuous, explosive, interrupted. Less loud than coarse crackles, lower in pitch, and of shorter duration	Interstitial lung disease; heart failure; atelectasis
Wheeze		Continuous, of long duration, high pitched, musical, hissing	Narrowing of airway; bronchial asthma; COPD
Rhonchus		Continuous, of long duration, low pitched, snoring	Production of sputum (usually cleared or lessened by coughing or suctioning)
Pleural friction rub		Grating, rasping noise	Rubbing together of inflamed parietal linings; loss of normal pleural lubrication

Assessing respiratory patterns

Type	Waveform	Characteristics	Possible clinical condition
Eupnea		Normal rate and rhythm for adults and teenagers (12–20 breaths/min)	Normal pattern while awake
Bradypnea		Decreased rate (<12 breaths/min); regular rhythm	Normal sleep pattern; opiate or alcohol use; tumor; metabolic disorder
Tachypnea		Rapid rate (>20 breaths/min); hypoventilation or hyperventilation	Fever; restrictive respiratory disorders; pulmonary emboli
Hyperpnea		Depth of respirations greater than normal	Meeting increased metabolic demand (e.g., sepsis, MODS, SIRS, and exercise)
Apnea		Cessation of breathing; may be intermittent	Intermittent with CNS disturbances or drug intoxication; obstructed airway; respiratory arrest if it persists
Kussmaul's		Deep, rapid (>20 breaths/min), sighing, labored	Renal failure, DKA, sepsis, shock
Cheyne-Stokes		Alternating patterns of apnea (10–20 sec) with periods of deep and rapid breathing. Lesions located bilaterally and deep within cerebral hemispheres	CHF, opiate or hypnotic overdose, thyrotoxicosis, dissecting aneurysm, subarachnoid hemorrhage, IICP, aortic valve disorders; may be normal in older adults during sleep
Central neurogenic hyperventilation		Rapid (>20 breaths/min), deep, regular. Lesions of midbrain or upper pons thought to be source of pattern	Primary injury (ischemia, infarction, space-occupying lesion); secondary injury (IICP, metabolic disorders, drug overdose)

Continued.

Assessing respiratory patterns—cont'd

Type	Waveform	Characteristics	Possible clinical condition
Apneustic		Deep, prolonged inspiration, followed by 20-30 sec pause and short expiration. Lesion located in lower pons	Anoxia, meningitis, basilar artery occlusion
Cluster		Irregular breaths occurring in clusters with periods of apnea. Overall pattern irregular. Lesion located in lower pons or upper medulla	Primary and secondary injury as above may produce this respiratory pattern
Ataxic (Biot's)		Irregular deep or shallow breaths. No discernible pattern. Lesion located in medulla	Primary and secondary injury as above may produce this respiratory pattern

3 GLASGOW COMA SCALE

Parameter	Patient response	Score
Best eye opening response (record "C" if eyes closed due to swelling)	Spontaneously	4
	To speech	3
	To pain	2
	No response	1
Best motor response (record best upper limb response to painful stimuli)	Obeys verbal command	6
	Localizes pain	5
	Flexion—withdrawal	4
	Flexion—abnormal	3
	Extension—abnormal	2
	No response	1
Best verbal response (record "E" if endotracheal tube is in place or "T" if tracheostomy tube is in place)	Conversation—oriented $\times$ 3	5
	Conversation—confused	4
	Speech—inappropriate	3
	Sounds—incomprehensible	2
	No response	1

Total score	Interpretation
15	Normal
13-15	Minor head injury
9-12	Moderate head injury
3-8	Severe head injury
≤ 7	Coma
3	Deep coma or brain death

CRANIAL NERVES: FUNCTIONS AND DYSFUNCTIONS

Cranial nerve	Type	Functions	Dysfunctions
I Olfactory	Sensory	Smell	Anosmia
II Optic	Sensory	Sight	Blindness
		Visual acuity	Visual field deficits
		Visual fields	
		Fundus	
III Oculomotor	Motor	Pupillary constriction	Ptosis, diplopia, pupillary dilatation, strabismus
		Elevation of upper eyelid	
		Extraocular movements	
IV Trochlear	Motor	Downward and inward movement of eye	Eye will not move down or out
V Trigeminal	Sensory and motor	*Motor:* Temporal and masseter muscles (jaw clenching and lateral movement for mastication)	Paresis or paralysis of muscles of mastication, decreased facial sensation
		Sensory: Facial, scalp, anterior two thirds of tongue, lips, teeth, proprioception for mastication, corneal reflex	Loss of corneal reflex
VI Abducens	Motor	Lateral eye movement	Eye will not move laterally
VII Facial	Sensory and motor	*Sensory:* Taste in anterior two thirds tongue, proprioception for face and scalp	Loss of taste in anterior two thirds tongue
		Motor: Facial expression, lacrimal and salivary glands	Paresis or paralysis of facial muscles, facial droop, loss of secretion of submandibular, sublingual, and lacrimal glands
VIII Acoustic	Sensory	*Cochlear division:* Hearing	Tinnitus, deafness
		Vestibular division: Balance	Vertigo, nystagmus

		Function	Dysfunction
IX Glossopharyngeal	Sensory and motor	*Sensory:* Taste in posterior one third tongue; pain, touch, heat, cold in tongue, tonsils, soft palate, and pharynx. *Motor:* Elevation of the soft palate, movement of pharynx, secretion and vasodilatation of parotid glands for saliva; gag reflex	Loss of taste, pain, touch, heat, and cold in posterior one third tongue, tonsils, and soft palate. Paresis or paralysis of soft palate and pharynx, dysphagia, dysarthria, hoarseness, loss of gag reflex
X Vagus	Sensory and motor	*Sensory:* Muscles of pharynx, larynx, esophagus, and thoracic and abdominal viscera; external ear, mucous membranes of larynx, trachea, esophagus, thoracic and abdominal viscera; lungs (stretch receptors), aortic bodies (chemoreceptors), respiratory/GI tract (pain receptors) *Motor:* Muscles of pharynx, larynx, esophagus, thoracic and abdominal viscera; respiratory/GI tract (smooth muscle), pacemaker and cardiac atrial muscle	Similar to dysfunction of glossopharyngeal Loss of gag reflex and difficulty swallowing
XI Spinal accessory	Motor	Sternocleidomastoid and trapezius muscles	Paresis or paralysis of sternocleidomastoid and trapezius muscles Inability to turn head or shrug shoulders
XII Hypoglossal	Motor	Tongue movement	Paresis or paralysis of the tongue

5 MAJOR DEEP TENDON (MUSCLE-STRETCH) REFLEXES

Reflex	Innervation	Examination technique	Normal response
Biceps	C5, C6	Arm partially flexed at elbow, palm down. Place thumb or finger on biceps tendon. Strike finger with reflex hammer	Contraction of biceps muscle Flexion at elbow
Triceps	C6, C7	Arm flexed at elbow, palm toward body, arm pulled slightly across body. Strike triceps tendon with reflex hammer above elbow	Contraction of triceps muscle Extension of arm at elbow
Brachioradialis	C5, C6	Hand resting on abdomen, palm slightly pronated. Strike radius with reflex hammer 3-5 cm above wrist	Contraction of brachioradialis muscle. Flexion and supination of forearm
Achilles (Ankle jerk)	S1, S2	Leg flexed at knee, dorsiflex the foot. Strike Achilles tendon	Plantar flexion of foot
Quadriceps (Knee jerk)	L3, L4	Leg flexed at knee. Strike patellar tendon	Contraction of quadriceps muscle. Extension of knee

See "Grading of deep tendon reflexes" on next page.

GRADING OF DEEP TENDON REFLEXES

Scale (0 to 4+)	Interpretation
4+	Very brisk, hyperactive, repetitive, rhythmic flexion and extension (clonus); indicative of disease
3+	Brisker than average; may be normal for certain individuals or may indicate disease
2+	Average/normal
1+	Diminished response or low normal
0	No response

APPENDIX

6 MAJOR SUPERFICIAL (CUTANEOUS) REFLEXES

Reflex	Innervation	Examination technique	Normal response
Abdominals Above/upper Below/lower	T8, T9, T10 T10, T11, T12	Using tongue blade or wooden end of cotton-tipped applicator, lightly stroke abdomen in each quadrant, outer to inner direction, toward umbilicus	Contraction of abdominal muscles Umbilicus deviates (pulls) toward the stimulus
Bulbocavernous (male)	S3, S4	Pinch glans penis or apply pressure over bulbocavernous muscle behind scrotum	Scrotum will elevate toward the body
Corneal	Cranial nerves V and VII	Using wisp of cotton, lightly touch cornea	Eyelids will quickly close
Cremasteric (male)	L1, L2	Lightly stroke inner aspect of thigh	Testicle on side stroked will elevate
Gag	Cranial nerves IX and X	Using tongue blade, lightly touch posterior pharynx	Gagging or retching
Perianal	S3, S4, S5	Stroke tissue surrounding anus with blunt instrument, or examine rectum by gently inserting gloved finger	Anal puckering with external stimuli. Tightening of anal sphincter with internal examination

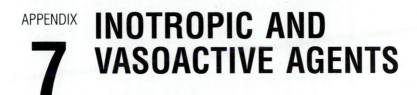

APPENDIX

7

INOTROPIC AND VASOACTIVE AGENTS

Agent	Effects				Dosage	Nursing implications
	(Preload)		(Afterload)			
	HR	PAWP	SVR	Contractility		
Inotropics/vasoactives						
dopamine hydrochloride (Intropin)	—↑	→	——	↑↑	Low dose 1-2 µg/kg/min	Affect cardiac contractility and vascular resistance
	—	—	↑↑	—	Moderate dose 2-10 µg/kg/min High dose >10 µg/kg/min	Major effect is increasing urine output; may potentiate effect of diuretics
dobutamine (Dobutrex)	—↑	—→	—	↑↑	2.5-10 µg/kg/min	Can cause tissue necrosis and sloughing if infiltration occurs; Overall effect is improved CO; may cause tachycardia and dysrhythmias as side effects
isoproterenol (Isuprel)	↑↑	—→	↓↓	↑↑	2-10 µg/kg/min	Significant increase in myocardial oxygen consumption; can produce ventricular tachycardia and fibrillation
norepinephrine (Levophed)	↓↑	↑	↑↑↑	↑	2-12 µg/min	Contraindicated when hypotension occurs secondary to hypovolemia. Can cause tissue necrosis and sloughing if infiltration occurs. Increased myocardial oxygen demand without increased coronary artery flow can cause myocardial ischemia and infarction

					Dose	Comments
epinephrine	⇈	↑	↓↑	⇈	0.5-1 mg for cardiac arrest 1-4 µg/kg/min for inotropic support	May induce ventricular ectopy
amrinone lactate (Inocor)	—↑	↓	↓	↑	2-20 µg/kg/min	Can exacerbate myocardial ischemia
Vasopressors						Main effect is vasoconstriction of peripheral blood vessels
methoxamine hydrochloride (Vasoxyl)	—	↑	⇈	—	3-5 mg	Used rarely; may increase myocardial oxygen demand
phenylephrine (Neo-Synephrine)	—	↑	⇈	—	0.1-0.5 mg	May cause dysrhythmias or trigger reflex bradycardia
Vasodilators						Main effect is dilatation of arterial and/or venous beds
sodium nitroprusside (Nipride)	—↑	↓	⇊	—	0.5-0.8 µg/kg/min	Drug is photosensitive; keep infusion container protected from light. Thiocyanate (a metabolite of nitroprusside) toxicity can occur after 72 h. Monitor thiocyanate levels daily, being alert to levels >10 mg/dl and for signs of metabolic acidosis (see p. 720)
nitroglycerin (Tridil, Nitrostat)	—↑	⇊	↓	—	0.5 µg/min	Absorbed by standard plastic IV tubing. Use special polyvinyl chloride tubing. Ensure that the drug is diluted for IV use

—, No effect; ↑, minimal effect; ⇈, moderate effect; ⇈⇈, major effect.

APPENDIX

8

INFECTION PREVENTION AND CONTROL

For several decades, infection prevention and control has focused on the use of barriers (e.g., gloves, gowns, and masks) to interrupt transmission of organisms among and between patients and health-care workers. These barriers are a major component of various systems of isolation precautions.

Systems of Isolation Precautions

Five different systems of isolation precautions (Table A-1) commonly have been used in hospitals. The Centers for Disease Control and Prevention (CDC) revised its guidelines for isolation precautions in 1995 to meet the following objectives: (1) to be epidemiologically sound, (2) to recognize the importance of all body fluids, secretions, and excretions in the transmission of nosocomial pathogens, (3) to ensure adequate precautions for infections transmitted by the airborne, droplet, and contact routes of transmission, (4) to be as simple and user friendly as possible, and (5) to use new terms to avoid confusion with existing infection control and isolation systems. The 1995 guideline contains two tiers of precautions (Table A-2): **Standard Precautions**, which are designed for the care of all patients in hospitals regardless of their diagnosis or presumed infection status, and **Transmission-based Precautions,** which are used for patients known to be or suspected of being infected or colonized with epidemiologically important pathogens that can be transmitted by airborne or droplet transmission or by contact with dry skin or contaminated surfaces.

The 1995 guideline replaces the 1983 guideline for isolation precautions in hospitals, which offered three options: a Category-Specific system, a Disease-Specific system, and a Hospital-Designed system. Body Substance Isolation (BSI) is a Hospital-Designed system that has been adopted by many hospitals in the United States and elsewhere. In 1987-1988, the CDC introduced Universal Precautions to reduce health-care workers' risk of being exposed to bloodborne pathogens. The 1995 Standard Precautions system synthesizes the major features of Universal Precautions and Body Substance Isolation and applies to (1) blood, (2) all body fluids, secretions, and excretions regardless of whether they contain visible blood, (3) nonintact skin, and (4) mucous

Text continued on p. 786.

TABLE A-1 Comparison of five systems of infection precautions in different situations§

Situation	Category-Specific*	Disease-Specific*	Body Substance Isolation (BSI)†	Universal Precautions (regulated by OSHA)‡	Standard Precautions§
Patient known to have HBV, HCV, HIV, or other bloodborne disease	The category of Blood and Body Fluid Precautions was replaced by Universal Precautions in 1987 (revised in 1988); superseded by Standard Precautions in 1995	Use Standard Precautions	Principles of BSI were incorporated into Standard Precautions in 1995	Use Standard Precautions	See Table A-2, Standard Precautions
Patient not known to have HBV, HCV, HIV, or other bloodborne disease	Use Standard Precautions	Use Standard Precautions	Use Standard Precautions	Use Standard Precautions	See Table A-2, Standard Precautions
Patient with diagnosed enteric disease (e.g., shigellosis)	Enteric Precautions, including sign on door, used until 1994; superseded by Standard Precautions in 1995	Precautions under named disease in 1983 CDC guideline and sign on door until 1994; superseded by Standard Precautions in 1995	Use of barriers based on interaction with patient's body substances, not patient's diagnosis; principles incorporated into Standard Precautions in 1995	Universal Precautions did not apply to feces unless visibly bloody; Universal Precautions were not intended for fecal-to-oral disease; Standard Precautions apply to feces, regardless	See Table A-2, Standard Precautions

Patient not known to have enteric disease	No special precautions due to absence of diagnosis; routine patient care practices followed; superseded by Standard Precautions in 1995, which apply to diagnosed and undiagnosed patients	No special precautions, because Disease-Specific Precautions were used only for diagnosed patients; superseded by Standard Precautions in 1995, which apply to diagnosed and undiagnosed patients	Same as above; BSI principles and practices apply to diagnosed and undiagnosed patients	of whether the patient is diagnosed with a fecal-to-oral disease Same as above	See Table A-2, Standard Precautions
Patient diagnosed with varicella (chickenpox)	Strict Isolation and sign on door used until 1994; superseded by Transmission-based Precautions in 1995	Precautions under named disease in 1983 CDC guideline; superseded by Transmission-based Precautions in 1995	Susceptible persons should not be assigned to care for patients; immune personnel can provide care with no precautions other than those for BSI; sign on door to restrict entry of persons; door closed; similar to 1995 Transmission-based Precautions: Airborne	Universal Precautions do not apply to airborne communicable diseases such as chickenpox	See Table A-2, Transmission-based Precautions: Airborne, and Transmission-based Precautions: Contact; susceptible persons should stay out of room

Continued.

TABLE A-1 Comparison of five systems of infection precautions in different situations—cont'd

Situation	Category-Specific*	Disease-Specific*	Body Substance Isolation (BSI)†	Universal Precautions (regulated by OSHA)‡	Standard Precautions§
Patient diagnosed with or suspected of having pulmonary or laryngeal tuberculosis (TB)	AFB Isolation, sign on door, door closed, room with special ventilation; superseded by Transmission-based Precautions: Airborne in 1995	Precautions under named disease in 1983 CDC guideline; superseded by Transmission-based Precautions: Airborne in 1995	Use Airborne Precautions; sign on door to restrict entry of persons; door closed; rooms need special ventilation; similar to 1995 Transmission-based Precautions: Airborne	Universal Precautions do not apply to airborne communicable diseases such as tuberculosis	See Table A-2, Transmission-based Precautions: Airborne

§Table based on CDC draft guidelines from: Draft guideline for isolation precautions in hospitals: notice of comment period, *Federal Register* 59(214):55552-55570, Nov 7, 1994.
Note: Final version may differ.
The article titles for the following references can be found in the Selected Bibliography at the end of this appendix.
*Centers for Disease Control: *Infection Control* 4:245-325, 1983.
†Jackson MM: *Crit Care Nurs Clin North Am* 4(3):401-409, 1992; Jackson MM, Lynch P: *Am J Infect Control*, 1995; Jackson MM, Lynch P: *Infect Control Hosp Epidemiol* 12:448-450, 1991; Jackson MM, Lynch P: *Am J Nurs* 90(10):65-73, 1990; Jackson MM, Lynch P: *Am J Nurs* 84:208-210, 1984; Jackson MM et al: *Am J Nurs* 87:1137-1139, 1987; Lynch P et al: *Ann Intern Med* 107:243-246, 1987; Lynch P et al: *Am J Infect Control* 18:1-12, 1990.
‡Centers for Disease Control: *MMWR* 37:377-388, 1988; Department of Labor, Occupational Safety and Health Administration: *Federal Register* 56:64003-64182, Dec 6, 1991.

Table A-2 Projected recommendations for isolation precautions in hospitals (CDC, 1995)§

	Standard Precautions	Transmission-based Precautions: Airborne	Transmission-based Precautions: Droplet	Transmission-based Precautions: Contact
When to use	All patients	Use in addition to Standard Precautions for patients known to be or suspected of being infected with microorganisms transmitted by airborne droplet nuclei (≤5 microns) of evaporated droplets containing microorganisms that can remain suspended in the air and can be widely dispersed by air currents	Use in addition to Standard Precautions for patient known to be or suspected of being infected with microorganisms transmitted by droplets (>5 microns) that can be generated during coughing, sneezing, talking, or performance of procedures	Use in addition to Standard Precautions for specified patients known to be or suspected of being infected or colonized with epidemiologically important microorganisms that can be transmitted by direct contact with patient, such as occurs during patient care activities, or by indirect contact, such as touching surfaces or equipment in patient's environment

Continued.

Table A-2   Projected recommendations for isolation precautions in hospitals (CDC, 1995)—cont'd

	Standard Precautions	Transmission-based Precautions: Airborne	Transmission-based Precautions: Droplet	Transmission-based Precautions: Contact
Handwashing	Wash hands after touching blood, body fluids, secretions, excretions, and contaminated items, regardless of whether gloves are worn; wash hands immediately after gloves are removed, between patient contacts, and to prevent transfer of microorganisms to other patients or environments			
Gloves	Wear nonsterile gloves when touching blood, body fluids, secretions, excretions, and contaminated items; put on clean gloves just before touching mucous membranes and nonintact skin; remove gloves promptly after use, before touching noncontaminated items, environmental surfaces, or going to another patient			In addition to glove use as described in Standard Precautions, wear gloves whenever providing direct patient care or having hand contact with potentially contaminated surfaces or items in patient's environment

Mask, eye protection, face shield	Wear mask and eye protection or face shield to protect mucous membranes of eyes, nose, and mouth during procedures and patient care activities likely to generate splashes or sprays	Wear respiratory protection when entering room of patient known to have or suspected of having tuberculosis (a type of particulate respirator is recommended) Do not enter room of patient known to have or suspected of having measles (rubeola) or varicella (chickenpox) if susceptible to these infections	Wear a mask when working within 3 ft of patient
Gown	Wear clean, nonsterile gown to protect skin and prevent soiling of clothing during procedures and patient care activities likely to generate splashes or sprays of blood, body fluids, secretions, or excretions, or to cause soiling of clothing; remove gown promptly when tasks are completed; wash hands		Wear clean, nonsterile gown if substantial contact is anticipated with patient, surfaces, or items in environment; wear gown if patient is incontinent, has diarrhea, an ileostomy, colostomy, or uncontained wound drainage; remove gown carefully when tasks are completed; wash hands

Continued.

Table A-2 Projected recommendations for isolation precautions in hospitals (CDC, 1995)—cont'd

	Standard Precautions	Transmission-based Precautions: Airborne	Transmission-based Precautions: Droplet	Transmission-based Precautions: Contact
Patient care equipment	Handle used patient care equipment in manner that prevents skin and mucous membrane exposures, contamination of clothing, and environmental soiling			When possible, dedicate use of noncritical patient care equipment to a single patient to avoid sharing between patients; if common equipment or items must be shared, adequately clean and disinfect them between uses
Linen	Handle, transport, and process used linen in manner that prevents skin and mucous membrane exposure, contamination of clothing, and environmental soiling			

| Patient placement | Place patient who contaminates environment or who does not (or cannot) assist in maintaining appropriate hygiene or environmental control in private room, if possible; consult infection control professionals for other alternatives | Place patient in private room that has (1) monitored negative air pressure in relation to surrounding areas, (2) a minimum of six air exchanges per hour, and (3) appropriate discharge of air outdoors or monitored high-efficiency filtration of room air before air is circulated to other areas of the hospital; keep room door closed when patient is in room. When a private room is not available, patient may be placed in room with another patient who has an active infection with the same microorganism; consult infection control professionals for alternatives | Place patient in private room when possible; when a private room is not available, maintain spatial separation of at least 3 ft between infected patient and other patients and visitors; consult infection control professional for other alternatives | Place patient in private room when possible; when a private room is not available, consult infection control professionals for selection of suitable roommates or other alternatives |

Continued.

Table A-2 Projected recommendations for isolation precautions in hospitals (CDC, 1995)—cont'd

	Standard Precautions	Transmission-based Precautions: Airborne	Transmission-based Precautions: Droplet	Transmission-based Precautions: Contact
Patient transport		Limit movement and transport of patient from room to essential purposes only; if transport or movement is necessary, minimize patient dispersal of droplet nuclei by placing surgical mask on patient, if possible	Limit movement and transport of patient from room to essential purposes only; if transport or movement is necessary, minimize patient dispersal of droplets by masking patient, if possible	Limit movement and transport of patient from room to essential purposes only; if transport is necessary, ensure that precautions are maintained to minimize contamination of environmental surfaces or equipment
Environmental control				Ensure that patient care items, bedside equipment, and frequently touched surfaces receive daily cleaning
Occupational Safety and Health Administration (OSHA) bloodborne pathogens standard (1991)	Take care to prevent injuries when using needles, scalpels, and other sharp instruments or devices; when handling sharp instruments after procedures; when cleaning used instruments; and when disposing of used needles Never recap used needles or otherwise manipulate			

them using both hands, or use any other technique that involves directing the point of a needle toward any part of the body

Use either one-handed "scoop" technique or mechanical device designed for holding needle sheath if recapping is required by procedure

Do not remove used needles from disposable syringes by hand; do not bend, break, or manipulate used needles by hand

Place used sharps in appropriate puncture-resistant containers located as close as practical to location of use

Use mouthpieces, resuscitation bags, or other ventilation devices as an alternative to mouth-to-mouth resuscitation methods in areas where need is predictable

§Table based on CDC draft guidelines from: Draft guideline for isolation precautions in hospitals: notice of comment period. *Federal Register* 59(214):55552-55570, Nov 7, 1994.
Note: Final version may differ.

membranes. Standard Precautions are designed to reduce the risk of transmission of microorganisms from both recognized and unrecognized sources of infection in hospitals.

The 1995 Transmission-based Precautions are designed for patients documented to be or suspected of being infected or colonized with organisms transmitted by the airborne route, by droplets, and by organisms that are epidemiologically important. Transmission-based Precautions replace the 1983 Category-Specific and Disease-Specific systems.

Thus, beginning in 1995, all hospitals are encouraged to review and consider adoption of Standard Precautions and Transmission-based Precautions and discontinue use of the older forms of isolation precautions. As always, the CDC offers hospitals the option of modifying the recommendations according to their needs and circumstances and as directed by federal, state, or local regulations. For example, the Occupational Safety and Health Administration's Bloodborne Pathogens Standard (1991) is still operable, and all facilities are required to comply with its provisions. The CDC's 1995 Standard Precautions incorporate all requirements of the OSHA Bloodborne Pathogens Standard.

Isolation Precautions for Patients with Pulmonary or Laryngeal TB

In response to the increasing incidence of pulmonary tuberculosis (TB) in the United States, the CDC in 1990 published guidelines for preventing the transmission of TB in the health-care setting. These guidelines were revised in 1994. A component of these guidelines is Airborne Precautions for persons diagnosed with or suspected of having pulmonary or laryngeal tuberculosis that can be transmitted to others *via* the airborne route. These guidelines focus on early identification and treatment of persons with a diagnosis or suspected diagnosis of active tuberculosis. In addition, the CDC defined requirements for special ventilation and use of masks that provide better filtration and a tighter fit than standard surgical masks. Masks of this type are called particulate respirators (PRs) and were originally developed for industrial use to protect workers from dust, fumes, and other hazardous substances that could affect the respiratory tract. The efficacy of PRs in protecting susceptible persons from infection with TB has not been demonstrated; however, research is in progress. In the meantime, OSHA is in the process of developing a Tuberculosis Control Standard for health-care settings that will include requirements for risk assessment, special ventilation, PRs, skin testing programs, exposure management, training programs, and other elements similar to those of OSHA's Bloodborne Pathogens Standard of 1991.

Management of Devices and Procedures to Reduce Risk of Nosocomial Infection

Use of barriers is but one of many strategies that can reduce the risk of nosocomial infection among patients and personnel. In fact, studies from the CDC show that significant gains can be made in reducing infection risks by focusing on the management of devices and procedures frequently used in patient care. For example, many patients need intravascular devices that deliver therapeutic medications, but they are put at risk for site infections and bacteremias when these devices are used. It is well known that rotating the access site at appropriate intervals reduces these risks to the patient, and new catheter materials that are more "vein friendly" also reduce trauma to the vascular system. In addition, use of needles to deliver medications and fluids to patients through these intravascular devices can put the health-care worker at risk for puncture injury. Needleless or needle-free IV access devices now are used to access line ports so that it is not necessary to use needles once the intravascular catheter has entered the vascular system. Thus the use of newer and safer intravascular devices and procedures can benefit both the patient and health-care worker by reducing their risk of nosocomial infection. Research studies of interventions to reduce nosocomial infection risks are published in general and specialty journals and presented at professional meetings each year. Infection control practitioners and hospital epidemiologists use these studies to make recommendations about changes in nursing and medical practice. The Joint Commission on Accreditation of Healthcare Organizations (JCAHO) requires that all accredited facilities have a person qualified to provide infection surveillance, prevention, and control services. The national associations for these professionals are the Association for Professionals in Infection Control and Epidemiology, Inc. (AIPC), which publishes the *American Journal of Infection Control,* and the Society for Healthcare Epidemiology of America (SHEA), which publishes the journal *Infection Control and Hospital Epidemiology.*

Selected Bibliography

Bennett JV, Brachman PS, editors: *Hospital infections,* ed 3, Boston, 1992, Little, Brown.

Centers for Disease Control and Prevention: Guidelines for preventing the transmission of *Mycobacterium tuberculosis* in health-care facilities, *MMWR* 43(No RR-13):1-133, 1994.

Centers for Disease Control and Prevention: Draft guideline for isolation precautions in hospitals: notice of comment period, *Federal Register* 59(214):55552-55570, Nov 7, 1994.

Centers for Disease Control: Guidelines for preventing the transmission of tuberculosis in health-care settings, with special focus on HIV-related issues, *MMWR* 39(RR 1-17), 1990.

Centers for Disease Control: Update: Universal Precautions for prevention of transmission of human immunodeficiency virus and other bloodborne pathogens in health-care settings, *MMWR* 37:377-388, 1988.

Centers for Disease Control: Recommendations for prevention of HIV transmission in health-care settings, *MMWR* 36(suppl 2):1-18, 1987.

Centers for Disease Control: Guideline for isolation precautions in hospitals, *Infect Control* 4:245-325, 1983.

Department of Labor, Occupational Safety and Health Administration: Occupational exposure to bloodborne pathogens; final rule, 29 CFR part 1910;1030, *Federal Register* 56:64003-64182, Dec 6, 1991.

Jackson MM: Infection prevention and control, *Crit Care Nurs Clin North Am* 4(3):401-409, 1992.

Jackson MM, Lynch P: Developing a numeric scale to assess health-care worker risk for bloodborne pathogen exposure, *Am J Infect Control,* 1995.

Jackson MM, Lynch P: An attempt to make an issue less murky: a comparison of four systems for infection precautions, *Infect Control Hosp Epidemiol* 12:448-450, 1991.

Jackson MM, Lynch P: In search of a rational approach, *Am J Nurs* 90(10):65-73, 1990.

Jackson MM, Lynch P: Infection control: too much or too little? *Am J Nurs* 84:208-210, 1984.

Jackson MM et al: Why not treat all body substances as infectious? *Am J Nurs* 87:1137-1139, 1987.

Lynch P et al: Implementing and evaluating a system of generic infection precautions: body substance isolation, *Am J Infect Control* 18:1-12, 1990.

Lynch P et al: Rethinking the role of isolation practices in the prevention of nosocomial infections, *Ann Intern Med* 107:243-246, 1987.

Martone WJ, Garner JS, editors: Proceedings of the Third Decennial International Conference on Nosocomial Infections, *Am J Med* 91(3B):1-333, 1991.

Pugliese G, Lynch P, Jackson MM, editors: *Universal Precautions: policies, procedures, and resources,* Chicago, 1990, American Hospital Publishing.

Wenzel RP: *Prevention and control of nosocomial infections,* ed 2, Baltimore, 1993, Williams & Wilkins.

ABBREVIATIONS USED IN THIS MANUAL

9

AAL: anterior axillary line
ABA: American Burn Association
ABG: arterial blood gas
ac: before meals
ACBaE: air contrast barium enema
ACE: angiotensin-converting enzyme
ACh: acetylcholine
AChR: acetylcholine receptors
ACI: acute cerebral infarct
ACLS: advanced cardiac life support
ACT: activated clotting time
ACTH: adrenocorticotropic hormone
ACV: assist-control ventilation
AD: autonomic dysreflexia
ADA: American Diabetes Association
ADH: antidiuretic hormone
ADL: activity of daily living
AFB: acid-fast bacillus
AIDS: acquired immunodeficiency syndrome
ALG: antilymphocyte globulin
ALL: acute lymphoblastic leukemia
ALP: alkaline phosphatase
ALS: amyotrophic lateral sclerosis
ALT: alanine aminotransferase
AMI: acute myocardial infarct
ANC: absolute neutrophil count
ANP: atrial natriuretic peptide
AP: anterior posterior
APR: abdominoperineal resection
ARC: AIDS-related complex
ARDS: adult respiratory distress syndrome
ARF: acute respiratory failure; acute renal failure
ASA: acetylsalicylic acid (aspirin)
AST: aspartate aminotransferase
ATCS: anterior tibial compartment syndrome
ATGAM: antithymocyte gamma globulin
atm: atmosphere (standard)

ATN: acute tubular necrosis
ATP: adenosine triphosphate
AV: atrioventricular; arteriovenous
AVM: arteriovenous malformation
BEE: basal energy expenditure
BP: blood pressure
bpm: beats per minute
BSA: body surface area
BSI: body substance isolation
BUN: blood urea nitrogen
bid: twice a day
C: cervical; Centigrade
Ca/C^{2+}: calcium
CABG: coronary artery bypass grafting
CAD: coronary artery disease
CAPD: continuous ambulatory peritoneal dialysis
CAVH: continuous arteriovenous hemofiltration
$C(a-v)o_2$: arteriovenous oxygen content difference
CBC: complete blood count
CCPD: continuous cycling peritoneal dialysis
CCU: coronary care unit
CDC: Centers for Disease Control and Prevention
CHF: congestive heart failure
CI: cardiac index
CK-MB: creatinine kinase–myocardial band
Cl: chloride
cm: centimeter
CMV: cytomegalovirus; controlled mechanical ventilation
CNS: central nervous system
CO: cardiac output; carbon monoxide
CO_2: carbon dioxide
COPD: chronic obstructive pulmonary disease
CPAP: continuous positive airway pressure
CPK: creatinine phosphokinase
CPP: cerebral perfusion pressure; coronary perfusion pressure
CPR: cardiopulmonary resuscitation
CRF: chronic renal failure
CSF: cerebrospinal fluid
CT: computed axial tomography
CVA: cerebrovascular accident; costovertebral angle
CVC: central venous catheter
CVP: central venous pressure
CVVH: continuous venovenous hemofiltration
CyA: cyclosporine
D_{50}: 50% dextrose
DBP: diastolic blood pressure
DI: diabetes insipidus
DIC: disseminated intravascular coagulation
DKA: diabetic ketoacidosis
dl: deciliter
DM: diabetes mellitus
Do_2: oxygen delivery

D₅NS: 5% dextrose in normal saline
DPL: diagnostic peritoneal lavage
DSA: digital subtractive angiography
DTR: deep tendon reflex
DTs: delirium tremens
DVT: deep vein thrombosis
D₅W: 5% dextrose in water
EACA: epsilon-aminocaproic acid
EBV: Epstein-Barr virus
ECF: extracellular fluid
ECFA: eosinophilic chemotactic factor of anaphylaxis
ECG: electrocardiogram
EEG: electroencephalogram
EMG: electromyography
EPS: electrophysiologic studies
ERCP: endoscopic retrocholangiopancreatography
ESR: erythrocyte sedimentation rate
ESRD: end-stage renal disease
ESWL: extracorporeal shock wave lithotripsy
ET: endotracheal
F: Fahrenheit
Fr: French
FBS: fasting blood sugar
FDA: Food and Drug Administration
FDP: fibrin degradation product
FEF: forced midexpiratory flow
FEV: forced expiratory volume
FFP: fresh-frozen plasma
FHF: fulminant hepatic failure
Fio₂: fraction of inspired oxygen
FRC: functional residual capacity
FRF: filtration replacement fluid
FSP: fibrin split product
FVC: forced vital capacity
g: gram
GBS: Guillain-Barré syndrome
GGTP: gamma-glutamyl transpeptidase
GI: gastrointestinal
GOT: glutamic-oxaloacetic transaminase
GU: genitourinary
h: hour
HAV: hepatitis A virus
HBIG: hepatitis B immune globulin
HBV: hepatitis B virus
HCl: hydrochloric acid
HCO₃: bicarbonate
H₂CO₃: carbonic acid
Hct: hematocrit
HCV: hepatitis C virus
HDL: high-density lipoprotein
HDV: hepatitis D virus
HELLP: hemolysis, elevated liver enzymes, low platelet count

HEV: hepatitis E virus
Hgb: hemoglobin
HHNS: hyperosmolar hyperglycemic nonketotic syndrome
HI: head injury
HIT: heparin-induced thrombocytopenia
HIV: human immunodeficiency virus
HOB: head of bed
HR: heart rate
hs: hour of sleep
HVWP: hepatic vein wedge pressure
IABP: intraaortic balloon pump
ICA: internal cerebral artery
ICD: implantable cardioverter-defibrillator
ICF: intracellular fluid
ICH: intracerebral hematoma
ICP: intracranial pressure
ICS: intercostal space
ICU: intensive care unit
IDDM: insulin-dependent diabetes mellitus
IE: infective endocarditis
IgA: immunoglobulin A
IgE: immunoglobulin E
IgG: immunoglobulin G
IgM: immunoglobulin M
IGT: impaired glucose tolerance
IICP: increased intracranial pressure
IL: interleukin
IM: intramuscular
IMA: internal mammary artery
I&O: intake and output
IPD: intermittent peritoneal dialysis; intracranial pressure dynamics
IPPB: intermittent positive pressure breathing
IRV: inverse ratio ventilation
ITP: idiopathic thrombocytopenic purpura
IU/iu: international unit
IV: intravenous
IVP: intravenous pyelogram
K/K$^+$: potassium
KCl: potassium chloride
kg: kilogram
KUB: kidney, ureter, bladder
L: liter; lumbar
LAD: left anterior descending (coronary artery)
LAP: left atrial pressure
LATS: long-acting thyroid stimulator
lb: pound
LCTs: long-chain triglycerides
LDH: lactate dehydrogenase; also abbreviated *LD*
LDL: low-density lipoprotein
LES: lower esophageal sphincter
LLQ: left lower quadrant
LMN: lower motor neuron

LOC: level of consciousness
LP: lumbar puncture
LUQ: left upper quadrant
LUT: lower urinary tract
LVEDP: left ventricular end-diastolic pressure
LVH: left ventricular hypertrophy
MAO: monoamine oxidase
MAP: mean arterial pressure
MAST: military antishock trousers
MCA: middle cerebral artery
MCHC: mean corpuscular hemoglobin concentration
MCL: modified chest lead; midclavicular line
MCTs: medium-chain triglycerides
MCV: mean corpuscular volume
mEq: milliequivalent
mg: milligram
MG: myasthenia gravis
Mg/Mg^{2+}: magnesium
MgSO$_4$: magnesium sulfate
MI: myocardial infarction
mi: mile
min: minute
ml: milliliter
mm Hg: millimeters of mercury
MMF: maximum midexpiratory flow
mmol: millimole
mo: month
MODS: multiple organ dysfunction syndrome
mOsm: milliosmole
MPAP: mean pulmonary artery pressure; also abbreviated *PAM*
MRI: magnetic resonance imaging
MS: multiple sclerosis
MSAP: mean systolic arterial pressure
MUGA scan: multiple-gated acquisition scan
μg: microgram
μm: micrometer
μm^3: cubic micrometer
N: nitrogen
Na/Na$^+$: sodium
NaCl: sodium chloride
NaHCO$_3$: sodium bicarbonate
NCV: nerve conduction velocity
ng: nanogram
NG: nasogastric
NH$_3$: ammonia
NH$_4$$^+$: ammonium
NIDDM: non–insulin dependent diabetes mellitus
NMBA: neuromuscular blocking agent
NPO: nothing by mouth
NSAID: nonsteroidal antiinflammatory drug
NSS: normal saline solution
NTG: nitroglycerin

O$_2$: oxygen
OGTT: oral glucose tolerance test
OOB: out of bed
OR: operating room
ORIF: open reduction with internal fixation
OSHA: Occupational Safety and Health Administration
OT: occupational therapist
OTC: over the counter
oz: ounce
PA: pulmonary artery
P(A-a)o$_2$: alveolar-arterial oxygen tension difference
PAC: premature atrial complexes
Paco$_2$: partial pressure of dissolved carbon dioxide in arterial blood
PAD: pulmonary artery diastolic
PAo$_2$: partial pressure of alveolar oxygen
Pao$_2$: partial pressure of dissolved oxygen in arterial blood
PAP: pulmonary artery pressure
PAS: pulmonary artery systolic
PASG: pneumatic antishock garment
PAT: paroxysmal atrial tachycardia
PAWP: pulmonary artery wedge pressure
PBV: percutaneous balloon valvuloplasty
pc: after meals
PCA: patient-controlled analgesia
PCM: protein-calorie malnutrition
PCP: *Pneumocystis carinii* pneumonia
PE: pulmonary embolus
PEEP: positive end-expiratory pressure
PEG: percutaneous endoscopic gastrostomy
PET: positron emission tomography
pg: picogram
pH: hydrogen ion concentration
PJC: premature junctional complexes
PMI: point of maximal impulse
PO: by mouth
PO$_4$: phosphorus
PPF: plasma protein fraction
PPN: peripheral parenteral nutrition
PR: particulate respirator
PRBCs: packed red blood cells
prn: as needed
PSV: pressure support ventilation
PT: physical therapy; physical therapist; prothrombin time
PTCA: percutaneous transluminal coronary angioplasty
PTH: parathyroid hormone
PTHC: percutaneous transhepatic cholangiogram
PTT: partial thromboplastin time
PUL: percutaneous ultrasonic lithotripsy
PVC: premature ventricular complexes, peripheral venous catheter
PVD: peripheral vascular disease
PVR: pulmonary vascular resistance
q: every

qid: four times a day
qt: quart
RAP: right atrial pressure
RBC: red blood cell
RDA: Recommended Daily Allowance; Recommended Dietary Allowance
REE: resting energy expenditure
RIA: radioimmunoassay
RL: Ringer's lactate
RLA: Rancho Los Amigos
RLQ: right lower quadrant
ROM: range of motion
RPE: rate perceived exertion
RQ: respiratory quotient
RR: respiratory rate
RRT: renal replacement therapy
RUQ: right upper quadrant
RVP: right ventricular pressure
S: sacral
SA: status asthmaticus
SAARD: slow-acting antirheumatic drug
SAH: subarachnoid hemorrhage
SANS: sympathetic/autonomic nervous system
Sao$_2$: saturation of hemoglobin by oxygen
SAS: subarachnoid space
S-B: Sengstaken-Blakemore
SBP: systolic blood pressure
SC: subcutaneous (also abbreviated *SQ*)
SCI: spinal cord injury
sec: second
SGOT: serum glutamic-oxaloacetic acid transaminase
SGPT: serum glutamic pyruvic transaminase
SIADH: syndrome of inappropriate antidiuretic hormone
SIMV: synchronized intermittent mandatory ventilation
SIRS: systemic inflammatory response syndrome
SNS: sympathetic nervous system
SOB: shortness of breath
Spo$_2$: peripheral arterial oxygen saturation
SRSA: slow-reacting substances of anaphylaxis
stat: immediately
SV: stroke volume
SVI: stroke volume index
Svo$_2$: mixed venous oxygen saturation
SVR: systemic vascular resistance
SVT: supraventricular tachycardia
T: thoracic
TB: tuberculosis
TBSA: total body surface area
TE: thrombotic emboli
TEE: total energy expenditure; transesophageal echocardiography
TENS: transcutaneous electrical nerve stimulation
TIA: transient ischemic attack

tid: three times a day
TKO: to keep open
TMP: transmembrane pressure
TNA: total nutrient admixtures
TOF: train-of-four
TPA: tissue plasminogen activator
TPN: total parenteral nutrition
TPR: temperature, pulse, respirations
TSF: triceps skinfold thickness
TTP: thrombotic thrombocytopenic purpura
U/u: unit
UA: urinalysis
UMN: upper motor neuron
URI: upper respiratory infection
UTI: urinary tract infection
UUN: urine urea nitrogen
VAD: venous access device; ventricular assist device
VC: vital capacity
VF: ventricular fibrillation
VLDL: very low-density lipoprotein
VMA: vanillylmandelic acid
Vo_2: oxygen consumption
VS: vital signs
VT: ventricular tachycardia
WB: whole blood, Western blot
WBC: white blood cell
WHO: World Health Organization
wk: week
WOB: work of breathing
yr: year

INDEX

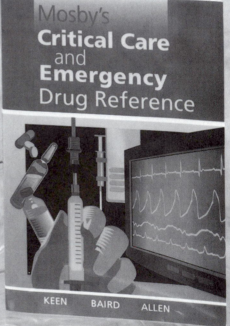
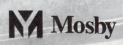